**Cerebral Palsy in Infancy**

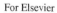

For Elsevier

Content Strategist: *Rita Demetriou-Swanwick*
Content Development Specialist: *Catherine Jackson*
Project Manager: *Caroline Jones*
Designer/Design Direction: *Christian Bilbow*
Illustration Manager: *Jennifer Rose*
Illustrator: *Kinesis Illustration*

# Cerebral Palsy in Infancy

## Targeted Activity to Optimize Early Growth and Development

Edited by

Roberta B. Shepherd EdD, MA, Dip Phty, FACP

Foundation Chair of Physiotherapy, Honorary Professor, Faculty of Health Sciences
The University of Sydney
Sydney, NSW, Australia

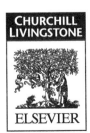

Edinburgh London New York Oxford Philadelphia St Louis Sydney Toronto

**ELSEVIER**
CHURCHILL
LIVINGSTONE

ISBN 978-0-7020-5099-2

**British Library Cataloguing in Publication Data**
A catalogue record for this book is available from the British Library

**Library of Congress Cataloging in Publication Data**
A catalog record for this book is available from the Library of Congress

**Notices**
Knowledge and best practice in this field are constantly changing. As new research and experience broaden our understanding, changes in research methods, professional practices, or medical treatment may become necessary.

Practitioners and researchers must always rely on their own experience and knowledge in evaluating and using any information, methods, compounds, or experiments described herein. In using such information or methods they should be mindful of their own safety and the safety of others, including parties for whom they have a professional responsibility.

With respect to any drug or pharmaceutical products identified, readers are advised to check the most current information provided (i) on procedures featured or (ii) by the manufacturer of each product to be administered, to verify the recommended dose or formula, the method and duration of administration, and contraindications. It is the responsibility of practitioners, relying on their own experience and knowledge of their patients, to make diagnoses, to determine dosages and the best treatment for each individual patient, and to take all appropriate safety precautions.

To the fullest extent of the law, neither the Publisher nor the authors, contributors, or editors, assume any liability for any injury and/or damage to persons or property as a matter of products liability, negligence or otherwise, or from any use or operation of any methods, products, instructions, or ideas contained in the material herein.

 your source for books, journals and multimedia in the health sciences
**www.elsevierhealth.com**

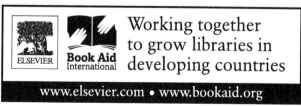

# Contents

**PART 3** Impairments and Neuromuscular Adaptations to
Impairments and Inactivity ...............................................................85

## 14 Constraint-induced therapy and bimanual training in children with unilateral cerebral palsy .......................................... 305
*Andrew M. Gordon*

## 15 Interactive technologies for diagnosis and treatment in infants with cerebral palsy........................................................... 323
*Jens Bo Nielsen*

Colour plate section

# Preface

The overall purpose of this book is to argue for early, targeted activity for infants with cerebral palsy that is focused on increasing muscle activation, training basic actions to stimulate learning, and minimizing (or preventing) maladaptive changes to muscle morphology and function. The authors present recent scientific findings in brain science, movement science (developmental biomechanics, motor control mechanisms, motor learning, exercise science) and muscle biology. This knowledge provides the rationale for active intervention, underpins the need for an early referral to appropriate services and suggests directions for future research.

The lifelong adaptability of brain and body systems is of critical importance to our existence and is largely activity-dependent. Adaptation may have either positive or negative effects. While enhanced and targeted physical activity enable us to learn new skills as well as to recover after injury and regain lost skills, inactivity results in muscle weakness, soft tissue contracture, and loss of fitness and skill.

So it is with a newborn infant. A baby's birth heralds an intense period of adaptation. The infant has the challenge of learning how to move in and interact with a complex, gravitational environment. This involves intensive self-initiated practice that enables the development of the fundamental characteristics of upper and lower limb control and of balancing a growing body mass over a small base of support. These basic abilities are normally learned/acquired over the first 18 months of life.

We now have a clearer understanding that the infant's own activities drive the organizational processes in brain and neuromuscular system in the process of learning commonly referred to as maturation or development. Motor control processes and muscle characteristics adapt and strengthen in response to the infant's rapidly increasing physical activity, and this exercise, particularly when weight-bearing, is known to stimulate bone growth. However, when the brain is damaged during the prenatal or perinatal period, the infant's attempts to move are hampered by poor muscle activation, muscle weakness and disordered motor control. Repeated attempts at movement result in the infant learning a small number of ineffective, inefficient and stereotypic movements and developing disuse-associated changes in muscle structure and function. Maladaptive movement and muscle changes probably arise much sooner than has been realized, and negatively affect attempts at motor training, particularly when they are not intensive and when muscles have already lost their extensibility.

My working hypothesis in planning this book was that non-productive changes to muscle architecture, muscle extensibility, and muscle–tendon relationships, to muscle spindle sensitivity, and to the mechanics of inter-segmental and inter-limb co-ordination, may be minimized or in some cases prevented by an early start to training and exercise. This programme, while stimulating learning processes and optimizing development of task-relevant motor control should also focus on actively preserving the extensibility and through-range contractility of muscles.

It is likely that to be effective such intervention must start very early, within the first few months, and in recent times early referral has been made possible by the development of diagnostic tools such as magnetic resonance imaging and the general movements assessment. For an infant activity programme to be effective, therapists and other exercise professionals must be knowledgeable in the movement sciences and skilled at using the environment to drive specific actions. For a programme to be sufficiently intensive to mimic the repetitive activity of the normally developing infant requires assistance for parent and child from interactive technologies, and from electronic devices and exercise equipment (such as treadmill, robotic limb trainers) that give the infant entertaining feedback and 'drive' the practice of basic actions of upper and lower limbs.

Medical intervention has focused on treatment of spasticity and correction of contracture.

However it is likely that the major impediments to the development of effective motor control and performance are the structural, mechanical and functional maladaptations that occur very early as the infant with muscle weakness and impaired motor control mechanisms attempts to move about. Targeted motor training for very young infants may stimulate and guide postnatal brain and corticospinal (re)organization. The result may be an increase in muscle activation and motor control, leading to more effective and efficient motor development in terms of goal achievement and energy expenditure, at a time when it may be particularly important. Such a programme provides an opportunity for an infant to practice and learn that may not otherwise exist for infants with CP. Structured, repetitive and task-driven activity in an interesting environment may actually be remedial.

The book provides guidelines for training and exercise in several chapters and annotations. The rationale for such intervention is outlined in the Introduction in Part 1. The other contributors, well known for their significant research in various fields, have written wisely and succinctly about their topics, making their work relevant in the context of cerebral palsy and intervention. Each chapter has extensive referencing for further study. In Part 2, Janet Eyre and Mary Galea discuss in their chapters the fundamentals of neuromotor plasticity and development and the negative effects of limited motor activity on brain (re)organization and corticospinal tract development. They are followed in Part 3 by a chapter in which Adel Alhusaini focuses on the functional effects of neural impairments and adaptations, with insights into the relationship between increased muscle stiffness and stretch reflex hypersensitivity. A discussion on pathophysiology, evaluation and intervention by

Nicolas Bayle and Jean-Michel Gracies follows. Descriptions of the functional mechanisms and adaptability of muscle, are provided in two seminal chapters by Richard Lieber and Lucas Smith, Martin Gough and Adam Shortland. In Part 4 Giovanni Cioni and colleagues discuss the general movement assessment that can provide early diagnosis and prognosis, and facilitate very early referral from paediatric specialists to training programmes. Diane Damiano writes on the effects of motor activity on brain and muscle, reflecting the importance of targeting specific motor activities, and David Anderson and colleagues provide a compelling argument for the significance of independent locomotion to brain and psychological development.

These discussions lead into the final section in which various methods of training are described. My chapter on training basic aspects of lower limb performance emphasizes methods of minimizing adverse changes to muscle and of stimulating critical task-specific muscle activity and joint movement. It is followed by Linda Fetters' Annotation on the development and use of a kicking device to promote specific use of lower limbs that enables infants to independently adapt their action to achieve a particular goal under variable conditions. This is followed by a discussion of the effects of treadmill training on sensory and motor function by Caroline Teulier and colleagues. In their chapters, Roslyn Boyd and her colleagues and Andrew Gordon raise interesting issues related to contemporary task-related training interventions for upper limbs. The book finishes with Jens Bo Nielsen's discussion of the place of new interactive technologies in enhancing home-based training sessions carried out by the infant's family.

Roberta B. Shepherd

# Acknowledgements

In the early stages of putting together the framework of this book, discussions with several colleagues and friends helped me to understand the current status of early intervention for infants with lesions affecting the brain. Thanks are due to Dr Roslyn Boyd (Queensland Cerebral Palsy Research Centre, The University of Queensland), Ann Lancaster (Sydney Children's Hospital Network, Randwick), Bronwyn Thomas (Brain Injury Service, Kids Rehab, The Children's Hospital at Westmead) and Cathy Morgan (Cerebral Palsy Alliance, Sydney). Dr Phu Hoang (Neuroscience Research Australia) shared his insights into muscle function and his research findings in discussions of muscle adaptability. Debbie Evans of Therapies for Kids, Sydney provided the opportunity for photography sessions. Parents and children enabled me to collect the photographs included in Chapters 1 and 11, and I am most grateful for their help. Two adult friends, Helen and Jason, one of whom I have known since infancy, the other since she was a young woman, gave me insights into living with disability from birth through their active and successful lives. They taught me more than they probably realize.

As editor, I am exceedingly grateful to the contributors. They accepted the challenge of explaining the scientific rationale for very early intervention, described new interventions and presented evidence of effects from their own and others' research. They presented the results of their research and their insights in a readable and interesting form and delivered their chapters on time.

For my own chapters, the idea of basing training and exercise methods on the biomechanics of critical everyday actions and motor learning as means of optimizing the development of motor control and functional performance, and the details of training methods, originated in the collaborative work of Dr Janet Carr (Faculty of Health Science, The University of Sydney) and me over several decades in adult neurorehabilitation and in the production of research papers and several textbooks. Particular thanks are due to Dr Carr for many stimulating and helpful discussions over the years and for her careful reading of several chapters of this book. Her criticisms and suggestions for Chapters 1 and 11 have been invaluable.

Finally, thanks are also due to Elsevier staff: Catherine Jackson, Caroline Jones and members of the art department, for their assistance in preparing the manuscript for publication, and Rita Demetriou-Swanwick, Content Strategist, for her continuing literary support.

*Roberta B. Shepherd, Editor*

# Contributors

**Adel Abdullah Alhusaini** PhD, MSc, PT
Assistant Professor, Department of Rehabilitation
Sciences, CAMS, King Saud University, Riyadh,
Saudi Arabia; Department Chair, Medical Rehabilitation
Department, King Abdulaziz University Hospital,
Riyadh, Saudi Arabia

**David I. Anderson** PhD
Professor, Department of Kinesiology,
San Francisco State University, San Francisco, California,
USA

**Marianne Barbu-Roth** PhD
Researcher, The Centre National de la Recherche
(CNRS), Université Paris Descartes, Paris, France

**Nicolas Bayle** MD
Arts et Métiers ParisTech, Laboratoire de Biomécanique,
Paris; Université Paris Est Créteil (UPEC); AP-HP, Service
de Médecine Physique et de Réadaptation, Unité de
Neurorééducation, Groupe Hôspitalier Henri Mondor,
Créteil, France

**Vittorio Belmonti** PhD, MD
Post-doc researcher, Stella Maris Scientific Institute,
University of Pisa, Pisa, Italy

**Roslyn Boyd** PhD, MSc (PT)
Professor of Cerebral Palsy Research, Queensland
Cerebral Palsy and Rehabilitation Research Centre,
School of Medicine, The University of Queensland,
Herston, Queensland, Australia

**Joseph J. Campos** PhD
Professor, Department of Psychology, University of
California, Berkeley, California, USA

**Giovanni Cioni** MD
Chair, Department of Developmental Neuroscience, Stella
Maris Scientific Institute and Professor of Child Neurology
and Psychiatry, University of Pisa, Pisa, Italy

**Audun Dahl** MPhil
Graduate Student Researcher, Department of
Psychology, University of California, Berkeley, California,
USA

**Diane L. Damiano** PhD, PT
Chief, Functional and Applied Biomechanics Section,
National Institutes of Health, Bethesda, Maryland, USA

**Christa Einspieler** PhD
Institute of Physiology, Center for Physiological Medicine,
Medical University of Graz, Graz, Austria

**Janet Eyre** BSc, MB, ChB, DPhil, FRCPCH
Professor of Paediatric Neuroscience, Institute of
Neuroscience, Newcastle University, Newcastle upon
Tyne, UK

**Linda Fetters** PhD, PT, FAPTA
Professor and Sykes Family Chair in Pediatric
Physical Therapy, Health and Development, Division
of Biokinesiology and Physical Therapy, The Herman
Ostrow School of Dentistry, University of Southern
California, Los Angeles, California, USA

**Mary P. Galea** BAppSci (Physio), BA, PhD
Professorial Fellow, Department of Medicine (Royal
Melbourne Hospital), The University of Melbourne,
Parkville, Victoria, Australia

**Andrew M. Gordon** PhD
Department of Biobehavioral Sciences, Teachers
College, Columbia University, New York, USA

**Martin Gough** MCh, FRCSI (Orth)
Paediatric Orthopaedic Surgeon,
Guy's & St Thomas' NHS Foundation Trust, London, UK

**Jean-Michel Gracies** MD, PhD
Université Paris Est Créteil (UPEC); AP-HP, Service
de Rééducation Neurolocomotrice, Unité de
Neurorééducation, Hôpitaux Universitaires Henri Mondor,
Créteil, France

**Andrea Guzzetta** PhD, MD
Senior Research Fellow, Stella Maris Scientific Institute,
University of Pisa, Pisa, Italy

**Richard L. Lieber** PhD
Professor and Vice Chair, Departments of Orthopedic
Surgery and Bioengineering, San Diego, La Jolla,
California

**Jens Bo Nielsen** MD, PhD, M.Sci.
Department of Exercise and Sports Science and
Department of Neuroscience and Pharmacology, Panum
Institute, University of Copenhagen, Denmark

**Micah Perez** MOTSt, BSc (Biomed)
PhD Scholar, Queensland Cerebral Palsy and
Rehabilitation Research Centre, School of Medicine, The
University of Queensland, Herston, Queensland, Australia

**Monica Rivera** MS, DPTSc(C)
Adjunct Assistant Professor, Physical Therapy
Department, Samuel Merritt University, Oakland
California

**Roberta B. Shepherd** EdD, MA, Dip Phty, FACP
Foundation Chair of Physiotherapy, Honorary Professor,
Faculty of Health Sciences, The University of Sydney,
Sydney, New South Wales, Australia

**Adam P. Shortland** PhD
Honorary Senior Lecturer, Imaging Science and
Biomedical Engineering, King's College London, UK;
Member of the Institute of Physics and Engineering and
Medicine

**Lucas R. Smith** PhD
Department of Anatomy and Cell Biology, University of
Pennsylvania, Philadelphia, Pennsylvania

**Carolino Toulior** PhD
Assistant Professor, Complexity Innovation and Motor
and Sport Activities Laboratory (CIAMS) , University of
Paris-Sud, France

**Ichiro Uchiyama** PhD
Professor, Faculty of Psychology, Doshisha University,
Kyoto, Japan

# PART 1

## Introduction

# The changing face of intervention in infants with cerebral palsy

Roberta B. Shepherd

## CHAPTER CONTENTS

This chapter examines some of the issues that are most relevant in a book that argues for early and specifically targeted activity training for infants with cerebral palsy (CP), from earliest infancy to 18 months of age. Early task-oriented training directed at stimulating muscle activation, sensory and motor control processes and motor learning may encourage optimal growth and development, and minimize maladaptive and deforming changes to the neuro-musculoskeletal system. Functional motor performance may, as a result, develop to be more effective and energy efficient. Whether it is possible that augmented and specifically targeted physical activity early in infancy can ameliorate or overcome the effects of the neural lesion is not known, but basing intervention on this hypothesis seems justified

at this time given the scientific knowledge available. There is now evidence that targeted training can bring about positive changes in motor behaviour and may therefore be both remedial and preventative (see Garvey et al., 2007). However, development and testing of infant training programmes requires at-risk infants to receive an early referral for intervention. The issues raised in this chapter are discussed in more detail throughout the book.

## Historical view

Looking back at the history of intervention in CP it is clear that significant advances have been made over the past half century, at least in countries with well-developed health facilities. However, currently it is evident that therapeutic intervention may start months after birth or later, and that the focus of treatment may still be on decreasing spasticity, stretching contractures and correcting deformity after they have developed, using drug therapy, surgery, splinting and orthoses. When the infant with CP is referred for physical therapy, the emphasis has commonly been on facilitation of movement by the therapist and passive stretching techniques to decrease spasticity. A method of intervention used in many centres is neurodevelopmental or Bobath therapy developed 50 years ago. Its current emphasis is on 'normalizing' movement and improving the 'quality' of movement, with the therapist facilitating and controlling the infant's movements. Under these conditions the infant may have little chance to experience his or her own attempts to achieve a goal, little chance of knowing who was responsible for the movement, or learning how to control self-initiated and independent limb and body movement. Learning by trial and error may not be a feature of intervention when the therapist controls the child's movements. There is little evidence that this form of therapy might be effective – methods are not based on a modern understanding of biomechanics, neuromotor control or learning.

New brain imaging methods support the view that the focus in early infancy should be, as it increasingly is in adult neurorehabilitation, on the infant's own self-initiated activity and on developing methods of driving exploratory, self-initiated and goal- or task-directed movements in an encouraging, challenging environment that allows for intensive practice. Investigations of such programmes are showing promising results (see Chapters 11 to 14; Andersen et al., 2011; Jorgensen et al., 2010) and suggest that such intervention may actually be remedial.

Since the 1980s, new developments in rehabilitation after acute brain lesion such as stroke, described in detail in textbooks and journals, have resulted from a contemporary understanding of the sciences related to movement and of the methods by which skill is developed (Carr and Shepherd, 2000, 2010; Magill, 2010; Shumway-Cook and Woollacott, 2011). The areas of particular interest to paediatric professionals, since they provide the theoretical background to clinical practice for children as well as adults, include neuroscience and muscle biology; functional anatomy; biomechanics of motor performance and changes occurring as the child develops and grows; relationships between cognition, vision, tactile sense receptors (such as plantar load receptors) and self-initiated action; the environmental (including gravitational) effects that drive the development of both structure and function; and the methods that drive learning and the acquisition of skills. The neural sciences provide the bases for understanding the mechanisms of neural impairments, but also of adaptability and of learning, two processes that go on through life with positive or negative effects (Kandel et al., 2000). More recently, investigations of factors that influence brain reorganization after a lesion using new imaging and other technologies, investigations of biomechanical changes during motor development and of muscle changes that occur over time are also stimulating the development and testing of new methods of intervention.

# Understanding impairments and adaptations and their effects on learning and motor performance

The results of lesions in the motor system must depend initially on the location and extent of the damage. In infants with CP, specifically those who develop diplegia or hemiplegia, who are the major targets of this book, it seems likely that the major impediments to the development of effective movement in the early months are *weakness* due to impaired muscle activation and *lack of motor control* (see Chapter 5). Both can interfere with subsequent development and learning. Both can worsen over time as the infant grows and body weight increases, but also as a result of inactivity, repetitive, stereotypic activity and subsequent maladaptive reorganizational processes.

*Spasticity* (increased sensitivity of stretch receptors) may not play a major role in physical disability in these infants and, since it appears to develop over time, may be related more to changes in the muscles, particularly length-associated changes, than to the brain lesion. There is no evidence that stretch reflex hyperactivity is a major cause of functional disability or that reducing it results in improved functional performance (Rameckers et al., 2008), although there has been little investigation. The presence of spasticity is often assumed, adequate methods of testing it are not always utilized and the nature of what is called spasticity is therefore unclear.

*Co-contraction* is commonly reported in electromyography (EMG) studies of children with CP during actions such as walking. It is a common manifestation of poor motor control – a natural phenomenon that occurs in the able-bodied person in the early stages of learning a new and difficult skill, decreasing as skill level increases (Enoka, 1997). Such co-contraction is also a natural feature of early postnatal development (O'Sullivan et al., 1998). A significant correlation has been reported between muscle weakness and the degree of co-contraction and motor disability (Chae et al., 2002a, 2002b). A decrease in motor unit firing rate results in decreased muscle tension. Additional motor units may be recruited to enable greater force development. Stiffening the lower limb in standing can prevent limb collapse but it may also prevent movement (see Fig. A.2B). Co-contraction can also occur to an excessive degree as a result of prolonged muscle activation, for example, carried over from agonist to antagonist phase in a reciprocal movement such as flexion–extension of the elbow (Kamper and Rymer, 2001). It is possible that development of disabling co-contraction can be minimized by an exercise and training programme designed to train basic actions (see Chapter 11) with emphasis on motor control but also targeting the preservation of the natural length of muscles (Gracies, 2005).

Of major significance in CP are the secondary (adaptive) *morphological and mechanical adaptations* of soft tissues that develop over time, in particular changes in muscle such as diminished extensibility and increased stiffness that must result to some extent from muscle inactivation and/or stereotyped muscle activity. These changes reflect the effects of growth and the level and type of infant activity. Muscle growth and development, including the muscle's architecture, are seriously affected by inactivation of muscle and disordered contraction patterns since muscle length reflects the muscle's 'history' of movement. Changes occurring to muscle spindle receptors may underlie the development of stretch reflex hyperactivity. Recent advances in the study of muscle changes in children and adults with CP are described in Chapters 4, 6 and 7. Muscle represents a classic biological example of the relationship between structure and function. A muscle's length reflects the range of lengths it is subject to throughout daily life and is therefore subject to change if our habitual activity changes. Contracture of one muscle group, e.g., hip flexors, can also affect another group, hip internal rotators (Delp et al. 1999).

The history of the development of these secondary phenomena is not known in infants during their first year, but they are likely to start early and develop over time, associated with the infant's physical inactivity and repetitive and stereotypic attempts at movement, together with skeletal growth. These secondary and maladaptive changes increase the disability caused by impaired muscle activation and motor control, and impact negatively on motor training, particularly if it starts late.

Currently, findings from investigations in two different areas of science, one examining post-lesion brain function, the other muscle adaptation, support the view that what an individual actually does after a brain lesion, i.e., the amount and relevance of physical and mental activity early after the lesion occurs, is important. It is therefore possible to hypothesize that targeted physical and mental activity in earliest infancy might 'direct' neural reorganization and motor development. To stimulate from earliest infancy a learning process that leads to enhanced development of motor control requires the training of purposeful and effective movement. Experience in early infancy of active exercise and meaningful use of upper and lower limbs, plus experience of standing upright and weight-bearing through the feet, in actions that actively lengthen muscles known to be prone to contracture, may be critical, not only to the development of balanced movement in a gravitational environment but also to the minimizing of maladaptive changes to muscle resulting from disuse (see Chapter 11). Practice of reach, grasp and manipulation, and of weight-bearing and pushing through the hands, may not only prevent one arm substituting for the other but also prevent the development of muscle contractures. However, the opportunity for early intervention that may be both remedial and preventative can only exist for infants with CP if they are referred in the first few months after birth to the appropriate services, and if those services exist.

New methods of intervention are being developed for infants and children with CP, based on a solid foundation in contemporary science and with some evidence of positive effects on motor performance and activity levels. However, there seems a lack of determination to find out whether or not it is possible to prevent or at least minimize the effects of initial impairments and of subsequent maladaptive changes on motor development by early referral to active training programmes in infancy. The focus in literature on CP is on investigation and treatment of established problems: for example, the effects of drug therapy on spasticity. There appears to be little or no focus on primary impairments such as weakness and lack of motor control, or on the development and testing of intensive activity-based programmes, and few investigations into the early history of maladaptive changes in the musculoskeletal system that must occur early in infancy, magnified by bone growth. A recent report from Sweden suggests that calf muscle contracture starts very early in susceptible infants, with the fastest increase before the age of 5–6 years (Hagglund and Wagner, 2011). Our current understanding of the plasticity of the brain and neuromuscular system now provides the stimulus to change the focus in paediatrics to address methods of stimulating neural drive, muscle activation and the processes of learning, and the minimization or prevention of maladaptations (see Chapter 2, Eyre, 2003, Garvey et al., 2007).

## New methods of intervention for infants: task-oriented and activity-based training and exercise

Motor development and the bone and soft tissue growth that goes with it are driven in healthy babies by their own active attempts to 'master' the movement of their limbs, i.e., to learn how to use them to achieve their goals. They 'exercise' their limbs with increasingly varied movements, in this way preserving an optimal or functional length of muscles, and increasing their strength as the body mass increases in size and weight and as the actions they practice require more forceful contractions.

Developments in our understanding of infant development have led to the current view of infants as learners and therapy as training. This has required the development of new methods of training, with therapists and parents developing their abilities as teachers, using methods that have been shown to be effective in bringing about motor learning in children and adults. Part 3 of this book addresses the issue of how to organize a learning environment for the infant and create the practice possibilities for learning to control muscle force and limb movement for effective motor performance. Structured exercise and activity, designed to aid motor learning and skill acquisition, with the positive effects of vigorous and challenging activity, are the treatments of choice at this time, since they have potentially remedial and preventative effects; activity-specific training and exercises have the potential to increase muscle activation and strength and motor control.

It is hypothesized, but as yet untested, that maladaptive changes to muscle morphology–architecture, stiffness (viscosity and elasticity) and length, muscle–tendon relationships, muscle spindle sensitivity, and changes to the mechanics of intersegmental and interlimb co-ordination, may be minimized or prevented with targeted programmes. These programmes, while stimulating motor learning processes and optimizing development of activity-specific motor control, also focus on preserving active length and through-range contractility of muscles. However, the changes that occur in muscles in infants with CP are complex and further investigation is necessary before effective interventions can be identified (see Delp, 2003). In the meantime it is possible that a targeted activity programme may have beneficial effects on muscle development if pursued from infancy and with sufficient intensity.

Early experience of bearing weight through the feet during varied physical activities, emphasizing the through-range activity of muscles, are critical for achieving balance but are also significant for bone and muscle growth. Weight-bearing pressure (load) and mechanical strain are powerful stimulants of bone formation and growth and physical activity, particularly while weight-bearing, increases bone density in children (Chad et al., 1999; LeVeau and Bernhardt, 1984; Moyer-Mileur et al., 2000; Specker and Binkley, 2003) and in adults (Slemender et al., 1991). Conversely, inactivity leads to resorbtion of bone and decreased bone mineral density (Kuperminc and Stevenson, 2008).

Training programmes for young infants should aim to mimic the flexible but also repetitive and intense activity of the normally developing infant in order to minimize negative/non-productive adaptations, to drive brain organization and motor learning. Parents are taught simple activities and task-specific exercises that are incorporated into play; community-based infant 'exercise' classes can encourage exploration and activity, and promote learning. Devices to 'drive' upper and lower limb activities are being designed so that an infant, once set up, can practice independently exploring the environment—for example, interactive devices encourage and reward kicking actions (Chen et al., 2002; Thelen, 1994; see Chapter 15 and Annotation C). Treadmill training, commonly used and effective in adult neurology, can encourage stepping in infants and strengthen muscles (Bodkin et al., 2003; Ulrich et al., 2001; see Chapters 10 to 12), and can induce changes in the modulation of short latency reflexes during gait in children with CP (Hodapp et al., 2009). Treadmill training and cycling induced by functional electrical stimulating has been shown to be feasible in infants (Trevisi et al., 2012). It is possible that, as in older children, treadmill stepping and walking may also increase the endurance and cardiorespiratory fitness of infants. The use of limb constraint can be effective in both adults and children and is also used in infancy in conjunction with bimanual training (see Chapter 14). Effective for adults after stroke, a suspended harness can provide support

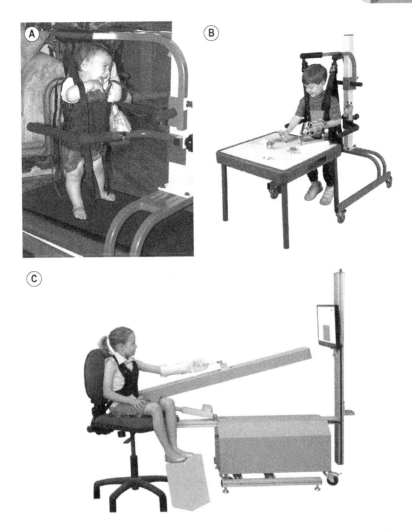

**Figure 1.1** • The advantage of a harness held by the parent or therapist or suspended from a ceiling grill or apparatus is in giving the infant the opportunity to practice weight-bearing on the feet and balancing in standing. Although the harness prevents a fall, it does not prevent movement, so the infant has to make postural adjustments to self-initiated movements as he plays. A harness can also be used for walking practice. For infants who cannot bear weight, the harness can take some weight, but the feet must be flat on the floor. **(A)** Treadmill with harness LiteGait®, with permission from LiteGait®, Mobility research, Tempe, AZ, USA; **(B)** walkable LiteGait®, with permission from LiteGait®, Mobility research, Tempe, AZ, USA; **(C)** non-robotic training device (the Sensorimotor Active Rehabilitation Training Arm Neurotrac 5, Verity Medical Ltd). [Courtesy of Dr Ruth Barker, James Cook University, Townsville, Australia.]

and prevent a fall during practice of balancing activities in infancy (Fig. 1.1A,B). A small harness enables an infant with CP to experience standing on the feet and develop the ability to balance while moving the body. Robotic and non-robotic limb trainers (Fig. 1.1C) and virtual reality systems are in development (Sveistrup, 2004; Wu et al., 2011). It is preferable for the infant to be actively engaged in the experience of balancing rather than being held supported in sitting or standing; the ability to balance, critical for all our actions, requires practice of self-initiated movement while unsupported.

The complex set of internal processes called motor learning has for some time been the focus of interventions designed to optimize motor performance in neurorehabilitation (Carr and Shepherd, 2010; Gentile, 2000; Magill, 2010). Clinicians are increasingly aware that knowledge

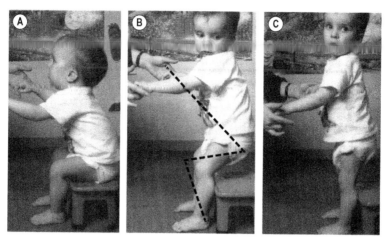

**Figure 1.2** • This little boy with diplegia cannot stand up independently from a seat. In **(A)** his feet should be back under the seat at 75°. In **(B)** he does not rotate his upper body forward enough to move his body mass over his feet (the next base of support), i.e., hip flexion is insufficient. He will fall back if he is not held. The dotted line represents optimal segmental alignment. In **(C)**, his weight is still too far back and he is not able to stand independently. In large part, this is the functional legacy of lack of training and ↓ calf muscle extensibility. [From Shepherd RB 1995 Physiotherapy in Paediatrics 3rd ed. with permission from Elsevier.]

of biomechanics provides the foundation for understanding how we move the body's segmental linkage and remain balanced as we acquire skill (Knutzen and Martin, 2002). Without knowledge of linked segment dynamics the clinician has only observation upon which to base analysis and training of motor actions, and several clinical studies have shown the inaccuracy of such observations. In observation of movement it is necessary to know what to look for, what matters and what does not (Eastlake et al., 1991; Malouin, 1995; Wall, 1999) and this knowledge comes from an understanding of biomechanics and functional anatomy. For example, the infant in Figure 1.2 can stand up, but only with assistance. Observation of the topology (shape) of the movement (dotted line) shows that he has started to extend into standing while his centre of body mass (COM) is too far behind his feet—if unsupported he would fall backward. If the infant's feet were further back at the start, guiding his knees forward with gentle pressure down toward the feet may enable him to do the rest of the movement himself (see Fig. 11.3A). Raising the seat would also make it easier and enable him to practice repetitions of the basic kinematic components of the standing up/sitting down action. Training of this critical action can be started in early infancy as described in Chapter 11.

## Effectiveness and efficiency

The focus of training and testing outcomes should be on improving the effectiveness of functional motor performance not the 'quality' of movement. There is increasing recognition among physiotherapists that the terms 'quality' of movement and 'normal' movement have no concrete meaning and cannot be tested in any meaningful way. Optimization is a useful term, inferring that movement is both as effective (successful in achieving a goal) and efficient (with least energy expenditure) as possible. Effectiveness, efficiency and biomechanical parameters can be tested; for example, kinematics and kinetics provide data about changes in angular displacements, velocities and forces before and after a period of training/exercise. For an action to be optimal, it must obey the laws of mechanics. Certain critical kinetic and kinematic features must occur and it is these biomechanical imperatives that can be targeted in training.

While the clinical focus is on motor learning processes and the mechanics of intersegmental movement, intervention also takes into account the impairments associated with the lesion (primarily, weakness and disordered motor control) and of the adaptive changes that occur when muscles are inactive or muscle activity is uncontrolled. Increasingly there are new findings related to the mechanisms underlying impairments and on adaptive muscle changes. As an example, focus of intervention after stroke in adults is moving away from spasticity (or reflex hyperactivity) as the major problem underlying disability, to the problems of impaired muscle activation and motor control, and of secondary adaptive soft tissue changes associated with inactivity (Carr and Shepherd, 2010). For infants and children with CP, interventions should be similarly focused. Although spasticity seems to attract most attention, clinically it may be confused with decreased extensibility of soft tissue (increased stiffness, decreased length). Furthermore, it is tested in the clinic and the laboratory by passive movement so its effect on active movement is not understood. In some children changes to the stretch reflex may be adaptive phenomena associated with changes to muscle fibres. Treatment of spasticity includes drug therapy that adds to the already present muscle weakness and may not be as effective as functional training (Rameckers et al., 2008; see Chapter 4).

Our understanding of the importance of early and active intervention, directed toward muscle weakness and lack of motor control, is increasing and we have a better understanding of the potential effects of inactivity on an immature neuromuscular system (Clowry, 2007; Eyre, 2003; Martin et al., 2007) and on developing perceptuo-cognitive function (see Chapter 10).

## Goals and methods of motor training

The goal of training in infants and children with CP is therefore to optimize the development of skilled motor performance (Shepherd, 1995). Ways to achieve these goals include physical activity targeted at the basic actions that are normally mastered by 18 months as part of an infant's functional skill acquisition: flexion and extension of hips, knees and ankles while weight-bearing; weight-bearing through the upper limbs and pushing and pulling actions; reaching and manipulation; balancing the body mass (Fig. 1.3). Active trunk and hip extension in prone is particularly important in young infants now there are guidelines for preventing cot death that avoid the prone position for sleeping. In general the methodology comprises:

- Fostering specific actions by manipulating the infant's environment to provide opportunity and challenge, using environmental constraints to guide and direct movement

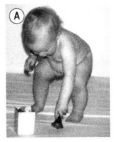
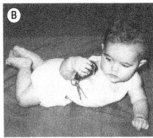
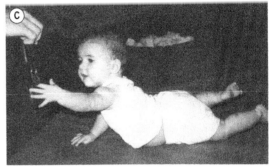
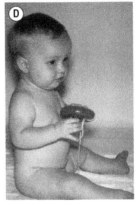
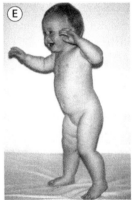

**Figure 1.3** • Basic movements that underlie and are critical for functional motor performance are learned in the infant's first year and should be the focus of early intervention (see Chapter 11). They include: **(A)** flexion and extension of lower limbs in standing; **(B)** weight-bearing through the arm and extending the head and spine in supine; **(C)** pushing and weight-bearing through the hands; **(D)** balancing in sitting with hips flexed; **(E)** balancing the body mass over the feet in standing. [From Shepherd RB 1995 Physiotherapy in Paediatrics 3rd ed. with permission from Elsevier.]

- Activity-related, task- and context-oriented training designed to promote acquisition of specific skill and optimal (effective) motor performance in changing environments, focusing on:
  - Exercises to stimulate muscle contractility and active stretching to preserve optimal length of soft tissues

○ Repetitive and varied practice of exercises to build up muscle strength and endurance, and stimulate learning

○ Training of actions, particularly in standing and sitting, but also in four-point kneeling and half-kneeling, to develop balance and motor control under these conditions

○ Methods of driving the use of a weak limb or limbs

Emphasis in this type of training programme is on maximizing the amount of time the infant or child spends in what could be called 'practice'—that is, 'on task'.

These activity-based methods of motor training have been developed over several decades for rehabilitation of adults after stroke (e.g., Carr and Shepherd, 2010) and in children with CP (Damiano, 2006; Fetters, 1991; Shepherd, 1995), and are described in Part 3. Positive effects of activity-based programmes on functional performance have been reported in adults (Dean and Shepherd, 1997; Dean et al., 2000; Eng et al., 2003; Marigold et al., 2005; Sherrington et al., 2008; Wevers et al., 2009) and in children with CP (e.g., Blauw-Hospers and Hadders-Algra, 2005; Echols et al., 2002; Ketelaar et al., 2001; Liao et al., 2007; Schneiberg et al., 2010). These investigations include a pilot study with children aged 3–8 years old that showed significant improvements in muscle strength, performance of sit-to-stand and walking after a four-week programme of lower limb exercise and action-specific training (Blundell et al., 2003). Several training and exercise programmes are being developed out of a similar theoretical background. Although they have various names (Box 1.1), they are basically driven by the need to get the infant as active as possible and all could be considered activity-based. Infants with CP who are less than 18 months are not commonly referred for physical intervention, and there has therefore been little investigation of the effects on infants of this type of intervention.

In summary, for therapists the scientific background for development of targeted activity training is provided in at least six major areas of scientific research, the findings of which have the potential to drive earlier referral of infants with suspected CP. These areas of science must be included in undergraduate and graduate educational programmes for physiotherapists and exercise practitioners:

• Adaptation of brain, neuromotor and cardiovascular systems and muscles in response

## Box 1.1

### Examples of training and exercise programmes

• Hand–arm bimanual intensive therapy or HABIT (Charles and Gordon, 2006)

• Coping with and caring for infants with special needs or COPCA (Blauw-Hospers et al. 2011)

• Action observation training or AOT based on modelling (Ertelt et al. 2007)

• Infant-modified version of AOT—an upper limb version for early intervention with infants, called UP-BEAT (see Chapter 14)

• Child-modified version of AOT or UP-CAT (Sgandurra et al. 2011)

• Constraint-induced movement training or CIMT (see Chapter 13)

to activity and patterns of use; the processes of brain reorganization and skill acquisition

• Mechanisms of primary impairments resulting from the neural lesion and their functional effects

• Biomechanics of movement and mechanisms of neuromuscular control; experiential development of movement, action, skill

• Specificity of neuromuscular control and, therefore, of exercise and training

• Mechanisms of motor learning, i.e., acquisition of skill, and the critical importance of repetitive, varied and intensive practice

• Exercise science: building up muscle extensibility and joint flexibility, muscle strength and endurance, cardiorespiratory fitness.

Many developments in interactive technologies including robotics and other interactive devices (Fig. 1.1C), in virtual reality, in orthotics and prosthetics, and in the use of brain scanning to guide treatment choice (Clowry, 2007) have the potential to impact increasingly on physical therapies and exercise science now and in the future (see Chapter 15 and Annotation C).

## New methods of diagnosis and prediction

Central neural damage can occur preterm or in the immediate perinatal period. It may be associated with prematurity, hypoxic brain damage, periventricular white matter (PWM) damage, or intraventricular haemorrhage. The sequelae are referred to as CP. The European Cerebral Palsy Study (Flodmark et al., 2003) found approximately 50% of the babies with CP who were studied had central neural damage occurring in the perinatal period. Central neural damage also occurs postnatally in association with traumatic brain injury or stroke.

A major problem for physicians, therapists and parents has been difficulty predicting which infants are likely to develop significant impairments that may impact on the infant's development. As a result, physicians have been understandably reluctant to refer infants for activity-based physiotherapy programmes before they could be confident, using neurological testing, that such a programme is necessary. Traditional neurological testing may not, however, be sensitive or specific enough to enable a reliable diagnosis or prognosis. No correlations have been found between any of these signs and the severity of later impairment (Ferrari et al., 2003).

However, it is likely that failure to intervene until soft tissue adaptations have occurred and ineffective patterns of motor behaviour have become well established is a major obstacle to the optimization of the infant's development. Early and reliable predictors allow for early intervention, and technological and theoretical advances currently being made will enable more accurate and earlier predictions (Ferrari et al., 2003). Two ongoing developments that should stimulate earlier referral are in neonatal neuroradiology and in the evaluation of infant movements.

**Developments in neonatal neuroradiology,** particularly in functional magnetic resonance imaging (fMRI) and the use of transcranial magnetic stimulation (TMS) are clarifying the causes and nature of brain injury and improving the predictability of impairments and disability (see Chapters 2 and 3). Neonatal neuroradiology has shown that certain patterns of brain damage depend on the selective vulnerability of various parts of the brain during development and maturation of the brain (Flodmark et al., 2003). Damage to PWM, for example, is the response to insults occurring between 24 and 34 gestational weeks. The analysis of 180 MRI scans as part of the European Cerebral Palsy Study showed that PWM damage was the most common cause of CP, often but not always causing diplegia. Partial hypoxia was correlated with widespread cortical damage. Hemiplegia was commonly the result of cortical/

subcortical damage. Quadriplegia and dyskinesis was caused by basal ganglia damage.

**Developments in clinical diagnosis** include investigations into the predictive capacity of the infant movement evaluation developed by Prechtl (2001) a decade ago based on observation of spontaneous motor activity, and called general movements (GMs). It has been suggested that the nature of endogenously generated motor activity may be a better indicator of the integrity of motor function than items of the neurological examination based mainly on reactivity to sensory stimuli (Ferrari et al., 2003; see Chapter 8).

General movements typical of able-bodied and healthy infants are characterized by complexity, fluency and variation (Hadders-Algra, 2004; Hadders-Algra et al., 2004). Newborn infants with brain lesions show spontaneous motility that does not differ in quantity but loses its elegance, fluency, and complexity. A standardized form of this evaluation has been found to have inter-rater reliability and reliable predictive value for CP and other developmental disorders such as minor neurological dysfunction. The range of abnormalities observable in GMs includes hypokinesis (reduced movement), poor repertoire of movements, abnormal or absent fidgety movements and chaotic and cramped synchronized GMs.

A study of 84 high-risk preterm infants examined the infants five to ten times from birth to 60 weeks' postmenstrual age (Ferrari et al., 2003). In addition, at age 2 years, the children were tested using the Griffith Developmental Scale. Infants with consistent or predominantly cramped synchronized GMs developed CP (33 infants), and the earlier they were observed the more severe the impairment. Absence or abnormality of fidgety movements at age 47–60 weeks' post-menstrual age was a reliable predictor for later neurological impairment. A poor repertoire of GMs in the absence of fidgety movements appears to be predictive of mild impairment. Figure 1.4 is from a study of the changes in movement occurring in a low-risk infant compared with a high-risk infant (Hadders-Algra et al., 2004). Movements such as kicking that lacked complexity and variation at 2–4 months' post-term were found to be highly predictive of CP and an indication of the need for early intervention.

Until recently, attitudes toward motor training and exercise in very young infants have not been particularly positive due to lack of investigative

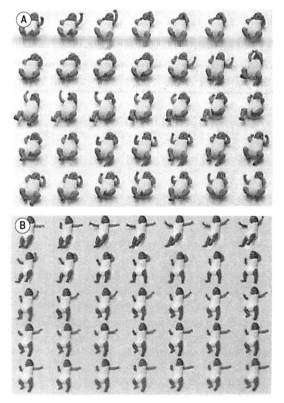

**Figure 1.4** • General Movements Assessment: analysing movements on the basis of the amount of complexity and variation. The video-frames are of two infants at fidgety GM age. Read the frames from R to L. The infant in **(A)** shows normal 'fidgety' GMs with rich spatial and temporal variation of movements. The infant in **(B)** shows abnormal GMs with lack of variation. [From Hadders-Algra M 2004 General movements: a window for early identification of children at high risk for developmental disorders. J Pediatr 145 (Suppl 2):12–18, with permission from Elsevier.]

power and knowledge of how the neuromotor system develops, of the mechanisms driving development, of motor learning processes, or of the potential for intensive physical and mental activity to drive post-lesion remedial processes. We are now aware that physical and mental activity affect brain organization through active, self-generated and meaningful physical and sensory perceptual engagement, and that lack of activity and diminished opportunity for learning can also affect brain organization. We understand the possibility that motor development may not be due to innate deterministic and maturational processes but occur largely as a result of the infant's experiences. Physical activity also drives the development and

growth of muscle, and when activity is diminished, muscles adapt and lose their capacity to generate force effectively (see Chapters 6 and 7).

In summary, for remedial training in paediatrics to be effective, infants need to be referred as early as possible to enable an early start to a targeted training programme. Increased muscle activation levels, strength and motor control, effectiveness of performance and variability of movement are the goals, using methods that may stimulate motor learning, promote muscle development and preserve muscle contractility and length. A major obstacle to referral for early intervention has been the lack of reliable ways of recognizing early signs of brain injury and of assessing infants. However, this is changing. Increased understanding of the mechanisms of brain and corticospinal tract organization in infancy provides support for referral to early and specifically targeted training programmes. Research and development collaborations are enabling the development of interactive devices for infants to encourage active self-directed movement (see Figs 10.3, 10.4). The next obstacle to be overcome will be educational- updating the knowledge base and clinical skills in undergraduate and postgraduate education and in continuing professional education for paediatricians, physiotherapists, occupational therapists and those who work in infant development.

# Background

## Brain plasticity

Chapters 2 and 3 present the current state of knowledge on brain plasticity as it relates to infants and young children, those who are able-bodied and those with a brain lesion. A brief introduction to this topic, and the research that has taken place over several decades, is presented here.

The capacity to adapt and reorganize is an intrinsic property of the neuromotor system. Adaptation is rapid, widely distributed and reversible. Cellular populations within the brain are dynamically organized with the possibility for variability in structure and function according to behavioural needs (Edelman, 1987). Regulation of both transient and long-term effectiveness of synapses occurs daily throughout life, determined by experience and its usefulness to the individual. Synaptic transmission becomes stronger or weaker according to use. It is tempting to consider that adaptation may be underpinned by mechanisms that are important more generally in motor learning and development of motor skill. After a part of the brain is damaged, the function of other interconnected structures must be affected. Part of the adaptive process therefore involves these undamaged structures functioning in novel ways that do not depend on functioning of the damaged tissue. Adaptive changes also involve the generation of new circuitry, and such anatomical changes as dendritic arborization, apparently in response to use (Kolb, 2003).

Studies of environmental effects on the brain demonstrate the dependence of central nervous system (CNS) connectivity on functional activity. Rats that were raised in an enriched environment that demanded motor skill acquisition showed expansion of motor areas of cerebral cortex (Kleim et al., 1997). Humans in an intellectually enriching environment showed increases in dendrite and synapse formation in areas of cortex involved in verbal understanding compared with subjects from a less specialized background (Scheibel et al., 1990).

New brain imaging techniques are confirming that the neural system is continuously remodelled throughout life, and also after injury, in response to experience, activity and learning (Jenkins et al., 1990; Johansson, 2000; Johnston, 2009; Martin et al., 2007). Nudo et al. (2001) summarized the complex organization of the primary motor cortex, with its extensive overlapping of muscle representations, individual corticospinal neurons diverging to multiple motoneuron pools, and horizontal fibres interconnecting distributed representations. They suggested this complex organization may provide the foundation for functional plasticity in the motor cortex. Merzenich et al. (1991) described a continual competition between neural groups for the domination of neurons on their mutual borders. This competition appears to be use-dependent, those movements that are the most effective at achieving a goal being the most successful. For example, in an animal experiment the use of the three middle fingers to obtain food was associated with expansion of the area of cortex that serves these fingers (Jenkins et al., 1990).

Studies of people with particular skills have helped the understanding of changes in the brain as a result of patterns of use. For example, blind Braille readers show an expanded sensorimotor

cortical representation (map) of the reading finger (Pascuol-Leone and Torres, 1993) that fluctuates according to reading activity (Pascuol-Leone et al., 1995). Right-handed string-players show increased cortical representation of flexor and extensor muscles for fingers of left but not the right hand, and the area remains large with regular performance (Elbert et al., 1995). These changes appear to be provoked by active, repetitive training, by continued practice of the activity and also, in the case of the musicians, by the sounds generated. Conversely, restriction of activity induces decreases in cortical motor representation. This has been found after only four to six weeks of ankle immobilization (Liepert et al., 1995). After a survey of investigations into brain plasticity due to visual deprivation in infancy, Noppeney (2007), discussing experience-dependent plasticity, concluded that visual deprivation can induce changes not only in the visual system but also in the sensorimotor system; that sensory experience shapes functional and structural brain organization during development (see Chapter 10).

There are similar findings from rehabilitation studies of both animals and humans. In monkeys with an ischaemic infarct, no intervention led to further loss of hand representation in an area adjacent to the lesion (Nudo and Milliken, 1996), suggesting that plasticity of perilesional tissue is an important substrate for the provision of functional recovery. A follow-up study showed that tissue loss was prevented when the monkeys had daily repetitive training in skilled use of the impaired hand with the unimpaired hand restrained (Nudo et al., 1996) and there was a 10% increase in the hand area adjacent to the lesion. Human studies after stroke have shown similar results associated with task-oriented training: that is, with meaningful use of the limb (Liepert et al., 2000; Nelles et al., 2001). These and other studies suggest that active use of a limb is critical for the survival of undamaged neurons and that practice and training need to be intensive. They show that there is considerable scope for use-dependent functional reorganization in the adult brain after an acute lesion such as stroke and recently this has also been observed in young infants with CP (Eyre, 2003, 2007; Eyre et al., 2000, 2001; Jang et al., 2005).

In the perinatal period the motor system is particularly vulnerable to damage (Johnston, 1998). Abnormal or decreased input from the corticospinal pathway during this critical perinatal period will secondarily disrupt development of spinal motor centres (Berger, 1998). Diplegia in which the lower limbs are most severely affected is the commonest type of CP and its prevalence is increasing due in part to improved survival rates of premature infants. Diplegia is caused by injury to the PWM and a characteristic feature is disruption of corticospinal axons. Cortical pyramidal projection neurons remain intact and subsequently make aberrant intracortical axonal projections, and it is in this period that there is likely to be a high degree of plasticity (Eyre et al., 2000).

The corticospinal system is critical for controlling skilled movements and develops during the late prenatal and early postnatal periods. It is a focus of research since it largely develops postnatally. In cats, inactivity and preventing use of a limb prevents the late developmental growth of corticospinal axon terminals and presynaptic sites and leads to motor control impairments that do not resolve without intervention. The finding that activity- and use-dependent processes in the cat can be harnessed to re-establish corticospinal connection and function suggests that this may also be possible early in infants with CP (Martin et al., 2007). It is possible that physiotherapy that stimulates purposeful use of the limbs and task-specific exercise can boost activity in residual corticospinal innervation to reinforce appropriate synaptic connections, with added excitation from TMS or pharmacology, as hypothesized by Clowry (2007). A recent study (Acerra et al., 2011) has reported that, at the conclusion of a period of task-specific training, a group of adults with stroke showed reduced activation in the contralesional sensorimotor cortex, pre-motor cortex and anterior cingulate cortex compared to a generalized practice group, together with increased activation in the ipsilateral cerebellum. The authors suggested that task-specific training (with a dose of 400 movements daily for three days) can facilitate motor learning and neuroplastic change compared to generalized increased arm use.

Technological developments, particularly the use of fMRI in neuroradiology and TMS, are providing insights into the organization and adaptations following brain injury in children. Central motor reorganization has been observed in children with hemiplegic CP (Carr et al., 2003) using focal magnetic stimulation of the motor cortex and multi-unit EMG. Novel ipsilateral motor pathways from undamaged motor cortex to hemiplegic hand were noted, with no ipsilateral projections from

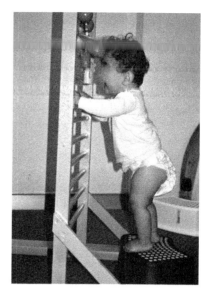

**Figure 1.5** • Play equipment can offer chances for exploratory movements and many challenges for the infant. This ladder provides opportunities for support in standing, practice of sit-to-stand, step-up exercises, reaching to grasp and hold, and climbing.

the damaged cortex. In one group of subjects who had mirror movements, corticospinal axons had branched abnormally to homologous motoneuron pools on both sides of the spinal cord. In subjects without mirror movements there was no evidence of such branching. In other studies, using TMS to test motor-evoked potentials, abnormally strong cortical projections to soleus and medial gastrocnemius muscles in adults with CP were demonstrated (Brouwer and Ashby, 1991). In addition, a common neural drive was observed between tibialis anterior and soleus. These results offer some insight into mechanisms underlying muscle hyperactivity and abnormal patterns of muscle activation. They illustrate how the neural lesion may result in a loss of specificity of corticospinal connections due to disruption of the emergence of a normal pattern of motor cortical projections (see Chapter 2).

In infancy, we know from our observations that motor performance adapts to the state of the system, to pressures from the environment, and it depends on what appears to the infant to work best. That is, an infant's changing patterns of movement reflect the infant's exploratory and problem-solving behaviour and repetitive practice in new and challenging environments (Fig. 1.5). Gradually, patterns of movement change as the

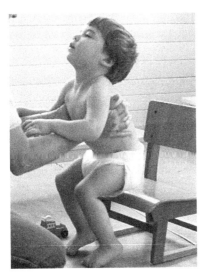

**Figure 1.6** • This little boy with diplegia cannot extend his legs when he tries to stand up. He cannot take weight through plantigrade feet or push down through his feet to stand up. He has weak lower limb extensor muscles and weak extensibility of calf muscle, with knee and hip flexion contractures. He does not have the ability to co-ordinate hip, knee and ankle movements. He should practice lower limb flexion and extension exercises with feet on the floor, starting with hip, knee and ankle joints flexed and increasing active range of motion.

Musculoskeletal adaptations (particularly hypoextensibility) arise to a large extent from lack of varied physical activity, from repetition of a limited repertoire of stereotypic, inflexible movements and from lack of concentric and eccentric muscle activity throughout the necessary joint range. These musculoskeletal adaptations may occur earlier and be far more significant for motor development, neural organization and future disability than has been realized. However, there has been surprisingly little investigation of these phenomena in the developing infant with CP between birth and 12–18 months. For example, it is not clear when the predominant pattern of ankle dorsiflexion in early infancy changes to plantarflexion and to walking on the toes in infants with diplegia, or when lack of extensibility of calf muscles develops in infants with hemiplegia or diplegia.

An important driving force in developing new methods of intervention is therefore our increasing understanding of the flexibility and adaptability of the neuromotor system, the innate plasticity of the system, and of what interventions might drive reorganizational and developmental changes after a brain lesion (see Chapters 2 and 3).

## Motor development

An understanding of motor development includes an awareness of the impact on brain organization and musculoskeletal growth of what the infant experiences and does actively and the environment in which he/she does it. This includes the impact of child-rearing practices (Adolph et al., 2010) and of therapeutic intervention. But what part does experience play in early life? According to Martin et al. (2007) 'Genetically-timed sequences of motor pathway and circuit development could set the stage for an *experience-independent* elaboration of controlled movements' (p. 1126) seen in early postnatal life. The late-developing corticospinal tracts could mediate more complex movements as learning occurs and early development of motor systems may then rely on active learning and experience to enable the structural changes taking place.

Over the last couple of decades a major shift has occurred in our understanding of motor development. It is no longer considered to be dependent solely on innate maturational processes but is dependent also on the influences of the

infant finds some movements more effective than others. These effective movements become more refined with practice, and flexibility and complexity increase. In this way skill is acquired.

In the infant with a brain lesion, however, movement patterns reflect the infant's attempts to achieve a goal in the presence of impaired motor control, muscle weakness and increasing muscle imbalance over time as adaptive length-associated changes develop (Figs 1.2 and 1.6). Without an organized and targeted training programme these inadequate movements may become more stereotyped and habitual—well learned but not skilled—as they are repetitively practiced. When this happens, as shown in the figure, training will be very difficult. A major goal of early intervention must be to test ways of preventing this cycle by an early start, targeting specific muscle activation and limb control and taking advantage of neural plasticity. Eyre (2003) pointed out that 'functional and anatomical evidence supports the view that spontaneous plasticity can be potentiated and shaped by activity … in enriched environments' (p. 102).

infant's discoveries in a new and gravitational environment and the infant's behaviour in that environment. The acquisition of balance control and stability, for example, are driven by the mechanical demands of gravity and the requirements of specific actions or tasks. Infants must adapt their movements to variations in their environment and changes in their bodies (Berger and Adolf, 2007); that is, to the affordances offered by action and context. Affordances is a term used by Gibson (1979) to denote the quality of an object or environment that allows an individual to perform any action that is physically possible; a cord affords pulling, a button on a key pad affords pressing. This view opens up the possibility for targeted therapy to have a significant effect by manipulating the infant's environment and experiences to enable or 'drive' actions and interactions that would otherwise be too difficult given muscle weakness and motor dyscontrol.

We have to consider the possible functional effects of a young infant practicing and 'learning' a limited repertoire of relatively ineffective movements that will be hard to 'unlearn' and may never be replaced by effective and energy-efficient performance once soft tissue changes contribute to the problem. Such movements may be satisfactory for the achievement of the limited goals of early infancy but not for optimal interactions with objects and people (the environment) when goals become more complex. In addition, with increased understanding of the rapidity with which body systems adapt, we can be much more proactive in attempts to target muscle activation both to stimulate and strengthen weak muscles and to minimize muscle stiffness and other soft tissue changes that occur in response to diminished or stereotyped movement.

To some extent views expressed in clinical practice are still influenced by 'old' ideas. For example, an earlier view of motor development considered brain function to be organized hierarchically. This view was associated with a theory of invariant sequential progression, i.e., a developmental sequence:

- Reflexive to voluntary control, as in reflex stepping to walking
- Cephalo-caudal development of motor control
- Proximal to distal development of motor control
- Lying to sitting to crawling to walking
- Stability before mobility
- Gross motor skills to fine motor skills

The theory of a deterministic developmental progression has guided clinical practice until quite recently. However, this view is no longer tenable given the current understanding of the brain and neuromotor system as a highly complex, interactive system, functioning in a distributed manner (dynamic interactive systems). It takes into account the influence of environmental and cultural experiences, of the system functioning by dynamic action-specific interactions between many subsystems (see Thelen and Smith, 1994). Hence, the above oversimplifications have been replaced by an understanding that, while there may be some motor behaviours (e.g., stepping) that may appear to be 'innate' or 'reflexive', movement emerges as a result of environmental as well as internal factors, the CNS utilizing the naturally occurring mechanics of a multi-segmental musculoskeletal system interacting with gravity and task demands. In utero, infants respond to that environment by pushing with the feet against the uterine wall, in a similar pattern to stepping.

The development of prehension skills (reaching, grasping, manipulation, unimanual and bimanual actions and the ability to grade grip force) normally proceeds through the first year and the rate of progress is influenced by the opportunities offered the infant (Forssberg et al., 1991, 1992). Prehension abilities enable the infant to explore and learn about the environment. Purposeful grasping is seen around 4 to 5 months (von Hofsten, 1984), and it appears that the characteristics of objects themselves, such as size and shape, enable infants to judge the type of grasp to be used. This illustrates the importance of being able to judge the relationship between the affordance of an object and one's own abilities (Olmos et al., 2000). Sgandurra et al. (2012) summarize the findings of studies of prehension development so far available. Their own investigation demonstrates the importance of toy selection and of infant position in activity or task-based training. For example, infants who have poor balance should sit supported during upper limb training in order to concentrate on reaching and prehension play. A recent study of children aged 6 to 11 years has shown the benefits of training reaching with the trunk/upper body constrained (Schneiberg et al., 2010). Practice of actions in sitting aimed at improving balance control can be trained, together with reaching to grasp, and included among a variety of actions during play and other interactions with family members.

Before birth, infants develop strong leg movements within the confines of the uterus (Milani Comparetti, 1980) and after birth they soon regain this kicking ability in the new, gravitational environment. Exploration to find solutions to new task demands, with adaptation to changes in the environmental context are assumed to be critical parts of motor learning and therefore of motor development. Prechtl (2001) has pointed out that one of the most fundamental new insights from research in developmental neurology is the concept of 'ontogenetic adaptation'. According to this concept, 'during the development of the individual the functional repertoire of the developing neural structure must meet the requirements of the organism and its environment'.

This change in theoretical perspective drives the present day re-examination of the relevance of testing reflexes as a means of determining the integrity or impairment of the infant nervous system. As Prechtl (2001) states, concepts of the reflex and of stimulus–response mechanisms have long dominated the interpretation of the function of the infant nervous system. It is the heritage from classic neurophysiology, but one that lingers on among physicians and therapists. Nevertheless, this new theoretical perspective, by providing us with much clearer guidelines for developing therapeutic interventions, is currently driving the major changes slowly taking place in clinical therapy practice. Modern descriptions of motor development are available in many texts (Berger and Adolf, 2007; Piek, 2006; Shepherd, 1995; Thelen and Smith, 1994). Biomechanical analyses of mature motor performance of everyday actions such as walking, reaching to grasp, and standing up, and of developmental and applied biomechanics, are found in textbooks and journal articles (Carr and Shepherd, 2000, 2003, 2010; Forssberg, 1985; Olney and Wright, 2006; Sutherland et al., 1980; Winter, 1987).

## Child rearing practices

Since motor development has long been considered a maturational phenomenon distinct from environmental influences (Hopkins and Westra, 1988), Western child-rearing practices have been largely based on this view, guided by studies of motor development carried out decades ago on limited numbers of babies in the Euro-American culture (e.g., McGraw, 1945). Our current understanding of developmental neurology has been greatly enhanced by studies of infants brought up in different child-rearing environments (Adolph et al., 2010). Several aspects of motor development have been shown to differ according to culture, i.e., what the infant experiences. The importance of environmental effects and experience on motor development, particularly in the first 18 months, is evident in comparative studies of development in a range of different cultures (Bril, 1986). These studies show what spontaneous 'parent-initiated' and 'environment-specific' training and practice can accomplish in infants.

Babies of African descent have been shown to be ahead of Caucasian babies specifically in sitting, standing alone and walking (Hopkins and Westra, 1988; Konner 1977). Similar results have been found for manipulation. Babies in the Yucatan, Mexico have advanced hand skills, including early development of a pincer grip, but are relatively delayed in walking. The infants studied were rarely placed on the floor and, when they were, there was little for them to hold on to (Solomons and Solomons, 1975). Kenyan Kipsigis mothers believed it was important to 'train' sitting and they set up the conditions by scooping out a hole in the soil in which the infant was placed (Super, 1976). In some tribes in Papua New Guinea, babies do not go through a crawling stage (Wong, 2009). They are carried until they can walk. When necessary, mothers put infants in the sitting position and the preferred way of getting about was scooting. Other cultures are said to have similar child-rearing methods, avoiding putting infants on the ground in order to protect them. Babies born in England to Jamaican mothers were found to be superior at independent sitting when compared with babies of English mothers. The Jamaican mothers trained sitting from age 3–4 months. Parents' expectations appear to be important considerations. The Jamaican mothers learned their child-rearing practices from their mother, the English from reading child care books. Both the predicted and the actual age of sitting and walking were significantly earlier in the Jamaicans compared to the English (Hopkins and Westra, 1988).

In an intracultural study, Zelazo and colleagues (1972, 1983) found that neonatal stepping can be trained, and the ability maintained through to independent walking; i.e., trained babies did not go through the period of locomotor inactivity reported for Western-reared babies. It has been shown that neonatal stepping has similar characteristics to

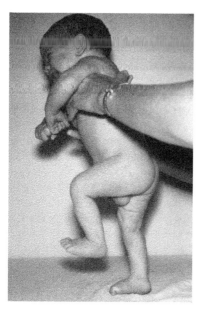

**Figure 1.7** • Many newborn babies when supported can straighten their legs, push up into standing and, if tilted forward, take a few steps.

mature walking and is a precursor to independent walking and not a reflex (Fig. 1.7). Thelen and Cooke (1987) suggested this transition from infant stepping to walking occurred due to the effect of training on muscular development: that is, the trained babies were stronger because the exercises would increase muscle mass.

## Motor learning and the acquisition of skill

We make the assumption that the acquisition of skill, involving practice and exercise, is a manifestation of those internal processes that make up what is called 'motor learning'. Motor learning itself cannot be directly observed but can be *inferred* from observation of a relatively consistent improvement in performance of an action as a result of practice of that action. This is why we measure certain characteristics of motor performance at the start of training and at various stages throughout and after training (Magill, 2010).

We can assume that motor development in infancy occurs, as does skill acquisition, through a process of learning: for example, learning how best to interact with the environment to achieve a certain goal. The infant explores the use and

control of gravitational forces and the interactional forces generated by movement itself. Movement of the limbs appears a fascination to the young infant. At first the arms and legs are waved about, then they become a focus of attention as the infant reaches out with hands or feet to touch what lies within reach and is attractive. Vigorous and apparently random movements of the arms become more organized to enable reaching for an object, grasping the feet, and so on. In very young infants, early movements such as kicking represent explorations of the possibilities offered by the linked segments of the lower limbs and gravity. This exploratory behaviour changes from apparently random kicks, to the use of the feet for a purpose: for example, touching a toy and manipulating its movement (see Fig. C.1) (Chen et al., 2002; Thelen, 1994).

Similar behaviours are seen as an infant develops more effective use of the upper limb. Thelen's study of 3-month-old infants in 1994 illustrated the remarkable capacity of the young infant to organize and control limb movements to learn a novel task (activating a mobile). She concluded that infants are participants in their own skill acquisition; that developmental change is engendered through the infant's everyday problem-solving activities (p. 284). In clinical practice, therapists might keep this in mind and avoid excessive hands-on. Holding and supporting the child too much can prevent an infant from trying out a variety of movement combinations in order to achieve a goal. Movement does not need to conform to an ideal 'normal' motor pattern/movement but it does have to obey the laws of mechanics, and the infant needs to know whether or not the attempt was successful. It can be difficult training young infants without holding on to them. However, a firm strap to save an infant from falling, fingertip control to guide the infant's own movements and environmental manipulation (see Fig. A.10B), including a harness, are preferable to a firm hold as they interfere less with the infant's self-initiated movements.

Young infants have to learn not only how to initiate an appropriate movement but also how to control interactional forces once movement has started, and the major impetus to this learning process is the need to achieve a specific goal. Once movement is successful, the infant will repeat and vary this action over and over again, preferring to do what works and is most successful. Motor performance becomes more effective as skill develops and adapts throughout growth, as morphology changes, and as new goals emerge.

Skill has been defined as any activity that has become more organized and more effective as a result of practice (Annett, 1971) and also as the ability to consistently attain a goal with some economy of effort (Gentile, 2000). For several decades, scientists have investigated the process of acquiring skill, typically with young healthy adults as they learn a novel task or train to improve a specific skill, and increasingly with people with motor disability. Everyday actions such as standing up and sitting down are skills; i.e., complex actions made up of segmental movements linked together in the appropriate spatial and temporal sequence to achieve a particular goal (see Chapter 11).

In acquiring skill, learning is said to take place in overlapping stages—an early cognitive stage, an intermediate associative stage and a final or autonomous stage (Fitts and Posner, 1967). Gentile (2000) described these stages as first getting the idea of the movement, then developing the ability to adapt the movement pattern to environmental demands. Note in both descriptions that the initial stage is cognitive; it is in this stage that the infant gets the idea of the action, learns to pay attention to critical features, and is actively engaged in practice. Vision and imitation play important roles at this stage. The infant imitates what a parent or sibling does, and later on will observe and copy other young children.

Awareness of the characteristics of each stage of learning enables the therapist to provide appropriate practice conditions to optimize performance (Carr and Shepherd, 2003). In clinical practice, the infant learner's focus of attention shifts as muscle strength, motor control and skill increase. In walking, for example, it may shift from how to balance on the legs to what possibilities are offered by the surrounding environment; focus in learning sit-to-stand may change from standing up without falling to carrying a favourite object while rising to walk.

As skill develops, the effort required decreases. Performance of an action that is effective in consistently achieving a specific goal with some economy of effort is said to be skilled. However, an infant with diplegic CP may practice, and get better at, an action that ultimately will not be effective, e.g., walking on the toes with small steps. This method of walking may be reasonably effective for a short time but as the child grows

and body mass increases and contractures of calf muscles, hip flexors, adductors and internal rotator muscles develop, the amount of energy required to balance and walk may become too great. A wheeled apparatus may be preferable and surgery may become necessary to overcome the contracted muscles. Writing of the development of manipulative skills, Seashore (1940) hypothesized that skills are acquired by a rather haphazard process of trial and error in such a way that the first fairly successful attempt at a complex action such as doing up a button will become established in the learner's repertoire. Other methods might exist which are faster and more reliable, or involve less effort, but the first method learned may remain.

As Damiano points out in Chapter 9, 'the dilemma with many infants with CP is that they may not be able to initiate a specific movement to be able to practice it at all or effectively. As a result, these children often develop compensatory strategies to accomplish a specific functional goal in the short term that ultimately limits movement efficiency and flexibility in the long term. In the absence of intervention (or if intervention is not appropriate), this less than optimal strategy is then reinforced through repetition.' New methods of identifying infants with poor muscle activation and of stimulating muscle activation and training effective limb control in infancy need to be developed and used in order to address the problems raised in this chapter and in Chapter 9.

Understanding the critical biomechanical characteristics of walking and applying this information in infant training may be critical if the infant is to learn to walk effectively and efficiently enough to preserve this walking pattern through childhood and adult life. This knowledge may enable future exercise and training programmes to change the typical walking of diplegia to a more effective method, or by starting early in infancy, to prevent it developing. For example, understanding the relationship of muscle length to angular displacement through stance and swing phases of walking should result in therapists starting a programme of exercises for an infant with diplegia that targets the necessary extensibility and strength. Delp et al. (1999) has demonstrated the widespread effects on hip adduction and rotation of persistent hip flexion. Yet, in therapy sessions, hip extension beyond the midline may not be a focus of training early in infancy or during the early weeks of independent standing and walking in infants with diplegia or hemiplegia. When the infant is walking, overground or on a treadmill, weak and limited hip extension may be masked by the forward tilt of the pelvis that results from hip flexor contracture.

To learn a more effective and energy-efficient way of walking, it is necessary to ensure that exercises practiced throughout infancy and early childhood are practiced with the load distributed appropriately over the surface of both feet. A recent study of children with hemiplegia and diplegia has reported that the area of the plantar surface that is in contact with the floor when walking is significantly different to that used by able-bodied and age-matched children (A. Nsenga, pers. comm., 2012).

Schmidt (1988) defined motor learning as 'a set of processes involving practice and exercise leading to a relatively stable change in motor behaviour'. The aim of intervention is to bring about stability but also flexibility of performance: that is, the optimization of motor performance; i.e., the most effective performance of the motor actions of daily life that is possible for that individual. A training programme can assist the infant and child to practice an action sufficiently intensively to ensure it can be performed more than once or twice in the clinic. A stable change in behaviour means that the action of, for example, standing up and sitting down, can be reliably and effectively performed on every similar occasion. This implies that learning has occurred. By making small changes to environmental demands, by raising or lowering the seat, for example, the infant learns to be flexible, to adapt the action according to external demands and internal goals. Although standing up and sitting down may share similar biomechanical characteristics, the demands placed on the control system and muscles by each action are different; for example, the extensor muscle work involved in eccentric contractions (sitting down) is different to that in concentric contractions (standing up).

Brain mapping techniques, used in conjunction with biomechanical and spatiotemporal measures of motor performance, may shed some light on the process of motor learning itself. These studies show use-dependent brain reorganization occurs throughout life and after injury in response to activity and learning. Several studies have shown that intervention methods can affect (both positively and negatively) brain reorganization (see Chapters 2 and 3). Positive effects seem to be related to practice of meaningful activities (goal-directed) in task-oriented and intensive (repetitive) training. In general, findings support Lemon's suggestion that the mechanisms underlying adaptation are also the mechanisms of motor learning and motor development. It helps to keep in mind that:

> The behaviour that dominates our daily lives is directed toward the accomplishment of goals. It is aimed at a specific purpose or end that we are trying to achieve. It is intentional, linked to outcomes we are attempting to produce. It has the quality of perseverance. Goal-directed behaviour is guided by the consequences it produces—by feedback as to how close or how far away we are from accomplishing our objective.
>
> Gentile, 2000, p112

## Implicit and explicit learning

In 1998, Gentile proposed that two interdependent learning processes mediate the acquisition of functional skills. They 'operate in parallel, change at different rates as a consequence of practice, and are differentially accessible to conscious awareness' (p. 7) (Gentile, 1998).

*Explicit learning* is primarily responsible for rapid improvement and success at achieving the goal of the action seen during initial practice. With practice a correspondence develops between the learner's morphology and the regulatory environmental conditions (the topology of the movement; see Fig. 11.8B,C), and in the specification of appropriate movement parameters that match task-constraints. The movement is 'good enough' to meet the demands of the task and achieve the goal but is not efficient—the movement may not be smooth flowing or energy-efficient.

*Implicit learning* is responsible for changes in movement organization that lead to efficient performance Movement organization changes in at least three ways with practice:

- Regulating intersegmental force dynamics
- Blending successive movement components
- Coupling simultaneous components

In other words, practice (usually over a long period of time) results in fine-tuning of these motor control processes, suggesting that motor control and learning should not be considered separate events (Willingham, 1992). Only with prolonged practice does the learner develop movement patterns that are smooth and efficient and characteristic of skilled performance.

These changes take place outside conscious awareness. They appear to occur 'automatically'. Reorganization processes are reinforced when minimization of cost (e.g., energy) occurs.

Studies of children and young adults as they learn and become skilled have explored such factors as the learner's focus of attention; imitating the performance of others or of oneself; the effects of contextual information on motor performance; the learner's perceived locus of control; and the effects of interactive practice (Shea and Wulf, 1999). There are increasing studies of children but few studies of infants. If we understand the infant is a learner, we can focus therapy on a more active training model, and this involves being up to date in methods of stimulating learning. Research into how people acquire skill has largely been on older children and adults rather than infants. This stems in part from belief that motor development in infancy is largely due to innate maturational processes. However, changes in our understanding of development and the processes of learning and the role of experience and opportunity in infant development have arisen out of investigations into motor behaviour and what guides it. Some examples of methods used in training motor performance and stimulating the processes of learning, both for 'beginners' at the earliest stages of learning an action and for those whose action needs fine-tuning, are provided below. For many of the common tasks of daily life, fine-tuning may not occur, even in the able-bodied individual, until the child is much older.

## Concrete versus abstract

Concrete tasks differ from abstract in the degree to which the required act is directed toward controlling physical interaction with the environment or the person's own body as opposed to producing movement for its own sake. In general, the more concrete the task the richer the perceptual information for guiding the movement (Fig. 1.8A,B). There have been several studies with adults (Leont'ev and Zaporozhets, 1960; Sietsma et al., 1993; van Vliet et al., 1995; Wu et al., 2000), but few with children or infants. However, one study of nine children with hemiplegia with a mean age of 5 years (van der Weel and van der Meer, 1991) showed significantly greater supination–pronation range of movement of the upper limb in a concrete 'beat the drum' task (turning the arm and drumstick into supination/

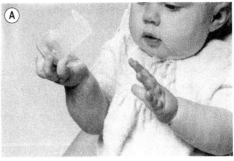

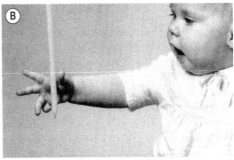

**Figure 1.8 •** Learning to handle objects, exploring their characteristics and the possibilities they offer.
**(A)** Exploring the possibilities of supination and pronation.
**(B)** Presenting a long rod vertically requires reaching combined with supination of the forearm. At this early stage of learning to reach and grasp, opening the fingers to grasp is accompanied by a similar action with the other hand, or combined with opening of the mouth.
[From Shepherd RB 1995 Physiotherapy in Paediatrics 3rd ed. with permission from Elsevier.]

pronation), compared to an abstract task (pronation/supination of the arm).

## Observational learning: imitation and modelling

Most human behaviour is learned by observation of another, through modelling and imitating. Many studies have addressed this issue in adults and children. An overview of existing data on imitation in infancy has suggested that imitation of different kinds of behaviour emerges at different ages (Jones, 2009), but with little evidence that infants used imitation until their second year. Several studies of self-modelling (Dowrick, 1999) used repeated observation of the learner on videotapes showing only the desired target behaviour and deleting the rest. One study examined school children (average age 12 years) learning volleyball serve and overhand pass (Zetou et al., 1999). The group that observed a videotape of an expert model improved their performance on the two aspects of the game more than the group who observed their own movements (self-modelling). These results suggest that a skilled model might command greater attention than an unskilled model, leading to greater learning, and so, for the infant, an older child or adult, or the infant's own 'best' performance, can be the skilled model.

Studies of children learning a new skill have shown that younger children can perform best with verbal self-instruction/rehearsal, and that verbal rehearsal strategies aid children's ability to attend selectively to relevant task components and to remember the specific execution order of a skill (Weiss and Klint, 1987). A combination of verbal cues and modelling may also effective. Modelling may be particularly effective with young infants in providing visual cues to the 'effective' performance of actions being trained. The AOT programme emphasizes modelling as a method of stimulating learning and improving functional performance. Visual information (from modelling) may be superior to auditory information when the task requires positional or spatial components.

## Focusing attention

There is increasing evidence with children and adults that directing a learner's attention to the effects of their movements, i.e., whether or not the goal has been achieved, may be more effective than attending to the movement itself (Wulf et al., 1999a, 1999b). It is also likely to be so for infants, and designers of infants' playthings know this when they build toys that give pleasurable feedback when touched or handled, toys that require or attract the infant's visual attention. Toys need to be selected for the possibilities they offer for exploration and experimentation but they can also be selected to force a particular grip or movement. How the toy is presented can also drive a particular action (Fig. 1.8B). Toys that are too large for the infant's hand should not be chosen unless the infant has the opportunity to take it with both hands (Fig. 1.9). Selection of toys for training specific functions is discussed in a literature review by Greaves et al. (2011).

Interactive technological devices, such as the mobile with control panel that allows the infant to control the mobile by touching the panel with a foot (Chen et al., 2002), will increasingly be used as training aids and to drive actions that are critical,

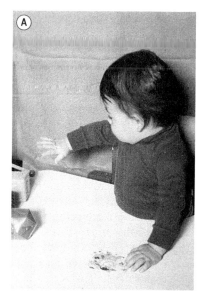

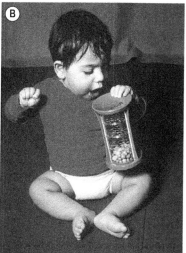

**Figure 1.9 •** Objects and their placement drive motor performance. Training upper limb actions needs the environment to be organized to optimize the learner's attempts at achieving the goal. In **(A)** there is no toy within reach that requires supination, so he reaches out in pronation, as he habitually does (Fig. 1.8B shows how to encourage supination). In **(B)** due to the effort required to hold on with one hand to an object that is too large, his right arm flexes. Associated movements occur when a task is difficult but this boy's arm movement is stereotyped and habitual behaviour. Toys and everyday objects must be carefully chosen for both their attractiveness and their graspability. Sessions of constraint-induced movement therapy with carefully selected toys may help him overcome the stereotypy and to learn to use his hand. [From Shepherd RB 1995 Physiotherapy in Paediatrics 3rd ed. with permission from Elsevier.]

at the biomechanical level, for the development of effective walking, and other actions involving flexion/extension of lower limbs (see Chapters 10 to 12 and Annotation C). Further development of the interactive mobile may also stimulate upper limb use in infants. A new interactive computer-based training system, delivered to the child's home through the internet with the aim of encouraging intensive practice at home, has recently been developed: *Move It To Improve It (MiTii)*. The system has been tested in children with CP who trained over a 20-week period with 30 minutes practice each day. Training resulted in significant improvement in the trained motor and cognitive functions (Bilde et al., 2011, Chapter 15). Similar programmes could be developed that would be suitable for infants.

## Practice

Improvement in a particular action requires practice of that action: i.e., the infant has to practice in order for performance to become effective. As the infant gets older, improving power generation to speed up an action and to hop and jump are major performance goals. However, for those whose muscle strength and motor control are below a certain threshold, such practice may not be possible. Infants and children normally find their own ways to challenge their strength and balance. The role of the teacher or coach for an infant in the clinic and at home involves developing ways to enable practice, with exercises to increase strength and control, concentrically and eccentrically, together with practice of the action under modified conditions: for example, standing up from a higher seat, which requires less extensor muscle force generation than a lower seat (see Chapter 11). The responsibility for increasing the opportunities for practice during the day must fall on the family. With able-bodied infants parents naturally provide these opportunities with play sessions, special toys and household objects, and spaces where the infant is free and safe to roam and explore. It is more difficult with an infant who has motor disability and to overcome this problem requires the development of interactive devices that can drive or reinforce the infant's own attempts. A good example of one such development is described in Annotation C.

## Repetition

Repetition seems to be a critical aspect of practice both for learning and for increasing muscle strength,

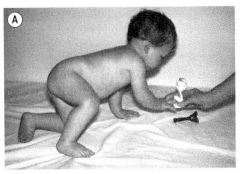
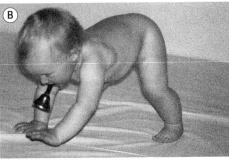
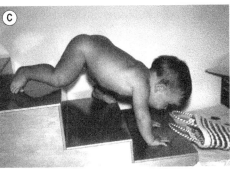

**Figure 1.10** • The drive to move about is strong in the months leading up to independent walking. Infants move about on the floor, exploring the possibilities (and limitations) of locomotion in prone.

and it may take thousands of repetitions before a person develops an optimal way of performing the action. However, as Whiting (1980) pointed out, acquiring skill does not only mean to repeat and consolidate but also to invent and to progress, also termed 'repetition without repetition' by Bernstein (1967). When an able-bodied infant is in an enriched environment of parents, siblings and home, each new skill can be practiced with many repetitions and in varied ways (Fig. 1.10). It seems important to motor learning at all ages that the actions attempted bring benefits that are obvious and meaningful.

Paediatric physiotherapists are becoming increasingly aware of infants and young children as active learners rather than as passive recipients of therapeutic facilitation, and significant changes in training are occurring. These changes are due to our increasing knowledge of how people learn and relearn motor skills, of the biomechanics and muscle activations that result in effective motor performance, of methods of strength training, and of the major impairments and adaptations that make successful performance difficult to attain.

In conclusion, the scientific knowledge and training skills to upgrade clinical physiotherapy practice for infants and young children with CP are available. We have better understanding of the effects on brain organization and motor development of what an infant does and experiences. Training methods appropriate for infants are driven by increased knowledge of neural control mechanisms, biomechanics of movement, and of the nature of impairments; of the challenging, intensive exercise that drives motor learning; and the assistive technologies available. The attitude of paediatricians and neonatologists is critical to enable an early referral for specialized intervention of infants whose brain scan and/or poverty of movement suggest the possibility of CP.

It is likely that targeted and intensive motor training and exercise can be therapeutic and preventative, driving the organizational processes necessary after a brain lesion in developing infants. In infants with CP, it is probable that the first 12 months of life may be significant in setting the foundation for future motor development. We need to acknowledge the primacy of and the potential for stimulating and training motor activity and refocus our interventions on to poor muscle activation and weakness, poor motor control, and the effects of limited physical activity on muscle growth and development. We should be more proactive with young infants in finding ways both to minimize the onset of negative adaptations that have the potential to augment disability, and to optimize the infants' chances of developing effective and flexible motor function.

# References

Acerra, N., Vidoni, E., Wessell, B., et al., 2011. Does task-specificity matter for motor sequence learning after stroke? Insights from fMRI. Physiotherapy Suppl. S1, 97.

Adolph, K.E., Karasik, L.B., Tamis-LeMonda, C.S., 2010. Motor skill. In: Bornstein, M.H. (Ed.), Handbook of Cultural Developmental Science Taylor & Francis, New York, pp. 61–88.

Andersen, L.L., Zeeman, P., Jorgensen, J.R., et al., 2011. Effects of intensive physical rehabilitation on neuromuscular adaptations in adults with poststroke hemiparesis. J. Strength Cond. Res. 25, 2808–2817.

Annett, J., 1971. Acquisition of skill. Br. Med. Bull. 27, 266–271.

Berger, S., Adolph, K.E., 2007. Learning and development in infant locomotion. In: von Hofsten, C., Rosander, K. (Eds.), From Action to Cognition Elsevier, Amsterdam, pp. 237–255.

Berger, W., 1998. Characteristics of locomotor control in children with cerebral palsy. Neurosci. Biobehav. Res. 22, 579–582.

Bernstein, N., 1967. The Coordination and Regulation of Movement. Pergamon Press, London.

Bilde, P.E., Klim-Due, M., Rasmussen, B., et al., 2011. Individualized, home-based interactive training of cerebral palsy children with cerebral palsy delivered through the Internet. BMC Neurol. 11, 32. doi: 10.1186/1471-2377-11-32.

Blauw-Hospers, C.H., Dirks, T., Hulshof, L.J., et al., 2011. Pediatric physical therapy in infancy: from nightmare to dream? A two-arm randomized trial. Phys. Ther. 91, 1323–1338.

Blauw-Hospers, C.H., Hadders-Algra, M., 2005. A systematic review of the effects of early intervention on motor development. Dev. Med. Child Neurol. 47, 421–432.

Blundell, S.W., Shepherd, R.B., Dean, C.M., et al., 2003. Functional strength training in cerebral palsy: a pilot study of a group circuit training class for children aged 4–8 years. Clin. Rehabil. 17, 48–57.

Bodkin, A.W., Baxter, R.S., Heriza, C.B., 2003. Treadmill training for an infant born preterm with a grade III intraventricular haemorrhage. Phys. Ther. 83, 1107–1118.

Bril, B., 1986. Motor development and cultural attitudes. In: Whiting, H.T.A., Wade, M.G. (Eds.), Themes in Motor Development. Martinus Nijhoff, Dordrecht.

Brouwer, B., Ashby, P., 1991. Altered corticospinal projections to lower limb motoneurons in subjects with cerebral palsy. Brain 114, 1395–1407.

Carr, J.H., Shepherd, R.B. (Eds.), 2000. Foundations for Physical Therapy in Rehabilitation, second ed. Aspen, Rockville, MD.

Carr, J.H., Shepherd, R.B., 2003. Stroke Rehabilitation Guidelines for Exercise and Training to Optimize Motor Skill. Butterworth-Heinemann, Oxford.

Carr, J.H., Shepherd, R.B., 2010. Neurological Rehabilitation:

Optimizing Motor Performance, second ed. Butterworth-Heinemann, Oxford.

Carr, L.J., Harrison, L.M., Evans, A.I., et al., 2003. Patterns of central motor organization in hemiplegic cerebral palsy. Brain 116, 1223–1247.

Chad, K.E., Bailey, D.A., McKay, H.A., et al., 1999. The effect of a weight-bearing physical activity programme on bone mineral content and estimated volumetric density in children with spastic cerebral palsy. J. Pediatr. 135, 115–117.

Chae, J., Yang, G., Park, B.K., et al., 2002a. Delay in initiation and termination of muscle contraction, motor impairment, and physical disability in upper limb paresis. Muscle Nerve 25, 568–575.

Chae, J., Yang, G., Park, B.K., et al., 2002b. Muscle weakness and contraction in upper limb paresis: relationship to motor impairment and physical disability. Neurorehabil. Neural Repair 16, 241–248.

Charles, J., Gordon, A.M., 2006. Development of hand-arm bimanual intensive training (HABIT) for improving bimanual coodination in children with hemiplegic cerebral palsy. Dev. Med. Child Neurol. 48, 931–936.

Chen, Y.-P., Fetters, L., Holt, K.G., et al., 2002. Making the mobile move: constraining task and environment. Infant. Behav. Dev. 25, 195–220.

Clowry, G.J., 2007. The dependence of spinal cord development on corticospinal input and its significance in understanding and treating spastic cerebral palsy. Neurosci. Biobehav. Rev. 31, 1114–1124.

Damiano, D.L., 2006. Activity, activity, activity: rethinking our physical therapy approach to cerebral palsy. Phys. Ther. 86, 1534–1540.

Dean, C.M., Shepherd, R.B., 1997. Task-related training improves performance of a seated reaching tasks after stroke: a randomised controlled trial. Stroke 28, 722–728.

Dean, C.M., Richards, C.L., Malouin, F., 2000. Task-related training improves performance of locomotor tasks in chronic stroke. A randomised controlled pilot trial. Arch. Phys. Med. Rehabil. 81, 409–417.

Delp, S.L., 2003. What causes increased muscle stiffness in cerebral palsy? Muscle Nerve 27, 131–132.

Delp, S.L., Hess, W.E., Hungerford, D.S., et al., 1999. Variation of rotational arms with hip flexion. J. Biomech. 23, 493–501.

Dowrick, P.W., 1999. A review of self-modeling and related interventions. Appl. Prevent. Psychol. 8, 23–39.

Eastlake, M.E., Arvidson, J., Snyder Macklin, L., et al., 1991. Interrater reliability of videotaped observational gait—analysis assessments. Phys. Ther. 71, 465–472.

Echols, K., DeLuca, S.C., Ramey, S.L., et al., 2002. Constraint-induced movement therapy versus traditional therapeutic services for young children with cerebral palsy: a randomised controlled trial. Dev. Med. Child Neurol. 91 (Suppl. 9).

Edelman, G.M., 1987. Neuronal Darwinism: The Theory of Neuronal Group Selection. Basic Books, New York.

Elbert, T., Pantev, C., Wienbruch, C., et al., 1995. Increased cortical representation of the fingers of the left hand in string players. Science 270, 305–307.

Eng, J.J., Chu, K.S., Kin, C.M., 2003. A community-based group exercise programme for persons with chronic stroke. Med. Sci. Sports Exerc. 35, 1271–1278.

Enoka, R.M., 1997. Neural strategies in the control of muscle force. Muscle Nerve 5 (Suppl.), S666–S669.

Ertelt, D., Small, S., Solodkin, A., et al., 2007. Action observation has a positive impact on rehabilitation of motor deficits after stroke. NeuroImage 36, T164–T173.

Eyre, J.A., 2003. Development and plasticity of the corticospinal system in man. Neur. Plast. 10, 93–106.

Eyre, J.A., 2007. Corticospinal tract development and its plasticity after perinatal injury. Neurosci. Biobehav. Rev. 31, 1136–1149.

Eyre, J.A., Miller, S., Clowry, G.J., et al., 2000. Functional corticospinal projections are established prenatally in the human fetus permitting involvement in the development of spinal motor centres. Brain 123, 51–64.

Eyre, J.A., Taylor, J.P., Villagra, F., et al., 2001. Evidence of activity-dependent withdrawal of corticospinal projections during human development. Neurology 57, 1543–1554.

Ferrari, F., Cioni, G., Einspieler, C., et al., 2003. General movements in preterm infants as a marker for later cerebral palsy. Dev. Med. Child Neurol. Suppl. 94 (45), 32–33.

Fetters, L., 1991. Measurement and treatment in cerebral palsy: an argument for a new approach. Phys. Ther. 71, 244.

Fitts, P.M., Posner, M.I., 1967. Human Performance. Brook/Cole, Belmont, CA.

Flodmark, O., Krageloh-Mann, I., Bax, M., et al., 2003. Brain imaging studies of individuals with cerebral palsy. Dev. Med. Child Neurol. Suppl. 94 (45), 33–34.

Forssberg, H., 1985. Ontogeny of human locomotor control I: infant stepping, supported locomotion and transition to independent locomotion. Exp. Brain Res. 57, 480–493.

Forssberg, H., Eliasson, A.C., Kinoshita, H., et al., 1991. Development of human precision grip.I: basic coordination of force. Exp. Brain Res. 85, 451–457.

Forssberg, H., Kinoshita, H., Eliasson, A.C., et al., 1992. Development of human precision grip.II: anticipatory control of isometric forces targeted for object's weight. Exp. Brain Res. 90, 393–398.

Garvey, M.A., Giannetti, M.L., Alter, K.E., et al., 2007. Cerebral palsy: new approaches to therapy. Curr. Neurol. Neurosci. Rep. 7, 147–155.

Gentile, A.M., 1998. Implicit and explicit processes during acquisition of functional skills. Scand. J. Occup. Ther. 5, 7–16.

Gentile, A.M., 2000. Skill acquisition. Action, movement and neuromotor processes. In: Carr, J.H., Shepherd, R.B. (Eds.), Movement Science. Foundations for Physical Therapy in Rehabilitation, second ed. Aspen, Rockville, MD, pp. 111–180.

Gibson, J.J., 1979. The Ecological Approach to Visual Perception. Houghton Mifflin, Boston, MA.

Gracies, J.M., 2005. Pathophysiology of spastic paresis 1: emergence of muscle overactivity. Muscle Nerve 31, 552–571.

Greaves, S., Imms, C., Krumlinde-Sundholm, L., et al., 2011. Bimanual behaviours in children aged 8–18 months: a literature review to select toys that elicit the use of two hands. Res. Dev. Disabil. 33, 240–250.

Hadders-Algra, M., 2004. General movements: a window for early identification of children at high risk for developmental disorders. J. Pediatr. 145 (Suppl 2), 12–18.

Hadders-Algra, M., Mavinkurve-Groothuis, A.M.C., Groen, S.E., et al., 2004. Quality of general movements and the development of minor neurological dysfunction at toddler and school age. Clin. Rehabil. 18, 287–299.

Hodapp, M., Vry, J., Mall, V., et al., 2009. Changes in soleus H-reflex modulation after treadmill training in children with cerebral palsy. Brain 132, 37–44.

Hagglund, G., Wagner, P., 2011. Spasticity of the gastrosoleus muscle is related to the development of reduced passive dorsiflexion of the ankle in children with cerebral palsy. Acta Orthop. 82, 744–748.

Hopkins, B., Westra, T., 1988. Maternal handling and motor development: an intracultural study. Genet. Soc. Gen. Psychol. Monogr. 114, 379.

Jang, S.H., You, S.H., Hallet, M., et al., 2005. Cortical reorganization and associated functional motor recovery after virtual reality in patients with chronic stroke. Arch. Phys. Med. Rehabil. 86, 2218–2223.

Jenkins, W.M., Marzenich, M.M., Ochs, M.T., et al., 1990. Functional reorganization of primary somatosensory cortex in adult owl monkeys after behaviourally controlled tactile stimulation. J. Neurophysiol. 63, 82–104.

Johansson, B.B., 2000. Brain plasticity and stroke rehabilitation: the Willis lecture. Stroke 31, 223–230.

Johnston, M.V., 1998. Selective vulnerability in the neonatal brain [editorial]. Ann. Neurol. 44, 155–156.

Johnston, M.V., 2009. Plasticity in the developing brain: implications for rehabilitation. Dev. Disabilities. Res. Rev. 15, 94–101.

Jones, S.S., 2009. The development of imitation in infancy. Phil. Trans. R. Soc. B. doi: 10.1098/rstb.2009.0045

Jorgensen, J.R., Bech-Pedersen, D.T., Zeeman, P., 2010. Effect of intensive outpatient physical training on gait performance and cardiovascular health in people with hemiparesis after stroke. Phys. Ther. 90, 527–537.

Kamper, D.G., Rymer, W.Z., 2001. Impairment of voluntary control of finger motion following stroke: role of inappropriate coactivation. Muscle Nerve 24, 673–681.

Kandel, E.R., Schwartz, J.H., Jessell, T.M. (Eds.), 2000. Principles of Neural Science, fourth ed. McGraw-Hill, New York.

Ketelaar, M., Vermeer, A., Hart, H., et al., 2001. Effects of a functional therapy programme on motor abilities of children with cerebral palsy. Phys. Ther. 81, 1534–1545.

Kleim, J.A., Vij, K., Ballard, D.H., et al., 1997. Learning-dependent synaptic modifications in the cerebellar cortex of the adult rat persist for at least four weeks. J. Neurosci. 17, 717–721.

Knutzen, K.M., Martin, L.A., 2002. Using biomechanics to explore children's movement. Pediatr. Exerc. Sci. 14, 222–247.

Kolb, B., 2003. Overview of cortical plasticity and recovery from brain injury. Phys. Med. Rehab. Clin. N. Amer. 14, S4–S25.

Konner, M., 1977. Maternal care and infant behavior and development among the Kalahari Desert San. In: Lee, R., deVore, I. (Eds.), Kalahari Hunter Gatherers. Harvard University Press, Cambridge, MA.

Kuperminc, M.N., Stevenson, R.D., 2008. Growth and nutrition disorders in children with cerebral palsy. Dev. Disabil. Res. Rev. 14, 137–146. doi: 10.1002/ddrr.14.

LeVeau, B.F., Bernhardt, D.B., 1984. Developmental biomechanics. Effects of forces on the growth, development and maintenance of the human body. Phys. Ther. 64, 1874–1882.

Leont'ev, A.N., Zaporozhets, A.V., 1960. Rehabilitation of Hand Function. Pergamon Press, London.

Liao, H.-F., Liu, Y.-C., Liu, W.-Y., et al., 2007. Effectiveness of loaded sit-to-stand resistance exercise for children with mild spastic diplegia: a

randomized clinical trial. Arch. Phys. Med. Rehabil. 88, 25–31.

Liepert, J., Tegenholt, M., Malin, J.P., 1995. Changes of cortical motor area size during immobilization. Electroenceph. Clin. Neurol. 97, 382–386.

Liepert, J., Bauder, H., Miltner, W., et al., 2000. Treatment-induced cortical reorganization after stroke in humans. Stroke 31, 1210–1216.

Magill, R., 2010. Motor Learning and Control: Concepts and Applications, 12th ed. McGraw-Hill, New York.

Malouin, F., 1995. Observational gait analysis. In: Craik, R., Oates, C.A. (Eds.), Gait Analysis. Theory and Applications. Mosby, St Louis, pp. 112–124.

Marigold, D.S., Eng, J.J., Dawson, A.S., et al., 2005. Exercise leads to faster postural reflexes, improved balance and mobility, and fewer falls in older persons with chronic stroke. J. Am. Geriatr. Soc. 5, 416–423.

Martin, J.H., Friel, K.M., Salimi, I., et al., 2007. Activity- and use-dependent plasticity of the developing corticospinal system. Neurosci. Biobehav. Rev. 31, 1125–1235.

McGraw, M.B., 1945. The Neuromuscular Maturation of the Human Infant. Columbia University Press, New York.

Merzenich, M.M., Allard, T.T., Jenkins, W.M., 1991. Neural ontogeny of higher brain function: implications of some recent neurophysiological findings. In: Franzen, O., Westman, I. (Eds.), Information Processing in the Somatosensory System. Macmillan, London.

Milani-Comparetti, A., 1980. Pattern analysis of normal and abnormal development: the fetus, the newborn, the child. In: Slaton, D.S. (Ed.), Development of Movement in Infancy. University of South Carolina Press, Chapel Hill, SC.

Moyer-Mileur, L., Brunstetter, V., McNaught, T.P., et al., 2000. Daily physical activity programme increases bone mineralisation and growth in preterm very low birth weight infants. Pediatrics 106, 1088–1092.

Nelles, G., Jentzen, W., Jueptner, M., et al., 2001. Arm training induced plasticity in stroke studied with serial positron emission tomography. NeuroImage 13, 1146–1154.

Noppeney, U., 2007. The effects of visual deprivation on functional and structural organization of the human brain. Neurosci. Biobehav. Rev. 31, 1169–1180.

Nudo, R.J., Milliken, G.W., 1996. Reorganization of movement representation in primary motor cortex following focal ischemia infarcts in adult squirrel monkeys. J. Neurophysiol. 75, 2144–2149.

Nudo, R.J., Wise, B.M., SiFuentes, F., et al., 1996. Neural substrates for the effects of neurorehabilitation on motor recovery after ischaemic infarct. Science 272, 1791–1794.

Nudo, R.J., Plautz, E.J., Frost, S.B., 2001. Role of adaptive plasticity in recovery of function after damage to motor cortex. Muscle Nerve 8, 1000–1019.

Olmos, M., Carranza, J.A., Ato, M., 2000. Force-related information and exploratory behavior in infancy. Infant. Behav. Dev. 23, 407–419.

Olney, S.J., Wright, M.J., 2006. Cerebral palsy. In: Campbell, S.K., Vander Linden, D.W., Palisano, R.J. (Eds.), Physical Therapy for Children, third ed. Elsevier, New York.

O'Sullivan, M.C., Miller, S., Rames, V., et al., 1998. Abnormal development of biceps brachii phasic stretch reflex and persistence of short latency heteronymous reflexes from biceps to triceps brachii in spastic cerebral palsy. Brain 121, 2381–2395.

Pascuol-Leone, A., Torres, F., 1993. Plasticity of the sensorimotor cortex representation of the reading finger in Braille readers. Brain 116, 39–52.

Pascuol-Leone, A., Wasserman, E.M., Sadato, N., et al., 1995. The role of reading activity on the modulation of motor cortical inputs to the reading hand in Braille readers. Ann. Neurol. 38, 910–915.

Piek, J., 2006. Infant Motor Development. Human Kinetics, New York.

Prechtl, H.F.R., 2001. General movement assessment as a method of developal neurology: new paradigms and their consequences. Dev. Med. Child Neurol. 43, 836–842.

Rameckers, E.A.A., Speth, L.A.W.M., Duysens, J., et al., 2008. Botulinum toxin-A in children with congenital

spastic hemiplegia does not improve upper extremity motor-related function over rehabilitation alone: a randomised controlled trial. Neurorehabil. Neural Repair 23, 218–225.

Scheibel, A.B., Conrad, T., Perdue, S., et al., 1990. A quantitative study of dendrite complexity in selected areas of the human cerebral cortex. Brain Cong. 87, 85–101.

Schmidt, R.A., 1988. Motor Control and Learning, second ed. Human Kinetics, Champaign, IL.

Schneiberg, S., McKinley, P.A., Sveistrup, H., et al., 2010. The effectiveness of task-oriented intervention and trunk restraint on upper limb movement quality in children with cerebral palsy. Dev. Med. Child Neurol. 52, e245–e253.

Seashore, R.H., 1940. An experimental and theoretical analysis of fine motor skills. Am. J. Psychol. 53, 86–98.

Sgandurra, G., Ferrari, A., Cossu, G., et al., 2011. Upper limb children action-observation training (UP-CAT): a randomised controlled trial in hemiplegic cerebral palsy. Bio. Med. Central Neurol. 11, 1–19.

Sgandurra, G., Cecchi, F., Serio, S.M., et al., 2012. Longitudinal study of unimanual actions and grasping forces during infancy. Infant Behav. Dev. 35 (2), 205–214.

Shea, C.H., Wulf, G., 1999. Enhancing training efficiency and effectiveness through the use of dyad practice. J. Motor. Behav. 31, 119–125.

Shepherd, R.B., 1995. Physiotherapy in Paediatrics, third ed. Butterworth-Heinemann, Oxford.

Sherrington, C., Pamphlet, P.I., Jacka, J., et al., 2008. Group exercise can improve participant's' mobility in an outpatient rehabilitation setting: a randomised controlled trial. Clin. Rehabil. 22, 493–502.

Shumway-Cook, A., Woollacott, M.H., 2011. Motor Control. Translating Research into Practice. Lippincott Williams Wilkins, Philadelphia.

Sietsma, J.M., Nelson, D.L., Mulder, R.M., et al., 1993. The use of a game to promote arm reach in persons with traumatic brain injury. Am. J. Occup. Ther. 47, 19–24.

Slemender, C.W., Miller, J.Z., Hui, S.L., 1991. Role of physical activity in the development of skeletal mass

in children. J. Bone Mineral Res. 6, 1227–1233.

Solomons, G., Solomons, H.C., 1975. Motor development in Yucatecan infants. Dev. Med. Child Neurol. 17, 41.

Specker, B., Binkley, T., 2003. Randomized trial of physical activity and calcium supplementation on bone mineral content in 3–5-year-old children. J. Bone Mineral Res. 18, 885–892.

Super, C.M., 1976. Environmental effects on motor development: the case of 'African infant precocity'. Dev. Med. Child Neurol. 18, 561.

Sutherland, D.H., Olshen, R., Cooper, L., et al., 1980. The development of mature gait. J. Bone Joint. Surg. Am. 62A, 336–353.

Sveistrup, H., 2004. Motor rehabilitation using virtual reality. J. Neuro. Eng. Rehabil. 1, 10. doi: 10.1186/1743-0003-1-10.

Thelen, E., 1994. Three-month-old infants can learn task-specific patterns of interlimb coordination. Psychol. Sci. 5, 280–285.

Thelen, E., Cooke, D.W., 1987. Relationship between newborn stepping and later walking: a new interpretation. Dev. Med. Child Neurol. 29, 380–393.

Thelen, E., Smith, L.B., 1994. A Dynamic Systems Approach to the Development of Cognition and Action. MIT Press, Cambridge, MA.

Trevisi, E., Gualdi, S., De Conti, C., 2012. Cycling induced by functional electrical stimulation in children affected by cerebral palsy: case report. Eur. J. Phys. Rehabil. Med. 48, 135–145.

Ulrich, D.A., Ulrich, B.D., Angulo-Kinzler, R.M., et al., 2001. Treadmill training of infants with Down syndrome: evidence-based development outcomes. Pediatrics 108, E84.

von Hofsten, C., 1984. Developmental changes in the organization of pre-reaching movements. Dev. Psychol. 20, 378–388.

van Vliet, P., Kerwin, D.G., Sheridan, M., et al., 1995. The influence of goals on the kinematics of reaching following stroke. Neural Rep. 19, 11–16.

van der Weel, F.R., van der Meer, A.L., Lee, D.N., 1991. Effect of task on movement control in cerebral palsy:

implications for assessment and therapy. Dev. Med. Child Neurol. 00, 110 120.

Wall, J.C., 1999. Walking. In: Durwood, B., Baer, G.D., Rowe, P.J. (Eds.), Functional Human Movement: Measurement and Analysis. Butterworth-Heinemann, Oxford.

Weiss, M.R., Klint, K.A., 1987. Show and tell in the gymnasium: an investigation of developmental differences in modelling and verbal rehearsal of motor skills. Res. Quart. Exerc. Sport 58, 234–241.

Wevers, L., van der Port, I., Vermue, M., et al., 2009. Effects of task-oriented circuit training class training on walking competency after stroke: a systematic review. Stroke 40, 2450–2459.

Whiting, H.T.A., 1980. Dimensions of control in motor learning. In: Stelmach, G.E., Requin, J. (Eds.), Tutorials in Motor Behavior. North Holland, New York, pp. 537–550.

Willingham, D.B., 1992. Systems of motor skill. In: Squire, L.A., Butters, N. (Eds.), Neuropsychology of Memory, second ed. Guilford Press, NY, pp. 166 178.

Winter, D.A., 1987. The Biomechanics and Motor Control of Human Gait. University of Waterloo Press, Waterloo, Ont.

Wong, K., 2009. Crawling may be unnecessary for normal child development. Scient. Am. 30 June.

Wu, C., Trombly, C.A., Lin, K., et al., 2000. A kinematic study of contextual effects on reaching performance in persons with and without stroke: influences of object availability. Arch. Phys. Med. Rehabil. 81, 95–101.

Wu, Y.-N., Hwang, M., Ren, Y., et al., 2011. Combined passive stretching and active movement rehabilitation of lower-limb impairments in children with cerebral palsy using a portable robot. Neurorehabil. Neural Repair 25, 378–385.

Wulf, G., McNevin, N., Shea, C., 1999a. Learning phenomena: future challenges for the dynamical systems approach to understanding the learning of complex motor skills. Int J. Psychol. 30, 531–557.

Wulf, G., Lauterbach, B., Toole, T., 1999b. The learning advantage of an external focus of attention in golf. Res. Quart. Exerc. Sport 70, 120–126.

Zelazo, P.R., 1983. The development of walking: new findings and old assumptions. J. Motor Behav. 15, 99–137.

Zelazo, P.R., Zelazo, N.A., Kolb, S., 1972. 'Walking' in the newborn. Science 176, 314.

Zetou, E., Fragouli, M., Tzetzis, G., 1999. The influence of star and self-modelling on volleyball skill acquisition. J. Hum. Movt. Stud. 37, 127.

# Annotation A
## Aspects of motor training

Roberta B. Shepherd

Training and exercise for infants should focus on critical motor behaviours, those basic actions that are required for functional independence. In general, these actions comprise behaviours in sitting and standing that involve support, moving and balancing the body mass over the feet, e.g., actions such as squatting, sitting down and standing up (Fig. A.1), various forms of locomotion, and reaching out to grasp and manipulate objects. By working early in infancy to provide opportunities for repetitive practice of these basic actions, as occurs normally in the first year, one can expect some transfer or 'generalizability' into other actions that have similar underlying biomechanical characteristics as the infant explores the possibilities of the environment. Focusing on these basic actions early in infancy is likely to increase muscle activation and force production (strength) and preserve soft tissue flexibility and extensibility throughout the early period of bone and soft tissue growth. Modern concepts of motor development free us from the constraints of keeping within the boundaries of a sequential progression, e.g., rolling→sitting→crawling→standing→walking, proximal-to-distal.

## Targeted training and exercise

The American College of Sports Medicine (2012) defines strength training as a systematic programme of exercises designed to increase an individual's ability to exert or resist force. Strength is the capacity to produce the muscle forces necessary to carry out a particular action. It is relative to that action. Inherent in the word 'strength' is not only the amount and timing of force but also the ability to control it so that the muscles necessary to produce an action, that may involve one, two or more joints, work together co-operatively. Strength is a neuromuscular phenomenon, activity-specific and therefore functionally specific.

Currently, there is increased interest in the importance of strength training in children and

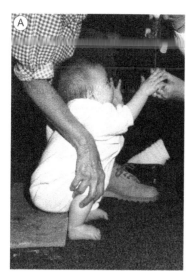
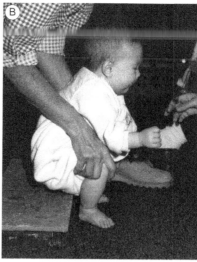

**Figure A.1 •** Training a small infant to stand up and sit down. The therapist has placed the feet back and the infant is persuaded to stand up to take the toy, then sit down to put it on the floor, with repetitions and with reducing assistance. [From Shepherd RB 1995 Physiotherapy in Paediatrics 3rd ed. with permission from Elsevier.]

adults with brain lesions (American College of Sports Medicine et al., 2009), perhaps because of the long overdue recognition of the significance of poor muscle function and weakness as a major cause of functional disability. Muscle weakness is initially due to impairments affecting descending fibres to the spinal cord with decreased activation of motor units. However, weakness also occurs secondary to lack of physical activity imposed by the brain lesion and may eventually be more debilitating for the individual than the direct effects of the injury. It is possible that these secondary changes to the neuromuscular system may be preventable or reversible if active training starts in early infancy. This hypothesis has not been tested and there is a lack of investigation into strength (or muscle activation) in infants less than 18 months old with or without cerebral palsy (CP).

Inadequate muscle activation (weakness) and poor motor control co-exist, and training should involve intensive active exercise both to strengthen muscles and to increase muscle control within the framework of a functional action. The strength required to perform basic motor actions is activity dependent (i.e., relative), and an able-bodied infant develops the necessary strength and control of the limbs during repetitive practice of a variety of novel actions. An infant normally finds many ways to practice moving the body mass about on the floor and over the feet in standing as part of

the learning process (see Fig. 1.10). The activity-dependent strength of lower limb muscles gradually increases in response to practice of standing up from crouching and sitting, cruising sideways along the furniture, and in response to increasing load as the infant grows and body dimensions change. This vigorous and challenging practice may not occur for the infant with brain lesion unless it is planned. It is evident that we should be embarking on an exploration of ways to give young infants the early, intensive and varied practice they need but seldom get.

Children with poor muscle function affecting lower limbs may not learn to bear weight and push down through the whole foot in standing up or in stance phase of walking, or to use the feet for balance and propulsion. This may, in part, be due to lack of experience in infancy of bearing weight through the feet in propulsive actions such as standing up and walking, and by the early development of calf muscle contracture (Fig. A.2A). Sitting with feet on the floor also needs to be practiced early to enable balance through the lower limbs while reaching in sitting and while standing up. The lower limbs play a significant role in balancing the body mass; hence the importance of ensuring sufficient active lengthening and force-generating ability of muscles that cross ankles, knees and hips and providing opportunities to develop appropriate

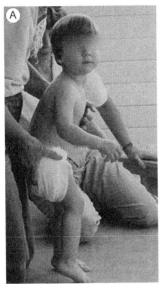

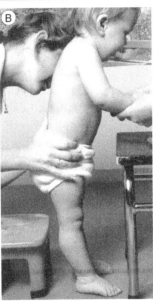

**Figure A.2** • These two little boys with diplegia have not learned to take weight on their feet, flex forward at the hips, push their feet to the floor, and stand. **(A)** This boy has decreased extensibility of hip flexors and adductors, hamstrings, and calf muscles so he cannot extend his knees and hips or dorsiflex his ankles. **(B)** This boy has stiffened his legs; his ankles are not dorsiflexed so he will fall backward if not held. Exercises targeting these problems with training of functional lower limb actions are described in Chapter 11. [From Shepherd RB 1995 Physiotherapy in Paediatrics 3rd ed. with permission from Elsevier.]

foot alignment when weight-bearing. If this is not targeted early, over time small rearrangements of joints in the foot and abnormal growth of bones in the foot may make it impossible to distribute force appropriately over the plantar foot surface (Nsenga and Doutrellot, 2012), with negative effects on balance and lower limb alignment.

Actions that require weight-bearing through the plantar surface of the feet and propulsive force involved in pushing down through the feet may be critical to development of an appropriate relationship between plantar load receptors and motor control. Proprioceptive afferents from load detectors in the lower limb extensor muscles and ankle dorsiflexors (and perhaps the Golgi tendon organs) and exteroceptive afferents from mechanoreceptors in the plantar surface of the feet (plantar load receptors) appear to play a critical role in balance and walking (Dietz and Duysens, 2000). Extensor load receptors probably signal changes in the projection of the centre of body mass (CBM) with respect to the feet. Infants with diplegia or hemiplegia, for example, may persistently stand on the toes or fail to bear weight through the feet and push into the floor (Fig. A.2A,B). As part of training weight-bearing and balancing activities, crouching and standing up can be practiced using shoes attached to a flat surface as those shown in Figure A.3B. In this way the feet are held with heels on floor. Once the child gets the idea of pushing down through the feet, and flexing and extending hips, knees and ankles over the feet, he can practice without the shoes. Similarly, use of the upper limb for bearing weight and pushing into the support surface needs to be specifically targeted early in infancy (Figs A.4 and 1.3B, C).

The current view of strength training is that it must involve increasing repetition and increasing load (resistance). Carr and Shepherd (2010) provide an extensive review and discussion of issues related to strength training in adult neurorehabilitation, much of which is also relevant in paediatric practice. Below are some guidelines for strength training. The programme may need to continue throughout growth as movement control has to adapt to increasing height and weight.

- Basic exercises to train step-ups, squats, push-ups, pulling, pushing, reaching
- Task/activity-oriented exercises: standing up/sitting down, stepping/walking up and down stairs, reaching towards targets, reaching to

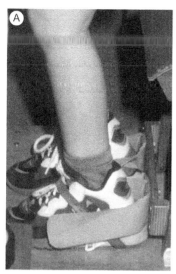
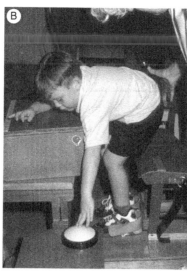

**Figure A.3 • (A)** The shoe holder keeps the feet plantigrade while **(B)** the child practices squatting to press a light switch (one of the workstations in a circuit training class). The holder constrains the child's foot so he cannot plantarflex and rise on to his toes. He can concentrate on flexing and extending his legs to increase strength and limb control. The exercise provides an active stretch to the calf muscles. Number of repetitions is monitored. i.e., he does as many as he can in the time allotted.

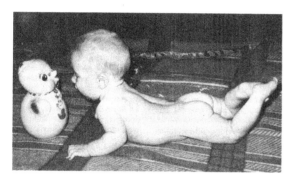

**Figure A.4 •** This normally developing infant shows a typical posture in prone, resting on the forearms, spine extended.

manipulate, manipulating objects of different sizes, textures, for different purposes
- Select actions that present a challenge to the infant: climbing a ladder, picking up a heavy object
- Grade resistance/load and number of repetitions to the infant's ability: as a general rule a maximum number of repetitions (<10) repeated three times
- Utilize resistance/load from body weight, elastic bands, treadmill incline, pushing a heavy trolley according to infant's capacity.

(See figures in Chapter 11)

Damiano et al. (2002) have made a convincing case for muscle strengthening in children with CP. They have shown that these children have substantial and generalized muscle weakness that can contribute to bony deformity as well as motor dysfunction

(Wiley and Damiano, 1998). Exercise principles for strength training are based on well-established scientific evidence and guidelines are readily available and modified for a disabled population and for children (American College of Sports Medicine et al., 2009; American College of Sports Medicine, 2012). Applying these principles to infant exercise is useful as a practical guide, but in practice some methods may be impractical until the infant reaches a certain stage. Exercise programmes must target specific goals, e.g., targeting strength, endurance or power training should lead to increased strength, or endurance, or power, but will not necessarily improve an individual's cardiorespiratory endurance or energy cost unless the exercises are organized to stress aerobic capacity and efficiency (Damiano and Abel, 1998; Faigenbaum, 2000; Faigenbaum et al., 1999; MacPhail and Kramer, 1995). Older children are reported to have poor levels of fitness (Provost et al., 2007) and programmes should be developed to enable children with CP to be sufficiently and vigorously active to increase or maintain their fitness as they grow (Damiano, 2003), e.g., treadmill locomotion with or without harness, or water activities, or cycle ergometry.

A small clinical study (Blundell et al., 2003) investigated the effects of lower limb strength training incorporated into task training in young children (aged 3–8 years) with diplegia, hemiplegia or quadriplegia. The children took part in a four-week group circuit training programme consisting of weight-bearing exercise designed to increase lower limb functional strength, balance through the feet, walking

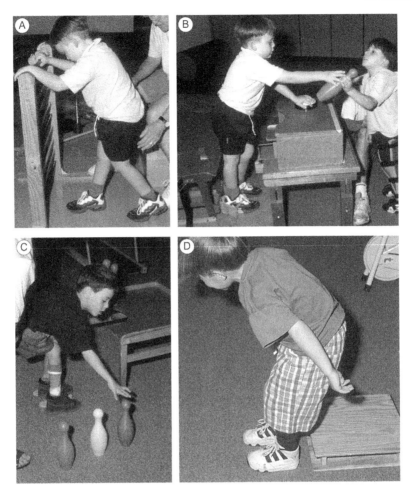

**Figure A.5** • A circuit training class showing different workstations where children practice specific actions designed to increase lower limb strength and control. At each station the action can be made more challenging as the child improves. **(A)** Balancing with one leg in front of the other. He practices extending his left knee and hip with heel on ground, stepping back and forth with right leg while keeping the left hip extended. When he is ready he will take his hands off the table. In **(B)** both boys are trying to balance without using their hands for support. The boy on the right has soft splints to constrain his knees so he gets the 'feel' of weight-bearing without his knees collapsing; the boy on the left stops using the table for support when he is able. **(C)** Practice of crouch-to-stand and **(D)** stand ups from increasingly lower seats, keeping weight evenly distributed. This can be monitored by feedback from pressure-sensitive devices under each foot.

and sit-to-stand performance (Fig. A.5A–D). The exercises had similar biomechanical characteristics to many actions that involve the lower limbs in support, balance and propulsion. The exercises took into account the specificity principle in that muscle force generated was directly related to the functions being trained. Isometric muscle strength, performance of walking and sit-to-stand were significantly improved by the end of the programme and the effect was still present at the eight-week follow-up.

Many other studies of children and adults with CP have found beneficial effects of strength training and several systematic reviews provide evidence that strength training can be effective (Bale and Strand 2008; Dodd et al., 2002, 2003; Liao et al., 2007; McBurney et al., 2003; Monkford and Coulton, 2008; Ryan et al., 2011; Taylor et al., 2005). What type of strength training is most effective depends on a number of factors, including the degree of weakness and a muscle's strength relative to a specific action. In a recent study, 5–12-year-old children with mild diplegia (gross motor function classification system [GMFCS] 1 and 11) took part in a programme of loaded sit-to-stand (STS) resistance training, three times per week for six weeks. At the end of the programme their repetition maximum (RM) STS, scores on the Physical Cost Index, and gross motor function measure (GMFM) goal dimension score, were all significantly better than the control group. Interestingly, isometric (static) quadriceps strength and gait speed did not differ significantly from the control group, a result that supports the notion of specificity as the muscles were exercised isotonically (Liao et al., 2007). This study appears to be one of the first to specifically target the strength of an action, e.g., hip, knee and ankle extension and flexion (with feet on floor). It also targets the specific training of a major functional action instead of a complete physiotherapy programme, and therapists followed a set of guidelines, providing a good model for future studies of exercise effects.

## Relationship between strength and function

Although it is intuitive that a relationship between strength and function exists, we do not know what type of strength training has the best effects on functional performance and there appears to be no published investigations of infants under 12–18 months. From Buchner's work with very weak adults (Buchner et al., 1996) it appears that, below a certain threshold of strength, exercise can result in some improvement in task performance (e.g., in walking). Above that threshold, however, function may not improve unless strength training is incorporated into skill training (e.g., increasing incline and speed in walking training and increasing load in STS training). Above a certain threshold, strength is task-dependent, i.e., the relative strength required for successful and stable performance of a particular action, such as, standing up from a seat, is not the same as absolute strength, the maximum load that can be lifted by the knee extensor muscles.

One of the advantages of task-oriented exercise and training in young infants is that emphasis is not only on muscle activation and the production of muscle force but also on the control of that force, particularly the time it takes to build up peak force. Inability to generate force fast enough

(lack of power) in lower limb muscles is probably a major factor underlying the inability to walk fast, run, jump and hop seen in children with CP, even in children who are independently mobile. Olney et al. (1991) have reported a positive correlation in adults with stroke between gait speed and the magnitude of push-off power[*] by the hemiparetic leg. The ability to time major power bursts is critical when walking, enabling, for example, increased speed, and a switch into running.

Training, even for infants in the latter half of their first year, needs to incorporate variations in speed of movement and actions that require rapid force production for success (throwing, pushing, pulling, jumping, stair-climbing, increasing walking speed), i.e., exercises directed at power as well as strength. A major emphasis in infants should be on preserving the length and activation levels of calf muscles and hip and knee extensors for bearing weight through the feet in standing. These muscles can be exercised at the joint angle at which a major burst is required in specific functional actions; for example, as noted by Olney et al. (1988), muscles required for walking, concentric and eccentric ankle plantarflexion, can be exercised between about 10° dorsiflexion and 20° plantarflexion.

Clinical studies in adults and children have failed to support the assumption that strengthening exercise might increase spasticity. Rather, strength training can result not only in increased muscle strength but also in improved functional motor performance, decreased resistance to passive movement and reductions in hyperreflexia (Bateman et al., 2001; Brown and Kautz, 1998; Damiano et al., 2001; Davies et al., 1996; Sharp and Brouwer, 1997; Teixeira-Salmela et al., 1999). Furthermore, strength training has positive effects on bone and muscle growth (Wilmshurst et al., 1996), and on muscle size and composition (Ryan et al., 2011).

## Endurance and fitness

Children and adults with CP may have poor muscle endurance, a major factor in ambulatory decline and cessation (Bottos et al., 2001), and low levels of cardiorespiratory fitness (Damiano, 2003; Tobimatsu et al., 1998; Unnithan et al., 1998). The age at which a decline in cardiorespiratory fitness and of endurance is evident is not known in these children. However, it may start earlier

---

[*]Power = force × angular velocity.

than expected. The growing trend for training on treadmill (with harness support if necessary) and functional electrical stimulation (FES)-cycling machines, cycle ergometers and recumbent bicycles may help promote endurance training in children with CP, together with growing opportunities for exercise programmes and sporting activity (e.g., Provost et al., 2007; Ulrich et al., 2008; Unnithan et al., 2006). Some of these machines can be adapted for use by infants and small children, enabling them not only to increase control over their limbs but also to be vigorously active and to help them maintain or increase their fitness as they grow (see Figs 1.1 and 11.10 A–C).

## Concentric–eccentric muscle activity

Functional strength training has the added advantage of exercising muscles in both lengthening (eccentric) and shortening (concentric) contractions as they naturally occur in real-life activities. Shifting between concentric and eccentric muscle activity is difficult at an early stage of developing motor control in all children, especially when weight-bearing. It is apparent from the observation of young children that concentric actions are relatively easier to learn to control at first than eccentric actions. For example, children learn to walk up a step independently before they can walk down, and they can stand up from crouch or from a seat but may need support or gentle pressure to bend the knees when lowering the body into crouch and sitting. Standing up independently occurs before sitting down, and falling into the sitting position is common until control over the lower limbs increases. There can be difficulty in switching between concentric and eccentric activity, especially when weight-bearing.

The force-producing capacity (tension regulation) of muscle differs according to whether the contraction is concentric or eccentric (Pinneger et al., 2000). Voluntary eccentric contractions produce greater force than concentric contractions yet involve lower rates of motor unit discharge than concentric contractions (Tax et al., 1990). In able-bodied adults, it has been shown that exercises involving concentric and eccentric contractions produce better gains in strength than exercises with concentric contractions alone. Figures 11.15–11.17 demonstrate exercises and activities for the lower

limbs that involve switching between concentric and eccentric muscle contractions.

When a muscle is actively stretched in an eccentric contraction, tension in the series elasticity component increases and the stored elastic energy is used in the subsequent concentric contraction (Svantessen and Sunnerhagen, 1997). Eccentric movements have to be practiced for skill in controlling such actions to be gained (Fig. A.3B). The effect of what is called *the stretch-shortening cycle* is seen when an eccentric contraction immediately precedes a concentric contraction, as in the brief flexion counter-movement seen in performance of the vertical jump. The concentric phase generates more force when it follows the flexion movement and the person jumps higher. A similar mechanism probably exists in walking (Komi, 1986) and in standing up (Shepherd and Gentile, 1994). The brief flexion at the knees in standing up, occurring at movement onset, provides a stretch to the knee extensor muscles, immediately prior to limb extension. In adult stroke patients, it is reported that a significantly larger concentric force occurred during limb loading in standing up after eccentric exercise on an isokinetic dynamometer (Engardt et al., 1995). From their research into changes in the mechanical properties of muscles in the affected limb after stroke, Svantessen et al. (2000) suggest that training activities in rehabilitation that emphasize eccentric–concentric exercise may result in more normal function and enhance recovery.

It follows that functional weight-bearing exercises, practiced repetitively, can provide a focus for training control of the limb at the same time as providing an action-specific strength training stimulus. These exercises directly address the weakness and lack of motor control which are major neural impairments in CP, compounded over time by the adaptive effects of disuse, stereotyped movement patterns and immobility. Preparatory and ongoing balance adjustments are also made during practice of weight-bearing exercises so the infant is also practicing the skill of balancing the body mass over the feet while moving.

## Specificity and transfer

It is evident that a major factor in developing skilled motor performance is training of the action itself and practice that is specific to the task and the different contexts in which it takes place (Magill, 2010). The infant needs verbal and visual guidance from a therapist/parent/sibling, who plans practice to ensure flexibility of performance in different environmental conditions. It has been an unspoken assumption in the neurofacilitation therapies that originated in the 1950s (e.g., Bobath's neurodevelopment therapy) that movement facilitated by a therapist transfers or carries over to improved functional performance (Blauw-Hospers et al., 2007), but there is no evidence that this is so or that non-specific exercise will result in functional gain (Blauw-Hospers and Hadders-Algra, 2005). The body adapts specifically to the demands imposed upon it, for example, to the challenge to balance when we move our arms in standing. Whenever the therapist holds on to the infant as she/he tries to stand independently, the challenge to balance disappears and the infant cannot learn what must be done to move independently. Experiments have clearly shown that holding on to a support in standing changes the balance demands and therefore the pattern of muscle activation and joint movement (Fig. 11.4; Cordo and Nashner, 1982).

Research over the years on the effects of motor training, including strength training in adults, has shown that exercise effects tend to be specific to task and context, i.e., what is practiced and where (Morrissey et al., 1995; Rutherford, 1988), with the greatest changes occurring in the training exercise itself. There is evidence, however, that transfer can occur between actions that share similar biomechanical characteristics (Buchner et al., 1996; Carr and Shepherd, 2003). The motor control system appears to use simplifying strategies. For example, the lower limbs are the focus in many activities that are performed while bearing weight through the feet. The basic pattern of intersegmental co-ordination is one of flexion and extension with the feet as a base of support (see Fig. 11.1). This pattern of co-ordination is seen in a number of actions significant to daily life that share major biomechanical characteristics, for example, standing up and sitting down, crouch-to-standing, stair ascent/descent (Fig. A.6A,B; see Chapter 11).

It is therefore possible that there can be some transfer from practice of one action to another. Two studies have exemplified this point: a study of children with CP by Liao et al. (2007) described earlier, and a study of adults after stroke by Dean and Shepherd (1997). In this study, seated subjects reached forward to grasp an object placed at the limit of reachability. The results showed that repetitive practice of various long-distance reaching tasks not only improved the distance that could be reached in sitting and the speed of reaching

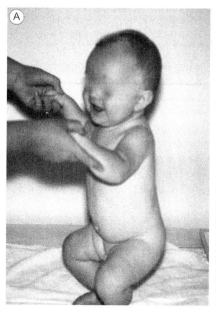
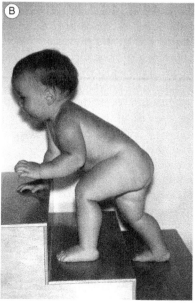

**Figure A.6** • Flexion and extension at hips, knees and ankles form the basic pattern of intersegmental movement of lower limbs in many common actions.

but also STS performance, yet STS had not been practiced. Perhaps it is not too surprising. The two actions share similar biomechanical characteristics in that both involve an initial horizontal momentum as body weight is shifted forward over the feet, with flexion at hips, knees and ankles. In training, subjects reached forward far beyond their arm length so that horizontal and vertical ground reaction forces generated through the lower limbs as the body moved forward would have been similar to those generated in the first phase of sitting to standing (Fig. 11.8B). The fact that speed of walking, unrelated to the action practiced, showed no change illustrates the significance of the specificity principle in exercise and training.

## Specificity of sensory inputs

Sensation also is specific to an action and where it is performed. Although we are normally bombarded with internal inputs and with inputs that originate from external sources to ourselves (e.g., somatosensory, proprioceptive, mechano-receptive, auditory, visual inputs), the system appears to select for attention only the information that is relevant to the action we are about to perform or are already performing. Sensory information is essential to the control of movement and particularly for manual dexterity and balancing the body mass over the lower limbs and feet. In infancy, the active experience of a variety of movements is a critical stimulus to sensory as well as motor development. Ensuring the infant is active and that actions practiced are self-generated provides the critical sensory information for the control of those actions.

For example, when training infants in lower limb activities with the feet on the floor, the *plantar pressure receptors* provide information critical to each action. The pressure under the feet moves in different directions as the body mass moves, giving information relevant to the muscles that maintain support and preserve balance. It may be helpful to have the infant pay attention to the feet, for example 'push down through your feet and stand up', and the therapist should avoid giving conflicting inputs that will divert the infant's attention.

Loss of tactile and pressure sensory discrimination also has major effects on the learning of manipulative tasks and dexterity. In precision grip during a grip and lift task, *tactile* information enables the adjustment of fingertip forces to the object's weight

and tendency to slip (Johansson and Westling, 1984; Westling and Johansson, 1984). The object's *texture* is known to affect grip force, probably due to the perception of slippage (Cadoret and Smith, 1996). Johansson and Westling (1990) provided critical information for the training of object manipulation in their analyses of the role of tactile sensation in manipulation. It is clear that an infant's early experiences should be organized to provide opportunities for the development of sensory discrimination along with motor performance.

Singer (1982) noted that animal and human observations of *vision* suggest that experience-dependent maturation of sensory functions is set up by attentional mechanisms, and visual signals stimulate the development of normal receptive fields in the visual cortex of kittens only when the kittens are alert and attend to those signals. In terms of vision, the developing brain can screen incoming retinal signals and enable only selected patterns to alter cortical connections.

Several decades ago, a series of interesting studies by von Hofsten (1982) showed that neonates can make extensive and complex arm movements. When they reached for a target they were more accurate when they looked at it than when they looked elsewhere. When von Hofsten videotaped newborns well-supported in a specially designed seat, he found that the arm was aimed closer to the target when the infants looked at it (Fig. A.7). By 2 months old, infants reached toward

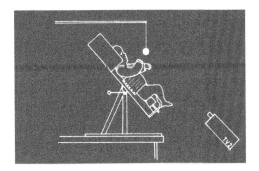

**Figure A.7 •** The specially designed infant seat built for a reaching experiment. When training an infant in functional arm movements it is a good idea to follow the methods used in order to optimize performance in the experiment: the infant is *well-supported*, reaching to capture an *attractive, graspable object* that *moves across the infant's field of vision* relatively *close*. [From von Hofsten C 1984 Developmental changes in the organization of pre-reaching movements. Develop Psychol 20:378–388, with permission from the American Psychological association].

the target vigorously with arm extended and hand fisted; by 3 months, when looking at the object the infant opened the hand when reaching and the number of reaching attempts increased, apparently under visual control (von Hofsten, 1984).

Binocular sensitivity develops rapidly between 3–5 months of age, as well as visually guided grasping, the infant watching the hands as they move into the visual field (Birch et al., 1982). By 6 months of age, the pattern of reaching appeared more like the adult, with an initial ballistic transportation phase followed by a slower fine adjustment manipulation phase. An infant as young as 5 months old can orient the hand appropriately before it reaches the object (von Hofsten and Fazel-Zandy, 1984), and can adjust the opening of the hand relative to object size by 9–13 months (von Hofsten and Rondquist, 1988).

von Hofsten and Lindhagen (1979) reported that infants of 18 weeks old appeared to have the ability to judge the speed of movement of an object and estimate its location. In this experiment, the infants were able to reach for, intercept and catch quite rapidly moving objects (30 cm/s). How can this be so? The conditions for this experiment are interesting to note as a guide to successful training methods. The test environment was set up to optimize the infant's chance of success (Fig. A.7). The setting itself was probably critical in making the reach and grasp action effective, and the setting gives us clues for training disabled infants:

* Infants were semi-reclined in a seat that supported head and trunk, allowing free movement of the arms
* The target object was brightly coloured and of graspable size and shape
* The object moved across the infant's field of vision at a distance of 12 cm from the eye.

## Preservation of soft tissue compliance

Muscle growth and development in infants occurs in response to activity of that muscle. A muscle's length is dependent upon the joint range(s) of movement over which it shortens and lengthens, i.e., muscle length is relative. Muscle activation and joint movement are critical for the preservation of a muscle's integrity. Lack of active contraction affects the passive and contractile properties of muscle

and tendon. Low levels of muscle activity and joint movement are known to result in anatomical, metabolic, mechanical and functional changes in muscle at any age. These changes are likely to be particularly significant in the growing and developing infant. Although in children with CP the primary UMN insult is not progressive, the resulting muscle pathology that develops secondary to disuse/misuse does progress (Smith et al., 2011; see Chapters 6 and 7). As well as maladaptive changes, there may also be a failure of growth (Foran et al., 2005; Smith et al., 2009). A build-up of connective tissue (collagen) in muscle can contribute to increased muscle stiffness as the child grows. It can affect a muscle's mechanical properties, increase stretch reflex activity and affect growth (Booth et al., 2001).

Weightlessness and joint immobility are associated with decreased metabolic demand that may have particularly negative effects in young infants in terms of growth and development. Skeletal muscles have a remarkable capacity for accommodating changes in demand. As part of the adaptive process they acquire characteristics that appear better suited to the new functional requirements. This adaptive capacity has the potential to impact both positively and negatively. If demands are limited, if for example, a muscle only generates force in a small part of range, that muscle acquires characteristics suited to the demand.

An interesting explanation of the lower limb flexion/internal rotation/adduction posture of the lower limbs, typically seen in children with diplegia, and an illustration of the potential mechanical effects of excessive hip flexion comes from a biomechanical and modelling study of the moment arms of hip rotator muscles (Delp, 2003; Delp et al., 1999). The investigators found that, with the hip held progressively more in flexion, some muscles switch their action from external rotation to internal rotation, e.g., the anterior compartments of gluteus maximus, and gluteus medius, gluteus minimus, and piriformis. This means that persistent hip flexion in infancy can exacerbate internal rotation deformity at the hip as well as adduction (Fig. A.8A–C).

Delp and colleagues also found that gluteus maximus has a large capacity for *external* rotation with the hip at 0 degree. A clinical implication from this work is that activities to promote hip extension in prone, standing and walking in infancy designed to strengthen gluteus maximus as a hip extensor (and external rotator) with the hip in

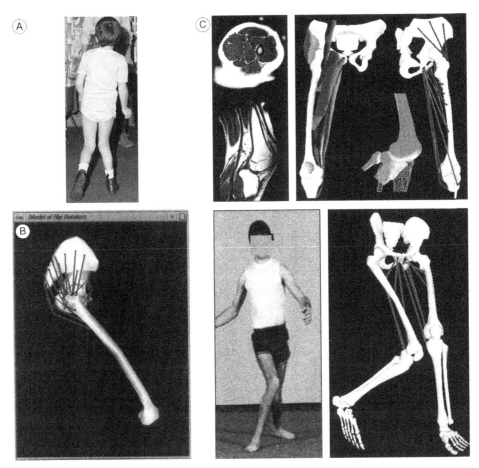

**Figure A.8 • (A)** This boy with diplegia shows a common method of independent walking with flexed, internally rotated, adducted hips and decreased knee extension. The goal from early infancy should be to strengthen hip, knee and ankle extensors by training basic functional movements, at the same time actively preserving extensibility of muscles that can be predicted to develop contracture (see Chapter 11). **(B)** A musculoskeletal model used to estimate moment arms of muscles that overlie and can rotate hip joint. Individual muscles and muscle compartments represented by lines, with dots for location of muscle insertions. **(C)** Hip rotation moment arms during crouched, internally rotated gait. Model from MRI and kinematic data of hips and knees of individuals with CP. Internal rotation arms of some muscles increase with flexion; the external moment arms of other muscles decrease. Some muscles turn from external rotation to internal rotation with the hip in flexion. [(B) From Delp S et al. 1999 Variation of rotational arms with hip flexion. J Biomech 23:493–501, with permission from Elsevier; (C) from Arnold AS and Delp SL 2005 Computer modelling of gait abnormalities in cerebral palsy: application to treatment planning. Theoretical Issues in Ergonomic Science 6:305–312, with permission from Taylor and Francis.]

extension may be critical from earliest infancy as a means of preventing disabling hip flexion and internal rotation deformity (see Chapter 11). Clinical methods, including strength training weight-bearing exercises in standing, games played in prone position and treadmill walking, may prevent the tendency toward persistent hip flexion, with its associated adduction and internal rotation of the hip by hip flexors, adductor and internal rotator muscle contractures, and ultimately hip deformity. Strapping applied posterolaterally

over the hip, to shorten the gluteus maximus and medius, may stimulate hip extension/external rotation while the infant steps, walks and stands.

The preservation of muscle extensibility and contractility by physical means depends upon raising levels of activation, with active challenging exercises involving concentric (shortening) and eccentric (lengthening) contractions of muscle over the specific joint range necessary to the action (consider the effect of crouch-standing-crouch, performed with feet flat on the support

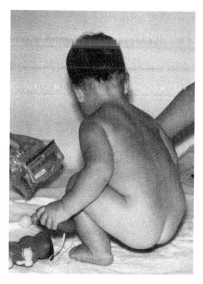

**Figure A.9** • With feet on the floor, a full squat actively stretches soleus muscle to nearly its full length as it contracts eccentrically.

surface, on the length and contractility of soleus muscle) (Fig. A.9). Exercises to stimulate muscle activation, force production and control of a limb in standing, described in more detail in Chapter 11, may minimize the weakness that increases as the infant grows and body weight increases. It is surely the effect of supporting the increasing body weight through the legs with insufficient lower limb extensor muscle strength that leads the young child to sink into the flexed, internally rotated and adducted posture typical of diplegia (Fig. A.8).

Weakness, not spasticity, is the problem on which to focus; increased sensitivity of stretch receptors in muscle may be secondary to weakness and contracture. In children with motor system impairments, stretch reflex hyperactivity, increased muscle stiffness and length-associated changes appear to be most evident in muscles that are weakest and when activity levels are low.

## Overcoming contractures

The main method used in physiotherapy to prevent or to overcome established contractures has been passive stretching and splinting. Medical interventions include drug therapy and surgery. There have been many outcome studies and at the present time there is no evidence that passive stretching is effective beyond the short term in children (Wiart et al., 2008).

Instead, it is likely that it is the *active* stretching that occurs normally throughout the day during active movement that is critical to muscle length because it shapes extensibility of the muscle and is a stimulus for muscle growth. Muscle represents a classic biological example of the relationship between structure and function. A muscle's length reflects the range of lengths it is subjected to throughout our lives and is therefore subject to change if our lifestyle changes. Some sporting activities require greater muscle extensibility than we need in our daily lives, so we prepare for the sport by doing exercises to lengthen these muscles and avoid the pain of torn muscle fibres. In the growing child contracture can also occur due to failure of muscle growth to keep up with bone growth. Emphasis in infant clinical practice should be on active lengthening of muscle during the performance of actions such as standing up and sitting down and crouch-to-standing, and exercises targeting muscle length such as heels raise and lower (see Chapter 11).

## Driving limb use

Intensive meaningful practice is likely to be particularly significant for infants with CP. We therefore need to find ways of providing young infants with sufficient opportunity to practice the actions they require for effective performance and less opportunity to practice stereotyped ineffective actions. The burden of practice typically falls on parents, but in reality no parent can provide enough practice time for an infant to overcome the effects of all the time spent inactive or repetitively practicing stereotyped movements. Group work provides support and companionship for infant and parent (Knis-Matthews et al., 2011). Technological advances enable us to develop new methods. Apparatus to drive and guide a variety of kicking movements in early infancy is being developed (Chen et al., 2002; see Annotation C). Interactive technologies aim to assist parents by providing online support (see Chapter 15). Some infants may be assisted by supportive clothing, soft splints such as knee supports (Fig. A.10A) or a harness or grab belt (Figs. A.10B and Fig. 1.1) so they can practice balancing while weight-bearing in standing, as healthy infants do.

There are promising reports in older children of the effectiveness of *computerized training systems*, using games operated by specially designed manipulanda (e.g., an early study by Krichevets et al., 1995; Fig. A.11). These investigations should

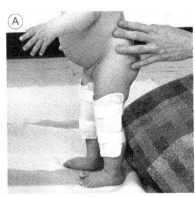

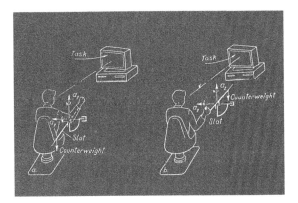

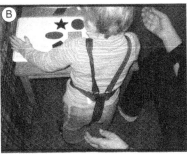

**Figure A.10 • (A)** Soft leg splints are useful when an infant does not extend the knees in standing; they can be worn for practice of sideways walking and for learning to balance during self-initiated movements in standing. **(B)** Harness with grab belt can be used to enable standing and walking practice—it enables the development of balance, allows the infant to correct a stumble, but prevents a fall.

**Figure A.11 •** The objective of creating a special training device was to test the possibility of increasing active arm movement of a 13-year-old boy with Erb's palsy. At the start he had minimum active movement. The specific aims were to break down the stereotypic movement that involved hitching his shoulder and to strengthen main muscle groups of the arm, starting with external rotation, which was absent. The task for the boy was to move a sighting beam to cover (and blow up) a submarine. The game took one hour and was played two to three times each week. There were two methods of manipulating the beam depending, on the particular aim. The details of training should be studied for their relevance to training any individual who has first to unlearn an ineffective and stereotyped motor behaviour. [From Krichevets AN et al. 1995 Computer games as a means of movement rehabilitation. Disabil Rehabil 17:100–105, with permission from Informa Healthcare.]

lead to the development of interactive games designed for infants and small children that 'drive' particular actions by providing an irresistible visual and/or auditory stimulus (see Chapter 12).

## Treadmill walking

With or without supporting harness, treadmill walking (TW) is a way of 'driving' the movements that make up walking, and it is increasingly recommended for children as a means of training walking and, using physiological principles, for improving cardiorespiratory fitness (Damiano, 2003; Shepherd, 1995). There is evidence that TW can be used effectively for infants and children (Barbeau, 2003; Blundell et al., 2003; Bodkin et al., 2003; Richards et al., 1997; Song et al., 2003; Ulrich et al., 2001) (Figs. A.12 and 11.10A–C). Treadmill walking may also involve virtual reality systems to

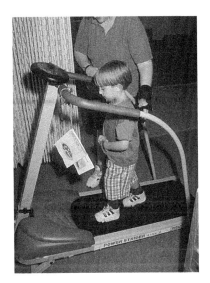

**Figure A.12 •** Treadmill walking was one of the work-stations in the circuit training class. This boy has progressed to walking without holding on. [Courtesy of SW Blundell.]

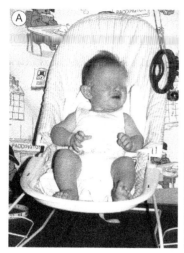
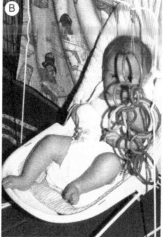
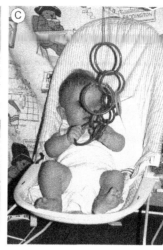

**Figure A.13** • A version of CIMT. **(A)** This infant has signs of hemiplegia. **(B)** Wearing a mitten, he was encouraged to play different games with different (graspable) objects using his paretic left limb. **(C)** After a session with the mitten, he started handling objects, sometimes playing with both hands. [From Shepherd RB 1995 Physiotherapy in Paediatrics 3rd ed. with permission from Elsevier.]

provide a realistic visual environment (Kott et al., 2009; Rahman et al., 2010). Treadmill training is described in more detail in Chapters 10 to 12.

## Constraint

There is a body of research showing that the combination of *constraint of the non-paretic upper limb and active, intensive and meaningful exercise and activity* of the paretic limb (constraint-induced movement therapy, CIMT) (Fig. A.13) can be effective in enabling children with hemiplegic CP to improve the functional use of their paretic limb (Charles et al., 2006; Eliasson et al., 2005; Huang et al., 2009). Two interesting small studies reported cortical reorganization changes after CIMT (Juenger et al., 2007; Sutcliffe et al., 2007). One single subject study of an 8-year-old boy with hemiplegia, using fMRI and magnetoencephalography, found increased sensory input as a result of increased use of the affected hand leading to increased recruitment and activity of the contralateral somatosensory cortex (Sutcliffe et al., 2007). The results of a Cochrane review in 2007 were equivocal, with reviewers critical of methodology of studies so far (Hoare et al., 2007). Whether the positive effects transfer into improved bimanual performance is not clear. There have been few studies of the use of constraint for infants under

12–18 months (Cope et al., 2008; deLuca et al., 2003), and studies usually include a broad range of ages and degrees of severity, with no reference to individual results. Cope et al. (2008) reported a study of an infant aged 12 months with encouraging results. Findings were positive, with improvements in upper limb function that were sustained for at least six months, and with no adverse events.

Most of what we do with our upper limbs involves bimanual arm use, both limbs working symmetrically, e.g., pushing and pulling actions, or asymmetrically with each limb carrying out different parts of the task, e.g., reaching to pick up a jar and unscrewing the lid. Whether or not improvements in the paretic arm use will transfer into effective bimanual limb use is not clear, but it may be unlikely given the complex and task-specific limb interactions required (Fig. A.14). It is possible that there is only a small window of opportunity for an infant to develop/ learn the complexities of bimanual interactions with objects in the environment. An example of this complexity is demonstrated by a biomechanical study of the arms during a bimanual action in an adult—reaching to open a can (Castiello et al., 1993). Figure A.15A illustrates the differences in velocity and acceleration as each hand reaches forward to perform a different action; the left hand has the more precise task (grasping and pulling a tab with a pincer grasp) while the other reaches to take hold of the can

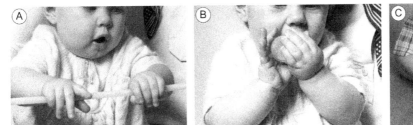

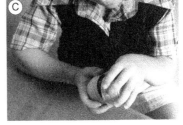

**Figure A.14 •** Developing skill in bimanual actions requires the ability to use the two limbs interactively and co-operatively. Each task affects specific temporal relationships between the two arms and between the hand and arm, depending on the task each hand performs. Tasks attempted and practiced are concrete and meaningful within an environment that has opportunities for the infant to explore other tasks.

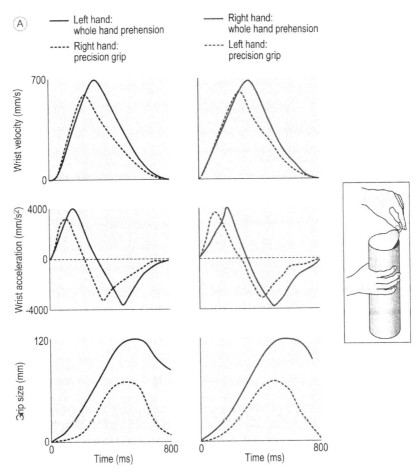

**Figure A.15 • (A)** A single trial of a bilateral task performed by an adult—reaching to open a can with the right hand grasping the can and the left hand lifting the tab. Both hands start the movement together and reach the can at a similar time but with distinct differences in timing and relative speed. From Castiello U et al. 1993 The bilateral reach-to-grasp movement. Behav Brain Res 56:43–57; reprinted from Carr and Shepherd, 2003, with permission of Elsevier.

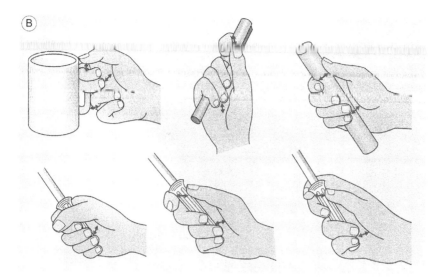

**Figure A.15 • (B)** Task- and object-related grasps with arrows showing the different 'oppositions' used in holding different tools for specific tasks. From Iberall et al. 1986. Opposition space as a structuring concept for the analysis of skilled hand movements. Exp Brain Res 15, 158–173, with permission of Springer Science + Business Media; reprinted from Carr and Shepherd, 2010.

with the whole hand. Figure A.15B illustrates how type (configuration) of grasp is dependent upon both the object and what might be done with it.

It is evident that bilateral and activity-related limb training must accompany sessions of constraint-induced unimanual training (Gordon et al., 2008). Various methods of training bimanual actions in infancy are being developed (Charles and Gordon, 2006; Gordon et al., 2007; Hung et al., 2010) and this is discussed in Chapter 14. The underlying science is compelling. It is likely that infants with hemiplegia will, if left to their own devices, learn to use the limb that is the most effective and will learn *not* to use the affected limb. The exclusive use of the non-paretic limb by infants with hemiplegia illustrates the phenomenon of 'learned non-use' described by Taub (1980), and 'driving' use of the affected limb early in life may prevent non-use being established in the infant's movement repertoire and difficult to 'unlearn'. However, there needs to be more information about the possibility of negative effects on brain organization of constraining the use of a limb in very young infants for this method to be considered (see Chapters 3 and 14).

## Electrical stimulation

Little is known about the effects of electrical stimulation applied in infants or children. Neuromuscular electrical stimulation (NMES)

is advocated as an adjunct to a physiotherapy programme that emphasizes task specificity and motor learning, and positive effects have been reported. It provides input while the child is engaged in a motivating, goal-directed activity. The decision about which muscles to stimulate is based on an understanding of the biomechanics and EMG patterns during effective performance of the action. The child is an active participant and is encouraged to initiate movement. A single-case study reports that a boy aged 6.7 years learned to perform a number of tasks, including tying his shoelaces, after 24 sessions of NMES to wrist extensors, finger flexors and extensors, with resisted exercises and task training (Carmick, 1997). A period of wearing a dorsal wrist splint made of orthoplast was included to help him with his task practice. This study shows that such intervention is feasible with children and can be remedial.

Whether or not ES in infancy would affect corticospinal drive and increase muscle activation is not known but should be investigated. In a small study reported at a conference in Canada (Juneau et al., 2003), three children with diplegia and one with hemiplegia, aged 3–6 years, had 15 minutes of NMES to their plantarflexors for eight weeks. For individual children, the results showed increases in range of movement, strength of plantarflexors (3/4), and GMFM scores (2/4), with increased heel-contact frequency when walking (4/4) and decreased stair-climbing time. There was also decreased resistance to passive stretch (2/4). At follow-up eight weeks later, range of movement, strength, muscle stiffness and GMFM had maintained improvement but only one child maintained heel contact when walking. Findings from group studies remain equivocal. A study of functional electrical stimulation applied to wrist extensor muscles found improvements in hand use (Wright and Granit, 2000) and another study of children with diplegia found an increase in walking speed and muscle strength (Stackhouse et al., 2007). A wireless distributed FES system is in development (Jovicic et al., 2012) and EMG-triggered FES is used in adult rehabilitation.

## Soft splinting: orthotic garments

Several types of garment, some made-to-measure, have been developed as aids to improving limb position, limb control, standing posture, and mobility (Lycra, Neoprene). They may be worn on the trunk or a limb, or the whole body. A study of the effects of an orthotic TheraTog™ garment (http://www.theratogs.com/descriptions.html), worn by children aged 7–13 years (GMFCS1-2), found that children's performance on two functional scales was significantly improved (Flanagan et al., 2009).

Children wore the garment for 12 weeks, 10–12 hours per day. At the end of this period kinematic analysis showed that peak hip extension at the end of stance phase was significantly increased and had not deteriorated four months later.

There is a possibility that the constraint to movement provided by such garments may interfere with rather than assist infants with weak muscles, yet there have been few studies examining their effect on movement in able-bodied infants. A recent study by Groenen et al. (2010) in able-bodied infants has found that during the first few months after birth, when their leg muscles are weak, the materials worn on the lower limbs can change the amount and effectiveness of movement, even when it may not be observable. The effects were to decrease step frequency and the number of alternating steps produced. Alternative stepping, an action that would be a particular focus of training programme with developmentally delayed infants, was found to be particularly sensitive to external constraints.

An unpublished systematic review in 2006 found no evidence to support the use of such splints for the upper limb, and a possibility of adverse effects of body suits (Blackmore et al., 2006). Another study found few relevant research papers and concluded that Lycra garments may be useful as they can provide some stability to a joint or joints and thereby enhance functional abilities in some children, but that they are expensive and can be uncomfortable (Coghill and Simkiss, 2010). There needs to be more investigation of the effects of the body suits before they are in common use with infants with CP. However, the use of soft splints for local use to enable an infant to stand (see Fig. A.10A), or to hold a limb in an optimal position for practice of hand use, for example, may be a good idea for some infants.

Therapists and parents need to give thought to what an infant wears during exercise sessions and through the day—in general, the least fettered they are the more opportunity they have to be active. Many infants in Western societies are constrained during the day in seats that restrict their movement (Chapman, 2002) and parents need to consider this with an infant who needs more opportunity to move about spontaneously and be active.

# The organization of intervention: methods of delivery

Intervention to improve an infant's motor control and motor performance takes place in the home, the clinic and in the community. Intervention needs to be intensive at appropriate times, especially with young infants. Although it is basically one-to-one: parent + infant, therapist + infant, it may be more congenial when therapy is organized in a group. The therapist teaches the parents (and siblings), by demonstration, those methods of motor training and exercise described in this book, and the parents, with siblings to help, carry out simple programmes at home (Craft et al., 1990). The therapist visits the infant's home from time to time and parent and child visit the therapist as often as is practical. The young infant with CP may be difficult to hold and the therapist can make suggestions for handling and caring for the baby (Bower, 2009). Parents are taught carrying, positioning, feeding and dressing techniques (Olney and Wright, 2006). Learning these skills will enable parents to develop confidence and be at ease with their infant, and will have positive effects on the infant, reducing the influence of impairments and minimizing activity limitations.

Interaction between therapist and parent using the internet or telephone may become a useful methods of assisting parents with details of training, exercise, handling and play (Bilde et al., 2011)

## Community involvement

The community can play an important role, and in many countries there are new opportunities emerging for parent and baby to attend baby gyms and similar groups. These groups aim to engage parent and infant in activity programmes designed to be fun and experiential. They encourage active engagement, for both infant and parent, and stimulate infants and small children to learn different activities.

## Group practice

A clinic can offer group practice sessions, where infants and children move between *work stations* in a *circuit training* format, assisted by parents, therapist and therapy aide. These sessions have been shown to be feasible and effective for young children (Blundell et al., 2003; Trahan and Malouin, 2002; Ustad et al., 2009). Figure A.5A–D illustrates some of the exercises and activities that made up the 'workstations' in a lower limb circuit class for children aged 3–8 years in an Australian clinic.

## Intermittent intensive physiotherapy

Research findings suggest that children with CP may need to exercise and train intensively and intermittently throughout their lives. Trahan and Malouin (2002) investigated the effects of an intensive programme (four times a week for four weeks), each exercise period separated by a period of eight weeks without therapy, over a period of six months. The five children were young (10–37 months) and severely impaired (levels IV and V on the GMFM). The level of attendance was high, three out of five children improved significantly on GMFM and all remained stable over the no treatment period. Therapists reported the advantages of sessions four times a week, including their observation that close interaction with child and parent enabled the adaptation of short-term

goals day by day. It is notable that the children over the six-month period had fewer therapy sessions, 30 sessions compared to the 48 sessions they would normally have. In another investigation (Sorsdahl et al., 2010), children 3 to 9 years old, attended a group programme of three hours of goal-directed activity-focused physiotherapy for five days a week over a period of three weeks. Children showed significant improvements in GMFM-66 scores, with an implication that the children classified as GMFM 1-11 improved more than those classed as 111-V. PEDI scores in self-care were significantly improved.

Finally, many therapists are exploring different ways to organize the delivery of interventions to enable the child to be an active learner, with provision for small-group training sessions where infants and parents work together. Technological innovations in computer science, robotics and orthotics, and in brain scanning, have the potential to impact on rehabilitation, making possible the development of computer-aided task- and activity-oriented training methods. The recently developed SMART arm, a non-robotic training device that enables repetitive task-oriented practice of reaching (see Fig.1.1C), has been shown in adults after stroke to improve functional performance of the limb, and these improvements were associated with modifications to corticospinal reactivity as measured by motor-evoked potentials (Barker et al., 2008, 2009, 2012). Small modifications should enable this device to be used by infants and young children.

There are plans for developing and testing a reorganization of the methods of delivering intensive training and exercise from one-to-one therapy once or twice a week to short daily periods with family involvement following science- and evidence-based guidelines accessed from the clinic via the internet; ongoing computer- and mobile phone-based guidance to be provided by the therapist (see Chapter 15) (Bilde et al., 2011). This is the future of intervention in CP in infancy and childhood, with therapists and physicians collaborating with engineers, computer scientists, robotists and technicians to develop new ways of training motor control and providing exercise stimulus, particularly for young infants whose collaboration is not always easy to achieve.

# References

American College of Sports Medicine, 2012. Current Comment on Youth Training. <www.acsm.org/docs/current-comment/youthstrengthening.pdf>.

American College of Sports Medicine, Durstine, J.L., Moore, G., Painter, P., et al., 2009. ACSM's Exercise Management for Persons with Chronic Diseases & Disabilities, third ed.. Human Kinetics, eBook.

Bale, M., Strand, L.I., 2008. Does functional strength training of the leg in subacute stroke improve physical performance? A pilot randomised controlled trial. Clin. Rehabil. 22, 911–921.

Barbeau, H., 2003. Locomotor training in neurorehabilitation: emerging rehabilitation concepts. Neurorehab. Neural Repair 17, 3–11.

Barker, R.N., Brauer, S.G., Carson, R.G., 2008. Training of reaching in stroke survivors with severe and chronic upper limb paresis using a novel nonrobotic device: A randomised clinical trial. Stroke 39, 1800–1807.

Barker, R.N., Brauer, S.G., Carson, R.G., 2009. Training-induced changes in the pattern of triceps to biceps activation during reaching tasks after chronic and severe stroke. Exp. Brain. Res. 196, 483–496.

Barker, R.N., Brauer, S.G., Barry, B.K., et al., 2012. Training-induced modifications of corticospinal reactivity in severely affected stroke survivors. Exp. Brain. Res. 221, 211–221. doi: 10.1007/s00221-012-3163-z.

Bateman, A., Culpan, F.J., Pickering, A.D., et al., 2001. The effect of aerobic training on rehabilitation outcomes after recent severe brain injury: a randomised controlled trial. Arch. Phys. Med. Rehabil. 82, 174–182.

Bilde, P.E., Klim-Due, M., Rasmussen, B., et al., 2011. Individualized, home-based interactive training of cerebral palsy children with cerebral palsy delivered through the Internet. BMC Neurol. 11, 32. doi: 10.1186/1471-2377-11-32.

Birch, H.G., Gwiazda, J., Held, J., 1982. Stereoacuity development for crossed and uncrossed disparities in human infants. Vision Res. 22, 507–513.

Blackmore, A.M., Garbellini, S.A., Buttigieg, P., et al., 2006. A systematic review of the effects of soft splinting on upper limb function in people. An AACPDM Evidence Report.

Blauw-Hospers, C.H., Hadders-Algra, M., 2005. A systematic review of the effects of early intervention on motor development. Dev. Med. Child Neurol. 47, 421–432.

Blauw-Hospers, C.H., de Graaf-Peters, V.B., Dirks, T., et al., 2007. Does early intervention in infants at high risk for a developmental motor disorder improve motor and cognitive development? Neurosci. Biobehav. Rev. 31, 1201–1212.

Blundell, S.W., Shepherd, R.B., Dean, C.M., et al., 2003. Functional strength training in cerebral palsy: a pilot study of a group circuit training class for children aged 4–8 years. Clin. Rehabil. 17, 48–57.

Bodkin, A.W., Baxter, R.S., Heriza, C.B., 2003. Treadmill training for an infant born preterm with a grade III intraventricular haemorrhage. Phys. Ther. 83 (1107), 1118.

Booth, C.M., Cortina-Borja, M.J.F., Theologis, T.N., 2001. Collagen accumulation in muscles of children with cerebral palsy and correlation with severity of spasticity. Dev. Med. Child Neurol. 43, 314–332.

Bottos, M., Feliciangeli, A., Sciuto, L., et al., 2001. Functional status of adults with cerebral palsy and implications for treatment for children. Dev. Med. Child Neurol. 43, 516–528.

Bower, E., 2009. Finnie's Handling the Young Child with Cerebral Palsy at Home, fourth ed. Elsevier, Oxford.

Brown, D.A., Kautz, S.A., 1998. Increased workload enhances force output during pedalling exercise in persons with poststroke hemiplegia. Stroke 29, 598–606.

Buchner, D.M., Larson, E.B., Wagner, E.H., et al., 1996. Evidence for a non-linear relationship between leg strength and gait speed. Age Ageing 25, 386–391.

Cadoret, G., Smith, A.M., 1996. Friction, not texture, dictates grip forces used during object manipulation. J. Neurophysiol. 75, 1963–1969.

Carmick, J., 1997. Use of neuromuscular electrical stimulation and a dorsal wrist splint to improve the hand function of a child with spastic hemiparesis. Phys. Ther. 77, 661–671.

Carr, J.H., Shepherd, R.B., 2010. Neurological Rehabilitation: Optimizing Motor Performance, second ed. Butterworth-Heinemann, Oxford.

Carr, J.H., Shepherd, R.B., 2003. Stroke Rehabilitation Guidelines for Exercise and Training to Optimize Motor Skill. Butterworth-Heinemann, Oxford.

Castiello, U., Bennett, K.M.B., Stelmach, G.E., 1993. The bilateral reach-to-grasp movement. Behav. Brain Res. 56, 43–57.

Chapman, D., 2002. Context effects on the spontaneous leg movements of infants with spina bifida. Pediatr. Phys. Ther. 14, 62–73.

Charles, J., Gordon, A.M., 2006. Development of hand-arm bimanual intensive training (HABIT) for improving bimanual coodination in children with hemiplegic cerebral palsy. Dev. Med. Child Neurol. 48, 931–936.

Charles, J.R., Wolf, S.L., Schneider, J.A., et al., 2006. Efficacy of a child-friendly form of constraint-induced movement therapy in hemiplegic cerebral palsy: a randomised control trial. Dev. Med. Child Neurol. 48, 635–642.

Chen, Y.-P., Fetters, L., Holt, K.G., et al., 2002. Making the mobile move: constraining task and environment. Infant. Behav. Dev. 25, 195–220.

Coghill, J.E., Simkiss, D.E., 2010. Question 1. Do Lycra garments improve function and movement in children with cerebral palsy? Arch. Dis. Child. 95, 393–395.

Cope, S.M., Forst, H.C., Bibis, D., et al., 2008. Modified constraint-induced movement therapy for a 12-month child with hemiplegia: a case report. J. Occ. Ther. 62, 430–437.

Cordo, P.J., Nashner, L.M., 1982. Properties of postural adjustments associated with rapid arm movements. J. Neurophysiol. 47, 287–302.

Craft, M.J., Lakin, J.A., Oppliger, R.A., et al., 1990. Siblings as change agents for promoting the functional status of children with cerebral palsy. Dev. Med. Child Neurol. 32, 1049–1057.

Damiano, D.L., 2003. Strength, endurance, and fitness in cerebral palsy. Dev. Med. Child Neurol. Suppl. 94, 8–10.

Damiano, D.L., Abel, M.F., 1998. Functional outcomes of strength training in spastic cerebral palsy. Arch. Phys. Med. Rehabil. 79, 119–125.

Damiano, D.L., Quinliven, J., Owen, B.F., et al., 2001. Spasticity versus strength in cerebral palsy: relations among involuntary resistance, voluntary torque, and motor function. Eur. J. Neurol. 8 (Suppl. 5), 40–49.

Damiano, D.L., Dodd, K., Taylor, N.F., 2002. Should we be testing and training muscle strength in cerebral palsy? Dev. Med. Child Neurol. 44, 68–72.

Davies, J.M., Mayston, M.J., Newham, D.J., 1996. Electrical and mechanical output of the knee muscles during isometric and isokinetic activity in stroke and healthy subjects. Disabil. Rehabil. 18, 83–90.

DeLuca, S.C., Echols, K., Ramey, S.L., et al., 2003. Pediatric constraint-induced movement therapy for a young child with cerebral palsy: two episodes of care. Phys. Ther. 83, 1003–1013.

Dean, C.M., Shepherd, R.B., 1997. Task-related training improves performance of seated reaching tasks after stroke: a randomised controlled trial. Stroke 28, 722–728.

Delp, S.L., 2003. What causes increased muscle stiffness in cerebral palsy? Muscle Nerve 27, 131–2003.

Delp, S.L., Hess, W.E., Hungerford, D.S., et al., 1999. Variation of rotational arms with hip flexion. J. Biomech. 23, 493–501.

Dietz, V., Duysens, J., 2000. Significance of load receptor input during locomotion: a review. Gait Posture 11, 102–110.

Dodd, K., Taylor, N., Damiano, D.L., 2002. A systematic review of the effectiveness of strength training programmes for people with cerebral palsy. Arch. Phys. Med. Rehabil. 83, 1157–1164.

Dodd, K.I., Taylor, N.F., Graham, H.K., 2003. A randomised clinical trial of strength training in young people with cerebral palsy. Dev. Med. Child Neurol. 45, 652–657.

Eliasson, A.C., Krumlinde-Sundholm, L., Shaw, K., et al., 2005. Effects of constraint-induced movement therapy in young children with hemiplegic cerebral palsy: an adapted model. Dev. Med. Child Neurol. 47, 266–275.

Engardt, M., Knutsson, E., Jonsson, M., et al., 1995. Dynamic muscle strength training in stroke patients: effects on knee extension torque, electromyographic activity, and motor function. Arch. Phys. Med. Rehabil. 76, 419–425.

Faigenbaum, A.D., 2000. Strength training for children and adolescents. Clin. Sports Med. 4, 593–619.

Faigenbaum, A.D., Westcott, W.L., Loud, R.L., et al., 1999. The effects of different resistance training protocols on muscular strength and endurance development in children. Pediatrics 104, e5.

Flanagan, A., Krzak, J., Peer, M., et al., 2009. Evaluation of short-term intensive orthotic garment use in children who have cerebral palsy. Pediatr. Phys. Ther. 21, 201–204.

Foran, J.R., Steinman, S., Barash, I., et al., 2005. Structural and mechanical alterations in spastic skeletal muscle. Dev. Med. Child Neurol. 47, 713–717.

Gordon, A.M., Schneider, J.A., Chinnan, A., et al., 2007. Efficacy of a hand-arm bimanual intensive therapy (HABIT) in children with hemiplegic cerebral palsy: a randomised control trial. Dev. Med. Child Neurol. 49, 830–838.

Gordon, A.M., Chinnan, A., Gill, S., et al., 2008. Both constraint-induced movement therapy and bimanual training lead to improved performance of upper extremity function in children with hemiplegia. Dev. Med. Child Neurol. 50, 957–958.

Groenen, A., Kruijsen, A.J.A., Mulvey, G.M., et al., 2010. Constraints on early movements styles, togo, and technology. Infant. Behav. Dev., 16 22.

Hoare, B., Imms, C., Carey, L., et al., 2007. Constraint-induced movement therapy in the treatment of the upper limb in children with hemiplegic cerebral palsy: a Cochrane systematic review. Clin. Rehabil. 21, 675–685. www.thecochranelibrary.com.

Huang, H.-H., Fetters, L., Hale, J., et al., 2009. Bound for success: a systematic review of constraint-induced movement therapy in children with cerebral palsy supports improve arm and hand use. Phys. Ther. 89, 1126–1141.

Hung, Y.-C., Charles, J., Gordon, A.M., 2010. Influence of accuracy constraints on bimanual coordination during a goal-directed task in children with hemiplegic cerebral palsy. Exp. Brain Res. 201, 421–428.

Johansson, R.S., Westling, G., 1984. Tactile afferent signals on the control of precision grip. In: Jeannerod, M. (Ed.), Attention and Performance. Erlbaum, Hillsdale, NJ, pp. 677–713.

Johansson, R.S., Westling, G., 1990. Tactile afferent signals in the control of precision grip. In: Jeannerod, M. (Ed.), Attention and Performance. Erlbaum, Hillsdale NJ, pp. 677–713.

Jovicic, N.S., Saranovac, L.V., Popovic, D.B., 2012. Wireless distributed functional electrical stimulation system. J. NeuroEng. Rehabil. 9, 54. doi: 10.1186/1743-0003-9-54.

Juenger, H., Linder-Lucht, M., Walther, M., et al., 2007. Cortical neuromodulation by constraint-induced movement therapy in congenital hemiparesis: an fMRI study. Neuropediatrics 38, 130–136.

Juneau, C., Roy, S., Richards, C.L., et al., 2003. Effects of neuromuscular electrical stimulation on muscle strength, range of motion, and locomotor ability in children with cerebral palsy. Dev. Med. Child Neurol. 2003 (Suppl. 94), 52.

Knis-Matthews, L., Falzarano, M., Baum, D., et al., 2011. Parents' experiences with services and treatment for their children diagnosed with cerebral palsy. Phys. Occup. Ther. Pediatr. 31, 263–274.

Komi, P.V., 1986. The stretch-shortening cycle and human power output. In: Jones, N.C. (Ed.), Human Muscle Power. Human Kinetics Publishers, Champaign, IL.

Kott, K., Lesher, K., DeLeo, G., 2009. Combining a virtual reality system with treadmill training for children with cerebral palsy. J. CyberTher. Rehabil. 2, 35.

Krichevets, A.N., Sirokina, E.B., Yevsevicheva, I.V., et al., 1995. Computer games as a means of movement rehabilitation. Disabil. Rehabil. 17, 100–105.

Liao, H.-F., Liu, Y.-C., Liu, W.-Y., et al., 2007. Effectiveness of loaded sit-to-stand resistance exercise for children with mild spastic diplegia: a randomized clinical trial. Arch. Phys. Med. Rehabil. 88, 25–31.

MacPhail, H.E., Kramer, J.F., 1995. Effect of isokinetic strength training on functional ability and walking efficiency in adolescents with cerebral palsy. Dev. Med. Child Neurol. 37, 763–775.

Magill, R., 2010. Motor Learning and Control: Concepts and Applications, 12th ed. McGraw-Hill, New York.

McBurney, H., Taylor, N.F., Dodd, K.J., et al., 2003. A qualitative analysis of the benefits of strength training for young people with cerebral palsy. Dev. Med. Child Neurol. 45, 658–663.

Monkford, M., Coulton, J.M., 2008. Systemic review of progressive strength training in children and adolescents with cerebral palsy who are ambulatory. Pediatr. Phys. Ther. 20, 38–333.

Morrissey, M.C., Harman, E.S., Johnson, M.J., 1995. Resistance training modes: specificity and effectiveness. Med. Sci. Sports Exerc. 27, 648–660.

Nsenga, A.N.L., 2012. Gait cycle and plantar pressure Personal communication.

Olney, S.J., Wright, M.J., 2006. Cerebral palsy. In: Campbell, S.K., Vander Linden, D.W., Palisano, R.J. (Eds.), Physical Therapy for Children, third ed. Elsevier, New York.

Olney, S.J., Jackson, V.G., George, S.R., 1988. Gait reeducation guidelines for stroke patients with hemiplegia using mechanical energy and power analyses. Physioth. Can. 40, 242–248.

Olney, S.J., Griffin, M.P., Monga, T.N., et al., 1991. Work and power in gait of stroke patients. Arch. Phys. Med. Rehabil. 72, 309–314.

Pinneger, G.J., Steele, J.R., Thorstensson, A., et al., 2000. Tension regulation during lengthening and shortening actions of the human soleus muscle. Eur. J. Appl. Physiol. 81, 375–383.

Provost, B., Dieruf, K., Burtner, P., et al., 2007. Endurance and gait in children with cerebral palsy after intensive body weight-supported treadmill training. Pediatr. Phys. Ther. 19, 2–10.

Rahman, S.A., Rahman, A., Shaheen, A.A., 2010. Virtual reality use in motor rehabilitation of neurological disorders: a systematic review. Middle-East J. Scientific Res. 7, 63–70.

Richards, C.L., Malouin, F., Dumas, F., et al., 1997. Early and intensive treadmill locomotor training for young children with cerebral palsy: a feasibility study. Pediatr. Phys. Ther. 9, 158–165.

Rutherford, O.M., 1988. Muscular coordination and strength training: implications for injury rehabilitation. Sports Med. 5, 196–202.

Ryan, A.S., Ivey, F.M., Prior, S., et al., 2011. Skeletal muscle hypertrophy and muscle myostatin reduction after resistive training in stroke survivors. Stroke 42, 416–420.

Sharp, S.A., Brouwer, B.J., 1997. Isokinetic strength training of the hemiparetic knee: effects on function and spasticity. Arch. Phys. Med. Rehabil. 78, 1231–1236.

Shepherd, R.B., 1995. Physiotherapy in Paediatrics, third ed. Butterworth-Heinemann, Oxford.

Shepherd, R.B., Gentile, A.M., 1994. Sit-to-stand: functional relationships between upper body and lower limb segments. Hum. Movt. Sci. 13, 817–840.

Singer, W., 1982. The role of attention in developmental plasticity. Hum. Neurobiol. 1, 41–43.

Smith, L.R., Ponten, E., Hedstrom, Y., et al., 2009. Novel transcription profiles in wrist muscles from cerebral palsy patients. BMC Med. Genomics 2, 44. doi: 10.1186/1755-8794-2-44.

Smith, L.R., Lee, K.S., Ward, S.R., et al., 2011. Hamstring contractures in children with spastic cerebral palsy result from a stiffer extracellular matrix and increased in vivo sarcomere length. J. Physiol. 589, 2625–2639.

Song, W.H., Sung, I.Y., Kim, Y.J., et al., 2003. Treadmill walking with partial body weight support in children with cerebral palsy. Arch. Phys. Med. Rehabil. 84, E2.

Sorsdahl, A.B., Moe-Nilssen, R., Kaale, H.K., et al., 2010. Change in basic motor abilities, quality of movement and everyday activities following intensive, goal-directed, activity-focused physiotherapy in a group setting for children with cerebral palsy. BMC Pediatr. 10, 26–36.

Stackhouse, S.K., Binder-McLeod, S.A., Stackhouse, C.A., et al., 2007. Neuromuscular electrical stimulation versus volitional isometric strength training in children with spastic diplegic cerebral palsy. Neurorehabil. Neural Repair 21, 475–485.

Sutcliffe, T.L., Gaetz, W.C., Logan, W.J., et al., 2007. Cortical reorganization after modified constraint-induced movement therapy in pediatric hemiplegic cerebral palsy. J. Child Neurol. 22, 1281–1287.

Svantessen, U., Sunnerhagen, K.S., 1997. Stretch-shortening cycle in patients with upper motor neuron lesion due to stroke. Eur. J. Appl. Physiol. 75, 312–318.

Svantessen, U., Takahashi, H., Carlsson, U., et al., 2000. Muscle and tendon stiffness in patients with upper motor neuron lesion following a stroke. Eur. J. Appl. Physiol. 82, 275–279.

Taub, E., 1980. Somatosensory deafferentation research with monkey: implications for rehabilitation medicine. In: Ince, L.P. (Ed.), Behavioral Psychology in Rehabilitation Medicine: Clinical Applications. Williams & Wilkins, New York, pp. 371–401.

Tax, A.A.M., Denier van der Gon, J.J., Erkelens, C.J., 1990. Differences in coordination of elbow flexors in force tasks and in movement. Exp. Brain Res. 81, 567–572.

Taylor, N., Dodd, K.J., Damiano, D.L., 2005. Progressive resistance exercise in physical therapy: a summary of systematic reviews. Phy. Ther. 85, 1208–1223.

Teixeira-Salmela, L.F., Olney, S.J., Nadeau, S., et al., 1999. Muscle strengthening and physical conditioning to reduce impairment and disability in chronic stroke survivors. Arch. Phys. Med. Rehabil. 80, 1211–1218.

Tobimatsu, Y., Nakamura Kusano, S., et al., 1998. Cardiorespiratory endurance in people with cerebral palsy measured using an arm ergometer. Arch. Phys. Med. Rehabil. 79, 991–993.

Trahan, J., Malouin, F., 2002. Intermittent intensive physiotherapy in children with cerebral palsy: a pilot study. Dev. Med. Child Neurol. 44, 233–239.

Ulrich, D.A., Ulrich, B.D., Angulo-Kinzler, R.M., et al., 2001. Treadmill training of infants with Down syndrome: evidence-based development outcomes. Pediatrics 108, E84.

Ulrich, D.A., Lloyd, M.C., Tieman, J.E., et al., 2008. Effects of intensity of treadmill training on developmental outcomes and stepping in infants with Down syndrome: a randomised trial. Phys. Ther. 88, 114–121.

Unnithan, V.B., Clifford, C., Bar-Or, O., 1998. Evaluation by exercise testing of the child with cerebral palsy. Sports Med. 26, 239–251.

Unnithan, V.B., Kenne, E.M., Logan, L., et al., 2006. The effect of body weight support on the oxygen cost of walking in children and adolescents with spastic cerebral palsy. Pediatr. Exerc. Sci. 18, 11–21.

Ustad, T., Sorsdale, A., Ljunggren, A., 2009. Effects of intensive physiotherapy in infants newly diagnosed with cerebral palsy. Pediatr. Phys. Ther. 21, 140–149.

von Hofsten, C., 1982. Eye–hand coordination in newborns. Dev. Psychol. 18, 450.

von Hofsten, C., 1984. Developmental changes in the organization of pre-reaching movements. Dev. Psychol. 20, 378–388.

von Hofsten, C., Fazel-Zandy, S., 1984. Development of visually-guided hand orientation in reaching. J. Exp. Child Psychol. 38, 208.

von Hofsten, C., Lindhagen, K., 1979. Observations on the development of reaching for moving objects. J. Exp. Child Psychol. 28, 158–173.

von Hofsten, C., Rönnqvist, L., 1988. Preparation for grasping an object: a developmental study. J. Exper. Psychol. Hum. Percep. Perfor. 14, 610–621.

Westling, G., Johansson, R.S., 1984. Responses in glabrous skin mechanoreceptors during precision grip in humans. Exp. Brain Res. 66, 128–140.

Wiart, L., Darrah, J., Kembhavi, G., 2008. Stretching with children with cerebral palsy: what do we know and where are we going? Pediatr. Phys. Ther. 20, 173–178.

Wiley, M.E., Damiano, D.L., 1998. Lower extremity strength profiles in spastic cerebral palsy. Dev. Med. Child Neurol. 40, 100–107.

Wilmshurst, S., Ward, K., Adams, J.E., et al., 1996. Mobility status and bone density in cerebral palsy. Arch. Dis. Child 75, 164–168.

Wright, P.A., Granit, M.H., 2000. Therapeutic effects of functional electrical stimulation of the upper limb of eight children with cerebral palsy. Dev. Med. Child Neurol. 42, 724–727.

# PART 2

## Neuromotor Plasticity and Development

# Corticospinal tract development and activity-dependent plasticity

2

Janet Eyre

## CHAPTER CONTENTS

Man is unrivalled in achieving complex language, remarkably skilled and flexible manual dexterity and adept bipedal gait, abilities that are dependent upon highly proficient neural control of motoneurons and muscles. The performance of skilled movements has been shown to rely upon the integrity of the corticospinal system and specifically on direct monosynaptic input from the motor cortex to spinal α-motoneurons (Armand et al., 1996; Bortoff and Strick, 1993; Kuypers, 1962, 1981; Lawrence and Hopkins, 1976; Porter and Lemon, 1993). In sub-human primates, direct corticomotoneuronal projections are largely restricted to the motoneurons of muscles controlling movements of the arm, hand, foot and tail and their density is related to the degree of skill achieved (Bortoff and Strick, 1993; Heffner and Masterton, 1983; Kuypers, 1981; Phillips and Porter, 1977; Porter and Lemon, 1993). Man is unique in possessing direct corticomotoneuronal projections to all motor nuclei so far investigated (Porter and Lemon, 1993), implying a greatly expanded role for the corticomotoneuronal system. In humans, skilled voluntary control of movements develops postnatally, with the initial rapid emergence of motor skills over the first 18–24 postnatal months. These skills are subsequently refined over a prolonged period, until early adulthood (Forssberg et al., 1991; Muetzel et al., 2008). While the maturation of many systems, including the visuomotor and sensorimotor systems, and the cognitive aspects of movement control such as selective attention and executive control will determine the expression of developing motor skills and the eventual level of dexterity achieved (Martins et al., 2012), these behavioural changes also undoubtedly reflect the prolonged maturation throughout childhood and adolescence of the corticospinal system.

If damage to the corticospinal system occurs in adulthood, great difficulty in learning new or relearning former sequences of skilled movements occurs (Brodal, 1973), emphasizing the role of the corticospinal system in the acquisition and maintenance of skill. When lesions occur in the perinatal period, not only is learning of skilled movements severely impaired but also such lesions can result in the development of cerebral palsy. In the immediate period after the lesion, however, babies who will develop cerebral palsy display only subtle, if any, abnormalities of movement control (Bouza et al., 1994; Nelson and Ellenberg, 1979; Prechtl et al., 1997). There follows over many months and years, the progressive development of a movement disorder, associated with significant secondary disruption of corticospinal and spinal motor centre development (Eyre et al., 2007; Leonard et al., 1991; Myklebust et al., 1982; O'Sullivan et al., 1998). This implies a further role for the corticomotoneuronal system in man, activity-dependent regulation of the development of the sensorimotor cortex, spinal motor centres and their connectivity.

Older concepts of developmental plasticity focused on the protective effect of a young age at the time of the brain damage (Kennard, 1936). In these views, a younger rather than an older age at onset was thought to produce fewer or less severe symptoms and a more rapid recovery. It is now clear that the specific effects of early brain damage produce complex and often severe patterns of impairment, which are different from those observed following lesions in the adult brain. Furthermore, although an understanding of the nature of neural plasticity in response to damage is critical to those attempting to augment recovery from neurological insults, it is misleading to treat the underlying mechanisms as self-reparative. The appreciation that these mechanisms evolved as an expedient for fine-tuning neurological circuitry during normal development by taking advantage of contextual information, and may only be available for response to damage as an incidental side effect, can help to focus on how best to augment the desirable and avoid any undesirable effects.

Seminal studies in the early 1960s by Wiesel and Hubel (1965) on the organization of ocular dominance columns signified the starting point of extensive basic research on developmental brain plasticity. The investigation of neuroplasticity has expanded rapidly over the past 10 years and has uncovered the remarkable capacity of the developing brain to be shaped by activity and environmental input. Knowledge of the time course and processes of normal development is essential both for a better understanding of current rehabilitation treatments and for the design of new strategies for the treatment of children who sustain brain damage early in life.

# Corticospinal tract development and plasticity in sub-primate mammals

The development of the corticospinal system has been studied most extensively in the rat. In the neonatal rat the corticospinal projection originates from the whole neocortex, including the visual cortex (O'Leary et al., 1992; Stanfield and O'Leary, 1985) (Fig. 2.1). Corticospinal projections in several mammalian species also have transient ipsilateral projections early in development that are predominantly eliminated when maturity is reached (O'Leary et al., 1992). Massive axonal withdrawal, coupled with modest corticospinal cell death, leads to complete elimination of the corticospinal projection from inappropriate regions of the cortex, a reduction in the number of corticospinal axons projecting from the primary sensorimotor cortex and almost complete withdrawal of the ipsilateral projection (Joosten et al., 1992; Oudega et al., 1994).

Substantial lesions of the sensorimotor cortex or corticospinal tract in sub-primate mammals early in postnatal life lead to hypertrophy of the undamaged motor cortex and corticospinal projection, which has an increased number of corticospinal axons (Hicks and D'Amato, 1970, 1977; Huttenlocher and Raichelson, 1989; Jansen and Low, 1996; Rouiller et al., 1991; Uematsu et al., 1996). These changes are associated with maintenance of an increased ipsilateral corticospinal projection from the undamaged hemisphere. The cells of origin of the aberrant ipsilateral axons are more widely distributed and distinct from the cells of origin of the crossed or contralateral corticospinal projection (Huttenlocher and Raichelson, 1989; Jansen and Low, 1996; O'Leary et al., 1992; Reinoso and Castro, 1989). There is no evidence for double labelling of corticospinal neurons in neonatally hemispherectomized animals that in adulthood had spinal cord injection of fluorescent tracers (Reinoso and Castro, 1989). Thus the ipsilaterally projecting corticospinal axons from the undamaged cortex do not arise solely as branches of the contralateral corticospinal projection, but arise also from neurons that extend axons into the ipsilateral spinal cord during development, and whose axons would normally be withdrawn. The distribution of aberrant ipsilateral axons within the spinal grey matter

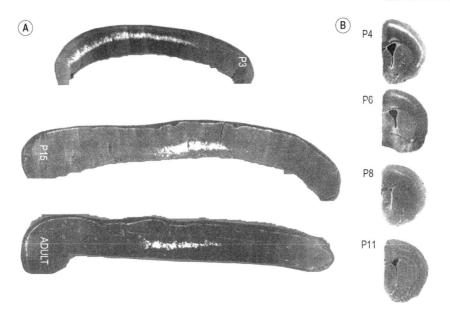

**Figure 2.1 • (A)** Sagittal sections through the cortex of a rat aged 3 postnatal days (P3), 15 postnatal days (P15) and in adulthood showing labelled cells following an injection of Fast blue at the high cervical level. **(B)** Coronal sections through the anterior parietal cortex in rats aged from 4 to 11 postnatal days (P4–P11) showing labelled cortical cells following injection of horseradish peroxidase into the high cervical spinal cord. [(A) Adapted from Schreyer D, Jones E. Growth and target finding by axons of the corticospinal tract in prenatal and postnatal rats. Neuroscience 1982;7:1837–1853, with permission from Elsevier. (B) Adapted from Bates C, Killackey H. The emergence of a discretely distributed pattern of corticospinal projection neurons. Brain Res. 1984;13:265–273, with permission from Elsevier.]

resembles that of the contralateral corticospinal projection (Barth and Stanfield, 1990; McClung and Castro, 1975)and synaptic contacts have been demonstrated (Leong, 1976; McClung and Castro, 1975). Ipsilateral forelimb movements are observed following stimulation of the intact cortex at abnormally low current thresholds, which are abolished by medullary pyramidotomy (Kartje-Tillotson et al., 1985, 1987).

# Corticospinal development and plasticity in sub-human primates

It has been proposed that corticospinal innervation in primates may not be governed by the same processes or have the degree of plasticity described in sub-primate mammals (Armand et al., 1997; O'Leary et al., 1992). However in the macaque monkey a halving of the area of the cerebral cortex from which corticospinal axons originate has been demonstrated during the first eight postnatal months, when brain volume overall increases by more than 30%. These changes

are associated with a threefold reduction in the number of retrogradely labelled cortical neurons, providing convincing evidence for an initially exuberant corticospinal projection and significant corticospinal axonal withdrawal (Galea and Darian-Smith, 1995). Although Kuypers (1962) and Armand et al. (1997) found no evidence for postnatal reduction in corticospinal synapses in the cervical spinal cord during the same period in macaque monkeys, this may reflect the methodology employed. Both studies used anterograde labelling of axons projecting from the hand area of the primary motor cortex. Such focal anterograde labelling would not detect projection and withdrawal of corticospinal axons and synapses from other areas of the cortex, including other areas of the motor cortex. It is from these other areas that the majority of supernumerary axons arise both in sub-primate mammals (Stanfield et al., 1982) and also in the macaque monkey (Galea and Darian-Smith, 1995). Furthermore, elimination of supernumerary synapses occurs in conjunction with the proliferation of synapses from the subset of axons that are maintained. It is the subset of axons that are maintained which would be labelled by anterograde tracers. Net increases in synaptic density have been observed during significant axonal withdrawal in other primate systems (LaMantia and Rakic, 1990, 1994).

Studies in monkeys have failed to reveal plasticity of corticospinal tract development following lesions; however, no study has yet replicated the circumstances in which plasticity has been demonstrated in sub-primate mammals and in humans (see below). Passingham et al. (1983) performed lesions too late, with all but one being between postnatal days 23 and 89. Rouiller et al. (1991) made very focal lesions in the motor cortex and demonstrated substantial reorganization of the surrounding motor cortex on the same side as the lesion. Reorganization of the ipsilateral projection from the undamaged hemisphere in sub-primate mammals has only been observed following large lesions such as ablation or extensive infarction of the motor cortex, or following pyramidotomy. Finally, Galea and Darian Smith (1997) performed a hemisection procedure of the cervical spinal cord in a monkey with the lesion located below the pyramidal decussation and involved the projections from both hemispheres. The detailed study did, however, exclude significant branching of corticospinal axons at spinal levels in response to early lesions of the corticospinal tract.

# Corticospinal development in humans

By eight weeks post-conceptional age (PCA) corticospinal axons reach the medulla (Humphrey, 1960; O'Rahily and Müller, 1994) and decussation occurs at about 15 weeks PCA. Corticospinal axons invade the axon tracts of the spinal cord from 17 to 29 weeks PCA (Altman and Bayer, 2001) and reach the lower cervical spinal cord by 24 weeks PCA (Fig. 2.2). Corticospinal innervation of the spinal motoneuronal pools can be demonstrated by at least 31 weeks PCA (Fig. 2.2C). There follows progressive innervation of the grey matter so that there is extensive innervation of spinal neurons, including motoneurons, prior to birth (Eyre, 2005; Eyre et al., 2000a, 2002). By 40 weeks PCA, corticospinal axons have begun to express neurofilaments and to undergo myelination (Fig. 2.3).

Detailed neurophysiological studies (Eyre et al., 2000a; Szelenyi et al., 2003) provided compelling evidence for the ability of the corticospinal axons in the term baby to conduct a coherent volley

and for the prenatal establishment of functional, corticospinal synapses with both α motoneurons and spinal interneurons influencing motoneuronal pool excitability. This early corticospinal innervation provides the capacity for activity in the corticospinal system to be intimately involved in shaping the development of the motor cortex, spinal motor centres and their connectivity through the corticospinal tract (Basu et al., 2010; Eyre, 2004, 2005, 2007; Eyre et al., 2000a, 2001), reflecting the uniquely dominant role of the corticomotoneuronal system in human movement control.

# Shaping of the efferent axonal projection from the neocortex

In maturity, cortical neurons projecting to specific subcortical targets are restricted to specialized areas of the neocortex. Thus, corticospinal neurons are largely limited to the primary sensorimotor cortex, whilst corticotectal neurons projecting to the superior colliculus are found primarily in the visual cortex. However, studies in sub-primate mammals reveal that neurons with subcortical projections initially project non-specifically to all subcortical target areas via axonal collateral branches. The mature, focused pattern is subsequently achieved by a selective pattern of withdrawal of the axonal collateral branches of neurons within each specialized projection area of the cerebral cortex (O'Leary and Koester, 1993; O'Leary and Stanfield, 1985; Stanfield et al., 1982).

This process is activity dependent, since rat pups exposed to the NMDA receptor antagonist MK-801 during the period of axonal refinement maintain a significantly increased corticospinal projection, which includes aberrant corticospinal projections from the occipital cortices (O'Donoghue et al., 1993). Thyroid hormone may also have a role in axonal withdrawal since pre- and postnatally hypothyroid rats also maintain inappropriate corticospinal projections from the occipital cortex (Li et al., 1995). Furthermore, if a portion of fetal rat occipital cortex is transplanted to the frontal region in newborn hosts, neurons in the transplant will maintain a corticospinal projection but withdraw their corticotectal projection. Conversely, fetal frontal cortex transplanted to the occipital region will withdraw corticospinal projections whilst maintaining projections to the

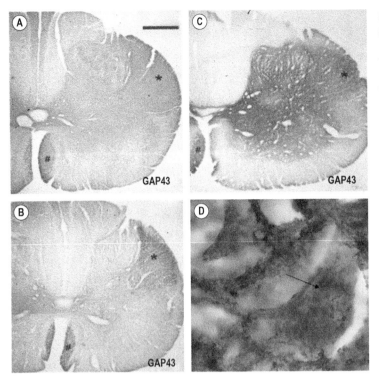

**Figure 2.2** • Horizontal sections of human spinal cord $C_{5-6}$. **(A)** 24 weeks PCA. GAP43 immunoreactivity is widespread in white and grey matter. **(B)** 27 weeks PCA. Corticospinal tracts are the only major axon tracts expressing GAP43 from which weaker immunoreactivity extends into the intermediate grey matter. **(C)** 31 weeks PCA. Immunoreactivity is also now intense in the intermediate grey matter and present in motoneuronal pools and dorsal horn. **(D)** 35 weeks PCA. Section counterstained with cresyl violet. #, Nissl-stained motoneuronal cell body; arrow, GAP43 expressing varicose axons. Motoneuron cell bodies are closely apposed by GAP43 immunoreactive varicose axons. (A–C), Scale bar, 500 μm. Stars mark the lateral and the anterior corticospinal tracts. (D) Scale bar, 20 μm. (Please refer to colour plate section). [From Eyre J, Miller S, Clowry G, Conway E, Watts C. Functional corticospinal projections are established prenatally in the human foetus permitting involvement in the development of spinal motor centres. Brain 2000;123:51–64, reprinted by permission of Oxford University Press.]

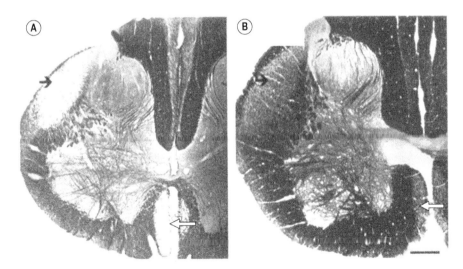

**Figure 2.3** • Onset of myelination of the human corticospinal tract in the lower cervical spinal cord. Sections of human spinal cord, level $C_{5,6}$. **(A)** 24 weeks PCA and **(B)** 40 weeks PCA stained for myelin. The black arrows mark the lateral corticospinal tract and the white arrows, the anterior corticospinal tract, both of which stand out clearly because of their lack of myelination relative to most other white matter tracts. From our studies of GAP43 immunoreactivity (Fig. 2.2), we know that corticospinal axons are present at 24 weeks PCA and it appears at this age that only occasional fibres within the tract may be myelinated. By birth, myelination is clearly underway although far from complete. [Reprinted from Eyre JA, Miller S, Clowry GJ. The development of the corticospinal tract in humans. In: Pascual-Leone A, Davey G, Rothwell J, Wasserman EM, editors. Handbook of Transcranial Magnetic Stimulation. London: Arnold, 2002, p. 235–49, with permission of Hodder UK Ltd.]

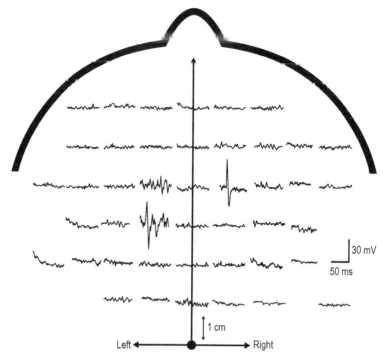

**Figure 2.4** • Mapping of the origin of responses evoked in right biceps brachii using transcranial magnetic stimulation (TMS) and a focal figure-of-eight coil. The coil was positioned using a 1 cm x 1 cm latex grid placed on the scalp. The subject was 3 weeks old. The filled circle marks the vertex. The electromyography traces are recorded in right biceps brachii. TMS was applied at the beginning of each trace. Responses were obtained in right biceps brachii following stimulation of both the ipsilateral and contralateral cortex.

tectum (O'Leary and Koester, 1993). Finally, occipital projections to the spinal cord persist in the newborn rat if a fetal tectum is transplanted to the spinal cord at birth and at the same time the host tectum is removed (Sharkey et al., 1986).

In longitudinal and cross-sectional studies of normal babies and children, neurophysiological findings are consistent with significant withdrawal of corticospinal axons occurring over the first 24 postnatal months (Basu et al., 2010; Eyre, 2007; Eyre et al., 2001, 2007). Axonal withdrawal has also been observed directly in studies of developing sub-human primates (Galea and Darian-Smith, 1995). We have demonstrated significant bilateral innervation of spinal motoneuronal pools from each motor cortex in neonates. Thus, focal transcranial magnetic stimulation (TMS) of the motor cortex evokes responses in ipsilateral and contralateral muscles that have similar thresholds and amplitudes but shorter onset latencies ipsilaterally, consistent with the shorter ipsilateral pathway length (Eyre et al., 2001, 2007) (Figs 2.4 and 2.5).

Rapid differential development of the ipsilateral and contralateral projections was observed so that the responses evoked at 2 years postnatal age in ipsilateral muscles are less frequent, significantly smaller, and have longer onset latencies and had higher thresholds than responses in contralateral muscles (Fig. 2.5). This differential development of the ipsilateral responses is consistent with a greater withdrawal of ipsilateral corticospinal projections than contralateral, as has been observed during development of the corticospinal tract in animals (Joosten et al., 1992; O'Leary et al., 1992). The small and late ipsilateral responses observed in older children and adults are consistent with the persistence of a small ipsilateral corticospinal projection, with slower conducting axons than contralateral projections. This conclusion is supported by anatomical studies in man and monkeys that demonstrate in maturity the corticospinal tract has approximately 8–15% of uncrossed axons (Armand et al., 1997; Galea and Darian-Smith, 1994; Nathan et al., 1990). These

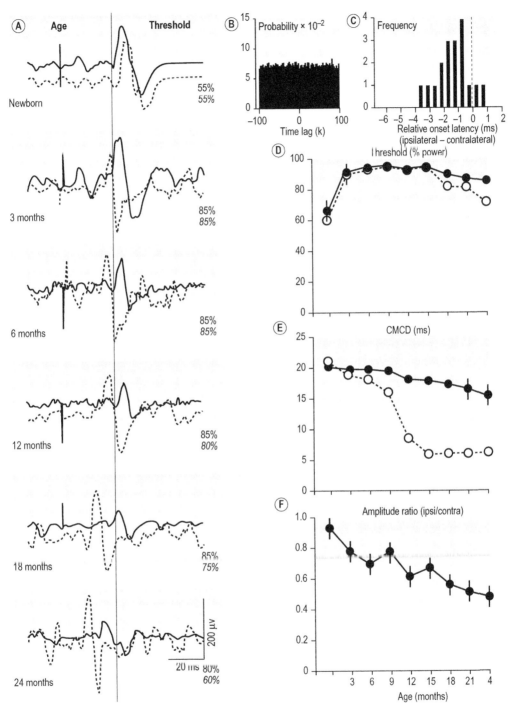

**Figure 2.5 • (A)** Serial ipsilateral and contralateral responses recorded in the electromyography (EMG) of biceps following transcranial magnetic stimulation (TMS) of the left cortex in the same normal subject at increasing ages. The continuous line traces are from ipsilateral (left) biceps and dashed line traces are from contralateral (right) biceps. The stimulus artefact marks the application of TMS. The vertical line indicates the onset of the ipsilateral response when the subject was newborn. Thresholds for the responses are recorded on the right above the traces. Those in italics are for contralateral responses. **(B)** Cross-correlogram of multi-unit EMGs from contracting right and left biceps in

◀ the same newborn subject illustrated in (A) demonstrating no evidence for common drive to the motoneuronal pools. **(C)** The relative onset latencies for the ipsilateral and contralateral responses in the 18 neonates studied, calculated by subtracting the onset of the ipsilateral response from that of the contralateral. These data demonstrate the significantly shorter onset latency of ipsilateral responses in the newborn period. **(D–F)** Longitudinal data from nine subjects, including the subject illustrated in (A) studied at three-monthly intervals. Filled symbols and continuous lines represent data from ipsilateral and open symbols and dashed lines from contralateral responses. The symbols represent the mean and the vertical lines the 95% confidence limits for mean. Threshold was measured as the per cent of maximum stimulator output. CMCD is the central conduction delay within the corticospinal tract. The amplitude ratio was calculated by dividing the peak-to-peak amplitude of the ipsilateral responses by that of the contralateral. The horizontal dashed line in (D) indicates a ratio of one where responses are of equal size. These data demonstrate differential development of ipsilateral and contralateral responses evoked by TMS so that by 15 months ipsilateral responses have significantly higher thresholds, longer CMCDs and smaller amplitudes compared to contralateral responses. [From Eyre J, Taylor J, Villagra F, Smith M, Miller S. Evidence of activity-dependent withdrawal of corticospinal projections during human development. Neurology 2001;57:1543–1554, with permission of Wolters Kluwer Health.]

ipsilaterally projecting axons have been shown in man and in sub-human primates to arise from similar areas of the cortex as the contralaterally projecting axons and to have a significant overlap in their areas of termination with the contralateral corticospinal projection from the other hemisphere both within spinal grey matter and motoneuronal pools (Galea and Darian-Smith, 1994; Lacroix et al., 2004; Liu and Chambers, 1964; Nathan et al., 1990).

Studies in animals reveal that, early in development, corticospinal axons initially occupy a larger terminal field within spinal grey matter and contact more spinal neurons than in the adult (Curfs et al., 1994; Martin et al., 1999). The elimination of the supernumerary synapses and refinement of the area of termination occurs during a process of axonal withdrawal in conjunction with the proliferation of synapses from the subset of axons that are maintained (Li and Martin, 2001, 2002).

In this way specificity in corticospinal connectivity is a dynamic process involving withdrawal of inappropriate connections and reinforcement and extension of appropriate connections, occurring at both the motor cortex and its subcortical projection sites including the spinal cord.

## Development of spinal reflexes

Many diverse studies in animals and in man establish that spinal cord development during a critical period early in development is also shaped by activity in descending motor pathways including the corticospinal tract (Wolpaw and Tennissen, 2001). Spinally mediated muscle stretch reflexes

and flexion withdrawal reflexes, which are poorly focused in the newborn, become precisely and appropriately focused during early life (Levinsson et al., 1999; McDonough et al., 2001; O'Sullivan, 1991; Seebach and Ziskind-Conhaim, 1994). Motoneuronal cell soma size, dendritic morphology and the pattern of synaptic input have been shown to be altered by activity deprivation during critical periods in early development (Commissiong and Sauve, 1993; Dekkers and Navarrete, 1998; Gibson et al., 2000; Inglis et al., 2000; Kalb, 1994; Kalb and Hockfield, 1992; McCouch et al., 1968; O'Hanlon and Lowrie, 1993, 1995). Crucial to the understanding of the sensorimotor deficits observed in cerebral palsy is the observation that perinatal lesions of the corticospinal tract leads also to abnormal development of spinal reflexes, evolving over months and years. This includes persistence of low threshold responses and excitatory connections to antagonist muscle groups, that do not emerge following adult stroke, even though survivors also suffer from spasticity (Gibson et al., 2000; Leonard et al., 1991; Levinsson et al., 1999; Myklebust et al., 1982; O'Sullivan et al., 1991, 1998; Wolpaw and Tennissen, 2001).

## Corticospinal system reorganization in man

There are now repeated observations in man that demonstrate substantial reorganization of the motor cortex and corticospinal projections following prenatal or perinatal lesions to the corticospinal system (Balbi et al., 2000; Basu et al., 2010; Benecke et al., 1991; Cao et al., 1994; Carr et al., 1993; Chu et al., 2000; Eyre et al., 2000b,

2001, 2007; Graveline et al., 1998; Hertz-Pannier, 1999; Holloway et al., 1999; Lewine et al., 1994; Maegaki et al., 1995; Muller et al., 1997, 1998; Nirkko et al., 1997; Staudt et al., 2004; Thickbroom et al., 2001; Wieser et al., 1999). In children and adults who have suffered unilateral injury to one corticospinal system early in development, significant bilateral corticospinal innervation of spinal motoneuronal pools persists from the undamaged hemisphere (Eyre et al., 2007). Thus focal TMS of the intact motor cortex evokes large responses in ipsilateral and contralateral muscles, which have similar latencies and thresholds (Fig. 2.6). These observations have been made following perinatal unilateral brain damage arising from a variety of pathologies including infarction, dysplasia, and arteriovenous malformations (Balbi et al., 2000; Basu et al., 2010; Benecke et al., 1991; Carr et al., 1993; Eyre et al., 2000b, 2001, 2007; Maegaki et al., 1995; Thickbroom et al., 2001). Short latency ipsilateral responses do not occur in normal subjects outside the perinatal period, nor do they occur in subjects who acquired unilateral cortical lesions in adulthood, establishing that fast ipsilateral responses are not simply unmasked by unilateral lesions (Eyre et al., 2001, 2007; Netz et al., 1997) (Fig. 2.6).

In both cross-sectional and longitudinal studies of children who have suffered perinatal brain damage, different patterns of corticospinal system development are observed after unilateral and bilateral lesions to the corticospinal tract (Basu et al., 2010; Eyre et al., 1989, 2000b; 2001, 2007) (Fig. 2.7). Following perinatal stroke, babies with contralateral motor evoked potentials (MEPs) evoked by TMS of the infarcted hemisphere immediately after the stroke, indicative of sparing of a critical residual of the corticospinal projection, subsequently lost these responses (Eyre et al., 2007) (Fig. 2.7B [unilateral infarct]). Progressive loss of responses from the infarcted hemisphere was associated with the rapid development in parallel of the contralateral and ipsilateral corticospinal projections from the undamaged hemisphere such that both had abnormally short onset latencies by 24 months of age (Fig.2.7B,D). In contrast, longitudinal study of subjects with extensive bilateral perinatal lesions of the motor cortex or subcortical white matter revealed an essentially normal pattern of development of the corticospinal projection with maintenance of a fast conducting contralateral and a slower conducting ipsilateral corticospinal projection from both hemispheres (Basu et al., 2010; Eyre et al., 2001, 2007) (Fig. 2.7B,D). The persistence of corticospinal projections in subjects with bilateral lesions establishes that reduction in or abnormality of the pattern of activity alone cannot explain the postnatal loss of corticospinal projections from the damaged cortex in subjects with unilateral perinatal lesions; rather, activity-dependent competition for spinal synaptic space during development between the overlapping less active contralateral corticospinal projection from the infarcted hemisphere and the more active ipsilateral from the other provides an explanation for these apparently contradictory results. This explanation is supported by significant hypertrophy of the corticospinal tract arising from the non-infarcted hemisphere. The hypertrophy has been observed not only indirectly from MRI measurements (Basu et al., 2010) (Figure 2.7A), but also directly from post-mortem material where the hypertrophy has been shown to be associated with significantly increased numbers of corticospinal axons projecting from the non-infarcted hemisphere (Scales and Collins, 1972; Verhaart, 1947, 1950).

Direct confirmation that such competition is likely to occur is provided by a series of studies by Martin (2005) in the cat. When the activity of neurons in one sensorimotor cortex is inhibited during development, it fails to maintain contralateral terminations in the spinal cord and its spinal synaptic space is taken over by increased ipsilateral axonal terminations from the normally active hemisphere (Martin and Lee, 1999). Confirmation that this process arises from activity-dependent competitive interaction between ipsilateral and contralaterally projecting axons from opposite hemispheres is provided by the observation that when both sensorimotor cortices are inhibited, a near-normal size and pattern of ipsilateral and contralateral terminations is maintained from both (Martin et al., 1999). Furthermore, unilateral electrical stimulation of the corticospinal tract during development leads to increased retention of ipsilateral terminations from the stimulated hemisphere, in a reciprocal manner with the pattern of loss of contralateral terminations from the non-stimulated side (Salimi and Martin, 2004).

In adults the findings of TMS within a week of a stroke are predictive of motor outcome, and demonstrate that motor recovery occurs only

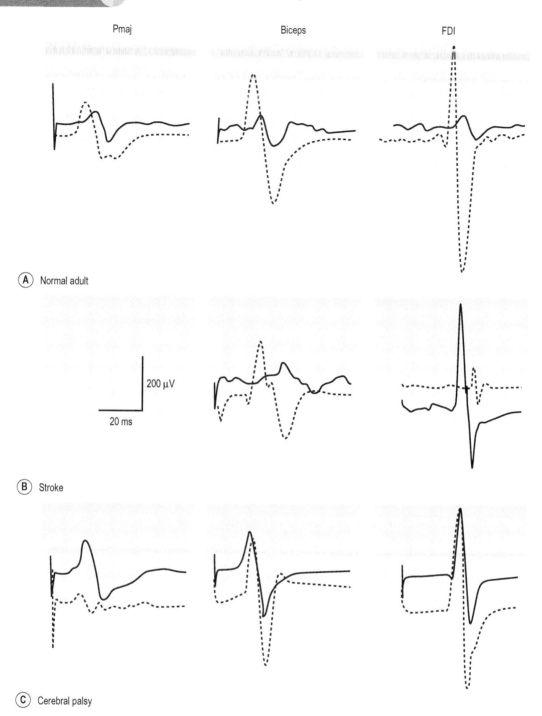

**Figure 2.6** ● Ipsilateral and contralateral responses recorded in the EMG of pectoralis major (Pmaj), biceps brachii (Biceps) and the first dorsal interosseus muscle (FDI) following TMS of **(A)** the left hemisphere in a normal adult and **(B)** the intact hemisphere in a subject with stroke that occurred in adulthood, and **(C)** a subject with hemiplegic cerebral palsy. The continuous traces in (A–C) are from ipsilateral muscles and dashed traces are from contralateral muscles. TMS was delivered at the onset of each trace. [From Eyre J, Taylor J, Villagra F, Smith M, Miller S. Evidence of activity-dependent withdrawal of corticospinal projections during human development. Neurology 2001;57:1543-1554, with permission of Wolters Kluwer Health.]

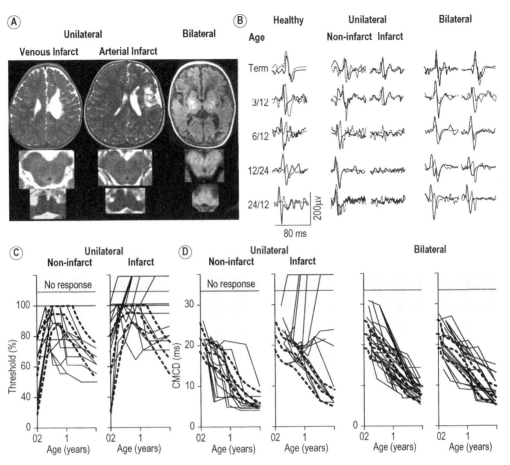

**Figure 2.7 • (A)** Axial magnetic resonance scans of subjects in the longitudinal study when aged 2 years showing sections at the level of the cortex (upper), cerebral peduncle (middle) and pyramid (lower): (unilateral venous infarct) left-sided venous infarction following perinatal intraventricular hemorrhage; (unilateral arterial infarct) left-sided perinatal middle cerebral artery infarct; (bilateral) extensive bilateral cortical and subcortical infarcts following birth asphyxia. **(B–D)** Development of corticospinal projections from each hemisphere. MEPs evoked in biceps following TMS of the cortex at term, 3, 6, 12 and 24 months. Black traces, EMG recorded from contralateral biceps; red traces, EMG recorded from ipsilateral biceps. (normal) TMS of the left hemisphere of a normal subject. (unilateral) TMS of the non infarcted hemisphere and the infarcted hemisphere of the subject with perinatal left hemisphere middle cerebral artery infarction illustrated in A. (bilateral) TMS of the right and left hemispheres, respectively, of the subject with bilateral cortical and subcortical infarctions illustrated in A. (C) The thresholds and (D unilateral) the CMCDs of MEPs evoked in contralateral biceps following TMS of the non-infarcted and infarcted hemispheres, respectively, in the 14 subjects followed longitudinally after unilateral perinatal stroke. (D bilateral) The CMCD of MEPs evoked in contralateral biceps following TMS of the right and left hemispheres, respectively, in the 25 subjects with bilateral lesions. Hashed lines indicate the mean and ±2 standard deviations for normal subjects. Solid lines join the results for individual subjects. No response indicates failure to evoke MEPs. [From Eyre J, Smith M, Dabydeen L, Clowry G, Petacchi E, Battini R, et al. Is hemiplegic cerebral palsy equivalent to amblyopia of the corticospinal system? Ann Neurol. 2007;62:493–503, with permission from John Wiley and Sons.]

when a critical residue of corticospinal system function has been spared by the stroke (Hendricks et al., 2002, 2003). The findings of TMS soon after perinatal stroke are not predictive, since sparing of a critical residue of corticospinal tract could equally be associated with good and poor motor outcomes (Eyre et al., 2007). However, persistence of corticospinal projections from the infarcted hemisphere at two years was associated with a good outcome in a manner similar to that observed in adults immediately after stroke at 24 months. Loss of corticospinal projections from the infarcted cortex and maintenance of fast ipsilateral projections from the non-infarcted hemisphere was strongly associated with a poor outcome (Eyre et al., 2007). These findings imply that the degree of motor impairment suffered after perinatal stroke depends not only on the extent of the acute loss of corticospinal projections from the initial insult but also on the degree to which the surviving corticospinal projections are later displaced. The consequences of a progressively diminishing corticospinal projection from the infarcted hemisphere over the first 18 months after birth would explain why the signs of hemiplegia are often not established until well into the second year of life and also the loss of previously acquired motor skills observed in some children (Bouza et al., 1994; Eyre et al., 2007). It appears counterintuitive that activity-driven maintenance of ipsilateral projections from the non-infarcted hemisphere is not associated with preservation of function. However, Martin and his colleagues similarly observed that cats who had unilateral sensorimotor cortex inhibition during development failed to develop skilled distal movements of the upper limb contralateral to the inhibited cortex, despite the terminations lost from the inhibited cortex being replaced by a similar number of terminations from the ipsilateral sensorimotor cortex (Martin, 2005).

A possible explanation of these findings lies in two observations in older children and adults who suffered unilateral perinatal brain lesions. First, the afferent sensory projection from the paretic arm does not show similar postnatal reorganization but always remains directed to the contralateral infarcted hemisphere (Thickbroom et al., 2001). Second, fast ipsilateral projections from the non-infarcted hemisphere may be associated with preserved hand and arm function but only if the lesion arises from a cortical malformation or occurs early in intrauterine development (Staudt et al., 2004). These two observations suggest that where the corticospinal reorganization occurs very early in development, the abnormal ipsilateral projections can establish appropriate linkage with the cortical and subcortical networks required for effective arm and hand control. However, where the reorganization occurs relatively late in development, the abnormal ipsilateral projections cannot access these networks, which are essential for space perception, the planning of movements and the guidance of actions (Culham and Valyear, 2006).

## Motor cortex reorganization

The visual cortex of those who are congenitally blind processes tactile and auditory sensations (Sadato, 2006), one of many observations revealing the potential for flexible, cross-modal plasticity within the cerebral cortex during development (Pallas, 2001). A young child (LJ) who suffered a presumed prenatal middle cerebral artery infarction provides the first evidence that plasticity of the cerebral cortex extends beyond reorganization within sensory modalities to re-specification of function across the rostral (motor output)/caudal (sensory input) divide (Basu et al., 2010). LJ suffered a stroke during early development, infarcting the cerebral cortical territory that would normally develop into left motor cortex. A primary motor area subsequently developed within the left occipital 'visual' cortex. We hypothesize that infarction of the left optic radiations isolated the immature left occipital cortex from afferent visual information. Concurrently infarction of the left sensorimotor cortex resulted in loss of its projection to the spinal cord. Plasticity at spinal cord level subsequently led to retention of the synapses from the normally transient occipitiocortical projection (O'Leary and Stanfield, 1985; Stanfield et al., 1982) through mechanisms such as reduction in activity-dependent competition for synaptic space (Eyre et al., 2007) and compensatory homeostatic (Chandrasekaran et al., 2007) reinforcement of remaining excitatory input to $\alpha$-motoneurons. If we are correct, the subsequent transformation of visual cortex into primary motor cortex implies that retrograde signals from the spinal cord and other efferent targets of cortical neuronal networks have a role in defining cortical areal structure and function.

## Summary

The observations on the marked plasticity of the corticospinal system in the perinatal period throw new light on 'cerebral palsy', a term originally used by William Osler in 1889 (Osler, 1889) to highlight the significant consequences on motor development of lesions to the brain which occur in the perinatal period. It is likely that William Osler's seminal observations identify the perinatal period, not only because of the special vulnerability of the motor system to damage at this time but also because abnormality or imbalance in the activity in the corticospinal system during this critical perinatal period will secondarily disrupt development of the motor cortex, corticospinal projections and spinal motor centres.

Over 40 years ago, Wiesel and Hubel (1965) first described in kittens the progressive loss of responsiveness by the primary visual cortex to an eye deprived of vision, thereby providing the premier physiological model of activity-dependent plasticity. It is very likely that during development similar mechanisms and consequences also apply to corticospinal development. If this is the case, it raises the exciting possibility that activity-dependent mechanisms might be harnessed to mitigate the effects of perinatal lesions and to optimize development of the corticospinal system in a manner analogous to successful interventions now in routine clinical practice to optimize visual development in children with visual impairment (Wu and Hunter, 2006). Functional and anatomical evidence exists that spontaneous plasticity can be potentiated and shaped by activity. Early interventions and the use of appropriately targeted

enriched environments are likely to mitigate the effects of lesions. Other potential but more invasive interventions might include repetitive TMS to alter levels of excitability of the corticospinal system (Garvey et al., 2003; Heide et al., 2006; Quartarone et al., 2005), targeted pharmacological interventions (Martin and Lee, 1999; Martin et al., 1999), or deep brain stimulation to augment the activity of the affected corticospinal system (Carmel et al., 2010; Martin, 2012; Salimi and Martin, 2004).

Control of dexterity does not mature until late adolescence (Garvey et al., 2003) and this mirrors a protracted period of development of the corticospinal system: for example, corticospinal axonal diameter and excitability have been shown to increase until late adolescence (Fig. 2.8) (Eyre, 2005; Eyre et al., 1991, 2000a; Giorgio et al., 2010; Muller and Homberg, 1992); sensorimotor cortex synaptic density decreases markedly in adolescence and does not plateau until young adulthood (Dickstein et al., 2007; Huttenlocher, 1979; 1990; Huttenlocher and Dabholkar, 1997); intracortical inhibition is not mature until

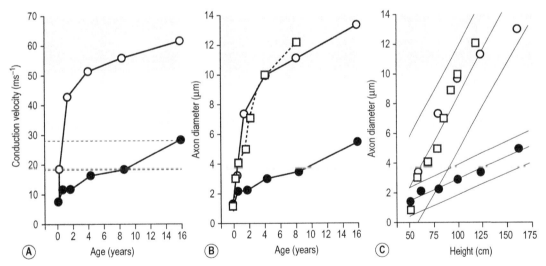

**Figure 2.8 • (A)** Development of corticospinal axon conduction velocities in (o) contralateral and (●) ipsilateral corticospinal projections in man. The conduction velocities are estimated from central motor conduction delays and estimates of the conduction distance within the corticospinal tract (see Eyre et al., 1991, 2000a). **(B, C)** The diameter of the largest corticospinal axons in human subjects in relation to age and mean body height, respectively. Open squares represent data obtained by direct measurement at the level of the pyramid in a newborn baby and in subjects aged 4, 8 and 18 months and 2, 3, 4 and 7 years, reported by Verhaart (1950) and in a subject aged 13 years reported by Häggqvist (1937). Open and closed circles represent the mean axonal diameters in the contralateral and ipsilateral corticospinal tract, respectively. The axonal diameters were estimated from the conduction velocities of the subjects in (A) using the ratio of 5.2 m/s/μm between the conduction velocity of corticospinal axons and their diameters in the medullary pyramid (Olivier et al., 1997).

adulthood (Mall et al., 2004; Walther et al., 2009); the morphological properties of α-motoneurons and their excitatory and inhibitory control only mature in adolescence (McDonough et al., 2001; O'Sullivan et al., 1991). The demonstration of activity-dependent development throughout the neuroaxis from the cerebral cortex to the spinal cord and the protracted time period of development of the corticospinal system will certainly provide a window of therapeutic opportunity.

# References

Altman, J., Bayer, S., 2001. Development of the Human Spinal Cord: An Interpretation Based on Experimental Studies in Animals. OUP, New York.

Armand, J., Olivier, E., Edgley, S.A., Lemon, R.N., 1996. The structure and function of the developing corticospinal tract. In: Wing, A.M., Haggard, P., Flanagan, J.R. (Eds.), The Neurophysiology and Psychology of Hand Movements. Academic Press, San Diego, pp. 125–145.

Armand, J., Olivier, E., Edgley, S.A., Lemon, R.N., 1997. Postnatal development of corticospinal projections from motor cortex to the cervical enlargement in the macaque monkey. J. Neurosci. 17, 251–266.

Balbi, P., Trojano, L., Ragno, M., Perretti, A., Santoro, L., 2000. Patterns of motor control reorganization in a patient with mirror movements. Clin. Neurophysiol. 111, 318–325.

Barth, T.M., Stanfield, B.B., 1990. The recovery of forelimb placing behaviour in rats with neonatal unilateral cortical damage involves the remaining hemisphere. J. Neurosci. 10, 3449–3459.

Basu, A., Graziadio, S., Smith, M., Clowry, G., Cioni, G., Eyre, J., 2010. Developmental plasticity connects visual cortex to motoneurons after stroke. Ann. Neurol. 67, 132–136.

Benecke, R., Meyer, B.U., Freund, H.J., 1991. Reorganisation of descending motor pathways in patients after hemispherectomy and severe hemispheric lesions demonstrated by magnetic brain stimulation. Exp. Brain. Res. 83, 419–426.

Bortoff, G., Strick, P., 1993. Corticospinal terminations in two new world primates: further evidence that corticomotoneuronal connections provide part of the neural substrate for mannual dexterity. J. Neurosci. 13, 5105–5118.

Bouza, H., Dubowitz, L., Rutherford, M., Pennock, J., 1994. Prediction of outcome in children with congenital hemiplegia: a magnetic resonance imaging study. Neuropediatrics 25, 60–66.

Brodal, A., 1973. Self observations and neuro-anatomocal considerations after stroke. Brain 96, 675–694.

Cao, Y., Vikingstad, E.M., Huttenlocher, P.R., Towle, V.L., Levin, D.N., 1994. Functional magnetic resonance studies of the reorganisation of human sensorimotor area after unilateral brain injury in the perinatal period. Proc. Natl. Acad. Sci. 91, 9612–9616.

Carmel, J., Berrol, L., Brus-Ramer, M., Martin, J.H., 2010. Chronic electrical stimulation of the intact corticospinal system after unilateral injury restores skilled locomotor control and promotes spinal axon outgrowth. J. Neurosci. 30, 10918–10926.

Carr, L., Harrison, L., Evans, A., Stephens, J., 1993. Patterns of central motor reorganisation in hemiplegic cerebral palsy. Brain 116, 1223 1247.

Chandrasekaran, A., Shah, R., Crair, M., 2007. Developmental homeostasis of mouse retinocollicular synapses. J. Neurosci. 27, 1746–1755.

Chu, D., Huttenlocher, P., Levin, D., Towle, V., 2000. Reorganization of the hand somatosensory cortex following perinatal unilateral brain injury. Neuropediatrics 31, 63–69.

Commissiong, J.W., Sauve, Y., 1993. Neurophysiological basis of functional recovery in the neonatal spinalised rat. Exp. Brain Res. 96, 473–479.

Culham, J., Valyear, K., 2006. Human parietal cortex in action. Curr. Opin. Neurobiol. 16, 205–212.

Curfs, M.H.J.M., Gribnan, A.A.M., Dederen, P.J.W.C., 1994. Selective elimination of transient corticospinal projections in the rat cervical spinal grey matter. Brain Res. Dev. Brain Res. 78, 182–190.

Dekkers, J., Navarrete, R., 1998. Persistence of somatic and dendritic growth associated processes and induction of dendritic sprouting in motoneurons with neonatal axonal injury in rats. Neuroreport 9, 1523–1527.

Dickstein, D., Kabaso, D., Rocher, A., Luebke, J., Wearne, S., Hof, P., 2007. Changes in the structural complexity of the aged brain. Aging Cell 6, 275–284.

Eyre, J., 2004. Developmental plasticity of the corticospinal system. In: Boniface, S., Ziemann, U. (Eds.), Plasticity of the Human Brain. Cambridge University Press, Cambridge.

Eyre, J., 2007. Corticospinal tract development and its plasticity after perinatal injury. Neurosci Biobehav Rev 31, 1136–1149.

Eyre, J., Gibson, M., Koh, T., Miller, S., 1989. Corticospinal transmission excited by electromagnetic stimulation of the brain is impaired in children with spastic hemiparesis but not those with quadriparesis. J. Physiol. (Lond) 414, 9P.

Eyre, J., Miller, S., Clowry, G., Conway, E., Watts, C., 2000a. Functional corticospinal projections are established prenatally in the human foetus permitting involvement in the development of spinal motor centres. Brain 123, 51–64.

Eyre, J., Taylor, J., Villagra, F., Miller, S., 2000b. Exuberant ipsilateral corticospinal projections are present in the human newborn and withdrawn during development probably involving an activity-dependent process. Dev. Med. Child Neurol. 82, 12.

Eyre, J., Taylor, J., Villagra, F., Smith, M., Miller, S., 2001. Evidence of activity-dependent withdrawal of corticospinal projections during human development. Neurology 57, 1543–1554.

Eyre, J., Smith, M., Dabydeen, L., Clowry, G., Petacchi, E., Battini, R., et al., 2007. Is hemiplegic cerebral palsy equivalent to amblyopia of the corticospinal system? Ann. Neurol. 62, 493–503.

Eyre, J.A., 2005. Developmental aspects of corticospinal projections. In: Eisen, A. (Ed.), Motor Neuron Diseases. Elsevier, Amsterdam, pp. 27–56.

Eyre, J.A., Miller, S., Ramesh, V., 1991. Constancy of central conduction delays during development in man: investigation of motor and somatosensory pathways. J. Physiol. (Lond) 434, 441–452.

Eyre, J.A., Miller, S., Clowry, G.J., 2002. The development of the corticospinal tract in humans. In: Pascual-Leone, A., Davey, G., Rothwell, J., Wasserman, E.M. (Eds.), Handbook of Transcranial Magnetic Stimulation. Arnold, London, pp. 235–249.

Forssberg, H., Eliasson, A., Kinoshita, H., Johansson, R., Westling, G., 1991. Development of human precision grip. I: basic coordination of force. Exp. Brain. Res. 85, 451–457.

Galea, M., Darian-Smith, I., 1994. Multiple corticospinal neuron populations in the macaque monkey are specified by their unique cortical origins, spinal terminations, and connections. Cerebral Cortex 4, 166–194.

Galea, M.P., Darian-Smith, I., 1995. Postnatal maturation of the direct corticospinal projections in the macaque monkey. Cerebral Cortex 5, 518–540.

Galea, M.P., Darian-Smith, I., 1997. Corticospinal projection patterns following unilateral section of the cervical spinal cord in the newborn and juvenile macaque monkey. J Comp. Neurol. 381, 282–306.

Garvey, M., Ziemann, U., Bartko, J., Denckla, M., Barker, C., Wassermann, E., 2003. Cortical correlates of neuromotor development in healthy children. Clin. Neurophysiol. 114, 162–1670.

Gibson, C., Arnott, G., Clowry, G., 2000. Plasticity in the rat spinal cord seen in response to lesions to the

motor cortex during development but not to lesions in maturity. Exp. Neurol. 166, 422–434.

Giorgio, A., Watkins, K., Chadwick, M., James, S., Winmill, L., Douaud, G., et al., 2010. Longitudinal changes in grey and white matter during adolescence. NeuroImage 49, 94–103.

Graveline, C., Mikulis, D., Crawley, A., Hwang, P., 1998. Regionalized sensorimotor plasticity after hemispherectomy fMRI evaluation. Ped. Neurol. 19, 337–342.

Häggqvist, G., 1937. Faseranalytische studien uber die pyramidenbahn. Acta Psych. Neurol. 12, 457–466.

Heffner, R., Masterton, R., 1983. The role of the corticospinal tract in the evolution of human digital dexterity. Brain Behav. Evol. 23, 165–183.

Heide, G., Witte, O., Ziemann, U., 2006. Physiology of modulation of motor cortex excitability by low-frequency suprathreshold repetitive transcranial magnetic stimulation. Exp. Brain Res. 171, 26–34.

Hendricks, H., Zwarts, M., Plat, E., van Limbeek, J., 2002. Systematic review for the early prediction of motor and functional outcome after stroke by using motor-evoked potentials. Arch. Phys. Med. Rehabil. 83, 1303–1308.

Hendricks, H., Pasman, J., van Limbeek, J., Zwarts, M., 2003. Motor evoked potentials in predicting recovery from upper extremity paralysis after acute stroke. Cerebrovasc. Dis. 16, 265–271.

Hertz-Pannier, L., 1999. Plasticite au cours de la maturation cerebrale: bases physogiques et etude par IRM fontinelle. J. Neuroradiol. 26, IS66–IS74.

Hicks, S., D'Amato, C., 1970. Motor-sensory and visual behaviour after hemispherectomy in newborn and mature rats. Exp. Neurol. 29, 416–438.

Hicks, S., D'Amato, C., 1977. Locating corticospinal neurons by retrograde axonal transport of horseradish peroxidase. Exp. Neurol. 56, 410–420.

Holloway, V., Chong, W., Connelly, A., Harkness, W., Gadian, D., 1999. Somatomotor fMRI and the presurgical evaluation of a case of focal epilepsy. Clin. Radiol. 54, 301–303.

Humphrey, T., 1960. The development of the pyramidal tracts in human fetuses, correlated with cortical differentiation. In: Tower, D.B., Schade, J.B. (Eds.), Structure and Function of the Cortex Proceedings of the Second International Meeting of Neurobiologists. Elsevier, Amsterdam, pp. 93–103.

Huttenlocher, P., 1979. Synaptic density in the human frontal cortex—developmental changes and effects of aging. Brain Res. 163, 195–205.

Huttenlocher, P., 1990. Morphometric study of human cerebral cortex development 28, 517–527.

Huttenlocher, P., Dabholkar, A., 1997. Regional differences in synaptogenesis in human cerebral cortex. J. Comp. Neurol. 387, 167–178.

Huttenlocher, P.R., Raichelson, R.M., 1989. Effects of neonatal hemispherectomy on location and number of corticospinal neurons in the rat. Brain Res. Dev. Brain Res. 47, 59–69.

Inglis, F., Zuckerman, K., Kalb, R., 2000. Experience-dependent development of spinal motor neurons. Neuron 299–305. 2000.

Jansen, E.M., Low, W.C., 1996. Quantitative analysis of contralateral hemisphere hypertrophy and sensorimotor performance in adult rats following unilateral neonatal ischemic-hypoxic brain injury. Brain Res. 708, 93–99.

Joosten, E., Schuitman, R., Vermelis, M., Dederen, P., 1992. Postnatal development of the ipsilateral corticospinal component in rat spinal cord: a light and electron microscopic anterograde HRP study. J. Comp. Neurol. 326, 133–146.

Kalb, R., 1994. Regulation of motoneuron dendrite growth by NMDA receptor activation. Development 120, 3063–3071.

Kalb, R., Hockfield, S., 1992. Activity-dependent development of spinal motor neurons. Brain Res. Brain Res. Rev. 17, 283–289.

Kartje-Tillotson, G., Neafsey, E.J., Castro, A.J., 1985. Electrophysiological analysis of motor cortical plasticity after cortical lesions in newborn rats. Brain Res. 332, 103–111.

Kartje-Tillotson, G., O'Donoghue, D.L., Dauzvardis, M.F., Castro, A.J., 1987. Pyramidotomy abolishes the abnormal movements evoked by intracortical microstimulation in adult rats that sustained neonatal cortical lesions. Brain Res. 415, 172–177.

Kennard, M., 1936. Age and other factors in motor recovery for precentral lesions in monkeys. Am. J. Physiol. 115, 138–146.

Kuypers, H.G.J.M., 1962. Corticospinal connections: postnatal development in the rhesus monkey. Science 138, 678–680.

Kuypers, H., 1981. Anatomy of the descending pathways. In: Brookhart, J., Mountcastle, V. (Eds.), Handbook of Physiology—The Nervous System II. American Physiological Society, Bethesda, MD.

LaMantia, A.S., Rakic, P., 1990. Axonal overproduction and elimination in the corpus callosum of the developing rhesus monkey. J. Neurosci. 10, 2156–2175.

LaMantia, A.S., Rakic, P., 1994. Axon overproduction and elimination in the anterior commissure of the developing rhesus monkey. J. Comp. Neurol. 340, 328–336.

Lacroix, S., Havton, L., McKay, H., Yang, H., Brant, A., Roberts, J., et al., 2004. Bilateral corticospinal projections arise from each motor cortex in the macaque monkey: a quantitative study. J. Comp. Neurol. 473, 147–161.

Lawrence, D., Hopkins, D., 1976. The development of motor control in the rhesus monkey: evidence concerning the role of corticomotoneuronal connections. Brain 99, 235–254.

Leonard, C.T., Hirschfeld, H., Moritani, T., 1991. Myotactic reflex development in normal children and children with cerebral palsy. Exp. Neurol. 111, 379–382.

Leong, S.K., 1976. A qualitative electron microscopic investigation of the anomalous corticofugal projections following neonatal lesions in the albino rat. Brain Res. 107, 1–8.

Levinsson, A., Luo, X.-L., Holmberg, H., Schouenborg, J., 1999. Developmental tuning in a spinal nociceptive system: effects of neonatal spinalisation. J. Neurosci. 19, 10397–10403.

Lewine, J.D., Astur, R.S., Davis, L.E., Knight, J.E., Maclin, E.L., Orrison, W.W., 1994. Cortical organization in

adulthood is modified by neonatal infarct: a case study. Radiology 190, 93–96.

Li, C., Olavarria, J., Greger, B., 1995. Occipital cortico-pyramidal projection in hypothyroid rats. Brain Res. Dev. Brain Res. 89, 227–234.

Li, Q., Martin, J., 2001. Postnatal development of corticospinal axon terminal morphology in the cat. J. Comp. Neurol. 435, 127–141.

Li, Q., Martin, J., 2002. Postnatal development of connectional specificity of corticospinal terminals in the cat. J. Comp. Neurol. 447, 57–71.

Liu, C., Chambers, W., 1964. An experimental study of the cortico-spinal system in the monkey. The spinal pathways and preterminal distribution of degenerating fibres following discrete lesions of the pre- and postcentral gyri and bulbar pyramid. J. Comp. Neurol. 123, 257–284.

Maegaki, Y., Yamamoto, T., Takeshita, K., 1995. Plasticity of central motor and sensory pathways in a case of unilateral extensive cortical dysplasia. Investigation of magnetic resonance imaging, transcranial magnetic stimulation and short latency somatosensory evoked potentials. Neurology 45, 2255–2261.

Mall, V., Berweck, S., Fietzek, U., Glocker, F., Oberhuber, U., Walther, M., et al., 2004. Low level of intracortical inhibition in children shown by transcranial magnetic stimulation. Neuropediatrics 35, 120–125.

Martin, J., 2005. The corticospinal system: from development to motor control. Neuroscientist 11, 161–173.

Martin, J., 2012. Systems neurobiology of restorative neurology and future directions for repair of the damaged motor systems. Clin. Neurol. Neurosurg. 114, 515–523.

Martin, J.H., Lee, S.J., 1999. Activity-dependent competition between developing corticospinal terminations. Neuroreport 10, 2277–2282.

Martin, J.H., Kably, B., Hacking, A., 1999. Activity-dependent development of cortical axon terminations in the spinal cord and brain stem. Exp. Brain. Res. 125, 184–199.

Martins, I., Lauterbach, M., Luís, H., Amaral, H., Rosenbaum, G., Slade, P., et al., 2012. Neurological soft signs and cognitive development: a study in late childhood and adolescence. Child Neuropsychol. (Jun 14 [Epub ahead of print]).

McClung, J.R., Castro, A.J., 1975. An ultrastructural study of ipsilateral corticospinal projections after frontal cortical lesions in newborn rats. Anat. Rec. 181, 417–418.

McCouch, G.P., Austin, G.M., Liu, C.Y., 1968. Sprouting as a cause of spasticity. J. Neurophysiol. 21, 205–216.

McDonough, S., Clowry, G., Miller, S., Eyre, J., 2001. Reciprocal and Renshaw (recurrent) inhibition are functional in man at birth. Brain Res. 899, 66–81.

Muetzel, R., Collins, P., Mueller, B., Schissel, A., Lim, K., Luciana, M., 2008. The development of corpus callosum microstructure and associations with bimanual task performance in healthy adolescents. NeuroImage 39, 1918–1925.

Muller, K., Homberg, V., 1992. Development of speed repetitive movements in children is determined by structural changes in corticospinal afferents. Neurosci. Lett. 144, 57–60.

Muller, R.A., Rothermel, R.D., Behen, M.E., Muzik, O., Chakraborty, P.K., Chugani, H.T., 1997. Plasticity of motor organization in children and adults. Neuroreport 8, 3103–3108.

Muller, R.A., Watson, C.E., Muzik, O., Chakraborty, P.K., Chugani, H.T., 1998. Motor organization after early middle cerebral artery stroke: a PET study. Pediatr Neurol 19, 294–298.

Myklebust, B., Gottlieb, G., Penn, R., Agarwal, G., 1982. Reciprocal excitation of antagonist muscles as a differentiating feature in spasticity. Ann. Neurol. 12, 367–374.

Nathan, P., Smith, M., Deacon, P.V., 1990. The corticospinal tracts in man. Course and location of fibres at different segmental levels. Brain 113, 303–324.

Nelson, K., Ellenberg, J., 1979. Neonatal signs as predictors of cerebral palsy. Pediatrics 64, 225–232.

Netz, J., Lammers, T., Hömberg, V., 1997. Reorganization of motor output in the non-affected hemisphere after stroke. Brain 120, 1579–1586.

Nirkko, A.C., Rosler, K.M., Ozdoba, C., Heid, O., Schroth, G., Hess, C.W., 1997. Human cortical plasticity. Functional recovery with mirror movements. Neurology 48, 1090–1093.

O'Donoghue, D., Poff, C., Block, J., 1993. Chronic neonatal N-methyl-D-aspartate receptor antagonism with MK-801 increases the number of corticospinal cells retained into adulthood in the rat. Neurosci. Lett. 158, 143–146.

O'Hanlon, G., Lowrie, M., 1995. Nerve injury in rats causes abnormalities in motoneuron dendritic fields that differ from those that follow neonatal nerve injury. Exp. Brain Res. 103, 243–250.

O'Hanlon, G.M., Lowrie, M.B., 1993. Neonatal nerve injury causes long-term changes in growth and distribution of motoneuron dendrites in the rat. Neuroscience 56, 453–464.

O'Leary, D., Koester, S., 1993. Development of projection neuron types, axon pathways, and patterned connections of the mammalian cortex. Neuron 10, 991–1006.

O'Leary, D., Stanfield, B., 1985. Occipital cortical neurons with transient pyramidal tract axons extend and maintain collaterals to subcortical but not intracortical targets. Brain Res. 336, 326–333.

O'Leary, D., Schlaggar, B., Stanfield, B., 1992. The specification of sensory cortex: lessons from cortical transplantation. Exp. Neurol. 115, 121–126.

O'Rahily, R., Müller, F., 1994. The Human Embryonic Brain: an Atlas of Developmental Stages. Wiley-Liss, New York.

O'Sullivan, M., 1991. The development of the phasic stretch reflex in man and its pathophysiology in central motor disorders. PhD thesis, Newcastle University.

O'Sullivan, M., Eyre, J., Miller, S., 1991. Radiation of the phasic stretch reflex in biceps brachii to muscles of the arm in man and its restriction during development. J. Physiol. (Lond) 439, 529–543.

O'Sullivan, M.C., Miller, S., Ramesh, V., Conway, E., Gilfillan, K., McDonough, S., et al., 1998.

Abnormal development of biceps brachii phasic stretch reflex and persistence of short latency heteronymous excitatory responses to triceps brachii in spastic cerebral palsy. Brain 121, 2381–2395.

Olivier, E., Edgley, S., Armand, J., Lemon, R., 1997. An electrophysiological study of the postnatal development of the corticospinal system in the macaque monkey. J. Neurosci. 17, 267–276.

Osler, W., 1889. The cerebal palsies of children A clinical study from the Infirmary for Nervous Diseases. Blakiston, Philadelphia.

Oudega, M., Varon, S., Hagg, T., 1994. Distribution of corticospinal motor neurons in the postnatal rat: quantitative evidence for massive collateral elimination and modest cell death. J. Comp. Neurol. 347, 115–126.

Pallas, S.L., 2001. Intrinsic and extrinsic factors that shape neocortical specification. Trends Neurosci 24 (7), 417–423.

Passingham, R.E., Perry, R.E., Wilkinson, F., 1983. The long term effects of removal of sensorimotor cortex in infant and adult rhesus monkeys. Brain 106, 675–705.

Phillips, C., Porter, R., 1977. Corticospinal Neurones: their Role in Movement. Academic Press, New York.

Porter, R., Lemon, R., 1993. Corticospinal Function and Voluntary Movement. Oxford University Press, Oxford.

Prechtl, H., Einspieler, C., Cioni, G., Bos, A., Ferrari, F., Sontheimer, D., 1997. An early marker for neurological deficits after perinatal brain lesions. Lancet 349, 1361–1363.

Quartarone, A., Bagnato, S., Rizzo, V., Morgante, F., Sant'angelo, A., Battaglia, F., et al., 2005. Distinct changes in cortical and spinal excitability following high-frequency repetitive TMS to the human motor cortex. Exp. Brain Res. 161, 114–124.

Reinoso, B.S., Castro, A.J., 1989. A study of corticospinal remodelling using retrograde fluorescent tracers in rats. Exp. Brain Res. 74, 387–394.

Rouiller, E.M., Liang, F., Moret, V., Wiesendanger, M., 1991. Trajectory

of redirected corticospinal axons after unilateral lesion of the sensorimotor cortex in neonatal rat; a phaseolus vulgaris-leucoagglutinin (PHA-L) tracing study. Exp. Neurol. 114, 53–65.

Sadato, N., 2006. Cross-modal plasticity in the blind revealed by functional neuroimaging. Suppl. Clin. Neurophysiol. 59, 75–79.

Salimi, I., Martin, J., 2004. Rescuing transient corticospinal terminations and promoting growth with corticospinal stimulation in kittens. J. Neurosci. 24, 4952–4961.

Scales, D.A., Collins, G.H., 1972. Cerebral degeneration with hypertrophy of the contralateral pyramid. Arch. Neurol. 26, 186–190.

Seebach, B.S., Ziskind-Conhaim, L., 1994. Formation of transient inappropriate sensorimotor synapses in developing rat spinal cords. J. Neurol. 17, 4520–4528.

Sharkey, M., Lund, R., Dom, R., 1986. Maintenance of transient occipitospinal axons in the rat. Brain Res. 395, 257–261.

Stanfield, B.B., O'Leary, D.D., 1985. The transient corticospinal projection from the occipital cortex during postnatal development of the rat. J. Comp. Neurol. 238, 236–248.

Stanfield, B.B., O'Leary, D.D.M., Fricks, C., 1982. Selective collateral elimination in early postnatal development restricts cortical distribution of rat pyramidal tract neurones. Nature 298, 371–373.

Staudt, M., Gerloff, C., Grodd, W., Holthausen, H., Niemann, G., Krägeloh-Mann, I., 2004. Reorganization in congenital hemiparesis acquired at different gestational ages. Ann. Neurol. 56, 854–863.

Szelenyi, A., Bueno de Camargo, A., Deletis, V., 2003. Neurophysiological evaluation of the corticospinal tract by D-wave recordings in young children. Child's Nerv. System 19, 30–34.

Thickbroom, G., Byrnes, M., Archer, S., Nagarajan, L., Mastaglia, F., 2001. Differences in sensory and motor cortical organization following brain injury early in life. Ann. Neurol. 49, 320–327.

Uematsu, J., Ono, K., Yamano, T., Shimada, M., 1996. Development of corticospinal tract fibres and their plasticity. II. Neonatal unilateral cortical damage and subsequent development of the corticospinal tract in mice. Brain Dev. 18, 173–178.

Verhaart, J., 1947. On thick and thin fibres in the pyramidal tracts. Acta Psychiat. Neurol. 22, 271–281.

Verhaart, J., 1950. Hypertrophy of the pes pedunculi and pyramid as a result of degeneration of the contralateral corticofugal fibre tracts. J. Comp. Neurol. 92, 1–15.

Walther, M., Berweck, S., Schessl, J., Linder-Lucht, M., Fietzek, U., Glocker, F., et al., 2009. Maturation of inhibitory and excitatory motor cortex pathways in children. Brain Dev. 31, 562–567.

Wiesel, T., Hubel, D., 1965. Comparison of the effects of unilateral and bilateral eye closure on cortical unit responses in kittens. J. Neurophysiol. 28, 1029–1040.

Wieser, H., Henke, K., Zumsteg, D., Taub, E., Yonekawa, Y., Buck, A.,

1999. Activation of the left motor cortex during left leg movements after right central resection. J. Neurol. Neurosurg. Psychiatry 67, 187–191.

Wolpaw, J., Tennissen, A., 2001. Activity-dependent spinal cord plasticity in health and disease. Annu. Rev. Neurosci. 24, 807–843.

Wu, C., Hunter, D., 2006. Amblyopia: diagnostic and therapeutic options. Am. J. Ophthalmol. 141, 175–184.

# Re-thinking the brain: new insights into early experience and brain development

3

Mary P. Galea

## CHAPTER CONTENTS

The brain is a self-organizing system that adapts to its specific environment throughout pre- and postnatal life (Braun and Bock, 2011). Self-organization refers to the spontaneous formation of patterns and pattern change in open non-equilibrium systems. Edelman's theory of neuronal group selection (Edelman, 1989) highlights this process. Groups of neurons are 'selected' or organized into groups or networks that are dynamically organized through epigenetic factors and experience. Developmental selection occurs largely before birth. Processes such as cell division, differentiation and programmed cell death and the mechanisms of neuronal migration are regulated by epigenetic factors. While genetics provides a general blueprint for neural development, the developmental processes are not precisely pre-specified by genes, and produce unique patterns of neurons and neuronal groups in every brain. The result is a diverse pattern of connectivity forming primary repertoires of different neuronal groups. Structural diversity occurs through selective mechanical and chemical events regulated by cell and substrate adhesion molecules. A second process called experiential selection occurs postnatally through behavioural experience, resulting in modifications in the strength of synaptic connections, and creating diverse secondary repertoires. Finally, re-entrant signalling leads to the development of dynamic 'maps', an interconnected series of neuronal groups that independently receive inputs from the real world and create coherent perceptual constructs.

## Early development

After the initial proliferation of precursor cells and differentiation of neurons, the cells migrate from the site of origin to their final location where they extend neurites and grow in size. Synapses begin to form around this time (refer to Shepherd, 1994, for review). Maturation of the neurons into their final form and function is a process that may take several decades (de Graaf-Peters and Hadders-Algra, 2006). The development of neural connections in many regions of the central nervous system is characterized by an initial overproduction of neurons, axons and synapses, followed at certain periods by the selective elimination or pruning of excess numbers of these structures (see Purves and Lichtman, 1985, for review). A wave of programmed neuronal cell death occurs very early in the prenatal period during which up to 50% of neurons initially formed will die (Oppenheim, 1981). This process is a means of regulating cell numbers to match the capacity of the target structures, and corrects for some errors in positioning. A second wave of cell death occurs in postmitotic neurons and plays a critical role in shaping the nervous system. Cells that survive appear to be successful in competing for growth factors (see Lossi and Merighi, 2003, for review).

Constant trophic input is essential for appropriate nervous system function. Trophic support is provided by the target cells (other neurons, muscle) as well as from local glial cells. However there is also evidence that blood-borne hormonal-like growth factors may also be important. These include insulin-like growth factor-I (IGF-I), fibroblast growth factor-2 (FGF-2) or the neurotrophins (Torres-Aleman, 2000). The implications of these effects will be discussed in a later section.

There has been a prevailing view that neuronal connectivity is more diffuse during early stages of development and that the final shaping of the adult-like pattern of connectivity is achieved by activity-dependent processes that prune non-relevant connections during critical periods (Katz and Shatz, 1996). This view relied heavily on research describing the postnatal development of the ocular dominance columns in visual cortex (Le Vay et al., 1978, reviewed below). In contrast, there is considerable accuracy of connections early during development, as soon as axons first reach their target structures. This selective synapse formation is controlled by specific molecular cues, for example, the patterning of thalamocortical projections by ephrin–A5 (Vanderhaeghen and Polleux, 2004), the control of the laminar origin of the corticospinal tract by Fezf2 (Han et al., 2011) and differential patterns of Lmo4 in sensory neurons (Chen et al., 2005), that influence innervation of the homonymous spinal motoneurons by Ia afferents in the absence of activity (Frank and Jackson, 1986).

It has long been thought that activity-dependent mechanisms during critical periods in the postnatal phase were key factors in the development of motor and sensory systems. A classic example is the development of the ocular dominance system in the visual cortex. The visual system has been a frequently investigated model of sensory systems. Neurons in lamina IV of the primary visual cortex (V1) are segregated into columns dominated alternately by the right or left eye (Hubel et al., 1977). At birth there is considerable overlap of the afferents from the lateral geniculate nucleus (LGN) in V1 from each eye (Hubel et al., 1977), so that many of the neurons in lamina IV are driven by inputs from both eyes. The segregation of these afferents into alternating bands occurs gradually by rearrangement of synapses and is dependent on visual experience. Occlusion of vision of one eye for the first three months (the critical period) leads to a change in the effectiveness of the occluded eye to drive neurons in V1, with a corresponding reduction in the size of the column for the occluded eye, and an expansion of the column for the non-occluded eye.

Newer investigative methods have led to a clarification about the development of ocular dominance columns. It is now realized that development involves two separate phases: an establishment phase, and an activity-dependent remodelling phase (Crowley and Katz, 2002). It appears that the initial establishment of the columns occurs considerably earlier than the critical period. In macaque monkeys, it has been shown that the projections carrying input from both eyes become segregated during the second half of gestation and become partially separated in the cortex about three weeks before birth, i.e., before visual experience (Horton and Hocking, 1996; Rakic, 1976). Development of the ocular dominance columns is relatively rapid and precise, occurring before the cortex responds to visual stimulation, i.e., before the onset of what has been described as the critical period (Crowley and Katz, 2000). Thus Edelman's primary repertoires are clearly complex and detailed patterns of connectivity. The ocular dominance columns do not develop independently, but in relation to other aspects of visual cortex organization, such as retinotopic maps that arise in part from connections within the LGN, and which are related to the pattern of ocular dominance columns (Le Vay et al., 1985). It is highly probable, therefore, that molecular guidance mechanisms, which play an important role in the establishment of topographical connections within the brain, also affect the development of the ocular dominance columns. This does not negate the effect of visual experience, but rather highlights the fact that a considerable degree of specificity occurs well before the postnatal period, enabled through internally generated spontaneous activity (Katz and Shatz, 1996).

The development of the somatosensory system follows a similar template. The animal model often used is the development of the barrel fields in rodents. Barrels are the largest and probably the most behaviourally important sensory areas in the rodent neocortex. Information from the large facial whiskers arrayed on the snout is transferred via the trigeminal nerve to the ventrobasal nucleus of the thalamus. Thalamic afferents then project to layer IV of the somatosensory cortex to form the distinct barrel pattern observed in the barrel map (Inan and Crair, 2007). Gradients of specific molecules, including ephrin-A5 and EphA4, regulate the guidance of thalamocortical axons into their appropriate cortical areas (Dufour et al., 2003). Neuronal activity is required for topographical specification and refinement of these projections (Jensen and Killackey, 1987).

## Thalamocortical projections

The thalamus provides the passage of entry for all sensory information to the cerebral cortex, as well as for all correlated and processed information from the spinal cord, cerebellum, and basal ganglia, including the substantia nigra. The thalamus provides the cerebral cortex with the key information needed to represent both body space and extrapersonal space, i.e., the contextual information for all complex behaviour. A previously widely accepted model of the organization of the thalamocortical projections to the sensorimotor cortex was that each nucleus with its own unique subthalamic input in turn projects to a particular region of cortex. This model implied that the thalamus subserves a largely passive relay function. However, there is considerable territorial convergence of input from two or more thalamic nuclei to each localized zone of cortex. Each thalamic nucleus, specified by its cytoarchitecture and subthalamic input, projects to a quite extensive area of sensorimotor cortex which overlaps with the projections of adjacent thalamic nuclei (Darian-Smith et al., 1996).

There is evidence that early topographic maps between and within individual cortical areas are generated prenatally through the interaction of the guidance cues ephrin-A5 and EphA receptors. Ephrin-A5 in the cortex acts as a graded repulsive cue for thalamocortical axons expressing graded levels of EphA receptors (including EphA4) to generate a topographic somatosensory map (Dufour et al., 2003; Vanderhaeghen and Polleux, 2004).

Subplate neurons play an important role in the development of the thalamocortical projections. The subplate represents a transient layer in the developing cerebral cortex. It comprises a heterogeneous set of neurons located directly under the cortical plate. Subplate neurons have extensive dendritic arborization and widespread axonal projections, and they have substantial glutamatergic or GABAergic synaptic inputs from thalamic, intra-subplate and cortical plate sources. They synchronize neuronal activity by receiving incoming extrinsic and intrinsic signals and distributing them throughout the developing cortical plate (Kanold and Luhmann, 2010). They play a critical role in regulating the maturation of cortical inhibition, as well as in the organization of the functional columns that are the hallmark of all cortical architecture, especially in sensory areas (Kanold and Luhmann, 2010). Subplate neurons are prone to hypoxic injury in the perinatal period (McQuillen and Ferriero, 2005), and their loss will affect the maturation of thalamocortical and other projections. For example, damage of the subplate in visual cortex prevents the maturation of thalamocortical synapses, the maturation of inhibition in layer 4, the development of orientation selective responses and the formation of ocular dominance columns. Subplate removal also alters ocular dominance plasticity during the critical period. Damage to the subplate in other cortical areas is likely to have similar effects, though this has not been investigated fully. The consequences of such damage have been highlighted by modern imaging methods. For example, diffusion tensor imaging has identified a reduction in the posterior thalamocortical tracts associated with periventricular leukomalacia in children with spastic quadriplegia who had normal corticospinal tracts (Hoon et al., 2002).

## Corticospinal projections

Corticospinal projections are the only direct link between the sensorimotor cortex and the spinal cord. They comprise parallel, somatotopically organized projections to each level of the spinal cord with unique, though overlapping, patterns of termination. In addition to a dense projection from the motor cortex, corticospinal fibres arise from the premotor cortex, the postcentral cortex, especially the posterior parietal areas, the second somatosensory area and the caudal part of the insula. On the medial surface, there are extensive projections to the spinal cord from the supplementary motor area and the cortex within the cingulate sulcus (Dum and Strick, 1991; Galea and Darian-Smith, 1994). Corticospinal neuron populations thus transmit a complex orchestrated output from a number of different regions of the cerebral cortex to the neuron populations of every segment of the spinal cord.

During development, the first pioneering axons to advance down the spinal cord are those that will innervate the lumbar segments, and these then are followed by a bulk of later arriving fasciculating corticospinal fibres projecting to upper cord segments (Stanfield, 1992). As is the case with other major neural structures, the early development of the corticospinal tract is regulated by transcription factors that play important roles on the specification of corticospinal neurons (Chen et al., 2005), and molecules such as EphA4, which are important for guidance of corticospinal axons to their targets in the spinal cord (Coonan et al., 2001; Dottori et al., 1998). Other molecules are the neural cell adhesion molecule L1, a deficit of which causes failure of decussation at the medulla (Cohen et al., 1998), and netrin-1, which mediates the path finding of corticospinal axons from the cortex to the internal capsule (Richards et al., 1997).

Studies in rodents (Stanfield and O'Leary, 1985), cats (Martin, 2005) and monkeys (Armand et al., 1997; Galea and Darian-Smith, 1995) have highlighted that, although the descent of corticospinal axons to the most caudal parts of the spinal cord occurs before birth, maturation of the corticospinal tract occurs largely postnatally. In monkeys, functional connections with motoneurons which are critical for individuated finger movements are not established until manipulative skills emerge several months after birth (Olivier et al., 1997). Certainly, very few corticospinal terminals have extended into the dorsal and ventral horns at birth, and only by the eighth postnatal month is the terminal arborization comparable with

that observed in the mature animal (Galea and Darian-Smith, 1995; Kuypers, 1962). Concurrently there is a threefold reduction in the number of neurons projecting to the spinal cord (Galea and Darian-Smith, 1994, 1995) and a comparable regression of thalamocortical projections to the sensorimotor cortex (Darian-Smith et al., 1990a, 1990b). The spatial and temporal correspondence in the postnatal regression occurring in both the corticospinal neuron populations and in their subcortical inputs from the thalamus highlights the probable interactions between the two populations via the subplate.

Unilateral lesion of the corticospinal system during early postnatal life in cats and rats can result in aberrant corticospinal organization, with maintenance of exuberant projections from the non-damaged side (Castro, 1985; Hicks and D'Amato, 1970; Leonard and Goldberger, 1987b; Leong and Lund, 1973). Martin and colleagues have conducted a series of experiments investigating the role of activity in shaping the developing corticospinal projections in the kitten. Blocking neural activity in the motor cortex by continuous infusion of a GABA$_A$ agonist, muscimol, in postnatal weeks 3–7 resulted in sparse corticospinal terminations to the contralateral spinal cord from the silenced area of cortex, while those from the active cortex maintained an immature bilateral pattern (Martin et al., 2009). The animals showed significant errors in reaching and grasping using the limb contralateral to the infusion, and these behavioural deficits persisted despite further training and practice (Martin et al., 2000). Such infusions have also been found to affect limb locomotor activity and postural reflexes (Leonard and Goldberger, 1987a).

In subsequent experiments, limb use was blocked in kittens by injection of botulinum toxin A into several forearm muscles. As with inactivation of the motor cortex, preventing limb use prevents the maturation of the corticospinal axon terminals and results in the same aberrant pattern of contralateral projections (Martin et al., 2004). Moreover, once the effects of botulinum toxin wore off, the animals showed persistent impairments of grasping (Martin et al., 2004). Thus, activity-dependent refinement of corticospinal axon terminations during the early postnatal period is the mechanism whereby early motor experiences shape the structural and functional organization of the corticospinal system.

# Experience and the development of target structures

Activity is not only required for neural development but is also important for the development of target structures. Neuronal activity can influence the maturation of the neuromuscular junction, the development of motoneurons within the spinal cord, and the pattern of outgrowth of motor axons.

## Neuromuscular junction

During normal development, muscle fibres are often innervated by more than one motor axon. As postsynaptic development progresses, this polyinnervation is reduced to single innervation during the postnatal period, a process that is activity-dependent (Buffelli et al., 2003; Purves and Lichtman, 1985).

The formation of nerve–muscle contacts, intramuscular nerve branching, and neuronal survival require reciprocal signals from nerve and muscle to regulate the formation of synapses. Following the production of muscle fibres, clusters of acetylcholine receptors (AChRs) are concentrated in the central regions of the muscle fibres, pre-patterned independently of neuronal signals in developing muscle fibres. ACh released by branching motor nerves causes AChR-induced postsynaptic potentials and regulates the localization and stabilization of developing synaptic contacts. These 'active' contact sites may prevent AChRs clustering in non-contacted regions and prevent the establishment of additional contacts. A further neuronal factor, agrin, stabilizes the accumulation of AChR at synaptic sites (Witzemann, 2006).

Activity is important for the maintenance of the neuromuscular junction. Disuse, as in spinal cord injury (Burns et al., 2007) or ageing (Valdez et al., 2010), can result in structural changes in the neuromuscular synapse, including synaptic detachment. Children with cerebral palsy aged between 7 and 15 years have been reported to show an abnormal spread of AChRs beyond the confines of the neuromuscular junction, indicating a deficit in development of the neuromuscular synapse (Theroux et al., 2002). They also demonstrate abnormal structural changes, including non-apposition of the synaptic components, which were more numerous in more highly affected patients (Theroux et al., 2005).

## Motoneuron development

While many properties of motoneurons are developmentally regulated, patterned neuronal activity in early postnatal life can regulate axon terminal morphology and synaptic efficacy at the neuromuscular junction. Motoneurons undergo extensive anatomical, physiological and molecular changes during the early postnatal period. The Cat-301 cell surface proteoglycan is first detected on rodent motoneurons during this period. The expression of Cat-301 immunoreactivity on motoneurons is dependent on input relayed by large-diameter primary afferents (e.g., from muscle spindles) as well as from supraspinal sources (Kalb and Hockfield, 1990) and a normal pattern of activity of the neuromuscular unit in early postnatal life (Kalb and Hockfield, 1994). Differentiation also requires activation of the NMDA receptor over the same time period (Kalb and Hockfield, 1992). Normal motoneuron differentiation requires a normal pattern of neuronal activity. Tail suspension in rat pups, which prevents load bearing on the hindlimbs but does not prevent movement about the cage, results in significant impairment of motor performance that can persist into adulthood (Walton et al., 1992). It has been shown that three weeks of tail suspension prevents postnatal increases in the soleus motoneuron soma size and succinate dehydrogenase activity (a marker of mitochondrial activity) (Nakano and Katsuta, 2000). Restriction of movement of the hindlimbs during the early postnatal period has a similar effect on motoneuron size and development of the sciatic nerve (Stigger et al., 2011). Treadmill training provided after this period can reverse these changes.

## Muscle

Muscle fibre numbers reach a maximum value at, or shortly after, birth and remain unchanged throughout development (Goldspink, 1972). Increases in muscle size and weight are therefore due to changes in muscle fibre size. Primary fetal muscle fibres are relatively large, and are destined to become type I or slow oxidative fibres in fully differentiated adult muscles. At a later stage a second population of smaller and more numerous fibres develops. These become type II or fast oxidative glycolytic fibres (Alnaqeeb and Goldspink, 1987). Although specific muscle fibre types are differentiated early in the absence of innervation, subsequent expression of different isoforms of myosin heavy chain is affected by environmental factors, such as the degree of muscle stretch experienced by the muscle fibres (Vandenburgh et al., 1990), as well as loading, e.g., for postural support (Lowrie et al., 1989).

Muscle fibre size is known to be affected by the level of nutrition. A sheep model of late placental insufficiency intrauterine growth retardation has been used to demonstrate an inhibition of skeletal muscle growth in the fetus, possibly associated with poor nutrition (Thorn et al., 2009). Children born preterm may have impaired muscle growth (Hay and Thureen, 2010; Yau and Chang, 1993), which may be exacerbated by the lack of cortical drive as a result of reduced corticospinal input. This may limit the ability of muscle to perform sustained contraction that is necessary for the development of posture and ambulation.

Children with cerebral palsy aged between 4 and 15 years show consistent morphological and structural changes in muscle, specifically reductions in muscle volume, cross-sectional area, thickness and muscle belly length (Barrett and Lichtwark, 2010). They have a preponderance of type I muscle fibres (Rose et al., 1994; Sarnat, 1986) and are unable to activate their muscles maximally (Elder et al., 2003; Rose and McGill, 2005). More important for functional tasks is the ability to generate rapid force, which is also impaired (Moreau et al., 2012). Gait impairments emerge from the interaction of weakness, spasticity and contracture (Rodda et al., 2004).

## Perinatal injury

Margaret Kennard's pioneering studies (Kennard, 1942) examined the effects of removal of Brodmann areas 4 and 6 (excluding face regions) in infant and older macaque monkeys. Kennard concluded that there were quantitative differences in motor recovery in infants and adults, with a greater capacity for dendritic reorganization in undamaged cortical regions in the infant. The differential recovery following lesions in infants and

adults is known as the 'Kennard effect' or 'infant lesion effect'. Later studies did not support these findings (Passingham et al., 1978, 1983, Slope et al., 1983). Indeed, some patterns appeared to be more impaired by lesions in infancy than in adulthood (Bregman and Goldberger, 1983; Isaacson, 1975).

The developing brain is undergoing a sequence of developmental events and damage to it produces a cascade of post-injury changes that are different from adult injury (Kolb and Teskey, 2012). These events involve neurogenesis, neuronal migration, neuronal maturation, synaptogenesis, apoptosis and myelin formation. The precise cascade of post-injury changes therefore depends on the precise stage of development in which injury occurs.

If damage occurs during the peak of neurogenesis, the brain responds by increasing neurogenesis to replace lost neurons. For example, irradiation during the beginning of cerebral neurogenesis in rats (embryonic day 12) destroyed all of the cerebral neurons but was followed by further neurogenesis (D'Amato, 1982). Damage to the cerebral cortex in the first postnatal week in rats leads to extensive cell death and loss of dendritic arborization and produces severe motor, cognitive and other behavioural deficits (Kolb and Gibb, 2007). However, damage in the second postnatal week leads to an increase in astrocyte and stem cell proliferation, and a general hypertrophy of dendritic arborization of cortical pyramidal neurons. These changes are associated with enhanced functional outcome (Kolb and Gibb, 2007). The basis of the difference in outcome is that neurons are migrating and just beginning to mature in week 1, while week 2 is characterized by branching of dendrites and synapse formation.

## Experience and brain development

Brain development can be modified by prenatal experiences, which may be detrimental or beneficial. For example, decreased dendritic length and spine density have been associated with prenatal antipsychotic medication (Frost et al., 2009). Prenatal stress leads to altered gene expression and synaptic organization (Mychasiuk et al., 2011). Increased serum levels of pro-inflammatory cytokines in infants with necrotizing enterocolitis have been associated with poor growth and nervous system development (Lodha et al., 2010). In contrast, provision of complex housing to pregnant rats prenatally leads to reduced dendritic length and increased spine density in the pups (Kolb and Teskey, 2012).

It is the postnatal period that is most amenable to intervention. As described in the previous sections, the traditional concept is that there are critical or sensitive periods, during which specific experiences influence development. The most common example is the window for visual development in the postnatal period, as described previously. Rather than the term 'critical' period, Greenough et al. (1987) have proposed the term 'experience–expectant processes'. Thus, developing sensory and motor systems may reliably expect specific experiences through the environment to help shape their connectivity. The advantage of experience–expectant processes is that developing systems can develop much greater performance capabilities by taking advantage of experiences that could be expected to be available to young animals (Greenough et al., 1987). A refined pattern of connections can emerge through selective retention or elimination of synapses through competitive processes, usually involving neural activity. Because the brain is a dynamic system, abnormal experience will lead to an abnormal pattern of organization. The key distinguishing aspect of the effects of experience early in sensorimotor development is the degree to which they are age-dependent and probably irreversible. A lack of appropriate stimulation during the period from birth to pre-school age is likely to have serious and sustained effects. Experience-dependent processes underlie another form of plasticity typical of the adult brain. Such information is unique to the individual and will differ in timing and character from person to person.

## Interventions

### The premature infant as a model for effect of environment

Premature birth is associated with a number of medical complications which may affect development. It usually involves being removed from the mother and being nursed in a neonatal intensive care unit (NICU). The importance of maternal–infant bonding through close contact was highlighted by the classic studies of Bowlby (1969, 1973, 1980). Maternal contact regulates the infant's activity levels, sucking behaviour, oxygen consumption, sleep–wake cycles, as well as hormonal, cardiovascular, immune and neuroendocrine responses (Hofer, 1994). Separation from the mother clearly affects these processes. In addition, the effect of the physical environment of the NICU, including exposure to bright lights, high sound levels and frequent noxious interventions, may have deleterious effects on the immature brain and alter its subsequent development (Anand, 1998; Anand and Scalzo, 2000). As with other sensory pathways, the development of pain pathways is not complete at birth and is dependent on external factors such as neurotrophins and neural activity (Baccei and Fitzgerald, 2006). It is not surprising, therefore, that repeated exposure to noxious stimuli will affect the connectivity of this system. Repeated heel lances are known to elicit hyperalgesia, as shown by a reduced threshold for cutaneous reflexes (Fitzgerald et al., 1989). Abnormal or excessive noxious stimulation in early life may have the potential to cause long-term changes in somatosensory and pain processing (Baccei and Fitzgerald, 2006). Reports of higher somatic pain sensitivity in prematurely born children and adolescents (Buskila et al., 2003) support this view.

Since infants preferentially respond to their mother's voice, they might not be able to discriminate their mother's voice in an environment where there is loud and unpredictable noise. Furthermore, the exposure to constant light without the rhythmical contrast of day/night cycles affects visual development and prevents the establishment of sleep patterns. There have been attempts to reduce the impact of the constant noise and light in the NICU. Supportive bedding provides support of the shoulders, legs, trunk and head, and allows the infant to nestle into a flexed position and more easily to bring their hands together, to touch their face and to push against the bedding (Als, 1998). These strategies, based on the synactive model of infant development (Als, 1996), a theoretical framework that promotes physiological stability as the foundation for the organization of motor, behavioural state, and attentive and interactive behaviours in neonates, have been examined in a number of clinical trials (Als et al., 1994; Fleisher et al., 1995; Maguire et al., 2009; Peters et al., 2009;

Westrup et al., 2000). In a dynamic system, all the subsystems contribute to overall function. Despite a strong theoretical rationale, there is limited evidence for their effectiveness, mainly because of methodological limitations (Symington and Pinelli, 2006; Wallin and Eriksson, 2009).

In addition to controlling the visual, auditory and temperature environment, specific facilitation strategies include handling, positioning the infant in prone, supine and side-lying, and cradling the infant. The outcome measures include factors such as weight gain, length of hospital stay, length of mechanical ventilation, heart rate and oxygen saturation. Neurodevelopmental outcomes have been measured using standardized instruments such as the Bayley Scales of Infant Development or the Assessment of Preterm Infant's Behaviour at various periods post-intervention. The heterogeneity in content, frequency and focus of programmes provided post-discharge and commencing within the first 12 months have made it difficult to evaluate the benefits in terms of motor outcomes (Koldewijn et al., 2010; Spittle et al., 2007).

## Sensorimotor stimulation and environmental enrichment

One powerful effect on brain development is tactile stimulation. Daily tactile stimulation of normal rat pups and those with perinatal injury for the first two weeks of life leads to a facilitation of both motor and cognitive behaviours in adulthood. However, the morphological changes in the intact and injured brain are different. While tactile stimulation reduces spine density in intact animals, there is an increase in spine density in brain-injured animals (Kolb and Teskey, 2012). These observations highlight the fact that the intact and injured brains respond differently to the same experiences, presumably because brain damage imposes a constraint on development, through loss of tissue or trophic factors, that has altered the developmental process. This will depend on the timing of the injury, as well as the site of injury. Not only is the pattern of connectivity within the nervous system affected, but the target structures downstream—spinal motoneurons, neuromuscular junctions and muscles—are also affected. These structures are deprived of the expected experiences required for their own development. The nexus between the brain and the body is highlighted by the role of blood-borne hormonal-like growth factors which provide trophic support to the nervous system. An example is IGF-I, which is released by exercising muscles and acts as a metabolic proprioceptive signal to brain centers to adapt to changes in muscle mass and function (Torres-Aleman, 2000).

Post-injury experience is a potent modulator of recovery. Studies in laboratory animals have shown that placing animals in complex, stimulating environments can optimize functional recovery from various forms of experimental brain damage (see Kolb and Teskey, 2012 for review). Such environments not only afford opportunities for movement but also expose the animals to complex perceptual and spatial stimuli. It has been hypothesized that such environments may increase the synthesis of neurotrophic factors, which in turn facilitate synaptic plasticity (Johansson, 2000).

After perinatal injury, normalizing the environment may be an important factor in reducing stress and preventing further injury. The developmental care model developed by Als et al. (2004) views the infant as an active participant who seeks ongoing caregiver support for self-regulation and development. Counteracting the deprivation of maternal contact and poverty of movement in the NICU environment would therefore be of benefit. Interventions such as kangaroo care (skin-to-skin contact) have been shown to have beneficial effects on respiratory function and temperature regulation in preterm infants (Ludington-Hoe et al., 2004). Analysis of EEG-sleep patterns showed that infants who had care involving skin-on-skin contact had more mature EEG-sleep organization than control infants (Scher et al., 2009). Although a previous Cochrane review (Vickers et al., 2004) showed that the evidence for the developmental benefits of massage was weak, Guzzetta et al. (2011) showed that the provision of massage in healthy preterm infants, involving stroking of the body in the prone position and passive movements of the limbs in the supine position, resulted in a relative increase of EEG spectral power. Such an increase in preterm infants approaching term age is considered to be the expression of a maturation of cortical circuitry (Guzzetta et al., 2011). Whether such effects are likely in infants with brain damage is a question that remains to be investigated.

Activity-based therapeutic approaches have been implemented to treat the impairments associated with cerebral palsy. These involve task-specific, repetitive motor training, based on a solid neurophysiological rationale (Nudo et al., 1996; Plautz et al., 2000), and include constraint-induced movement therapy for the affected upper limb (Hoare et al., 2007), strength training for the lower limbs (Taylor et al., 2005) and treadmill training (Damiano and de Jong, 2009). It has been suggested that targeted activation of the spared corticospinal projections, using electrical stimulation of the brain, could lead to improved competitiveness for connections with spinal targets (Salimi et al., 2008). Active targets attract axonal connections (Richards et al., 1997).

Performance impairments in children with perinatal brain damage result from impaired development of both sensorimotor pathways and target tissues. Early brain damage exerts constraints on development of peripheral systems that are developing at the same time, and so the emergent neuromuscular system develops abnormally at multiple levels. Sensorimotor deprivation underlies this abnormal development. However, this is a potentially modifiable factor. Appreciation of the timing of specific developmental processes, particularly of target structures, should lead to a re-evaluation of the timing and content of early intervention. Does the environment afford appropriate afferent input, which is one factor necessary for the development of spinal motoneurons? Does it afford opportunities for stretch and loading of muscles so that differentiation of muscle fibre type can occur? Deficits in the development of target structures are likely to remain constraints on performance later in childhood, and will negatively affect functional outcomes of training programmes. Apart from this, what opportunities does the infant have for self-directed exploration of the environment in order to provide appropriate perceptual experiences? The deficit in anticipatory scaling of fingertip forces during object manipulation in children with cerebral palsy (Gordon and Duff, 1999) could be considered another effect of sensory deprivation. The integration of signals from tactile afferents and the motor responses in the fingers (Johansson and Westling, 1987) develops with experience of manipulation of objects of different weight, texture and size, resulting in an internal representation that enables adaptive control of grip forces. However this internal model is not only based on tactile signals. Kittens deprived of visual information about their limb movements failed to demonstrate normal visually guided behaviours in maturity (Held and Bauer, 1974). Martin et al. (2000) have suggested that prehension deficits resulting from sensorimotor cortex inactivation reflect a failure to integrate tactile and visual information with motor signals driving the emerging movements.

## Summary

Substantial changes take place in the central nervous system during infancy. Developing sensory and motor systems expect specific experiences through the environment to help shape their connectivity. Their target structures also depend on specific experiences to fully mature. The window for the critical period for sensorimotor development in the human infant has yet to be fully defined. However the evidence shows that the early postnatal period, and indeed the first year of life, is of particular importance.

## References

Alnaqeeb, M.A., Goldspink, G., 1987. Changes in fibre type, number and diameter in developing and ageing skeletal muscle. J. Anat. 153, 31–45.

Als, H., 1996. A synactive model of neonatal behavioural organization: framework for the assessment of neurobehavioural development in the premature infant and for support of infants and parents in the neonatal intensive care environment. Phys. Occup. Ther. Pediatr. 6, 3–55.

Als, H., 1998. Developmental care in the newborn intensive care unit. Curr. Opin. Pediatr. 10, 138–142.

Als, H., Lawhon, G., Duffy, F.H., McAnulty, G.B., Gibes-Grossman, R., Blickman, J.G., 1994. Individualized developmental care for the very low birthweight preterm infant. Medical and neurofunctional effects. JAMA 272, 853–858.

Als, H., Duffy, F.H., McAnulty, G.B., Rivkin, M.J., Vajapeyam, S., Mulkern, R.V., et al., 2004. Early

experience alters brain function and structure. Pediatrics 113, 846–857.

Anand, K.J., 1998. Clinical importance of pain and stress in preterm neonates. Biol. Neonate 73, 1–9.

Anand, K.J.S., Scalzo, F.M., 2000. Can adverse neonatal experiences alter brain development and subsequent behavior? Biol. Neonate 77, 69–82.

Armand, J., Olivier, E., Edgley, S.A., Lemon, R.N., 1997. Postnatal development of corticospinal projections from motor cortex to the cervical enlargement in the macaque monkey. J. Neurosci. 17, 251–266.

Baccei, M., Fitzgerald, M., 2006. Development of pain pathways and mechanisms. In: McMahon, S.B., Koltzenburg, M. (Eds.), Wall and Melzack's Textbook of Pain, fifth ed. Elsevier, London, pp. 143–158.

Barrett, R.S., Lichtwark, G.A., 2010. Gross muscle morphology and structure in spastic cerebral palsy: a systematic review. Dev. Med. Child Neurol. 52, 794–804.

Bowlby, J., 1969. Attachment and Loss. vol. 1: Attachment. Basic Books, New York.

Bowlby, J., 1973. Attachment and Loss. vol. 2: Separation: Anxiety and Anger. Basic Books, New York.

Bowlby, J., 1980. Attachment and Loss. vol. 3: Loss. Basic Books, New York.

Braun, K., Bock, J., 2011. Experience-dependent maturation of prefronto-limbic circuits and the origin of developmental psychopathology: implications for the genesis and therapy of behavioural disorders. Dev. Med. Child Neurol. 53, 14–18.

Bregman, B.S., Goldberger, M.E., 1983. Infant lesion effect: I. Development of motor behaviour following neonatal spinal cord damage in cats. Dev. Brain Res. 9, 103–117.

Buffelli, M., Burgess, R.W., Feng, G., Lobe, C.G., Lichtman, J.W., Sanes, J.R., 2003. Genetic evidence that relative synaptic efficacy biases the outcome of synaptic competition. Nature 424, 430–434.

Burns, A.S., Jawaid, S., Zhong, H., Yoshihara, H., Bhagat, S., Murray, M., et al., 2007. Paralysis elicited by spinal cord injury evokes selective disassembly of neuromuscular synapses with and without terminal sprouting in ankle flexors of the adult rat. J. Comp. Neurol. 500, 116–133.

Buskila, D., Neumann, L., Zmora, E., Feldman, M., Bolotin, A., Press, J., 2003. Pain sensitivity in prematurely born adolescents. Arch. Pediatr. Adolesc. Med. 157, 1079–1082.

Castro, A.J., 1985. Ipsilateral corticospinal projections after large lesions of the cerebral hemisphere in neonatal rats. Exp. Neurol. 46, 1–8.

Chen, B., Schaevitz, L.R., McConnell, S.K., 2005. Fezl regulates the differentiation and axon targeting of layer 5 subcortical projection neurons

in cerebral cortex. Proc. Natl Acad. Sci. USA 102, 17184–17189.

Cohen, N.R., Taylor, J.S.H., Scott, L.B., Guillery, P., Soriano, P., Furley, A.J.W., 1998. Errors in corticospinal axon guidance in mice lacking the neural cell adhesion molecule L1. Curr. Biol. 8, 26–33.

Coonan, J.R., Greferath, U., Messenger, J., Hartley, L., Murphy, M., Boyd, A.W., et al., 2001. The development and reorganization of corticospinal projections in EphA4 deficient mice. J. Comp. Neurol. 436, 248–262.

Crowley, J.C., Katz, L.C., 2002. Ocular dominance development revisited. Curr. Opin. Neurobiol. 12, 104–109.

Damiano, D.L., De Jong, S.L., 2009. A systematic review of the effects of treadmill training and body weight support in pediatric rehabilitation. J. Neurol. Phys. Ther. 33, 27–44.

Darian-Smith, C., Darian-Smith, I., Cheema, S.S., 1990a. Thalamic projections to sensorimotor cortex in the macaque monkey: use of multiple fluorescent tracers. J. Comp. Neurol. 299, 17–46.

Darian-Smith, C., Darian-Smith, I., Cheema, S.S., 1990b. Thalamic projections to sensorimotor cortex in the newborn macaque. J. Comp. Neurol. 299, 47–63.

Darian-Smith, I., Galea, M.P., Darian-Smith, C., Sugitani, M., Tan, A., Burman, K., 1996. The anatomy of manual dexterity. The new connectivity of the primate sensorimotor thalamus and cerebral cortex. Adv. Anat. Embryol. Cell Biol. 133.

De Graaf-Peters, V.B., Hadders-Algra, M., 2006. Ontogeny of the human central nervous system: what happens when? Early Hum. Dev. 82, 257–266.

Dottori, M., Hartley, L., Galea, M., Paxinos, G., Kilpatrick, T., Bartlett, P., et al., 1998. EphA4 (Sek 1) receptor tyrosine kinase is required for the development of the corticospinal tract. Proc. Natl Acad. Sci. USA 95, 13248–13253.

Dufour, A., Seibt, J., Passante, L., Depaepe, V., Ciossek, T., Frisen, J., et al., 2003. Area specificity and topography of thalamocortical projections are controlled by ephrin/Eph genes. Neuron 39, 453–465.

Dum, R.P., Strick, P.L., 1991. The origin of corticospinal projections from the premotor areas in the frontal lobe. J. Neurosci. 11, 667–689.

D'Amato, C.J., 1982. Regeneration and recovery in the fetal nervous system after radiation injury. Exp. Neurol. 76, 457–467.

Edelman, G.M., 1989. Neural Darwinism: The Theory of Neuronal Group Selection. Oxford University Press, Oxford.

Elder, G.C.B., Kirk, J., Stewart, G., Cook, K., Weir, D., Marshall, A., et al., 2003. Contributing factors to muscle weakness in children with cerebral palsy. Dev. Med. Child Neurol. 45, 542–550.

Fitzgerald, M., Millard, C., McIntosh, M., 1989. Cutaneous hypersensitivity following peripheral tissue damage in newborn infants and its reversal with topical anaesthesia. Pain 39, 31–36.

Fleisher, B.E., VandenBerg, K.A., Constantinou, J., Heller, C., Benitz, W.E., Johnson, A., et al., 1995. Individualized developmental care for very-low-birth-weight premature infants. Clin. Pediatr. (Phila) 34, 523–529.

Frank, E., Jackson, P.C., 1986. Normal electrical activity is not required for the formation of specific sensory-motor synapses. Brain Res. 378, 147–151.

Frost, D.O., Cerceo, S., Carroll, C., Kolb, B., 2009. Early exposure to haloperidol or olanzapine induces long-term alterations of dendritic form. Synapse 64, 191–199.

Galea, M.P., Darian-Smith, I., 1994. Multiple corticospinal neuron populations in the macaque monkey are specified by their unique cortical origins, spinal terminations and connections. Cereb. Cortex 4, 166–194.

Galea, M.P., Darian-Smith, I., 1995. Postnatal maturation of the direct corticospinal projections in the macaque monkey. Cereb. Cortex 5, 518–540.

Goldspink, G., 1972. Studies of postembryonic growth and development In: Bourne, G.H. (Ed.), The Structure and Function of Muscle, 1. Academic Press, New York.

Gordon, A.M., Duff, S.V., 1999. Relation between clinical measures and fine manipulative control in children with hemiplegic cerebral palsy. Devel. Med. Child Neurol. 41, 586–591.

Greenough, W.T., Black, J.E., Wallace, C.S., 1987. Experience and brain development. Child Dev. 58, 539–559.

Guzzetta, A., D'Acunto, M.G., Carotenuto, M., Berardi, N., Bancale, A., Biagoni, E., et al., 2011. The effects of preterm infant massage on brain electrical activity. Dev. Med. Child Neurol. 53 (Suppl. 4), 46–51.

Han, W., Kwan, K.Y., Shim, S., Lam, M.M.S., Shin, Y., Xu, X., et al., 2011. TBR1 directly represses Fezf2 to control the laminar origin and development of the corticospinal tract. Proc. Natl. Acad. Sci. USA 108, 3041–3046.

Hay, W.W., Thureen, P., 2010. Protein for preterm infants: how much is needed? How much is enough? How much is too much? Pediatr. Neonatol. 51, 198–207.

Held, R., Bauer Jr., J.A., 1974. Development of sensorially-guided reaching in infant monkeys. Brain Res. 71, 265–271.

Hicks, S.P., D'Amato, C.J., 1970. Motor-sensory and visual behaviour after hemispherectomy in newborn and mature rats. Exp. Neurol. 29, 416–438.

Hoare, B.J., Wasiak, J., Imms, C., Carey, L., 2007. Constraint-induced movement therapy and forced use in children with hemiplegic cerebral palsy. Cochrane Database Syst. Rev. 18, CD004149.

Hofer, M.A., 1994. Early relationships as regulators of infant physiology and behaviour. Acta Pediatr. Suppl. 397, 9–18.

Hoon, A.H., Lawrie, W.T., Melhem, E.R., Reinhardt, E.M., van Zijl, P.C.M., Solaiyappan, M., et al., 2002. Diffusion tensor imaging of periventricular malacia shows affected sensory cortex white matter pathways. Neurology 59, 752–756.

Horton, J.C., Hocking, D.R., 1996. An adult-like pattern of ocular dominance columns in striate cortex of newborn monkeys prior to visual experience. J. Neurosci. 16, 1791–1807.

Hubel, D.H., Wiesel, T.N., Le Vay, S., 1977. Plasticity of ocular dominance columns in the monkey striate

cortex. Phil. Trans. Royal Soc. London, Series B: Biol. Sci. 278, 377–409.

Inan, M., Crair, M.C., 2007. Development of cortical maps: perspectives from the barrel cortex. Neuroscientist 13, 49–61.

Isaacson, R.L., 1975. The myth of recovery from early brain damage. In: Ellis, N.R. (Ed.), Aberrant Development in Infancy. Human and Animal Studies. Lawrence Erlbaum & Associates, Hillsdale NJ, pp. 1–25.

Jensen, K.F., Killackey, H.P., 1987. Terminal arbors of axons projecting to the somatosensory cortex of the adult rat. I. The normal morphology of specific thalamocortical afferents. J. Neurosci. 7, 3529–3543.

Johansson, R.S., Westling, G., 1987. Signals in tactile afferents from the fingers eliciting adaptive motor responses during precision grip. Exp. Brain Res. 66, 141–154.

Johansson, B.B., 2000. Brain plasticity and stroke rehabilitation: the Willis lecture. Stroke 31, 223–230.

Kalb, R.G., Hockfield, S., 1990. Large diameter primary afferent input is required for expression of the Cat-301 proteoglycan on the surface of motor neurons. Neuroscience 34, 391–401.

Kalb, R.G., Hockfield, S., 1992. Activity-dependent development of spinal cord motor neurons. Brain Res. Rev. 17, 283–289.

Kalb, R.G., Hockfield, S., 1994. Electrical activity in the neuromuscular unit can influence the development of motor neurons. Dev. Biol. 162, 539–548.

Kanold, P.O., Luhmann, 2010. The subplate and early cortical circuits. Annu. Rev. Neurosci. 33, 23–48.

Katz, L.C., Shatz, C.J., 1996. Synaptic activity and the construction of cortical circuits. Science 274, 1133–1138.

Kennard, M.A., 1942. Cortical reorganization of motor function: studies on series of monkeys of various ages from infancy to maturity. Arch. Neurol. Psychiatr. 48, 227–240.

Kolb, B., Gibb, R., 2007. Brain plasticity and recovery from early cortical injury. Dev. Psychobiol. 49, 107–118.

Kolb, B., Teskey, G.C., 2012. Age, experience, injury, and the changing brain. Dev. Psychobiol. 54, 311–325.

Koldewijn, K., van Wassenaer, A., Wolf, M.-J., Meijssen, D., Houtzager, B., Beelen, A., et al., 2010. A neurobehavioural intervention and assessment program in very low birth weight infants: outcome at 24 months. J. Pediatr. 156, 359–365.

Kuypers, H.G.J.M., 1962. Corticospinal connections: postnatal development in the rhesus monkey. Science 138, 678–680.

Le Vay, S., Stryker, M.P., Shatz, C.J., 1978. Ocular dominance columns and their development in layer IV of the cat's visual cortex. J. Comp. Neurol. 79, 223–244.

Le Vay, S., Connolly, M., Houde, J., Van Essen, D.C., 1985. The complete pattern of ocular dominance stripes in the striate cortex and visual field of the macaque monkey. J. Neurosci. 5, 486–501.

Leonard, C.T., Goldberger, M.E., 1987a. Consequences of damage to sensorimotor cortex in neonatal and adult cats. I. Sparing and recovery of function. Brain Res. Dev. Brain Res. 32, 1–14.

Leonard, C.T., Goldberger, M.E., 1987b. Consequences of damage to sensorimotor cortex in neonatal and adult cats. II. Maintenance of exuberant projections. Brain Res. Dev. Brain Res. 32, 15–30.

Leong, S.K., Lund, R., 1973. Anomalous bilateral corticofugal pathways in albino rats after neonatal lesions. Brain Res. 62, 218–221.

Lodha, A., Asztalos, E., Moore, A.M., 2010. Cytokine levels in neonatal necrotizing enterocolitis and long-term growth and neurodevelopment. Acta Paediatr. 99, 338–343.

Lossi, L., Merighi, A., 2003. In vivo cellular and molecular mechanisms of neuronal apoptosis in the mammalian CNS. Prog. Neurobiol. 69, 287–312.

Lowrie, M.B., Moore, A.F.K., Vrbova, G., 1989. The effect of load on the phenotype of the developing rat soleus muscle. Pflüg Arch. 415, 204–208.

Ludington-Hoe, S.M., Anderson, G.C., Swinth, J.Y., Thompson, C., Hadeed, A.J., 2004. Randomized controlled trial of kangaroo care: cardiorespiratory and thermal effects on health preterm infants. Neonatal Net. 23, 39–48.

Maguire, C.M., Walther, F.J., Sprij, A.J., Le Cessie, S., Wit, J.M., Veen,

S., 2009. Effects of individualized developmental care in a randomized trial of preterm infants <32 weeks. Pediatrics 124, 1021–1030.

Martin, J.H., 2005. The corticospinal system: from development to motor control. Neuroscientist 11, 161–173.

Martin, J.H., Donarummo, L., Hacking, A., 2000. Impairments in prehension produced by early postnatal sensorimotor cortex activity blockade. J. Neurophysiol. 83, 895–906.

Martin, J.H., Choy, M., Pullman, S., Meng, Z., 2004. Corticospinal development depends on experience. J. Neurosci. 24, 2122–2132.

Martin, J.H., Friel, K.M., Salimi, I., Chakrabarty, S., 2009. Corticospinal development. In: Squire, L.R. (Ed.), Encyclopedia of Neuroscience. Academic Press, Oxford, pp. 202–214.

McQuillen, P.S., Ferriero, D.M., 2005. Perinatal subplate neuron injury: implications for cortical development and plasticity. Brain Pathol. 15, 250–260.

Moreau, N.G., Falvo, M.J., Damiano, D.L., 2012. Rapid force generation is impaired in cerebral palsy and is related to decreased muscle size and functional mobility. Gait Posture 35, 154–158.

Mychasiuk, R., Ilnytskyy, S., Kovalchuk, O., Kolb, B., Gibb, R., 2011. Intensity matters: brain, behaviour and the epigenome of prenatally stressed rats. Neuroscience 180, 105–110.

Nakano, H., Katsuta, S., 2000. Non-weight-bearing condition arrests the morphological and metabolic changes of rat soleus motoneurons during postnatal growth. Neurosci. Lett. 290, 145–148.

Nudo, R.J., Wise, B.M., SiFuentes, F., Milliken, G.W., 1996. Neural substrates for the effects of rehabilitative training on motor recovery after ischemic infarct. Science 272, 1791–1794.

Olivier, E., Edgley, S.A., Armand, J., Lemon, R.N., 1997. An electrophysiological study of the postnatal development of the corticospinal system in the macaque monkey. J. Neurosci. 17, 267–276.

Oppenheim, R.W., 1981. Neuronal cell death and some related regressive phenomena during neurogenesis:

a selective historical review and a progress report. In: Cowan, W.M. (Ed.), Studies in Developmental Neurobiology. Essays in Honor of Viktor Hamburger. Oxford University Press, New York.

Passingham, R.E., Perry, V.H., Wilkinson, F., 1978. Failure to develop a precision grip in monkeys with unilateral neocortical lesions made in infancy. Brain Res. 145, 410–414.

Passingham, R.E., Perry, V.H., Wilkinson, F., 1983. The long-term effects of removal of sensorimotor cortex in infant and adult rhesus monkeys. Brain 106, 675–705.

Peters, K.L., Rosychuk, J., Hendson, L., Coté, J.J., McPherson, C., Tyebkhan, J.M., 2009. Improvement of short- and long-term outcomes for very low birth weight infants: Edmonton NIDCAP trial. Pediatrics 124, 1009–1020.

Plautz, E.J., Milliken, G.W., Nudo, R.J., 2000. Effects of repetitive motor training on movement representation in adult squirrel monkeys: role of use versus learning. Neurobiol. Learn Mem. 74, 27–55.

Purves, D., Lichtman, J.W., 1985. Principles of Neural Development. Sinauer Associates, Sunderland, Massachusetts.

Rakic, P., 1976. Prenatal genesis of connections subserving ocular dominance in the rhesus monkey. Nature 261, 471–476.

Richards, L.J., Koester, S.E., Tuttle, R., O'Leary, D.D.M., 1997. Directed growth of early cortical axons is influenced by a chemoattractant released from an intermediate target. J. Neurosci. 17, 2445–2458.

Rodda, J.M., Graham, H.K., Carson, L., Galea, M.P., Wolfe, R., 2004. Sagittal gait patterns in spastic diplegia. J. Bone Joint Surg. 86, 251–258.

Rose, J., McGill, K.C., 2005. Neuromuscular activation and motor-unit firing characteristics in cerebral palsy. Dev. Med. Child Neurol. 47, 329–336.

Rose, J., Haskell, W.L., Gamble, J.G., Hamilton, R.L., Brown, D.A., Rinsky, L., 1994. Muscle pathology and clinical measures of disability in children with cerebral palsy. J. Orthop. Res. 12, 758–768.

Salimi, I., Friel, K., Martin, J.H., 2008. Pyramidal tract stimulation restores normal corticospinal tract

connections and visuomotor skill after early postnatal motor cortex activity blockade. J. Neurosci. 28, 7426–7434.

Sarnat, H.B., 1986. Cerebral dysgeneses and their influence on fetal muscle development. Brain Dev. 8, 495–499.

Scher, M.S., Ludington-Hoe, S., Kaffashi, F., Johnson, M.W., Holditch-Davis, D., Loparo, K.A., 2009. Neurophysiologic assessment of brain maturation after an eight-week trial of skin-to-skin contact on preterm infants. Clin. Neurophysiol. 120, 1812–1818.

Shepherd, G.M., 1994. Neurobiology, third ed. Oxford University Press, New York.

Sloper, J.J., Brodal, P., Powell, T.P., 1983. An anatomical study of the effects of unilateral removal of sensorimotor cortex in infant monkeys on the subcortical projections of the contralateral motor cortex. Brain 106, 707–716.

Spittle, A., Orton, J., Doyle, L.W., Boyd, R., 2007. Early developmental intervention programs post hospital discharge to prevent motor and cognitive impairments in preterm infants. Cochrane Database Syst. Rev. 18, CD005495.

Stanfield, B.B., 1992. The development of the corticospinal projection. Prog. Neurobiol. 38, 169–202.

Stanfield, B.B., O'Leary, D.D., 1985. The transient corticospinal projection from the occipital cortex during the postnatal development of the rat. J. Comp. Neurol. 238, 236–248.

Stigger, F., do Nascimento, P.S., Dutra, M.F., Couto, G.K., Ilha, J., Achaval, M., et al., 2011. Treadmill training induces plasticity in spinal motoneurons and sciatic nerve after sensorimotor restriction during early postnatal period: new insights into the clinical approach for children with cerebral palsy. Int. J. Dev. Neurosci. 29, 833–838.

Symington, A.J., Pinelli, J., 2006. Developmental care for promoting development and preventing morbidity in preterm infants. Cochrane Database Syst. Rev., CD001814.

Taylor, N., Dodd, K.J., Damiano, D.L., 2005. Progressive resistance exercise in physical therapy: a summary of systematic reviews. Phys. Ther. 85, 1208–1223.

Theroux, M.C., Akins, R.E., Barone, C., Boyce, B., Miller, F., Dabney, K.W., 2002. Neuromuscular junctions in cerebral palsy. Anesthesiology 96, 330–335.

Theroux, M.C., Oberman, K.G., Lahaye, L., Boyce, B., Duhadaway, D., Miller, F., et al., 2005. Dysmorphic neuromuscular junctions associated with motor ability in cerebral palsy. Muscle Nerve 32, 626–632.

Thorn, S.R., Regnault, T.R.H., Brown, L.D., Rozance, P.J., Keng, J., Roper, M., et al., 2009. Intrauterine growth restriction increases fetal gluconeogenic capacity and reduces messenger ribonucleic acid translation initiation and nutrient sensing in fetal liver and skeletal muscle. Endocrinology 150, 3021–3030.

Torres-Aleman, I., 2000. Serum growth factors and neuroprotective surveillance. Focus on IGF-1. Mol. Biol. 21, 153–160.

Valdez, G., Tapia, J.C., Kang, H., Clemenson, G.D., Gage, F.H., Lichtman, J.W., et al., 2010. Attenuation of age-related changes in mouse neuromuscular synapses by caloric restriction and exercise. Proc. Natl. Acad. Sci. USA 107, 14863–14868.

Vandenburgh, H.H., Hatfaludy, S., Karlisch, P., Shansky, J., 1990. Mechanically-induced alterations in cultured myotube growth. In: Pette, D. (Ed.), The Dynamic State of Muscle Fibres. De Gruyter, Berlin, pp. 151–164.

Vanderhaeghen, P., Polleux, F., 2004. Developmental mechanisms patterning thalamocortical projections: intrinsic, extrinsic and in between. Trends Neurosci. 27, 384–391.

Vickers, A., Ohlsson, A., Lacy, J.B., Horsley, A., 2004. Massage for promoting growth and development of preterm and low birth-weight infants. Cochrane Database Syst. Rev., CD000390.

Wallin, L., Eriksson, M., 2009. Newborn Individual Development and Assessment Program (NIDCAP): a systematic review of the literature. Worldviews Evid. Based Nurs. 6, 54–69.

Walton, K.D., Lieberman, D., Llinas, M., Begin, M., Llinas, R.R., 1992. Identification of a critical period for motor development in neonatal rats. Neuroscience 51, 763–767.

Westrup, B., Kleberg, A., von Eichwald, K., Stjernqvist, K., Lagercrantz, H., 2000. A randomized, controlled trial to evaluate the effects of the newborn individualized developmental care and assessment program in a Swedish setting. Pediatrics 105, 66–72.

Witzemann, V., 2006. Development of the neuromuscular junction. Cell Tissue Res. 326, 263–271.

Yau, K.-I., Chang, M.-H., 1993. Growth and body composition of preterm, small-for-gestational age infants at a postmenstrual age of 37–40 weeks. Early Hum. Dev. 33, 117–131.

# PART 3

## Impairments and Neuromuscular Adaptations to Impairments and Inactivity

# Functional effects of neural impairments and subsequent adaptations

4

Adel Abdullah Alhusaini

## Introduction

### Brief historical review

In 1861, William Little wrote the first medical descriptions of a disorder, named Little disease, that caused stiff, spastic muscles in the legs of affected young children (Bax et al., 2005; Jones et al., 2007; Shimony et al., 2008). Little disease is now known as the diplegia form of cerebral palsy (CP) (Pincus, 2000). A century later, Bax (1964) defined CP as 'a disorder of posture and movement due to a defect or lesion of the immature brain'. More recently Bax et al. (2005), through the American Academy for Cerebral Palsy and Developmental Medicine, proposed a new definition:

> Cerebral palsy (CP) describes a group of disorders of the development of movement and posture, causing activity limitation, that are attributed to non-progressive disturbances that occurred in the developing fetal or infant brain. The motor disorders of cerebral palsy are often accompanied by disturbances of sensation, cognition, communication, perception, and/or behaviour, and/or by a seizure disorder.

It is currently this definition that is most often used. CP is not a disease, per se, but rather, a term that describes a heterogeneous condition resulting in chronic motor impairment and other impairments. Although the brain lesion may be non-progressive, variable or progressive symptoms also occur due to the effects of growth and development (Eames et al., 1997; Klingbeil et al., 2004) and of adaptive changes occurring in the neuromusculoskeletal system (Carr and Shepherd, 1998; Gajdosik and Cicirello, 2001).

The movement disorders resulting from the lesion and from adaptive changes occurring as the infant grows and develops become more evident and more severe over time (Hanna et al., 2009). This progression seems to occur in particular as a result of adaptive changes occurring in muscle (Friden and Lieber, 2003; Malaiya et al., 2007; Mohagheghi et al., 2007).

Children with CP are already at a disadvantage, their levels of physical functioning having a lower starting point due to slowed development of muscle, bone and cardiorespiratory system following the insult to the brain (Damiano, 2006).

These children are usually less physically active than typically developing children, and their physical activity levels tend to decrease with increasing age (Maher et al., 2007).

## Prevalence and aetiology

Worldwide, CP is one of the most common causes of chronic disability in children. In Europe, the prevalence has risen from about 1.5 per 1000 live births in the 1960s to about 2.5 in the 1990s (Odding et al., 2006). However the overall prevalence of CP remains stable (Baxter, 2009), occurring in 2–2.5 individuals per 1000 live births in developed countries (Blair and Stanley, 1997; Hirtz et al., 2007; Odding et al., 2006; Sigurdardottir et al., 2009; Stanley et al., 2000). The worldwide cumulative incidence rate at 5–7 years was 2.7 cases of CP for 1000 birth cohorts, with approximately 36% of all CP occurring in infants weighing less than 2500 g at birth (Rosen and Dickinson, 1992). Improvement in the survival rate of infants with a low birth weight is accompanied by an increase in the rate of neurological impairment or disability among the survivors (Escobar et al., 1991; Kitchen et al., 1992). The prevalence of CP is higher among both the low birth weight children (Odding et al., 2006) and preterm-born children (Himpens et al., 2008).

Some form of motor impairment is present in all children with CP, with the majority (72–91%) reported to display spasticity (Odding et al., 2006). One study has found that 73% of children and adolescents with a spastic hemiplegic presentation also have soft tissue contractures (Odding et al., 2006). Multiple risk factors can be identified in over 70% of cases (Bialik and Givon, 2009; Jones et al., 2007). These risk factors cause injury to the developing brain and can occur in the prenatal (38%) or peri/neonatal (35%) periods (uncertain in 27%) in children born at term. In preterm children, brain injury is less frequent prenatally (17%) and more common in the perinatal period (49%) or occurs at an uncertain time (33%) (Himmelmann et al., 2005). Children with CP may have one or more risk factors, with the definitive cause difficult to determine (Jones et al., 2007). Prenatal risk factors are associated with infection, maternal drug or alcohol abuse, genetic causes, maternal epilepsy, mental retardation, hyperthyroidism, severe toxaemia, third trimester bleeding and low birth weight (less than

1500 g) (Pakula et al., 2009). Perinatal risk factors are associated with hypoxia or birth trauma such as brain haemorrhage during delivery and placental complications. Postnatal causes include head trauma, meningitis, encephalitis and brain infarcts (Bialik and Givon, 2009; Jones et al., 2007).

The evidence on lesion site from recent neuroimaging studies has consistently shown abnormalities in 70–90% of affected children, facilitating clinical classification into groups with early brain malformations, periventricular white matter injury, neonatal encephalopathies and focal ischaemic/haemorrhagic lesions (Hoon, 2005; Robinson et al., 2009; Wu et al., 2006). Using neuroimaging studies can assist clinicians in the early identification of injury before the establishment of marked motor deficits (Shimony et al., 2008) and has the potential to show a relationship between neuroanatomical structure and function (Feys et al., 2010).

## Classification of cerebral palsy

CP has multiple classification systems due to its heterogeneity (Bax et al., 2005). Using classification subcategories helps clinicians to build a better picture of the motor disorder which is important when comparing, predicting and evaluating any changes that occur over time. The traditional classification system for CP is based on topographical classification of motor impairment (the involvement of limbs, trunk and oropharynx). This classification focuses principally on the distributional pattern of the affected limbs (quadriplegia, diplegia, hemiplegia, monoplegia and triplegia) (Bialik and Givon, 2009).

Recently, a more comprehensive classification system (Bax et al., 2005; Bialik and Givon, 2009) has been proposed to obtain a complete picture of CP and is based on several components, including motor abnormalities, associated abnormalities, topographical distribution and neuroanatomical findings.

### Motor abnormalities

Motor abnormalities are divided into two themes based on the nature and type of the motor disorder, and functional motor abilities:

- The *nature and type of the motor disorder:* CP can be divided into two major physiologic classifications (Jones et al., 2007)—pyramidal and extrapyramidal, indicating the area of the brain that has been affected as well as the resulting predominant motor disorder. Pyramidal CP is the common subtype (Andersen et al., 2008; Himmelmann et al., 2006, 2005; Howard et al., 2005; Jain et al., 2008; McClelland et al., 2006) and results from defects or damage to the corticospinal pathways in the brain, also described as upper motor neuron damage. It is commonly associated with muscle weakness and loss of motor control, with spasticity illustrated by hyperreflexia, clonus, and extensor Babinski response. Extrapyramidal CP is caused by damage to nerve cells/neural pathways outside the pyramidal tracts in the basal ganglia or the cerebellum. It is typically divided into two subtypes, dyskinetic and ataxic.

- *Functional motor abilities*: Evaluating the functional consequences of CP is the key to treating children with CP. Several scales have been developed to measure function in all body areas. They include the *Gross Motor Function Classification System* (GMFCS), which is often used to evaluate children with CP and is internationally validated in relation to ambulation and activity limitations (Hanna et al., 2009; Palisano et al., 1997, 2006; Pfeifer et al., 2009; Rosenbaum et al., 2008). It is a five-level, age-categorized system developed to classify the severity of motor involvement in children with CP and is based on functional abilities and limitations. The scale has a section on infants that can be used to test those who are younger than 2 years of age. They can be given a provisional score until they are reviewed at 2 years old, as more clinical information becomes available (Gorter et al., 2009b). Infants are classified as level I when they move in and out of sitting and floor sit with both hands free to manipulate objects; they crawl on hands and knees, pull to stand and take steps holding on to furniture; and they walk between 18 months and 2 years of age without the need for any assistive mobility device. Infants at level V have physical impairments limiting voluntary control of movement; they are unable to maintain antigravity head and trunk postures in prone and sitting; and they require an adult's help to roll.

Other motor assessments for young children include the *Alberta Infant Motor Scale* (AIMS),

an observational assessment scale constructed to measure gross motor maturation in infants 1 month to the age of independent walking. Based upon the literature, 58 items were generated and organized into four positions: prone, supine, sitting and standing. Each item describes three aspects of motor performance—weight-bearing, posture and antigravity movements. The scale is unidimensional, and measures the construct of motor maturation (Piper et al., 1992, Piper and Darrah, 1994). The score for each position is summed to obtain a total raw score, then converted to an age-based percentile rank based on Canadian normative data. The AIMS has a high degree of test-retest, intra-rater and inter-rater reliability when it is used to measure typically developing infants (Cui et al., 2009; Jeng et al., 2000; Pin et al., 2010; Snyder et al., 2008).

The *Bayley Scales of Infant Development, second version* (BSID-II) was developed to assess the development of children between 1 and 42 months, and to discriminate typically from non-typically developing children. The BSID-II contains a motor scale (111 items, motor items), a mental scale (178 items) and a behavioural rating scale (30 items) (Bayley, 1993).

## Associated impairments

These include seizures, hearing and visual problems, cognitive and attentional deficits and emotional and behavioural issues. These impairments are classified as present or absent; if present, the extent to which they interfere with the individual's ability to function or participate in desired activity is noted.

## Topographical and neuroanatomical findings

Topographical classification is based on the parts of the body affected by motor impairments or limitations. Neuroanatomical findings evident on computed tomography or magnetic resonance imaging include ventricular enlargement, white matter loss, or brain anomaly. Recently developed functional neuroimaging tools now make it possible to study non-invasively several aspects of human brain functional reorganization in response to injury (Chugani et al., 1996; Maegaki et al., 1999; Staudt, 2010) (see Chapters 2 and 3).

# Motor impairments and muscle adaptations

In terms of daily living activities, children with motor impairments have less diversity and a slower rhythm in carrying out activities, with more time needed in activities and personal care (Beckung and Hagberg, 2002; Brown and Gordon, 1987; Ostensjo et al., 2004). Consequently, their participation in social engagements, active recreation, household tasks and activities away from home is reduced (Brown and Gordon, 1987). Although the activity and participation domains are more immediately relevant to the children and their parents, understanding CP at the impairment level clarifies whether an intervention is likely to be effective (Burridge et al., 2009) and to what extent the impairment, or combination of impairments, will limit activity in children with CP.

Upper motor neuron lesions, for example, those that occur in utero and in the perinatal period in infants with a potential to develop hemiplegia or diplegia, are categorized as having either positive or negative features (Barnes and Johnson, 2008; Kerr and Selber, 2003; Pandyan et al., 2005). The positive features, 'signs of presence', include increased reflex activity (hyperreflexia). The negative features, 'signs of absence', are weakness, delayed initiation or failure of muscle activation, reduced dexterity and co-ordination (i.e., reduced selective or task-specific motor control), sensory deficits and fatigue. Associated with these features are adaptive or secondary sequelae that occur over time. Some of the later-onset features relate to non-neurogenic, mechanical changes that develop as a consequence of the primary impairments (Turk et al., 2008) together with habitual patterns of active limb use or limb disuse. Morphological and mechanical changes include changes to muscle and tendon length (e.g., contractures) and changes in the mechanical properties of muscles and in connective tissues (Burridge et al., 2009; Mayer, 1997). Although the lesion that occurs in the developing brain is considered to be non-progressive, the secondary musculoskeletal pathology progresses over time (Boyd and Graham, 1997), as children grow and develop.

Currently we understand impairments and adaptations to be interrelated, at least in their cause and presentation, with activity limitations, but an understanding of which are the primary contributors to functional motor deficits is still in its infancy. Nevertheless, it seems certain that the neuromotor impairments with the greatest impact are decreased or impaired activation of muscles resulting in weakness and poor motor control/co-ordination. Clinicians have tended to concentrate on novel features of the upper motor neuron syndrome such as spasticity and have neglected to some extent the abnormalities of muscle activation and motor control together with the secondary or adaptive features. However, it is these combined features that lead to activity restrictions such as difficulty learning to walk and carrying out other activities of daily living (Turk et al., 2008). The focus in neurorehabilitation for both adults with stroke and children with CP is shifting to the lack of muscle activation, poor motor control, the subsequent loss of mobility, and their relation to the adaptive sequelae and function (Ada et al., 2006; Carr and Shepherd, 2003; Vaz et al., 2006).

## Impaired activation of motor neurons and poor motor control

Muscle weakness has been defined as a difficulty in generating and controlling the necessary voluntary muscle force for effective motor performance (Carr and Shepherd, 1998). Marked strength deficit is a major negative feature and has been well documented in children with CP compared to typically developing children (Damiano et al., 1995b; Eek and Beckung, 2008; Elder et al., 2003; Rose and McGill, 2005; Stackhouse et al., 2005; Wiley and Damiano, 1998). Inability to voluntarily activate the muscle to the appropriate level (i.e., to generate sufficient muscle force) is believed to be due to several different factors. Among those are loss of motor unit activation, changes in recruitment ordering, or changes in firing rates of agonist muscles, co-activation of antagonist muscles as well as morphological and mechanical changes in the muscles due to decreased physical activity or disuse (Damiano et al., 2000; Rose and McGill, 1998, 2005; Shepherd, 2001; Tedroff et al., 2008). In addition, muscle weakness may occur as a side effect of some pharmacological interventions such as botulinum toxin (BoNT-A) (Edgar, 2001; Saguil, 2005), although the latter is not typically given to infants under 2 years.

# Spasticity (reflexive response to stretch)

Spasticity is said to be the most common form of hypertonicity that affects the majority of children with CP (Sanger et al., 2003). It is defined as *'a motor disorder characterized by a velocity-dependent increase in tonic stretch reflexes with exaggerated tendon jerks, resulting from hyperexcitability of the stretch reflex, as one component of the upper motor neuron syndrome'* (Lance, 1980). Upper motor neuron syndrome is a clinical term used to indicate disruption of the corticospinal tract at any point along its course and may result in predominantly spastic types. The corticospinal tract descends through the corona radiata and internal capsule to reach the brainstem, midbrain, pons, then the medulla oblongata, and here it forms the pyramid (Filloux, 1996; Fitzgerald, 1992; Priori et al., 2006) and descends in the spinal cord.

The term spasticity is used to describe several different features and its use is frequently confusing. Typical tests of spasticity involve an examination of the muscle response to passive movement. Sanger et al. (2003) defined spasticity in terms of the features of the clinical examination as hypertonia in which one or both of the following signs are present: (1) resistance to externally imposed movement increases with increasing speed of stretch and varies with the direction of joint movement; and/or (2) resistance to externally imposed movement rises rapidly above a threshold speed or joint angle. Under the first criterion, an increase in stretch velocity does not mean a more exaggerated response to passive stretch (Powers et al., 1989). However, the resistance to passive movement must be different for high versus low speeds (Sanger et al., 2003).

The II (secondary) and Ia (primary) sensory neurons of the muscle spindle provide signals to the CNS about change in muscle length (tonic component) and the rate of change in length (phasic component), respectively. The synaptic connection between the Ia and II neurons with the alpha-motor neurone leads to stretch reflex activation (Matthew 1972 cited in Salazar-Torres et al., 2004). However, until now our understanding of spasticity is limited because spasticity is caused by several mechanisms which are more or less linked and associated with different clinical manifestations (Sindou, 2003).

From Lance's widely used definition, it is evident that the clinical symptom of spasticity is a velocity-dependent increase in tonic stretch reflexes at rest in response to passive movement. Gracies (2005b) simplified the wording of Lance's definition and presented it as 'a velocity-dependent increase in reflexes to phasic stretch, in the absence of volitional activity'(see Chapter 5). This definition emphasizes the exaggerated stretch reflex or hyperreflexia (triggered by phasic muscle stretch) as the prominent clinical sign of spasticity (Poon and Hui-Chan, 2009). The stretch reflex has a phasic and a tonic component (Alter, 2004). The phasic response is an initial burst of action potentials that results in a rapid rise of muscle tension, proportional to the velocity of the stretch. The tonic response is a later phase of slow (low-frequency) firing, lasting for the duration of the stretch, which is proportional to the amount of stretch.

In the past, spasticity was the focus of research and it was assumed that it can interfere with movement and positioning, contribute to the formation of contractures and musculoskeletal deformities over time, and be a source of discomfort by negatively impacting function, making caregiver tasks, such as transfers and dressing, more difficult (Cardoso et al., 2006; Koman et al., 2004; Petrillo and Knoploch, 1988; Suputtitada, 2000; Voerman et al., 2007). However, contracture is not necessarily linked to spasticity and reduction of spasticity may not prevent deformity. Tedroff et al. (2009) report the outcome of a prospective uncontrolled study on the long-term effect of BoNT-A on the lower limb muscles of children with pyramidal CP The study group is heterogeneous in terms of age (median 5 years 4 months, range 11 months to 17 years 8 months), GMFCS level (29% level I, 15% level II, 16% level III, 17% level IV, 23% level V), and topographical pattern (50% diplegic CP, 22% hemiplegic CP, 25% tetraplegic CP, 3% dyskinetic CP) Outcome measures were limited to the Modified Ashworth Scale (MAS) and joint range-of-motion measures to estimate muscle 'tone', made at a minimum before and 3 months after each injection. Injections were repeated, to a maximum of eight injections per muscle. They found a persistent reduction in muscle tone in the muscles injected but a progressive reduction in joint passive ranges, following an initial improvement. They found that BoNT-A can be effective in reducing muscle tone over a longer period, but not in preventing development of contractures in spastic muscles. They concluded that dissociation between the effects on muscle tone and range of motion (ROM) indicates that development of contractures is not coupled to increased muscle tone only, but might be caused by other mechanisms.

Until recently, little work had been done on the role of spasticity during active movement (Damiano et al., 2006) although passive stretch and active movement are likely to elicit different manifestations of spasticity (Fleuren et al., 2009). Spasticity is usually tested by reference to clinical measurements made while the patient lies in a relaxed position, although active voluntary movements such as walking are the target of clinical assessment and intervention (Burridge and McLellan, 2000). There are difficulties in studying reflex activity during active movement, possibly due to difficulty in differentiating it from voluntary muscle contraction (Fleuren et al., 2009). Spasticity during passive movement may be greater than, the same as, or less than during active voluntary movement. For this reason it is important not to assume that what is detected during passive examination will necessarily reflect what is happening during functional movements (Burne et al., 2005; Burridge and McLellan, 2000; Dietz, 2000; Fleuren et al., 2009).

Stretch reflex hyperexcitability has little functional consequence in spastic patients due to its disappearance during active movement in the agonist muscle although it may be manifest at rest (Ada et al., 1998; Burne et al., 2005; Morita et al., 2001; Nielsen et al., 2007). However, it should be pointed out that the functional significance of spasticity does not solely relate to the agonist muscle, but also to the antagonist muscles (Nielsen et al., 2007). Crenna (1998, 1999) carried out one of the very few investigations of reflex hyperactivity during active movement. He noted that abnormal stretch responses were more easily elicited during lengthening contractions around the time of ground contact of the stride than at other points in the cycle (Crenna, 1998). He attributed this to the floor contact as a critical event that may be more dependent on supraspinal rather than peripheral control, and the disruptions in movement in other parts of the cycle may be attributable to weakness, co-contraction and passive muscle properties, rather than to stretch responses. Dietz and Sinkjaer (2007)

showed in their review that oversensitive muscle stretch receptors (hyperreflexia) appear to make a relatively minor contribution to dysfunctional motor performance while secondary changes in mechanical muscle fibre properties have a major role in spastic movement disorder.

# Differentiation between neural (stretch reflex hypersensitivity) and mechanical factors

Clinicians and researchers frequently group the passive mechanical properties together with the neurally mediated phenomena and refer to them as spasticity. It is important to distinguish between reflex- and non-reflex-mediated stiffness in order to understand and reliably evaluate spasticity's mechanisms because it has consequences for treatment (Zhang et al., 2000). For example, Burridge and McLellan (2000) showed that stroke patients who had poor control of ankle movement and spasticity/reflex hyperactivity were more likely to respond well to functional electrical stimulation (FES), whereas those with mechanical resistance to passive movement and with normal muscle activation respond less well. Resistance to passive movement, however, occurs not only as a result of increased neuromuscular activity but also as a function of the passive mechanical properties of the muscle and its connective tissue content (passive stiffness) (Berger et al., 1984; Hufschmidt and Mauritz, 1985; Johnson, 2002; Sinkjaer et al., 1993). Therefore, these need to be differentiated from each other.

## Changes in reflex sensitivity as contracture develops

Research has shown that morphological modifications of muscle fibres due to disuse or immobilization lead to changes in their neural activation. In animal studies, Giroux et al. (2005) observed a loss of muscle weight and atrophy in both the soleus and peroneus longus of wistar female rats after four weeks of immobilization due to a reduction in mean fibre cross-sectional area (CSA). The morphological modifications were accompanied by an increase in the integrated EMG amplitude. Rosant et al. (2006) related the spindle discharges to stiffness of the muscle–tendon unit using a spindle efficacy index, defined as the ratio between spindle sensitivity and incremental stiffness. They verified that changes in muscle stiffness contribute to changes in spindle responses to stretch after 21 days of hindlimb unloading in rat soleus muscle.

There is a possibility that stretch reflex hypersensitivity may be an adaptive response evident sometime after injury and occurring in conjunction with length changes. The increased quantum of connective tissue found after immobilization in a shortened position reduces muscle compliance. This leads to an increase in the spindle response to a given amount of stretching force, as the pull is more efficiently transmitted to the spindles in a less extensible muscle (Gracies, 2005a, 2005b; Maier et al., 1972). Thus, when muscle fibres and spindles become short, sensitivity of the stretch reflex increases.

In human studies, although Blackburn et al. (2008) found that soleus stretch reflex latency and amplitude did not differ among individuals with high (men) or low (women) triceps surae stiffness, a significant number of authors were of a different opinion. Kamper et al. (2001) suggested that absolute muscle fibre length plays a highly significant role in the spastic reflex response to imposed movements of the elbow flexors in individuals with chronic spastic hemiplegia following stroke. In a similar way, Meinders et al. (1996) showed that stretch reflex activity varies with ankle position. Although the exact mechanisms responsible for the disuse-induced loss of neuromotor control are far from understood, it does seem that disuse results in reductions in motor performance that are likely related to adaptations in neurophysiologic parameters (Clark, 2009).

# Adaptive changes in passive mechanical properties of muscle

## Passive response to stretch (passive mechanical properties)

When a joint is moved passively by an external force to produce displacement, it simply resists the motion by exhibiting a measurable resistance even when skeletal muscles' motor neurons are quiescent and their myofibres are not actively contracting. This behaviour is called passive muscle stiffness (Schleip et al., 2006). The resistance is derived from the myotendinous unit and its

associated connective tissues, but also integrates resistance to motion provided by skin, the joint capsule and ligamentous structures.

## Muscle mechanical components

A muscle–tendon unit (MTU) is a composite structure that includes muscle fibres, the supportive connective tissues within and around the muscle belly, and dense regular connective tissue of the tendons that secure the MTU to bone (Gajdosik and Gajdosik, 2006). According to Hill's model (Fig. 4.1), these structures are arranged in three separate components and this explains the role of elastic energy in human movement (Hill 1938, cited in Wilson and Flanagan, 2008). They consist of a contractile component (CC), a series elastic component (SEC), and a parallel elastic component (PEC), each of which contributes to overall muscle tension and may be classified as either elastic or viscous (Alter, 2004).

The cross-bridge component is the active force-generating structure within the myofibrils and is composed of thousands of sarcomeres connected in series. The sarcomere is made of multiple actin and myosin filaments, and with their cross-bridges they produce contraction (Edman, 2003; Givli and Bhattacharya, 2009). The maximum force that can be generated by a muscle fibre or single sarcomere can be affected by the length of muscle, velocity of muscle contraction, type of contraction, frequency of stimulation, motor unit recruitment, and muscle fibre alignment and type (Trew and Everett, 2005). The active curve is obtained only indirectly

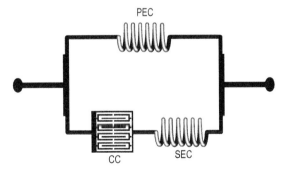

**Figure 4.1** • Hill's functional muscle model consists of a series elastic component (SEC), a contractile component (CC) and an elastic component (PEC) parallel to the CC.

[Adapted with slight modifications from Wilson and Flanagan (2008). The role of elastic energy in activities with high force and power requirements: a brief review. J Strength Cond Res, 22, 1705–1715, with permission from Wolters Kluwer Health.]

by subtracting the passive length–tension curve (measured in the absence of active simulation) from the total forces throughout the full length of the muscle (Gajdosik, 2001).

The series elastic component is a non-CC of muscle that lies in series with muscle fibres (Hill, 1950). It stores energy when stretched and makes a major contribution to the elasticity of the human skeleton (Hill, 1950). Tendons are the major representatives of the series elastic component, but the cross-bridges between actin and myosin, within the muscle fibre, may also contribute (Herzog, 1997). During passive stretch, the major deformation occurs more in the PEC than in the tendons (Wilson and Flanagan, 2008). The series elastic component's function is to transmit the forces of the contraction and to store and later release elastic energy (Lindstedt et al., 2002; Roberts, 2002; Wilson and Flanagan, 2008). Ishikawa et al. (2005) suggested that the elastic recoil takes place not as a spring-like bouncing but as a catapult action in natural human walking. It has been shown that the series elastic component adapts its properties according to the functional demand (Almeida-Silveira et al., 2000; Lindstedt et al., 2002; Roberts, 2002).

The PEC stores elastic energy in parallel to the CCs of a muscle. Passive elements, such as titin, act in parallel with both the contractile element and the series elastic component, or in parallel with only the contractile element (MacIntosh and MacNaughton, 2005). Increasing the muscle length, and stretching the PEC, increases the passive force or resting tension in muscle (passive force–length relationship) (Alter, 2004). Gajdosik (2001) suggested that the cytoskeleton of the sarcomere and intramuscular connective tissue constitute PECs that contribute to passive tension, modification of which could lead to a change in overall stiffness of the MTU.

## Sources of passive tension or stiffness

The structures that contribute the majority of the passive force at the MTU are not entirely known, but it is often assumed that connective tissue, its collagen content, titin filaments and desmin are a source of passive tension if the muscle is stretched beyond its resting length (Bensamoun et al., 2006; Gajdosik and Gajdosik, 2006; Lindstedt et al., 2002; Wang et al., 1993).

The connective tissues of muscle, divided into endomysium, perimysium and epimysium,

are usually considered to play a major role in the development of passive tension while not actively generating force (Gajdosik, 2001). The endomysium surrounds an individual muscle fibre (cell), the perimysium encircles a group of muscle fibres forming a fascicle, and the epimysium encircles all the fascicles to form the complete muscle (Purslow, 1989). The ensemble of these tissue sheaths, called the fascia, encloses the muscles and ultimately connects them at their ends to the tendons (Van Loocke, 2007). Overstretching of the muscle fibre bundles is prevented by the perimysium and is thought to be the major contributor to passive muscle resistance due to its relative abundance within all components of the connectives tissues (Gajdosik, 2001; Purslow, 1989).

The passive mechanical properties of muscle are dependent on the amount, type and architectural organization of collagen fibrils (Mockford and Caulton, 2010). Booth et al. (2001) have shown that collagen is increased in the spastic muscles of children with CP and that the amount of total collagen correlates with the severity of their disorder. The distribution of this increased collagen is consistent with it playing a role in increased muscle stiffness, and collagen content in muscle can change in response to altered use patterns (Herbert, 1988; Waterman-Storer, 1991) or pathologies (Booth et al., 2001).

Among the intracellular proteins, which include titin, nebulin, desmin, troponin and tropomyosin, titin and desmin are the most important contributors to the resistive force during passive muscle stretching (Balogh et al., 2005; Gajdosik and Gajdosik, 2006; Prado et al., 2005). The giant titin molecules' protein (also called connectin) is a subcellular component macromolecule that connects the ends of the myosin filament to the Z-disk and overlaps in the Z-disk and M-band of the sarcomere, forming a continuous elastic filament system inside the myofibre (Craig and Padrón, 2004; Maruyama and Kimura, 2000; Skeie, 2000). Consequently, titin is frequently assumed to be the main structural element responsible for the even distribution of sarcomeric length in non-activated muscle (Goulding et al., 1997; MacIntosh and MacNaughton, 2005).

Strain of the titin protein of the endosarcomeric cytoskeleton and of the desmin protein of the exosarcomeric cytoskeleton within the muscle fibre contribute to increased passive resistance during passive lengthening (Bartoo et al., 1997; Gajdosik et al., 2005; Wang et al., 1993). Anderson (2002) suggested that the presence of desmin is crucial and titin is unlikely to be responsible for the large increase in passive stiffness observed in whole soleus muscles when desmin is lacking. Desmin (also called skeletin) is an intermediate-size protein of the exosarcomeric cytoskeleton oriented in both the transverse and longitudinal planes of the muscle cell (Tokuyasu et al., 1983; Wang et al., 1993). It serves to interconnect myofibrils at the level of their Z-bands, and to connect Z-bands in series in a single myofibril and in parallel in adjacent myofibrils (Tokuyasu et al., 1983). This arrangement creates a mechanical structural framework of the serial and parallel mechanical connections to form a network for passive force transmission (Boriek et al., 2001; Gajdosik and Gajdosik, 2006). Desmin's protein will lengthen as the sarcomere is stretched. Hence, it is thought to contribute to the passive muscle stiffness when stretched (Gajdosik and Gajdosik, 2006).

Although muscle spasticity is neural in origin, there is strong evidence that spastic muscles are not normal and have an altered intrinsic mechanical structure secondary to spasticity (Foran et al., 2005; Friden and Lieber, 2003; Lieber and Friden, 2002; Smith et al., 2009), together with lack of or altered patterns of use. Sinkjaer and Magnussen (1994) suggested that the reduced maximal voluntary force generation in the spastic limb is not caused by changed contractile properties in the spastic muscles. Friden and Lieber (2003) found that muscle cells obtained from patients with spasticity had a decreased resting sarcomere length and nearly double the elastic modulus of the stress–strain relationship in fibres compared with normal muscle cells. They suggested that dramatic remodelling of intracellular (such as titin) or extracellular (such as collagen) muscle structural components were the structural basis for their observations of increased viscoelastic properties. Details of data demonstrating that titin is actually altered secondary to spasticity are lacking but there is circumstantial evidence to suggest that it is possible (Foran et al., 2005).

The passive mechanical properties of isolated muscle cells and small muscle fibre bundles are two structures that may be altered. Lieber et al. (2003) used single fibres and small bundles of muscle cells (5–50 fibres) ensheathed by the connective tissue matrix of the muscle tissue to demonstrate the difference in the mechanical properties of spastic

muscle tissue bundles compared with normal muscle fibre bundles. They found that the spastic single fibres were stiffer than the non-spastic single fibres, even though the non-spastic bundles were remarkably stiffer than the spastic bundles. They also found a large amount of poorly organized extracellular material in spastic bundles compared with normal bundles. In addition, in the spastic muscle bundles, 40% of the CSA was occupied by muscle fibres, compared to 95% in normal muscle bundles (Lieber et al., 2004). Malaiya et al. (2007) collected 3D ultrasound images of the medial gastrocnemius muscle belly in 16 children with pyramidal hemiplegic CP (mean age: 7.8 years; range: 4–12 years) and 15 typically developing children (mean age: 9.5 years; range: 4–13 years). They found reduced muscle volume and length of the paretic limb compared to the non-paretic limb without decrease in fascicle length. The authors attributed these changes to the lack of cross-sectional growth. Further investigation is necessary. Mirbagheri et al. (2008) suggested that using the non-paretic limb may not be an appropriate control for the study of neuromuscular properties in hemiparetics because it is not subject to the forces and usage found in a typically developing child.

In histological studies, Rose et al. (1994) showed that children with CP have abnormal variation in the size of muscle fibres and altered distribution of fibre types. Changes in muscle architecture are not limited to passive condition only, but also affect the contractile properties of muscle fascicles (Gao and Zhang, 2008). Ito et al. (1996) studied the histopathology of spastic muscles in nine children with pyramidal CP (age range: 6–18 years) using specimens obtained from the gastrocnemius muscles during orthopaedic operations. They found changes in fibre type distribution, i.e., type 1 fibre predominance and type 2B fibre deficiency. In agreement with previous observations, Marbini et al. (2002) performed muscle biopsy on adductor longus (16 cases) and triceps surae muscles (four cases) during tendon lengthening operations for 20 children with pyramidal CP aged from 4 to 16 years old (mean: 9.4 years). They showed mild myopathic changes, type 1 predominance, and type 1 and type 2 hypotrophy. Mohagheghi et al. (2008) found in an in vivo study of 18 children with diplegia (aged 2–15 years) and 50 typically developing children that children with diplegia had shorter fascicle lengths in the gastrocnemius muscle compared to those typically developing, irrespective of whether absolute or normalized (against leg length) fascicle lengths were compared. Shortland et al. (2002) reported architectural variables of the medial gastrocnemius in five normally developing adults (aged 24–36 years) and five typically developing children (aged 7–11 years), and in seven children with spastic diplegia (aged 6–13 years) who had plantarflexion contractures of greater than 10° with the knee extended. They showed a dependence of deep fascicle angle (increasing with increasing plantarflexion) and fascicle length (decreasing with increasing plantarflexion) on ankle joint angle. However, the architecture of the medial gastrocnemius (fascicle length) in normally developing children and children with spastic diplegia does not differ greatly at a common angle of 30° of plantarflexion or at the resting ankle angles.

## Stiffness, hysteresis and flexibility definitions

Stiffness is a term regularly used when referring to the passive mechanical properties of a muscle. Passive myotendinous stiffness (MTS) is defined as the mechanical response to a tensile load on the non-contracting muscle (Harlaar et al., 2000). It refers to the ratio of the change in tensile force to the change in myotendinous length associated with joint motion (Δ force/Δ length) (Blackburn et al., 2004; Herbert, 1993). In biomechanics, stiffness can be used to model the force/deformation relationship of many structures from a single muscle fibre to entire limbs (Wilson and Flanagan, 2008). The calf myotendinous unit, as with most

biological tissues, acts viscoelastically by exhibiting both elastic and viscous properties at the same time in the absence of neural activation (Alter, 2004; Davidoff, 1992; Taylor et al., 1990).

An elastic component deforms instantaneously when load is externally applied to it but resumes its original shape instantly when the applied loads are removed (Hosford, 2010). Therefore, the loading and unloading paths for an elastic material overlap and involve length changes in proportion to the applied force. Purely elastic materials do not dissipate energy (heat) when a load is applied, then removed (i.e., elastic implies the ability to deform reversibly without loss of energy) (Fig. 4.2) (Gosline et al., 2002). Viscous properties are characterized as time-dependent and rate change-dependent proportional to the applied force. They exhibit gradual deformation and recovery when subjected to loading and unloading (Fig. 4.2) (Alter, 2004; Levin and Wyman, 1927; Taylor et al., 1990).

Hysteresis is seen in a viscoelastic material as the difference between loading and unloading stress–strain relationships, which may be quantified as the area between the loading and unloading portions of the torque vs. range-of-motion curve (hysteresis loop). It is expressed in terms of newton-metres-degrees (Nm-deg) (Taylor et al., 1990; Trevino et al., 2004). This area between loading and unloading curves demonstrates the energy lost as heat due to internal damping, while the area under the unloading curve is the energy recovered in the elastic recoil (Hajrasouliha et al., 2005). In other words, if the hysteresis is low, the percentage of energy dissipated during sequential flexion and extension of a joint would be small (Kubo et al., 2005).

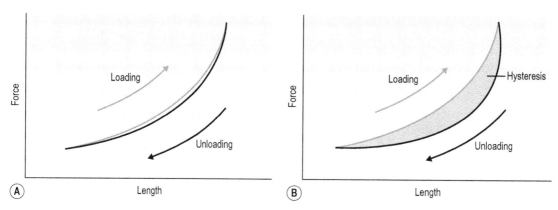

**Figure 4.2** • Hypothetical illustration of **(A)** elastic material and **(B)** viscoelastic material and typical hysteresis loop (the area within the loop) resulting from cyclical plantarflexion and dorsiflexion of ankle joint.

It is important to distinguish between 'muscle stiffness' and 'joint flexibility' as they are not the same and frequently cause confusion (Aquino et al., 2006). Flexibility, also referred to as muscle extensibility, is frequently taken to infer muscle length regardless of the force that causes the change in length (Aquino et al., 2006; Blackburn, 2004). On the other hand, passive muscle stiffness reflects the resistance of the myotendinous unit to the force that is attempting to change its length. The greater the stiffness, the more force required. This is quantified mechanically by measuring the rate of change of the joint angle with respect to change in torque [stiffness ($\kappa$) = $\Delta$ force/$\Delta$ length (Gavronski et al., 2007). Therefore, flexibility [$\Delta$ length] is a component of, but is not the same as, stiffness. Magnusson et al. (1996) reported an increase in the ROM for hamstring muscles after training, without reduction in the passive stiffness of the muscle–tendon unit. These authors concluded that the mechanism for improved joint ROM is an enhanced stretch tolerance rather than a change in muscle mechanical or viscoelastic properties (see Chapters 6 and 7).

### Stiffness measurement

Biomechanical measures, unlike most clinical scales, offer a more precise way to quantify the resistance offered by a muscle group at rest to an imposed limb displacement or muscle stretch (Calota and Levin, 2009; Johnson, 2002). This type of measurement allows torque and angle to be collected simultaneously as the joint is passively moved through its whole range (Moseley et al., 2001). Oscillatory rotations of the ankle joint in plantarflexion–dorsiflexion have been used in the past to provide an effective objective assessment of foot and ankle passive mechanical function (Agarwal and Gottlieb, 1977; Evans et al., 1983; Goddard et al., 1969; Gottlieb et al., 1978). The passive torque–angle relation curve at the ankle is a sigmoidal curve having C-shaped relations between torque and angle when the joint is moved between the two ends of its ROM by externally applied loads (Gottlieb and Agarwal, 1988; Kostyukov, 1998). Sinusoidal oscillation of the ankle joint can be generated with a complex torque motor such as Kin–Com isokinetic dynamometer (Bressel and McNair, 2001) or with more simple and portable measurement using the therapist's hand to perform the oscillation using, for example, the torque

ROM (TROM) device (Trevino et al., 2004) or the apparatus used in the experiments summarized in the Annotation B.

More information may be gained when biomechanical and neurophysiological, i.e. electromyography (EMG), measures are combined. One advantage of monitoring EMG signals is the possibility of detecting voluntary muscle activation that may interfere with the identification of, or influence, the reflex response. Several recent studies have recommended using a combination of electromyography and biomechanical measurements as a more accurate method of evaluating spasticity and its functional effects (Biering-Sorensen et al., 2006; Kim et al., 2005; Kumar et al., 2006; Malhotra et al., 2008).

## Clinical implications

One of the most prominent features of the central nervous system is plasticity and the ability to adapt to changes in the environment, store information in memory to help learn skills and capacity to reorganize and recover from injury (Dobkin, 2003; Johnston, 2004; Wittenberg, 2009). This neuronal plasticity is enhanced in the developing brain and children have the ability to learn motor skills or recover from certain brain injuries more quickly than adults (Johnston, 2009).

This adaptability is not limited to the central nervous system. Skeletal muscle is a very adaptable tissue in its response to its working environment (McComas, 1994; O'Dwyer et al., 1989; Smith et al., 2009). Hodapp et al. (2009) have shown in children with CP that treadmill training can induce changes in the modulation of short latency reflexes during gait. The neuromuscular system is adaptable and adaptation in one system may influence the other. For example, McComas et al. (1973) showed the trans-synaptic changes that take place after degeneration of corticospinal fibres that indicate a reduction in the number of functional motor units in adults after stroke. This leads to muscle wasting adaptively as a consequence of denervation. Skeletal muscle adaptations also occur over time due to disuse or training (functional requirements). The primary morphological adaptations to strength training, for example, involve an increase in the CSA of the whole muscle and of individual muscle fibres, which is due to an increase in myofibrillar size and number, hyperplasia (an increase in the number of muscle fibres), changes in fibre type, muscle architecture, and myofilament density, and also in the structure of connective tissue and tendons (Folland and Williams, 2007). Morphological adaptations depend on exercise intensity (Fry, 2004) and can be reversible with loss of training (Mujika and Padilla, 2000a, 2000b).

Understanding impairments and adaptations allows us to review the efficacy of diverse interventions (Shepherd, 2001), including BoNT-A injections. Skeletal muscle represents an example of the relationship between structure and function by adapting to the level of use imposed upon it (Lieber, 1988; Salmons and Henriksson, 1981; Stewart and Rittweger, 2006). Gao and co-workers (Gao and Zhang, 2008; Gao et al., 2009) found biomechanical changes at the joint originating from the muscle fascicles, and changes at the fascicle and joint levels were correlated in stroke survivors. These changes included decreased length and reduced pennation angle of the muscle fascicles, and decreased ROM and increased stiffness during dorsiflexion at the joint.

Although some studies have suggested that strengthening muscle is not effective in children and adolescents with CP, inasmuch as an increase in muscle volume is not transferable to improvement in function (McNee et al., 2009; Scholtes et al., 2010), many other recent studies have shown that strengthening exercises can be a useful adjunct to improve gait in patients with pyramidal CP, without significant adverse effects or increased muscle tone (Andersson et al., 2003; Damiano et al., 2002; Gorter et al., 2009a; Kanda et al., 2004; Kumar et al., 2010; Lee et al., 2008; Mattern-Baxter et al., 2009; Sterba, 2007; Verschuren et al., 2007; Williams and Pountney, 2007). Functional strength training may also enhance motor development in younger children and counteract deterioration in youth (Mockford and Caulton, 2008; Sorsdahl et al., 2010) and adult life. It is also likely to stimulate motor learning. Thus, strengthening exercises continue to be a major component of any rehabilitation programme (Givon, 2009) and it is likely that effectiveness in transferring increased strength to improved function depends on the type of exercise practiced: for example, functional strength training such as sit-to-stand with increasing load and repetitions (Liao et al., 2007) versus single joint weight-lifting exercise (see Chapter 11).

Exercises tested in children include progressive resistance exercise (Behm et al., 2008; Damiano et al., 1995a; Eek et al., 2008; Mockford and Caulton, 2008; Morton et al., 2005; Scholtes et al., 2008), eccentric exercises (Reid et al., 2010), task-oriented strength training directed toward optimizing the development of motor control (Blundell et al., 2003; Katz-Leurer et al., 2009; Liao et al., 2007; Salem and Godwin, 2009; Smith et al., 1999; Sorsdahl et al., 2010) and progressive treadmill training (Willoughby et al., 2009). The focus has shifted from spasticity reduction and movements facilitated by the therapist to exercise training, as improved strength and motor control are more related to motor function (Ross and Engsberg, 2007) and exercises have not been found to increase spasticity in children with CP (Fowler et al., 2001; Mockford and Caulton, 2008). There appear to be no studies of muscle strength in infancy but it may become possible in future studies to estimate strength in the very young by testing with ultrasound.

It is known that increased calf muscle stiffness of either neural or mechanical origin affects functional motor performance in children with CP. Premature and excessive activation of calf muscles has been reported in the stance phase of walking (Crenna, 1998), and premature activation of calf muscles in the terminal swing phase can cause excessive plantarflexion and varus (Brunt and Scarborough, 1988), with consequent functional restriction and an increased risk of tripping (Aiona and Sussman, 2004). However, walking problems in children with CP are not based solely on neural factors (spasticity). Dietz and Berger (1983) reported increased tension of the triceps surae during the stance phase of gait without an associated increase in EMG activity, and Dietz et al. (1981) observed reduced dorsiflexion during the swing phase in individuals with spasticity and rigidity. They postulated that this was not a result of abnormal stretch reflex activity either in the plantarflexors or from recruitment failure of the tibialis anterior muscle, but rather an increase in passive resistance in the plantarflexors. Increased passive muscle torque also increases the resistance to forward rotation of the tibia over the foot (i.e., dorsiflexion) during stance phase of gait in children with CP (Tardieu et al., 1989). Further, increased passive stiffness can potentially impair gait efficiency by changing the amount of elastic energy stored in and returned from the soft tissues in proportion to the resistance of these tissues to deformation (Fonseca et al., 2001).

Passive plantarflexor stiffness has been found to account for an additional 11% of the variance in walking speed (Salsich and Mueller, 2000) and is significantly correlated with balance control, ankle proprioception and evertor peak torque (Santos and Liu, 2008).

## Conclusions and statement of the problem

This chapter has reviewed aspects of the active and passive mechanical properties of lower limb muscles in children with CP. In addition to changes in involuntary (reflexes) and voluntary muscle activation, adaptations of the viscoelastic properties of muscles and connective tissue are significant factors with potential to interfere with motor development and functional performance. These changes need to be identified and described in order to plan and implement meaningful interventions. Chapter 11 describes interventions targeting muscle integrity as part of training lower limb weight-bearing and functionality. Chapters 6 and 7 provide an up-to-date overview of the status of research into muscle.

It is likely that future research will be directed toward documenting the longitudinal development of muscle changes from earliest infancy and answering questions of interest to those who plan and implement interventions for infants with CP. What are the characteristics of adaptive muscle changes? Are these changes related to deficiencies in growth and development of muscle? What part does physical inactivity and stereotyped, limited motor activity play in muscle changes? Are they preventable by targeted exercise and training programmes?

Increasing attention is being directed to the passive mechanical properties of the ankle plantarflexors in children with CP as an independent factor making a major contribution to functional disabilities. Investigation of the characteristics of non-reflexive components of muscle, independent of neural activation, has been part of ongoing examinations of spastic muscle in children. A series of four small investigations was completed recently with children aged 4 to 10 years, with hemiplegia or diplegia. A control group of age-matched able-bodied children was used for comparison. This work is the focus of Annotation B.

## References

Ada, L., Vattanasilp, W., O'Dwyer, N.J., Crosbie, J., 1998. Does spasticity contribute to walking dysfunction after stroke? J. Neurol. Neurosurg. Psychiatry. 64, 628–635.

Ada, L., O'Dwyer, N., O'Neill, E., 2006. Relation between spasticity, weakness and contracture of the elbow flexors and upper limb activity after stroke: an observational study. Disabil. Rehabil. 28, 891–897.

Agarwal, G.C., Gottlieb, G.L., 1977. Oscillation of the human ankle joint in response to applied sinusoidal torque on the foot. J. Physiol. 268, 151–176.

Aiona, M.D., Sussman, M.D., 2004. Treatment of spastic diplegia in patients with cerebral palsy: Part II. J. Pediatr. Orthop. B 13, S13–S38.

Almeida-Silveira, M.I., Lambertz, D., Perot, C., Goubel, F., 2000. Changes in stiffness induced by hindlimb suspension in rat Achilles tendon. Eur. J. Appl. Physiol. 81, 252–257.

Alter, M.G., 2004. Science of Flexibility. Human Kinetics, Champaign, IL.

Andersen, G.L., Irgens, L.M., Haagaas, I., Skranes, J.S., Meberg, A.E., Vik, T., 2008. Cerebral palsy in Norway: prevalence, subtypes and severity. Eur. J. Paediatr. Neurol. 12, 4–13.

Anderson, J., Joumaa, V., Stevens, L., Neagoe, C., Li, Z., Mounier, Y., et al., 2002. Passive stiffness changes in soleus muscles from desmin knockout mice are not due to titin modifications. Pflüg. Arch. Eur. J. Phy. 444, 771–776.

Andersson, C., Grooten, W., Hellsten, M., Kaping, K., Mattsson, E., 2003. Adults with cerebral palsy: walking ability after progressive strength training. Dev. Med. Child Neurol. 45, 220–228.

Aquino, C.F., Goncalves, G.G., Fonseca, S.T., Mancini, M.C., 2006. Analysis of the relation between flexibility and passive stiffness of the hamstrings. Rev. Bras. Med. Esporte 12, 175–179.

Balogh, J., Li, Z., Paulin, D., Arner, A., 2005. Desmin filaments influence myofilament spacing and lateral compliance of slow skeletal muscle fibers. Biophys. J. 88, 1156–1165.

Barnes, M.P., Johnson, G.R., 2008. Upper Motor Neurone Syndrome and Spasticity: Clinical Management and Neurophysiology. Cambridge University Press, Cambridge.

Bartoo, M.L., Linke, W.A., Pollack, G.H., 1997. Basis of passive tension and stiffness in isolated rabbit myofibrils. Am. J. Physiol. 273, C266–C276.

Bax, M., Goldstein, M., Rosenbaum, P., Leviton, A., Paneth, N., Dan, B., Executive Committee for the Definition of Cerebral Palsy, 2005. Proposed definition and classification of cerebral palsy, April 2005. Dev. Med. Child Neurol. 47, 571–576.

Bax, M.C., 1964. Terminology and classification of cerebral palsy. Dev. Med. Child Neurol. 6, 206-204.

Baxter, P., 2009. Preventing cerebral palsy: hidden improvements. Dev. Med. Child Neurol. 51, 335.

Bayley, S. 1993. Bayley scales infant development kit.

Beckung, E., Hagberg, G., 2002. Neuroimpairments, activity limitations, and participation restrictions in children with cerebral palsy. Dev. Med. Child Neurol. 44, 309-316.

Behm, D.G., Faigenbaum, A.D., Falk, B., Klentrou, P., 2008. Canadian Society for Exercise Physiology position paper: resistance training in children and adolescents. Appl. Physiol. Nutr. Metab. 33, 547-561.

Bensamoun, S., Stevens, L., Fleury, M.J., Bellon, G., Goubel, F., Ho Ba Tho, M.C., 2006. Macroscopic-microscopic characterization of the passive mechanical properties in rat soleus muscle. J. Biomech. 39, 568-578.

Berger, W., Horstmann, G., Dietz, V., 1984. Tension development and muscle activation in the leg during gait in spastic hemiparesis: independence of muscle hypertonia and exaggerated stretch reflexes. J. Neurol. Neurosurg. Psychiatry 47, 1029-1033.

Bialik, G.M., Givon, U., 2009. Cerebral palsy: classification and etiology. Acta Orthop. Traumatol. Turc. 43, 77-80.

Biering-Sorensen, F., Nielsen, J.B., Klinge, K., 2006. Spasticity—assessment: a review. Spinal Cord 44, 708-722.

Blackburn, J.T., 2004. The relationship between muscle stiffness and spinal stretch reflex sensitivity in the triceps surae. Ph.D., The University of North Carolina at Chapel Hill.

Blackburn, J.T., Riemann, B.L., Padua, D.A., Guskiewicz, K.M., 2004. Sex comparison of extensibility, passive, and active stiffness of the knee flexors. Clin. Biomech. (Bristol, Avon) 19, 36-43.

Blackburn, J.T., Padua, D.A., Guskiewicz, K.M., 2008. Muscle stiffness and spinal stretch reflex sensitivity in the triceps surae. J. Athl. Train. 43, 29-36.

Blair, E., Stanley, F.J., 1997. Issues in the classification and epidemiology of cerebral palsy. Ment. Retard. Dev. Disabil. Res. Rev. 3, 184-193.

Blundell, S.W., Shepherd, R.B., Dean, C.M., Adams, R.D., Cahill, B.M., 2003. Functional strength training in cerebral palsy: a pilot study of a group circuit training class for children aged 4-8 years. Clin. Rehabil. 17, 48-57.

Booth, C.M., Cortina-Borja, M.J., Theologis, T.N., 2001. Collagen accumulation in muscles of children with cerebral palsy and correlation with severity of spasticity. Dev. Med. Child Neurol. 43, 314-320.

Boriek, A.M., Capetanaki, Y., Hwang, W., Officer, T., Badshah, M., Rodarte, J., et al., 2001. Desmin integrates the three-dimensional mechanical properties of muscles. Am. J. Physiol. Cell Physiol. 280, C46-C52.

Boyd, R., Graham, H.K., 1997. Botulinum toxin A in the management of children with cerebral palsy: indications and outcome. Eur. J. Neurol. 4, S15-S21.

Bressel, E., McNair, P.J., 2001. Biomechanical behavior of the plantar flexor muscle–tendon unit after an Achilles tendon rupture. Am. J. Sports Med. 29, 321-326.

Brown, M., Gordon, W.A., 1987. Impact of impairment on activity patterns of children. Arch. Phys. Med. Rehabil. 68, 828-832.

Brunt, D., Scarborough, N., 1988. Ankle muscle activity during gait in children with cerebral palsy and equinovarus deformity. Arch. Phys. Med. Rehabil. 69, 115-117.

Burne, J.A., Carleton, V.L., O'Dwyer, N.J., 2005. The spasticity paradox: movement disorder or disorder of resting limbs? J. Neurol. Neurosurg. Psychiatry. 76, 47-54.

Burridge, J.H., McLellan, D.L., 2000. Relation between abnormal patterns of muscle activation and response to common peroneal nerve stimulation in hemiplegia. J. Neurol. Neurosurg. Psychiatry 69, 353-361.

Burridge, J.H., Turk, R., Notley, S.V., Pickering, R.M., Simpson, D.M., 2009. The relationship between upper limb activity and impairment in post-stroke hemiplegia. Disabil. Rehabil. 31, 109-117.

Calota, A., Levin, M.F., 2009. Tonic stretch reflex threshold as a measure of spasticity: implications for clinical practice. Top. Stroke Rehabil. 16, 177-188.

Cardoso, E.S., Rodrigues, B.M., Barroso, M., Menezes, C.J., Lucena, R.S., Nunes, D.B., et al., 2006. Botulinum toxin type A for the treatment of the spastic equinus foot in cerebral palsy. Pediatr. Neurol. 34, 106-109.

Carr, J.H., Shepherd, R.B., 1998. Neurological Rehabilitation: Optimizing Motor Performance. Butterworth-Heinemann, Oxford; Boston.

Carr, J.H., Shepherd, R.B., 2003. Stroke Rehabilitation: Guidelines for Exercise and Training to Optimize Motor Skill. Butterworth-Heinemann, Scotland; New York.

Chugani, H.T., Muller, R.A., Chugani, D.C., 1996. Functional brain reorganization in children. Brain Dev. 18, 347-356.

Clark, B.C., 2009. In vivo alterations in skeletal muscle form and function after disuse atrophy. Med. Sci. Sports Exerc. 41, 1869-1875.

Craig, R., Padrón, R., 2004. Molecular structure of the sarcomere. In: Engel, A.G., Franzini-Armstrong, C. (Eds.), Myology, third ed. McGraw-Hill, New York, pp. 129-166.

Crenna, P., 1998. Spasticity and 'spastic' gait in children with cerebral palsy. Neurosci. Biobehav. Rev. 22, 571-578.

Crenna, P., 1999. Pathophysiology of lengthening contractions in human spasticity: a study of the hamstring muscles during locomotion. Pathophysiology 5, 283-297.

Cui, W., Yucheng, X., Zhuo, L., 2009. Reliability study of the Alberta infant motor scale in normal infants. Chin. J. Rehabil. Med. 10, 012.

Damiano, D.L., 2006. Activity, activity, activity: rethinking our physical therapy approach to cerebral palsy. Phys. Ther. 86, 1534-1540.

Damiano, D.L., Kelly, L.E., Vaughn, C.L., 1995a. Effects of quadriceps femoris muscle strengthening on crouch gait in children with spastic diplegia. Physi. Ther. 75, 658-667. (discussion 668-671).

Damiano, D.L., Vaughan, C.L., Abel, M.F., 1995b. Muscle response to heavy resistance exercise in children with spastic cerebral palsy. Dev. Med. Child Neurol. 37, 731-739.

Damiano, D.L., Martellotta, T.L., Sullivan, D.J., Granata, K.P., Abel, M.F., 2000. Muscle force production and functional performance in spastic cerebral palsy: relationship of cocontraction. Arch. Phys. Med. Rehabil. 81, 895–900.

Damiano, D.L., Dodd, K., Taylor, N.F., 2002. Should we be testing and training muscle strength in cerebral palsy? Dev. Med. Child Neurol. 44, 68–72.

Damiano, D.L., Laws, E., Carmines, D.V., Abel, M.F., 2006. Relationship of spasticity to knee angular velocity and motion during gait in cerebral palsy. Gait Posture 23, 1–8.

Davidoff, R.A., 1992. Skeletal muscle tone and the misunderstood stretch reflex. Neurology 42, 951–963.

Dietz, V., 2000. Spastic movement disorder. Spinal Cord 38, 389–393.

Dietz, V., Berger, W., 1983. Normal and impaired regulation of muscle-stiffness in gait—a new hypothesis about muscle hypertonia. Exp. Neurol. 79, 680–687.

Dietz, V., Sinkjaer, T., 2007. Spastic movement disorder: impaired reflex function and altered muscle mechanics. Lancet Neurol. 6, 725–733.

Dietz, V., Quintern, J., Berger, W., 1981. Electrophysiological studies of gait in spasticity and rigidity. Evidence that altered mechanical properties of muscle contribute to hypertonia. Brain 104, 431–449.

Dobkin, B., 2003. The Clinical Science of Neurologic Rehabilitation. Oxford University Press, New York.

Eames, N.W.A., Baker, R.J., Cosgrove, A.P., 1997. Defining gastrocnemius length in ambulant children. Gait Posture 6, 9–17.

Edgar, T.S., 2001. Clinical utility of botulinum toxin in the treatment of cerebral palsy: comprehensive review. J. Child Neurol. 16, 37–46.

Edman, K., 2003. Contractile performance of skeletal muscle fibres. In: Komi, P.V. (Ed.), Strength and Power in Sport, second ed. Blackwell Science, Osney Mead, Oxford; Malden, MA.

Eek, M.N., Beckung, E., 2008. Walking ability is related to muscle strength in children with cerebral palsy. Gait Posture 28, 366–371.

Eek, M.N., Tranberg, R., Zugner, R., Alkema, K., Beckung, E., 2008. Muscle strength training to improve gait function in children with

cerebral palsy. Dev. Med. Child Neurol. 50, 759–764.

Elder, G.C., Kirk, J., Stewart, G., Cook, K., Weir, D., Marshall, A., et al., 2003. Contributing factors to muscle weakness in children with cerebral palsy. Dev. Med. Child Neurol. 45, 542–550.

Escobar, G., Littenberg, B., Petitti, D., 1991. Outcome among surviving very low birthweight infants: a meta-analysis. Arch. Dis. Child. 66, 204.

Evans, C.M., Fellows, S.J., Rack, P.M., Ross, H.F., Walters, D.K., 1983. Response of the normal human ankle joint to imposed sinusoidal movements. J. Physiol. 344, 483–502.

Feys, H., Eyssen, M., Jaspers, E., Klingels, K., Desloovere, K., Molenaers, G., et al., 2010. Relation between neuroradiological findings and upper limb function in hemiplegic cerebral palsy. Eur. J. Paediatr. Neurol. 14, 169–177.

Filloux, F.M., 1996. Neuropathophysiology of movement disorders in cerebral palsy. J. Child Neurol. 11 (Suppl. 1), S5–S12.

Fitzgerald, M.J.T., 1992. Neuroanatomy: Basic and Clinical. Baillière Tindall, London.

Fleuren, J.F., Snoek, G.J., Voerman, G.E., Hermens, H.J., 2009. Muscle activation patterns of knee flexors and extensors during passive and active movement of the spastic lower limb in chronic stroke patients. J. Electromyogr. Kinesiol. 19, e301–e310.

Folland, J.P., Williams, A.G., 2007. The adaptations to strength training: morphological and neurological contributions to increased strength. Sports Med. 37, 145–168.

Fonseca, S.T., Holt, K.G., Saltzman, E., Fetters, L., 2001. A dynamical model of locomotion in spastic hemiplegic cerebral palsy: influence of walking speed. Clin. Biomech. (Bristol, Avon) 16, 793–805.

Foran, J.R., Steinman, S., Barash, I., Chambers, H.G., Lieber, R.L., 2005. Structural and mechanical alterations in spastic skeletal muscle. Dev. Med. Child Neurol. 47, 713–717.

Fowler, E.G., Ho, T.W., Nwigwe, A.I., Dorey, F.J., 2001. The effect of quadriceps femoris muscle strengthening exercises on spasticity in children with cerebral palsy. Phys. Ther. 81, 1215–1223.

Friden, J., Lieber, R.L., 2003. Spastic muscle cells are shorter and stiffer than normal cells. Muscle Nerve 27, 157–164.

Fry, A.C., 2004. The role of resistance exercise intensity on muscle fibre adaptations. Sports Med. 34, 663–679.

Gajdosik, C.G., Cicirello, N., 2001. Secondary conditions of the musculoskeletal system in adolescents and adults with cerebral palsy. Phys. Occup. Ther. Pediatr. 21, 49–68.

Gajdosik, C.G., Gajdosik, R.L., 2006. Musculoskeletal development and adaptation. In: Campbell, S.K., Vander Linden, D.W., Palisano, R.J. (Eds.), Physical Therapy for Children, third ed. Saunders Elsevier, Philadelphia, PA.

Gajdosik, R.L., 2001. Passive extensibility of skeletal muscle: review of the literature with clinical implications. Clin. Biomech. (Bristol, Avon) 16, 87–101.

Gajdosik, R.L., Vander Linden, D.W., McNair, P.J., Riggin, T.J., Albertson, J.S., Mattick, D.J., et al., 2005. Viscoelastic properties of short calf muscle–tendon units of older women: effects of slow and fast passive dorsiflexion stretches in vivo. Eur. J. Appl. Physiol. 95, 131–139.

Gao, F., Zhang, L.Q., 2008. Altered contractile properties of the gastrocnemius muscle poststroke. J. Appl. Physiol. 105, 1802–1808.

Gao, F., Grant, T.H., Roth, E.J., Zhang, L.Q., 2009. Changes in passive mechanical properties of the gastrocnemius muscle at the muscle fascicle and joint levels in stroke survivors. Arch. Phys. Med. Rehabil. 90, 819–826.

Gavronski, G., Veraksits, A., Vasar, E., Maaroos, J., 2007. Evaluation of viscoelastic parameters of the skeletal muscles in junior triathletes. Physiol. Meas. 28, 625–637.

Giroux-Metges, M.A., Pennec, J.P., Petit, J., Morel, J., Talarmin, H., Droguet, M., et al., 2005. Effects of immobilizing a single muscle on the morphology and the activation of its muscle fibers. Exp. Neurol. 194, 495–505.

Givli, S., Bhattacharya, K., 2009. A coarse-grained model of the myofibril: overall dynamics and the evolution of sarcomere non-uniformities. J. Mech. Phys. Solids 57, 221–243.

Givon, U., 2009. Muscle weakness in cerebral palsy. Acta Orthop. Traumatol. Turc. 43, 87–93.

Goddard, R., Dowson, D., Longfield, M.D., Wright, V., 1969. The measurement of stiffness in human joints. Rheol. Acta 8, 229–234.

Gorter, H., Holty, L., Rameckers, E.E., Elvers, H.J., Oostendorp, R.A., 2009a. Changes in endurance and walking ability through functional physical training in children with cerebral palsy. Pediatr. Phys. Ther. 21, 31–37.

Gorter, J.W., Ketelaar, M., Rosenbaum, P., Helders, P.J.M., Palisano, R., 2009b. Use of the GMFCS in infants with CP: the need for reclassification at age 2 years or older. Dev. Med. Child Neurol. 51, 46–52.

Gosline, J., Lillie, M., Carrington, E., Guerette, P., Ortlepp, C., Savage, K., 2002. Elastic proteins: biological roles and mechanical properties. Philos. Trans. R. Soc. Lond. B, Biol. Sci. 357, 121–132.

Gottlieb, G.L., Agarwal, G.C., 1988. Compliance of single joints: elastic and plastic characteristics. J. Neurophysiol. 59, 937–951.

Gottlieb, G.L., Agarwal, G.C., Penn, R., 1978. Sinusoidal oscillation of the ankle as a means of evaluating the spastic patient. J. Neurol. Neurosurg. Psychiatry 41, 32–39.

Goulding, D., Bullard, B., Gautel, M., 1997. A survey of in situ sarcomere extension in mouse skeletal muscle. J. Muscle Res. Cell Motil. 18, 465–472.

Gracies, J.M., 2005a. Pathophysiology of spastic paresis. I: paresis and soft tissue changes. Muscle Nerve 31, 535–551.

Gracies, J.M., 2005b. Pathophysiology of spastic paresis. II: emergence of muscle overactivity. Muscle Nerve 31, 552–571.

Hajrasouliha, A.R., Tavakoli, S., Esteki, A., Nafisi, S., Noorolahi-Moghaddam, H., 2005. Abnormal viscoelastic behaviour of passive ankle joint movement in diabetic patients: an early or a late complication? Diabetologia 48, 1225–1228.

Hanna, S.E., Rosenbaum, P.L., Bartlett, D.J., Palisano, R.J., Walter, S.D., Avery, L., et al., 2009. Stability and

decline in gross motor function among children and youth with cerebral palsy aged 2 to 21 years. Dev. Med. Child Neurol. 51, 295–302.

Harlaar, J., Becher, J.G., Snijders, C.J., Lankhorst, G.J., 2000. Passive stiffness characteristics of ankle plantar flexors in hemiplegia. Clin. Biomech. (Bristol, Avon) 15, 261–270.

Herbert, R., 1988. The passive mechanical properties of muscle and their adaptations to altered patterns of use. Aust. J. Physiother. 34, 141–149.

Herbert, R., 1993. Preventing and treating stiff joints. In: Crosbie, J., McConnell, J. (Eds.), Physiotherapy Foundation for Practice: Key Issues in Musculoskeletal Physiotherapy. Butterworth-Heinemann, Oxford.

Herzog, W., 1997. What is the series elastic component in skeletal muscle? J. Appl. Biomech. 13, 443–448.

Hill, A.V., 1950. The series elastic component of muscle. Proc. R. Soc. Lond. B, Biol. Sci. 137, 273–280.

Himmelmann, K., Hagberg, G., Beckung, E., Hagberg, B., Uvebrant, P., 2005. The changing panorama of cerebral palsy in Sweden. IX. Prevalence and origin in the birth-year period 1995–1998. Acta Paediatr. 94, 287–294.

Himmelmann, K., Beckung, E., Hagberg, G., Uvebrant, P., 2006. Gross and fine motor function and accompanying impairments in cerebral palsy. Dev. Med. Child Neurol. 48, 417–423.

Himpens, E., Van Den Broeck, C., Oostra, A., Calders, P., Vanhaesebrouck, P., 2008. Prevalence, type, distribution, and severity of cerebral palsy in relation to gestational age: a meta-analytic review. Dev. Med. Child Neurol. 50, 334–340.

Hirtz, D., Thurman, D.J., Gwinn-Hardy, K., Mohamed, M., Chaudhuri, A.R., Zalutsky, R., 2007. How common are the 'common' neurologic disorders? Neurology 68, 326–337.

Hodapp, M., Vry, J., Mall, V., Faist, M., 2009. Changes in soleus H-reflex modulation after treadmill training in children with cerebral palsy. Brain 132, 37–44.

Hoon JR., A.H., 2005. Neuroimaging in cerebral palsy: patterns of brain dysgenesis and injury. J. Child Neurol. 20, 936–939.

Hosford, W.F., 2010. Mechanical Behavior of Materials. Cambridge University Press, Cambridge, New York.

Howard, J., Soo, B., Graham, H.K., Boyd, R.N., Reid, S., Lanigan, A., et al., 2005. Cerebral palsy in Victoria: motor types, topography and gross motor function. J. Paediatr. Child Health 41, 479–483.

Hufschmidt, A., Mauritz, K.H., 1985. Chronic transformation of muscle in spasticity: a peripheral contribution to increased tone. J. Neurol. Neurosurg. Psychiatry 48, 676–685.

Ishikawa, M., Komi, P.V., Grey, M.J., Lepola, V., Bruggemann, G.P., 2005. Muscle–tendon interaction and elastic energy usage in human walking. J. Appl. Physiol. 99, 603–608.

Ito, J., Araki, A., Tanaka, H., Tasaki, T., Cho, K., Yamazaki, R., 1996. Muscle histopathology in spastic cerebral palsy. Brain Dev. 18, 299–303.

Jain, S., Mathur, N., Joshi, M., Jindal, R., Goenka, S., 2008. Effect of serial casting in spastic cerebral palsy. Indian J. Pediatr. 75, 997–1002.

Jeng, S.F., Yau, K.I.T., Chen, L.C., Hsiao, S.F., 2000. Alberta infant motor scale: reliability and validity when used on preterm infants in Taiwan. Phys. Ther. 80, 168.

Johnson, G.R., 2002. Outcome measures of spasticity. Eur. J. Neurol. 9 (Suppl. 1), 10–16 (discussion 53–61).

Johnston, M.V., 2004. Clinical disorders of brain plasticity. Brain Dev. 26, 73–80.

Johnston, M.V., 2009. Plasticity in the developing brain: implications for rehabilitation. Dev. Disabil. Res. Rev. 15, 94–101.

Jones, M.W., Morgan, E., Shelton, J.E., Thorogood, C., 2007. Cerebral palsy: introduction and diagnosis (part I). J. Pediatr. Health Care 21, 146–152.

Kamper, D.G., Schmit, B.D., Rymer, W.Z., 2001. Effect of muscle biomechanics on the quantification of spasticity. Ann. Biomed. Eng. 29, 1122–1134.

Kanda, T., Pidcock, F.S., Hayakawa, K., Yamori, Y., Shikata, Y., 2004. Motor outcome differences between two groups of children with spastic diplegia who received different intensities of early onset physiotherapy followed for 5 years. Brain Dev. 26, 118–126.

Katz-Leurer, M., Rotem, H., Keren, O., Meyer, S., 2009. The effects of a 'home-based' task-oriented exercise programme on motor and balance performance in children with spastic cerebral palsy and severe traumatic brain injury. Clin. Rehabil. 23, 714–724.

Kerr, G.H., Selber, P., 2003. Musculoskeletal aspects of cerebral palsy. J. Bone Joint Surg. Br. 85, 157–166.

Kim, D.Y., Park, C.I., Chon, J.S., Ohn, S.H., Park, T.H., Bang, I.K., 2005. Biomechanical assessment with electromyography of post-stroke ankle plantar flexor spasticity. Yonsei Med. J. 46, 546–554.

Kitchen, W.H., Rickards, A.L., Doyle, L.W., Ford, G.W., Kelly, E.A., Callanan, C., 1992. Improvement in outcome for very low birthweight children: apparent or real? Med. J. Aust. 157, 154–158.

Klingbeil, H., Baer, H.R., Wilson, P.E., 2004. Aging with a disability. Arch. Phys. Med. Rehabil. 85, S68–S73. (quiz S74–75).

Koman, L.A., Smith, B.P., Shilt, J.S., 2004. Cerebral palsy. Lancet 363, 1619–1631.

Kostyukov, A.I., 1998. Muscle hysteresis and movement control: a theoretical study. Neuroscience 83, 303–320.

Kubo, K., Kanehisa, H., Fukunaga, T., 2005. Effects of viscoelastic properties of tendon structures on stretch—shortening cycle exercise in vivo. J. Sports Sci. 23, 851–860.

Kumar, A., Kabeer, S., Aikat, R., Juneja, M., 2010. Effect of strength training of muscles of lower limb of young children with cerebral palsy on gross motor function. Indian J. Physiother. Occup. Ther. 4, 4–7.

Kumar, R.T., Pandyan, A.D., Sharma, A.K., 2006. Biomechanical measurement of post-stroke spasticity. Age Ageing 35, 371–375.

Lance, J.W., 1980. Symposium synopsis. In: Feldman, R.G., Young, R.R., Koella, W.P. (Eds.), Spasticity: Disordered Motor Control. Symposia Specialists, Chicago.

Lee, J.H., Sung, I.Y., Yoo, J.Y., 2008. Therapeutic effects of strengthening exercise on gait function of cerebral palsy. Disabil. Rehabil. 30, 1439–1444.

Levin, A. & Wyman, J. 1927. The viscous elastic properties of muscle. Proceedings of the Royal Society of London. Series B, Containing Papers of a Biological Character 101, 218–243.

Liao, H.F., Liu, Y.C., Liu, W.Y., Lin, Y.T., 2007. Effectiveness of loaded sit-to-stand resistance exercise for children with mild spastic diplegia: a randomized clinical trial. Arch. Phys. Med. Rehabil. 88, 25–31.

Lieber, R.L., 1988. Comparison between animal and human studies of skeletal muscle adaptation to chronic stimulation. Clin. Orthop. Relat. Res., 19–24.

Lieber, R.L., Friden, J., 2002. Spasticity causes a fundamental rearrangement of muscle–joint interaction. Muscle Nerve 25, 265–270.

Lieber, R.L., Runesson, E., Einarsson, F., Friden, J., 2003. Inferior mechanical properties of spastic muscle bundles due to hypertrophic but compromised extracellular matrix material. Muscle Nerve 28, 464–471.

Lieber, R.L., Steinman, S., Barash, I.A., Chambers, H., 2004. Structural and functional changes in spastic skeletal muscle. Muscle Nerve 29, 615–627.

Lindstedt, S.L., Reich, T.E., Keim, P., Lastayo, P.C., 2002. Do muscles function as adaptable locomotor springs? J. Exp. Biol. 205, 2211–2216.

MacIntosh, B.R., MacNaughton, M.B., 2005. The length dependence of muscle active force: considerations for parallel elastic properties. J. Appl. Physiol. 98, 1666–1673.

Maegaki, Y., Maeoka, Y., Ishii, S., Eda, I., Ohtagaki, A., Kitahara, T., et al., 1999. Central motor reorganization in cerebral palsy patients with bilateral cerebral lesions. Pediatr. Res. 45, 559–567.

Magnusson, S.P., Simonsen, E.B., Aagaard, P., Sorensen, H., Kjaer, M., 1996. A mechanism for altered flexibility in human skeletal muscle. J. Physiol. 497 (Pt 1), 291–298.

Maher, C.A., Williams, M.T., Olds, T., Lane, A.E., 2007. Physical and sedentary activity in adolescents with cerebral palsy. Dev. Med. Child Neurol. 49, 450–457.

Maier, A., Eldred, E., Edgerton, V.R., 1972. The effects on spindles of muscle atrophy and hypertrophy. Exp. Neurol. 37, 100–123.

Malaiya, R., McNee, A.E., Fry, N.R., Eve, L.C., Gough, M., Shortland, A.P., 2007. The morphology of the medial gastrocnemius in typically developing children and children with spastic hemiplegic cerebral palsy. J. Electromyogr. Kinesiol. 17, 657–663.

Malhotra, S., Cousins, E., Ward, A., Day, C., Jones, P., Roffe, C., et al., 2008. An investigation into the agreement between clinical, biomechanical and neurophysiological measures of spasticity. Clin. Rehabil. 22, 1105–1115.

Marbini, A., Ferrari, A., Cioni, G., Bellanova, M.F., Fusco, C., Gemignani, F., 2002. Immunohistochemical study of muscle biopsy in children with cerebral palsy. Brain Dev. 24, 63–66.

Maruyama, K., Kimura, S., 2000. Connectin: from regular to giant sizes of sarcomeres. Adv. Exp. Med. Biol. 481, 25–33.

Mattern-Baxter, K., Bellamy, S., Mansoor, J.K., 2009. Effects of intensive locomotor treadmill training on young children with cerebral palsy. Pediatr. Phys. Ther. 21, 308–318.

Mayer, N.H., 1997. Clinicophysiologic concepts of spasticity and motor dysfunction in adults with an upper motoneuron lesion. Muscle Nerve Suppl. 6, S1–13.

McClelland, J.F., Parkes, J., Hill, N., Jackson, A.J., Saunders, K.J., 2006. Accommodative dysfunction in children with cerebral palsy: a population-based study. Invest. Ophthalmol. Vis. Sci. 47, 1824–1830.

McComas, A.J., 1994. Human neuromuscular adaptations that accompany changes in activity. Med. Sci. Sports. Exerc. 26, 1498–1509.

McComas, A.J., Sica, R.E., Upton, A.R., Aguilera, N., 1973. Functional changes in motoneurones of hemiparetic patients. J. Neurol. Neurosurg. Psychiatry 36, 183–193.

McNee, A.E., Gough, M., Morrissey, M.C., Shortland, A.P., 2009. Increases in muscle volume after plantarflexor strength training in children with spastic cerebral palsy. Dev. Med. Child Neurol. 51, 429–435.

Meinders, M., Price, R., Lehmann, J.F., Questad, K.A., 1996. The stretch reflex response in the normal and spastic ankle: effect of ankle position. Arch. Phys. Med. Rehabil. 77, 487–492.

Mirbagheri, M.M., Alibiglou, L., Thajchayapong, M., Rymer, W.Z., 2000. Muscle and reflex changes with varying joint angle in hemiparetic stroke. J. Neuroeng. Rehabil. 5, 6.

Mockford, M., Caulton, J.M., 2008. Systematic review of progressive strength training in children and adolescents with cerebral palsy who are ambulatory. Pediatr. Phys. Ther. 20, 318–333.

Mockford, M., Caulton, J.M., 2010. The pathophysiological basis of weakness in children with cerebral palsy. Pediatr. Phys. Ther. 22, 222–233.

Mohagheghi, A.A., Khan, T., Meadows, T.H., Giannikas, K., Baltzopoulos, V., Maganaris, C.N., 2007. Differences in gastrocnemius muscle architecture between the paretic and non-paretic legs in children with hemiplegic cerebral palsy. Clin. Biomech. (Bristol, Avon) 22, 718–724.

Mohagheghi, A.A., Khan, T., Meadows, T.H., Giannikas, K., Baltzopoulos, V., Maganaris, C.N., 2008. In vivo gastrocnemius muscle fascicle length in children with and without diplegic cerebral palsy. Dev. Med. Child Neurol. 50, 44–50.

Morita, H., Crone, C., Christenhuis, D., Petersen, N.T., Nielsen, J.B., 2001. Modulation of presynaptic inhibition and disynaptic reciprocal Ia inhibition during voluntary movement in spasticity. Brain 124, 826–837.

Morton, J.F., Brownlee, M., McFadyen, A.K., 2005. The effects of progressive resistance training for children with cerebral palsy. Clin. Rehabil. 19, 283–289.

Moseley, A.M., Crosbie, J., Adams, R., 2001. Normative data for passive ankle plantarflexion–dorsiflexion flexibility. Clin. Biomech. (Bristol, Avon) 16, 514–521.

Mujika, I., Padilla, S., 2000a. Detraining: loss of training-induced physiological and performance adaptations. Part I: short term insufficient training stimulus. Sports Med. 30, 79–87.

Mujika, I., Padilla, S., 2000b. Detraining: loss of training-induced physiological and performance adaptations. Part II: long term insufficient training stimulus. Sports Med. 30, 145–154.

Nielsen, J.B., Crone, C., Hultborn, H., 2007. The spinal pathophysiology of spasticity–from a basic science point of view. Acta Physiol. (Oxf.) 189, 171–180.

O'Dwyer, N.J., Neilson, P.D., Nash, J., 1989. Mechanisms of muscle growth related to muscle contracture in cerebral palsy. Dev. Med. Child Neurol. 31, 543–547.

Odding, E., Roebroeck, M.E., Stam, H.J., 2006. The epidemiology of cerebral palsy: incidence, impairments and risk factors. Disabil. Rehabil. 28, 183–191.

Ostensjo, S., Carlberg, E.B., Vollestad, N.K., 2004. Motor impairments in young children with cerebral palsy: relationship to gross motor function and everyday activities. Dev. Med. Child Neurol. 46, 580–589.

Pakula, A.T., Van Naarden Braun, K., Yeargin-Allsopp, M., 2009. Cerebral palsy: classification and epidemiology. Phys. Med. Rehabil. Clin. N. Am. 20, 425–452.

Palisano, R., Rosenbaum, P., Walter, S., Russell, D., Wood, E., Galuppi, B., 1997. Development and reliability of a system to classify gross motor function in children with cerebral palsy. Dev. Med. Child Neurol. 39, 214–223.

Palisano, R.J., Cameron, D., Rosenbaum, P.L., Walter, S.D., Russell, D., 2006. Stability of the gross motor function classification system. Dev. Med. Child Neurol. 48, 424–428.

Pandyan, A.D., Gregoric, M., Barnes, M.P., Wood, D., Wijck, V.A.N., Burridge, F., et al., 2005. Spasticity: clinical perceptions, neurological realities and meaningful measurement. Disabil. Rehabil. 27, 2–6.

Petrillo, C.R., Knoploch, S., 1988. Phenol block of the tibial nerve for spasticity: a long-term follow-up study. Int. Disabil. Stud. 10, 97–100.

Pfeifer, L.I., Silva, D.B.R., Funayama, C.A.R., Santos, J.L., 2009. Classification of cerebral palsy association between gender, age, motor type, topography and gross motor function. Arq. Neuropsiquiatr. 67, 1057–1061.

Pin, T.W., De Valle, K., Eldridge, B., Galea, M.P., 2010. Clinimetric properties of the Alberta infant motor scale in infants born preterm. Pediatr. Phys. Ther. 22, 278–286.

Pincus, D., 2000. Everything You Need to Know about Cerebral Palsy. Rosen Publishing Group, New York.

Piper, M.C., Darrah, J., 1994. Motor Assessment of the Developing Infant. Saunders, Alberta.

Piper, M.C., Pinnell, L.E., Darrah, J., Maguire, T., Byrne, P.J., 1992. Construction and validation of the Alberta infant motor scale (AIMS). Can. J. Public Health 83 (Suppl. 2), S46–S50.

Poon, D.M., Hui-Chan, C.W., 2009. Hyperactive stretch reflexes, co-contraction, and muscle weakness in children with cerebral palsy. Dev. Med. Child Neurol. 51, 128–135.

Powers, R.K., Campbell, D.L., Rymer, W.Z., 1989. Stretch reflex dynamics in spastic elbow flexor muscles. Ann. Neurol. 25, 32–42.

Prado, L.G., Makarenko, I., Andresen, C., Kruger, M., Opitz, C.A., Linke, W.A., 2005. Isoform diversity of giant proteins in relation to passive and active contractile properties of rabbit skeletal muscles. J. Gen. Physiol. 126, 461–480.

Priori, A., Cogiamanian, F., Mrakic-Sposta, S., 2006. Pathophysiology of spasticity. Neurol. Sci. 27, s307–s309.

Purslow, P.P., 1989. Strain-induced reorientation of an intramuscular connective tissue network: implications for passive muscle elasticity. J. Biomech. 22, 21–31.

Reid, S., Hamer, P., Alderson, J., Lloyd, D., 2010. Neuromuscular adaptations to eccentric strength training in children and adolescents with cerebral palsy. Dev. Med. Child Neurol. 52, 358–363.

Roberts, T.J., 2002. The integrated function of muscles and tendons during locomotion. Comp. Biochem. Physiol. A, Mol. Integr. Physiol. 133, 1087–1099.

Robinson, M.N., Peake, L.J., Ditchfield, M.R., Reid, S.M., Lanigan, A., Reddihough, D.S., 2009. Magnetic resonance imaging findings in a population-based cohort of children with cerebral palsy. Dev. Med. Child Neurol. 51, 39–45.

Rosant, C., Nagel, M.D., Perot, C., 2006. Adaptation of rat soleus muscle spindles after 21 days of hindlimb unloading. Exp. Neurol. 200, 191–199.

Rose, J., McGill, K.C., 1998. The motor unit in cerebral palsy. Dev. Med. Child Neurol. 40, 270–277.

Rose, J., McGill, K.C., 2005. Neuromuscular activation and motor-unit firing characteristics in cerebral palsy. Dev. Med. Child Neurol. 47, 329–336.

Rose, J., Haskell, W.L., Gamble, J.G., Hamilton, R.I., Brown, D.A., Rinsky, L., 1994. Muscle pathology and clinical measures of disability in children with cerebral palsy. J. Orthop. Res. 12, 758–768.

Rosen, M.G., Dickinson, J.C., 1992. The incidence of cerebral palsy. Am. J. Obstet. Gynecol. 167, 417–423.

Rosenbaum, P.L., Palisano, R.J., Bartlett, D.J., Galuppi, B.E., Russell, D.J., 2008. Development of the gross motor function classification system for cerebral palsy. Dev. Med. Child Neurol. 50, 249–253.

Ross, S., Engsberg, J., 2007. Relationships between spasticity, strength, gait, and the GMFM-66 in persons with spastic diplegia cerebral palsy. Arch. Phys. Med. Rehab. 88, 1114–1120.

Saguil, A., 2005. Evaluation of the patient with muscle weakness. Am. Fam. Physician 71, 1327–1336.

Salazar-Torres J., J.D.E., Pandyan, A.D., Price, C.I., Davidson, R.I., Barnes, M.P., Johnson, G.R., 2004. Does spasticity result from hyperactive stretch reflexes? Preliminary findings from a stretch reflex characterization study. Disabil. Rehabil. 26, 756–760.

Salem, Y., Godwin, E.M., 2009. Effects of task-oriented training on mobility function in children with cerebral palsy. NeuroRehabilitation 24, 307–313.

Salmons, S., Henriksson, J., 1981. The adaptive response of skeletal muscle to increased use. Muscle Nerve 4, 94–105.

Salsich, G.B., Mueller, M.J., 2000. Effect of plantar flexor muscle stiffness on selected gait characteristics. Gait Posture 11, 207–216.

Sanger, T.D., Delgado, M.R., Gaebler-Spira, D., Hallett, M., Mink, J.W., Task Force On Childhood Motor Disorders 2003. Classification and definition of disorders causing hypertonia in childhood. Pediatrics 111, e89–e97.

Santos, M.J., Liu, W., 2008. Possible factors related to functional ankle instability. J. Orthop. Sports Phys. Ther. 38, 150–157.

Schleip, R., Naylor, I.L., Ursu, D., Melzer, W., Zorn, A., Wilke, H.J., et al., 2006. Passive muscle stiffness may be influenced by active contractility of intramuscular connective tissue. Med. Hypotheses 66, 66–71.

Scholtes, V.A., Dallmeijer, A.J., Rameckers, E.A., Verschuren, O., Tempelaars, E., Hensen, M., et al., 2008. Lower limb strength training in children with cerebral palsy—a randomized controlled trial protocol for functional strength training based on progressive resistance exercise principles. BMC Pediatr. 8, 41.

Scholtes, V.A., Becher, J.G., Comuth, A., Dekkers, H., Van Dijk, L., Dallmeijer, A.J., 2010. Effectiveness of functional progressive resistance exercise strength training on muscle strength and mobility in children with cerebral palsy: a randomized controlled trial. Dev. Med. Child Neurol. 52, e107–e113.

Shepherd, R.B., 2001. Exercise and training to optimize functional motor performance in stroke: driving neural reorganization? Neural Plast. 8, 121–129.

Shimony, J.S., Lawrence, R., Neil, J.J., Inder, T.E., 2008. Imaging for diagnosis and treatment of cerebral palsy. Clin. Obstet. Gynecol. 51, 787–799.

Shortland, A.P., Harris, C.A., Gough, M., Robinson, R.O., 2002. Architecture of the medial gastrocnemius in children with spastic diplegia. Dev. Med. Child Neurol. 44, 158–163.

Sigurdardottir, S., Thorkelsson, T., Halldorsdottir, M., Thorarensen, O., Vik, T., 2009. Trends in prevalence and characteristics of cerebral palsy among Icelandic children born 1990 to 2003. Dev. Med. Child Neurol. 51, 356–363.

Sindou, M., 2003. History of neurosurgical treatment of spasticity. Neurochirurgie 49, 137–143.

Sinkjaer, T., Magnussen, I., 1994. Passive, intrinsic and reflex-mediated stiffness in the ankle extensors of hemiparetic patients. Brain 117 (Pt 2), 355–363.

Sinkjaer, T., Toft, E., Larsen, K., Andreassen, S., Hansen, H.J., 1993. Non-reflex and reflex mediated ankle joint stiffness in multiple sclerosis patients with spasticity. Muscle Nerve 16, 69–76.

Skeie, G.O., 2000. Skeletal muscle titin: physiology and pathophysiology. Cell. Mol. Life Sci. 57, 1570–1576.

Smith, G.V., Silver, K.H., Goldberg, A.P., Macko, R.F., 1999. 'Task-oriented' exercise improves hamstring strength and spastic reflexes in chronic stroke patients. Stroke 30, 2112–2118.

Smith, L.R., Ponten, E., Hedstrom, Y., Ward, S.R., Chambers, H.G., Subramaniam, S., et al., 2009. Novel transcriptional profile in wrist muscles from cerebral palsy patients. BMC Med. Genomics 2, 44.

Snyder, P., Eason, J.M., Philibert, D., Ridgway, A., McCaughey, T., 2008. Concurrent validity and reliability of the Alberta infant motor scale in infants at dual risk for motor delays. Phys. Occup. Ther. Pediatr. 28, 267–282.

Sorsdahl, A.B., Moe-Nilssen, R., Kaale, H.K., Rieber, J., Strand, L.I., 2010. Change in basic motor abilities, quality of movement and everyday activities following intensive, goal-directed, activity-focused physiotherapy in a group setting for children with cerebral palsy. BMC Pediatr. 10, 26.

Stackhouse, S.K., Binder-Macleod, S.A., Lee, S.C., 2005. Voluntary muscle activation, contractile properties, and fatigability in children with and without cerebral palsy. Muscle Nerve 31, 594–601.

Stanley, F., Blair, E., Alberman, E., 2000. Cerebral Palsies: Epidemiology and Causal Pathways. MacKeith, London.

Staudt, M., 2010. Reorganization after pre- and perinatal brain lesions. J. Anat. 217, 469–474.

Sterba, J.A., 2007. Does horseback riding therapy or therapist-directed hippotherapy rehabilitate children with cerebral palsy? Dev. Med. Child Neurol. 49, 68–73.

Stewart, C.E., Rittweger, J., 2006. Adaptive processes in skeletal muscle: molecular regulators and genetic influences. J. Musculoskelet. Neuronal Interact. 6, 73–86.

Suputtitada, A., 2000. Managing spasticity in pediatric cerebral palsy using a very low dose of botulinum toxin type A—Preliminary report.

Am. J. Phys. Med. Rehabil. 79, 320–326.

Tardieu, C., Lespargot, A., Tabary, C., Bret, M.D., 1989. Toe-walking in children with cerebral palsy: contributions of contracture and excessive contraction of triceps surae muscle. Phys. Ther. 69, 656–662.

Taylor, D.C., Dalton JR., J.D., Seaber, A.V., Garrett JR., W.E., 1990. Viscoelastic properties of muscle–tendon units. The biomechanical effects of stretching. Am. J. Sports Med. 18, 300–309.

Tedroff, K., Knutson, L.M., Soderberg, G.L., 2008. Co-activity during maximum voluntary contraction: a study of four lower-extremity muscles in children with and without cerebral palsy. Dev. Med. Child Neurol. 50, 377–381.

Tedroff, K., Granath, F., Forssberg, H., Haglund-Akerlind, Y., 2009. Long-term effects of botulinum toxin A in children with cerebral palsy. Dev. Med. Child Neurol. 51, 120–127.

Tokuyasu, K.T., Dutton, A.H., Singer, S.J., 1983. Immunoelectron microscopic studies of desmin (skeletin) localization and intermediate filament organization in chicken skeletal muscle. J. Cell Biol. 96, 1727–1735.

Trevino, S.G., Buford Jr., W.L., Nakamura, T., John Wright, A., Patterson, R.M., 2004. Use of a Torque-Range-of-Motion device for objective differentiation of diabetic from normal feet in adults. Foot Ankle Int. 25, 561–567.

Trew, M., Everett, T., 2005. Human Movement: An Introductory Text. Elsevier/Churchill Livingstone, Edinburgh; New York.

Turk, R., Notley, S.V., Pickering, R.M., Simpson, D.M., Wright, P.A., Burridge, J.H., 2008. Reliability and sensitivity of a wrist rig to measure motor control and spasticity in poststroke hemiplegia. Neurorehabil. Neural Repair 22, 684–696.

Van Loocke, M., 2007. Passive mechanical properties of skeletal muscle in compression. Ph.D., the University of Dublin.

Vaz, D.V., Cotta Mancini, M., Fonseca, S.T., Vieira, D.S., De Melo Pertence, A.E., 2006. Muscle stiffness and strength and their relation to hand function in children with hemiplegic cerebral palsy. Dev. Med. Child Neurol. 48, 728–733.

Verschuren, O., Ketelaar, M., Gorter, J.W., Helders, P.J., Uiterwaal, C.S., Takken, T., 2007. Exercise training program in children and adolescents with cerebral palsy: a randomized controlled trial. Arch. Pediatr. Adolesc. Med. 161, 1075–1081.

Voerman, G.E., Burridge, J.H., Hitchcock, R.A., Hermens, H.J., 2007. Clinometric properties of a clinical spasticity measurement tool. Disabil. Rehabil. 29, 1870–1880.

Wang, K., McCarter, R., Wright, J., Beverly, J., Ramirez-Mitchell, R., 1993. Viscoelasticity of the sarcomere matrix of skeletal muscles. The titin-myosin composite filament is a dual-stage molecular spring. Biophys. J. 64, 1161–1177.

Waterman-Storer, C., 1991. The cytoskeleton of skeletal muscle: is it affected by exercise? A brief review. Med. Sci. Sports Exerc. 23, 1240–1249.

Wiley, M.E., Damiano, D.L., 1998. Lower-extremity strength profiles in spastic cerebral palsy. Dev. Med. Child Neurol. 40, 100–107.

Williams, H., Pountney, T., 2007. Effects of a static bicycling programme on the functional ability of young people with cerebral palsy who are non-ambulant. Dev. Med. Child Neurol. 49, 522–527.

Willoughby, K.L., Dodd, K.J., Shields, N., 2009. A systematic review of the effectiveness of treadmill training for children with cerebral palsy. Disabil. Rehabil. 31, 1971–1979.

Wilson, J.M., Flanagan, E.P., 2008. The role of elastic energy in activities with high force and power requirements: a brief review. J. Strength Cond. Res. 22, 1705–1715.

Wittenberg, G.F., 2009. Motor mapping in cerebral palsy. Dev. Med. Child Neurol. 51 (Suppl. 4), 134–139.

Wu, Y.W., Lindan, C.E., Henning, L.H., Yoshida, C.K., Fullerton, H.J., Ferriero, D.M., et al., 2006. Neuroimaging abnormalities in infants with congenital hemiparesis. Pediatr. Neurol. 35, 191–196.

Zhang, L.Q., Wang, G., Nishida, T., Xu, D., Sliwa, J.A., Rymer, W.Z., 2000. Hyperactive tendon reflexes in spastic multiple sclerosis: measures and mechanisms of action. Arch. Phys. Med. Rehabil. 81, 901–909.

# Annotation B
## Findings from a series of studies of passive mechanical properties of muscle in young children with cerebral palsy

Adel Abdullah Alhusaini

## CHAPTER CONTENTS

Progressive plantarflexor muscle dysfunction is common, particularly in children with hemiplegia or diplegia and may result from changes in muscle activation, myotendinous length and stiffness (Becher et al., 1998). When a non-contracting (resting) muscle is stretched in a child with cerebral palsy (CP), any force opposing the movement is due to tension originating through the passive mechanical properties of the muscle, as well as any abnormal muscle activation evoked in spastic muscle. This resistance, however, is commonly recognized as primarily a manifestation of enhanced stretch reflex activity (Mirbagheri et al., 2000) that is often presented as the primary opponent to movement. Researchers frequently group passive myotendinous stiffness under a general label of spasticity/

contracture and may not treat it as a separate impairment. For a number of years the abnormal muscle activation evoked in muscle was considered to be the main contributor to the resistance to movement. However, work by Dietz and Berger (1983) was the first to suggest that muscle stiffness during locomotion in patients with spasticity was due more to changed passive mechanical properties of the muscle than to heightened stretch reflexes in both adults and children with spastic cerebral palsy.

The contributions of passive myotendinous stiffness to either passive or active joint motion are often unreported in children with CP, and inadequate knowledge of the adaptive nature of passive myotendinous stiffness may lead to poor functional outcomes and difficulty in producing significant therapeutic improvement. Expanding our knowledge in this area is critical for the ongoing development of effective rehabilitation practices and may increase our understanding of the role of these affected muscles during functional performance.

The following will review some studies which were held on this matter. Some studies were aimed at determining the relative importance of the passive mechanical properties of the myotendinous unit as a source of resistance to movement, a factor that is frequently under-reported in regard to lower limb function, particularly in children with CP.

## Methodology

All studies were approved through both the Hospital Ethics Committee of The Children's

Hospital at Westmead, Sydney, Australia and the Human Research Ethics Committee of the University of Sydney. Participants were recruited through the Child Assessment Centre in The Children's Hospital at Westmead and through open advertisement for typically developing children. All participants were aged between 4 and 10 years. Participants were consecutively selected based on inclusion and exclusion criteria, and their willingness to participate. Full details of the participants, including inclusion and exclusion criteria, demographic detail and clinical status are given for each study in the relevant publication.

A specially constructed ankle measurement device, similar to that described by Moseley et al. (2001) was used for this aspect of the studies (Fig. B.1). It consisted of a footplate hinged to a support bracket for the lower leg, with a rotary potentiometer (Model 157, RS Australia, Sydney) aligned with the lateral malleolus. The footplate and axis of rotation were adjustable to match the dimensions of the child. A 450 N load cell (XTRAN S1W, Applied Measurement Australia Pty, Oakleigh) was attached perpendicular to the footplate to measure resistance to movement. A handle was attached to allow manual oscillation of the footplate.

The angle signals were checked and calibrated by holding the footplate in a number of different static positions using rigid struts throughout the arc of motion and recording the electrical signal obtained from the potentiometer. The process was repeated five times. The calibration regression equation was consistent in each repetition and the correlation coefficient for angle to signal was 0.9998. In a similar fashion, the load cell was repeatedly calibrated over its relevant range through the application of a number of different known weights and recording of the output signal. Once again, the linear regression equation was identical in each set of tests and the correlation coefficient for force to signal was 0.9999.

High inter-rater and intra-rater reliability has previously been demonstrated for the measurement of passive torque and ankle displacement using similar techniques (intraclass correlation coefficient (ICC)>0.86) (Chesworth and Vandervoort, 1988) and the procedure has been shown to be highly responsive to change in soft tissue stiffness characteristics (Sinkjaer et al., 1988).

Applied torque values were calculated from the product of applied force and the perpendicular distance from the point of application of the force to the axis of rotation of the footplate. To correct for the effect of the footplate weight, a calibration equation was developed in which the torque due to the footplate was computed as a function of the angle of the footplate and its weight. This torque, which was positive or negative according to the footplate position, was added to the applied torque.

The load transducer measured uniaxial loading. This was consistent with the monoplanar rotation of the ankle and the application of force by means of a rod-like handle minimized any risk of 'off-perpendicular' force application. Torque and angle were sampled at 125 Hz.

Each child lay supine with the foot placed in the ankle apparatus and positioned, by visual approximation, such that the point midway between the lateral and medial malleolus in the

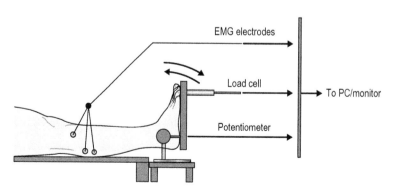

**Figure B.1** • Schematic of ankle measurement device and experimental procedure. EMG electrodes detect muscle activity in medial gastrocnemius, soleus and tibialis anterior. Applied torque is calculated from the product of the force measured through the load cell and the perpendicular distance to the axis of rotation (potentiometer). The lower leg is clear of the support surface.

sagittal plane was aligned with the axis of rotation of the device. The participant's foot was secured to the footplate with Velcro® straps, the knee was placed in an extended position, and light pressure was applied by the researcher's hand above the knee over the thigh to ensure that knee position was maintained. The calf was free of contact and clear of all surfaces and structures. In the children with CP, the affected or more affected leg was tested; in typically developing children, the leg tested was randomly selected. The researcher rotated the foot passively in a sinusoidal pattern around the ankle from full plantarflexion to full available dorsiflexion (determined visually by loss of heel contact). All children were instructed to keep their legs relaxed and to avoid assisting or resisting the motion during the sinusoidal rotation.

A warm-up and familiarization process, with two or three repetitions of full range movement of the rig, was applied before recording the data. For each child, a minimum of 10 passive stretch cycles were applied at a target frequency of 0.5 Hz. This sequence was repeated two more times to ensure relaxation and compliance on the part of the participant and to avoid the eliciting of reflex muscle activity. This allowed at least one full cycle of passive stretching and recovery for analysis. Joint displacements into dorsiflexion were taken as positive and those in the plantarflexion direction as negative. An ankle angle of 90° (plantigrade) was considered to be the neutral position and defined as zero.

Electromyographic (EMG) activity of the soleus, medial gastrocnemius and tibialis anterior muscles was recorded simultaneously with ankle rotation, using a telemetric 16-channel EMG unit (Telemyo 2400 R G2 system, Noraxon, Arizona) with a sampling rate of 3000 Hz. We used disposable, self-adhesive Ag/AgCl bipolar surface electrodes (Kendall Medi-Trace Mini 130 Foam ECG Electrodes, Neurotronics, Randwick, NSW), placing pairs of electrodes parallel with the muscle fibre direction with minimal inter-electrode distance. Before electrode placement, we cleaned the skin with isopropyl alcohol. The location of electrodes was based on contemporary recommendations (Hermens et al., 2000). EMG acquisition enabled monitoring of muscle activity during the test.

We collected force and angle data simultaneously at a frequency of 125 Hz using a 16-bit analogue-to-digital converter (DAQCard-6036E, National Instruments, Austin, Texas). The application software (PhysioDAQXS version 3.0, the University of Sydney) consisted of a graphical user interface designed using Borland C++ builder. Access to the data was gained by using National Instruments' call back functions to retrieve data collected by the data acquisition card. The graphical user interface supports the collection, display and storage of data in real time. The repeatability and linearity of the force and angle signals were confirmed before data collection.

The child's compliance with the instruction to keep the leg relaxed and to avoid assisting or resisting the motion was confirmed by the absence of EMG activity (Spike2 software version 2.09, Cambridge Electronic Design, Cambridge). During analysis of data in those studies in which passive mechanics were investigated, one complete loading and unloading cycle without evidence of EMG activity was chosen for analysis, ensuring that there was no reflex contribution to total stiffness. In the event of more than one cycle meeting this criterion, selection was random. Specific details of analytic conventions are given for each study in the relevant publication.

Torque values were extracted from the data at predetermined dorsiflexion angles (0°, 5° and 10°; Fig. B.2, points A, B and C, respectively). These provided an indication of the torque necessary to displace the ankle to comparable positions for each group tested. Stiffness was computed as the

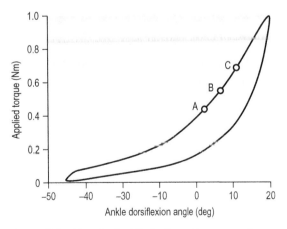

**Figure B.2** • Hypothetical illustration of torque–angle relationship of ankle. Data processing conventions for analysis of passive mechanical properties are defined in the text.

slope of the line between 0° and 5° of dorsiflexion. Hysteresis, expressing the energy absorbed by the muscle–tendon unit during the loading/unloading cycle, was calculated as the area enclosed between the loading and unloading curves of applied torque against ankle angle.

## Study 1: Non-reflex stiffness in children with CP

This study revealed that the plantarflexors of the children with CP were much less mechanically compliant than an age-matched group of typically developing children (Alhusaini et al., 2010a). Torques at predetermined joint angles, ankle stiffness (slope of curve) and hysteresis were almost three times as great in the children with CP compared with the typically developing group ($p < 0.001$).

These findings are important, particularly as we know that non-reflex stiffness in children with CP has not been described or quantified, nor have the effects been recognized of adaptive changes such as decreased muscle extensibility on motor development (Lambertz et al., 2003). This knowledge, therefore, has the potential to improve clinical practice by furthering what is known about the changes in the muscle's intrinsic properties and broadening physiotherapists' understanding about the effects of such changes in these children.

The attempt was made to expose the calf muscle to conditions similar to those found during normal gait by using a sinusoidal movement that was similar in angular velocity and range of motion to that encountered during the stance phase of walking (Ada et al., 1998; Becher et al., 1998), while also avoiding stimulation of reflex hyperactivity in the calf muscles. Although this criterion was not always easy to achieve, and the responses of the children did vary in their ability to relax, it was possible to produce at least one complete cycle in each test during which EMG activity was silent. This situation, therefore, fulfilled the requirement for measurement of the passive myotendinous characteristics. Torque–angle curves at velocities up to 70 degrees/second show the characteristic shape of tissue stretch only (van der Salm et al., 2005). In a study of adults exhibiting spastic hypertonia, it was reported that, even at stretch velocities of 120 degrees/second, only four of 15 people demonstrated reflex

responses in the triceps surae (Rabita et al., 2005). The sinusoidal movement speeds used in the experiments were felt to be adequate to measure the passive myotendinous stiffness parameters while not eliciting simultaneous reflex activity. Although the oscillation frequency was significantly different between groups, the children with CP, who were more likely to respond with hyper-reflexia, were stretched at the slightly lower rate, consistent with the subjective need to maintain a relaxed, passive movement.

## Study 2: Distinguishing between reflex and non-reflex stiffness in children with CP in a clinical scale

In another study, we highlighted the importance of distinguishing between reflex and non-reflex components of resistance to passive stretch and the usefulness of incorporating a tool for assessing soft tissue compliance in the clinical assessment of these children (Alhusaini et al., 2010b). Although the Ashworth Scale or its modified version is the most commonly used method for the assessment of spasticity in the clinical setting (Pandyan et al., 1999), its validity and reliability are under question (Alibiglou et al., 2008; Ansari et al., 2006; Mutlu et al., 2008; Pandyan et al., 1999; Yam and Leung, 2006). Indeed, a recent study by Fleuren et al. (2010) supports its discontinuation. Alhusaini et al. (2010b) support these positions and show that the Tardieu Scale is able to identify the presence and severity of contracture, enhancing its clinical usefulness. However, like the Ashworth Scale, it grades spasticity (stretch reflex hyperactivity) according to the resistance to passive movement (Kumar et al., 2006), a finding that can be confounded by changes in non-neurally mediated muscle stiffness (see Chapter 5, for an updated version of the Tardieu Scale).

In the clinical setting, clinicians need to be aware of the differences between neurally and non-neurally mediated muscle stiffness even though it is hard at this stage to distinguish between them using clinical scales. Therefore, what is needed is a new, simple and quantitative tool that is able to evaluate non-neurally mediated muscle stiffness exclusively without the stretch reflex activity associated with increased resistance to passive movement. This may be done by using a handheld dynamometer and goniometer, available in most clinics. The target joint can be move slowly and passively by the handheld dynamometer through predetermined ranges of motion and the torque values at these predetermined angles recorded. A simple computation of stiffness is then possible and could be compared to normative values. A previously reported, and simple, tool for assessing ankle motion might be adapted for this purpose (Moseley and Adams, 1991).

Measurement of the passive torque–angle relationships throughout dorsiflexion range is a more precise way to determine tissue stiffness than quantifying the passive range using a single point (Moseley et al., 2001), because passive torque increases more rapidly as the joint is moved towards its maximum range. The length of the plantarflexor muscles is difficult to measure in vivo; therefore, indirect measures of angular displacement in response to applied torque are taken as indicative of the force–length variables (Ada et al., 1998; Moseley et al., 2001). The protocol used in these experiments did not allow differentiation between the mechanical properties of the calf muscle and those of the Achilles tendon and other connective tissues. Nor could it exclude the contribution of other tissues, such as skin, ligament, joint capsule and cartilage. However, these last structures generally contribute to stiffness only at the extremity of the dorsiflexion range (Abellaneda et al., 2009). As the gradient of the loading curve was measured between plantigrade and 5° of dorsiflexion, well short of the limit of the participant's full dorsiflexion, values for stiffness probably excluded any substantive contribution of these ancillary tissues. Thus, the myotendinous unit can be considered the major impediment to passive ankle joint dorsiflexion (Riemann et al., 2001).

A number of variables were extracted from the data expressing both discrete (e.g., torque at three angles) and continuous (e.g., equation of the slope of the curve, hysteresis) measures of the passive stiffness of the plantarflexor muscles in an attempt to ensure that the analysis was as comprehensive as possible. It was reassuring to note that there were no inconsistencies in the results whether the data were scaled against available range of dorsiflexion or taken as absolute and discrete values at predetermined joint angles, supporting the conclusions regarding tissue compliance in children with CP.

# Study 3: Non-reflex stiffness can influence the motor performance of children with CP

The findings of a third investigation have drawn attention to the probability that increased passive calf muscle stiffness is a critical factor that can influence the performance of children with CP during walking and climbing stairs (Crosbie et al., 2012). In this study we have found that passive mechanical properties of the calf muscle, isometric muscle force and ankle joint range of motion are strongly and consistently associated with components of walking in children with CP.

The response of the calf muscle to passive stretch can provide some insight into control during lower limb functional performance and of the mechanisms responsible for muscle adaptations following brain insult such as that seen in children with CP. Normal human walking involves complex patterns of movement that require us to understand in detail how different parts within the neuromuscular system interact, particularly in the presence of pathological conditions such as CP. In cases like these the body has adapted the gait to accommodate various neuromuscular limitations, often resulting in new, less effective and less energy-efficient gait patterns. Passive mechanical properties play an important role in functional motor performance and its development.

In gait, for example, the compliance and strength of the calf muscle allow heel contact and control 'roll-over' of the ankle on the plantigrade foot. They contribute to forward propulsion of the body mass through stance phase and at heel-off since the ankle must be free to move into dorsiflexion without excessive resistance from soft tissues that would tend prematurely to lift the heel. Muscle extensibility also contributes to the storage and release of elastic energy (low hysteresis) that increases movement efficiency. Secondary changes in mechanical muscle fibre properties should not be considered as pathological, but rather as adaptive to a primary disorder to compensate for the loss of neuronal drive such as allows for the support of the body during walking (Dietz and Sinkjaer, 2007). Therefore, knowledge about the nature of these changes in muscle mechanics is fundamental to understanding of function and its limitations.

Exploration of the data from the children with hemiplegia to seek associations between the variables relating to muscle compliance, muscle weakness or spasticity and walking characteristics highlight the significant positive relationship between stiff calf muscles and walking ability (Crosbie et al., 2012). This study draws attention to an influence of muscle compliance on function that has not previously been addressed, particularly in children.

## Study 4: Effect of botulinum injections on non-reflex stiffness in children with CP

The findings from this investigation demonstrated that calf muscle stiffness remained relatively unchanged after botulinum A toxin (BoNT-A) injections and the muscles continued to offer substantial resistance to passive motion of the ankle, despite any reduction in stretch reflex hyperactivity. Therefore, additional treatment approaches are required to supplement the effects of BoNT-A injections when managing children with calf muscle spasticity. Alhusaini et al. (2011) showed that the passive intrinsic muscle stiffness and hysteresis in the plantarflexor muscles of children with mild CP were not decreased after BoNT-A injection, although there was a slight increase in total range of angular displacement. This study reinforces the need for a clearer understanding and recognition of the adaptive modifications in stiffness and length of the plantarflexor muscles occurring in early development. Thus, while BoNT-A clearly reduces stretch reflex hyperactivity, lack of response at the activity and participation levels may be related to the unchanged intrinsic stiffness of the muscle. Further studies are required to find the most functionally effective clinical method of minimizing the development of adaptive increases in intrinsic muscle stiffness and other adaptive muscle changes; for example, exercises and activities that target active stretch. In addition, more studies are needed to measure the effect of BoNT-A on muscle morphology, growth and development if we wish to optimize function in children with CP.

In this study, the impact of a smaller sample might have distorted the results. However, when a retrospective power analysis was undertaken to determine the likelihood of Type II error among the non-significant results, it was discovered that, to find a statistically significant differences between the pre- and post-BoNT-A results samples of between 500 and 3000 would be required and even then the effect size would not, in all probability, be considered of clinical importance.

## Suggestions for future studies

These research findings have particular clinical relevance to the field of paediatric rehabilitation. A number of issues which deserve investigation have been raised in these studies. Further studies are needed to explore the time frame of postnatal growth and development of muscles in infants and children with CP, and the adaptive effects of subsequent movement restriction on the muscle's passive mechanical properties, principally stiffness and hysteresis (see Chapters 5 and 6). These adaptations would negatively affect muscle development and the development of functional motor control. Recently, Pierce et al. (2010) suggested that passive stiffness may play a larger role than reflex activity as children with CP age. They also found a significant positive relationship between age and mean knee flexor passive torque in children with spastic diplegic CP. Skeletal muscles are highly adaptive in that they change functionally and morphologically in response to the level and type of use habitually imposed upon them. A better understanding of the adaptations and changes in the biomechanical properties of the myotendinous unit may help us gain insight into functional motor problems in children with CP and this may facilitate the development of novel and more specifically focused rehabilitation methods.

Modifications of the ankle device to fit infants and very young children will be considered in future work in order to follow the time course of adaptive changes occurring in muscle from early after birth throughout the period of growth and development. The feasibility and effectiveness of ongoing monitoring of soft tissue extensibility and passive muscle stiffness from infancy, together with more functional measurements such as the gross motor function measure (GMFM) and paediatric evaluation of disability inventory (PEDI), warrants further examination in future studies. It is important to gain more knowledge about the course of the functional status and correlated factors in order to predict future participation limitations, and to set training and exercise goals. Maintenance of soft tissue extensibility and prevention of excessive increases in passive stiffness should have a positive impact on the development of activities and participation.

This work provides a grounding for future studies centred around the specific nature of impairment and also for intervention studies. Future studies of underlying impairment and interventions might include the use of ultrasound to differentiate adaptive changes in muscle from those in tendon and other joint structures. Although the intention in the studies described here was to measure the myotendinous unit stiffness, a recent study by Zhao et al. (2009) has shown that the muscle belly, rather than the tendinous elements, offers the greater resistance to passive stretching. They found that, after stroke, the calf muscles on the impaired side became stiffer and shorter, leading to a proximal shift of the midpoint between the muscle and the Achilles tendon. Therefore, on the impaired side, the Achilles tendon elongates and become less stiff than that on the unimpaired side. Mohagheghi et al. (2007) assessed in vivo the gastrocnemius muscle architecture in the paretic and non-paretic legs of eight children with CP using ultrasound scans. They showed that the gastrocnemius muscle has shorter, thinner fascicles, although similar pennation angles, in the paretic limbs of children with CP, indicating a loss of both in-series and in-parallel sarcomeres in the affected muscles.

An early implementation of specific active exercise and training programmes designed to promote motor learning and development and musculoskeletal growth and development may reduce these adaptive changes in children. Given the difficulties in working with infants and very young children, such programmes might require the use of simple mechanical training aids.

There is a need for studies on the effect of different treatment modalities on passive stiffness as well as on muscle weakness starting in infancy, and on the impact of specific methods such as eccentric or isokinetic resistance training exercises. This certainly opens up avenues for future research if conducted for longer time durations to explore the relationship between passive mechanical changes and long-term strength training regimens.

## Conclusion

Skeletal muscle is not only characterized by its contractile properties but also by its viscoelastic properties that are often under-reported by researchers and clinicians. This series of studies has shown that the passive mechanical properties of the calf muscle were significantly different in children with CP compared to typically developing children and this has an effect on some aspects of function. Also, the studies have shown the importance of quantifying secondary, adaptive changes in muscle even though it is difficult to distinguish these clinically from the contribution of reflex hyperexcitability (using Ashworth or Tardieu scales). Therefore, evaluation techniques in the clinic need to be optimized, perhaps by combining biomechanical with electrophysiological measurements. Interventions for children with CP may need to focus earlier than usual and to a greater extent on the passive mechanical properties of muscle and not just motor neuron excitability. BoNT-A will be of little use in improving function if increased muscle resistance, rather than hyperreflexia, is the primary cause of the impairment.

## References

Abellaneda, S., Guissard, N., Duchateau, J., 2009. The relative lengthening of the myotendinous structures in the medial gastrocnemius during passive stretching differs among individuals. J. Appl. Physiol. 106, 169–177.

Ada, L., Vattanasilp, W., O'Dwyer, N.J., Crosbie, J., 1998. Does spasticity contribute to walking dysfunction after stroke? J. Neurol. Neurosurg. Psychiatry 64, 628–635.

Alhusaini, A., Crosbie, J., Shepherd, R., Dean, C., Scheinberg, A., 2010a. Passive mechanical properties of the calf muscles in children with cerebral palsy compared to healthy children. Dev. Med. Child Neurol. 52, e101–e106.

Alhusaini, A.A.A., Dean, C.M., Crosbie, J., Shepherd, R.B., Lewis, J., 2010b. Evaluation of spasticity in children with cerebral palsy using Ashworth and Tardieu scales compared with laboratory measures. J. Child Neurol. 25, 1242.

Alhusaini, A.A.A., Crosbie, J., Shepherd, R.B., Dean, C.M., Scheinberg, A., 2011. No change in calf muscle passive stiffness after botulinum toxin injection in children with cerebral palsy. Dev. Med. Child Neurol. 53, 553–558.

Alibiglou, L., Rymer, W.Z., Harvey, R.L., Mirbagheri, M.M., 2008. The relation between Ashworth scores and neuromechanical measurements of spasticity following stroke. J. Neuroeng. Rehabil. 5, 18.

Ansari, N.N., Naghdi, S., Moammeri, H., Jalaie, S., 2006. Ashworth Scales are unreliable for the assessment of muscle spasticity. Physiother. Theory Pract. 22, 119–125.

Becher, J.G., Harlaar, J., Lankhorst, G.J., Vogelaar, T.W., 1998. Measurement of impaired muscle function of the gastrocnemius, soleus, and tibialis anterior muscles in spastic hemiplegia: a preliminary study. J. Rehabil. Res. Dev. 35, 314–326.

Chesworth, B.M., Vandervoort, A.A., 1988. Reliability of a torque motor system for measurement of passive ankle joint stiffness in control subjects. Physiother. Can. 40, 300–303.

Crosbie, J., Alhusaini, A.A., Dean, C.M., Shepherd, R.B., 2012. Plantarflexor muscle and spatiotemporal gait characteristics of children with hemiplegic cerebral palsy: an observational study. Dev. Neurorehabil. 15, 114–118.

Dietz, V., Berger, W., 1983. Normal and impaired regulation of muscle stiffness in gait: a new hypothesis about muscle hypertonia. Exp. Neurol. 79, 680–687.

Dietz, V., Sinkjaer, T., 2007. Spastic movement disorder: impaired reflex function and altered muscle mechanics. Lancet Neurol. 6, 725–733.

Fleuren, J.F., Voerman, G.E., Erren-Wolters, C.V., Snoek, G.J., Rietman, J.S., Hermens, H.J., et al., 2010. Stop using the Ashworth Scale for the assessment of spasticity. J. Neurol. Neurosurg. Psychiatry 81, 46–52.

Hermens, H.J., Freriks, B., Disselhorst-Klug, C., Rau, G., 2000. Development of recommendations

for SEMG sensors and sensor placement procedures. J. Electromyogr. Kinesiol. 10, 001–0.14.

Kumar, R.T., Pandyan, A.D., Sharma, A.K., 2006. Biomechanical measurement of post-stroke spasticity. Age Ageing 35, 371–375.

Lambertz, D., Mora, I., Grosset, J.F., Perot, C., 2003. Evaluation of musculotendinous stiffness in prepubertal children and adults, taking into account muscle activity. J. Appl. Physiol. 95, 64–72.

Mirbagheri, M.M., Barbeau, H., Kearney, R.E., 2000. Intrinsic and reflex contributions to human ankle stiffness: variation with activation level and position. Exp. Brain Res. 135, 423–436.

Mohagheghi, A.A., Khan, T., Meadows, T.H., Giannikas, K., Baltzopoulos, V., Maganaris, C.N., 2007. Differences in gastrocnemius muscle architecture between the paretic and non-paretic legs in children with hemiplegic cerebral palsy. Clin. Biomech. (Bristol, Avon) 22, 718–724.

Moseley, A., Adams, R., 1991. Measurement of passive ankle dorsiflexion: procedure and reliability. Aust. J. Physiother. 373, 175–181.

Moseley, A.M., Crosbie, J., Adams, R., 2001. Normative data for passive ankle plantarflexion–dorsiflexion flexibility. Clin. Biomech. (Bristol, Avon) 16, 514–521.

Mutlu, A., Livanelioglu, A., Gunel, M.K., 2008. Reliability of Ashworth and modified Ashworth scales in children with spastic cerebral palsy. BMC Musculoskelet. Disord. 9, 44.

Pandyan, A.D., Johnson, G.R., Price, C.I., Curless, R.H., Barnes, M.P., Rodgers, H., 1999. A review of the properties and limitations of the Ashworth and modified Ashworth

Scales as measures of spasticity. Clin. Rehabil. 13, 373–383.

Pierce, S.R., Prosser, L.A., Lauer, R.T., 2010. Relationship between age and spasticity in children with diplegic cerebral palsy. Arch. Phys. Med. Rehabil. 91, 448–451.

Rabita, G., Dupont, L., Thevenon, A., Lensel-Corbeil, G., Perot, C., Vanvelcenaher, J., 2005. Quantitative assessment of the velocity-dependent increase in resistance to passive stretch in spastic plantarflexors. Clin. Biomech. (Bristol, Avon) 20, 745–753.

Riemann, B.L., Demont, R.G., Ryu, K., Lephart, S.M., 2001. The effects of sex, joint angle, and the gastrocnemius muscle on passive ankle joint complex stiffness. J. Athl. Train. 36, 369–375.

Sinkjaer, T., Toft, E., Andreassen, S., Hornemann, B.C., 1988. Muscle stiffness in human ankle dorsiflexors: intrinsic and reflex components. J. Neurophysiol. 60, 1110–1121.

Van Der Salm, A., Veltink, P.H., Hermens, H.J., Ijzerman, M.J., Nene, A.V., 2005. Development of a new method for objective assessment of spasticity using full range passive movements. Arch. Phys. Med. Rehabil. 86, 1991–1997.

Yam, W.K., Leung, M.S., 2006. Interrater reliability of modified Ashworth scale and modified Tardieu scale in children with spastic cerebral palsy. J. Child Neurol. 21, 1031–1035.

Zhao, H., Ren, Y.P., Wu, Y.N., Liu, S.Q., Zhang, L.Q., 2009. Ultrasonic evaluations of Achilles tendon mechanical properties poststroke. J. Appl. Physiol. 106, 843–849.

# The syndrome of deforming spastic paresis: pathophysiology, assessment and treatment

5

Nicolas Bayle, Jean-Michel Gracies

## CHAPTER CONTENTS

Central nervous system (CNS) lesions affecting central motor pathways involved in motor command execution lead to the syndrome of deforming spastic paresis, i.e., stretch-sensitive paresis associated with soft tissue shortening and stretch-sensitive muscle overactivity (Gracies, 2005a,b). Such lesions may be caused by disorders as common as infant paresis (a term we feel is more appropriate than cerebral palsy) but also adult disorders such as stroke, traumatic brain injury, multiple sclerosis, spinal cord injury, anoxic brain injury, primary lateral sclerosis and hereditary spastic paraparesis.

We proposed a simplification of the Lance et al. (1980) definition of spasticity as an 'increase in the velocity-dependent reflexes to phasic stretch' (Gracies, 2005b) This increase, measured at rest, is manifested by both a reduced threshold and an increased gain of the responses to stretch (Gracies, 2005b). As such, spasticity is probably not the most disabling type of muscle overactivity. The whole syndrome of deforming spastic paresis, however, causes limb deformities and motor limitations hindering social life, mobility and activities of daily living. This chapter reviews the triple phenomenology of deforming spastic paresis (stretch-sensitive paresis, soft tissue contracture and muscle overactivity) including the definition of the different types of muscle overactivity, methods of clinical evaluation, and therapeutic methods currently established through controlled protocols, particularly as it pertains to children with infant paresis.

# Phenomenology and taxonomy in deforming spastic paresis

Three fundamental phenomena occur after a lesion to the central pathways involved with motor command execution: stretch-sensitive paresis, soft tissue contracture and spastic muscle overactivity.

## Stretch-sensitive paresis

*Paresis*, i.e., the quantitative lack of voluntary command accessing agonist muscles when attempting to generate force or movement, is the first, immediate consequence of a CNS lesion involving the corticospinal pathway (Gracies, 2005a). This lack of voluntary activation involves insufficient synchronization, insufficient discharge frequency and higher firing threshold of the recruited motor units. The term *stretch-sensitive* paresis was coined to refer to further reduction of the ability to recruit motor units in an agonist effort when a contractured, spastic antagonist is stretched (Gracies, 2005b). This phenomenon occurs particularly for the less contractured of two muscles around a joint.

## Soft tissue contracture

As a consequence of paresis, some muscles and their surrounding soft tissues are left immobilized in a shortened position, relating to the influence of gravity when patients are left in a specific body posture most of the day (often reclined, or supine). Reciprocally, their antagonists are also submitted to immobilization due to paresis but in a normal or lengthened position. This is the first source of the asymmetry that will characterize muscle changes around joints, with some muscles (often lower limb extensors and upper limb flexors, internal rotators and pronators) undergoing contracture to a much greater extent than their antagonists. In a muscle left immobilized in a short position, muscle plasticity, characterized by gene changes and transcriptional events leading to protein synthesis modifications within muscle fibres (Baptista et al., 2010; Giger et al., 2009), initiates as soon as a few hours after immobilization onset. These modified transcriptional profiles have also been observed and analysed in children with infant paresis (Smith et al., 2009). These muscle changes are understood under the term *contracture*, which involves at least:

(a) physical shortening, which adapts soft tissue (muscles, tendons, ligaments, joint capsules, skin, vessels and nerves) to its newly imposed length; (b) reduced extensibility; and (c) modifications of muscle contractile properties, e.g., slow-to-fast changes of originally slow muscles (Baptista et al., 2010; Giger et al., 2009; Gracies, 2005a; Smith et al., 2009). These early transformations only intensify in the days and weeks that follow the onset of immobilization, if no or insufficient preventative treatment is implemented (Gracies, 2005b). They initiate the body deformities characteristic of deforming spastic paresis. When the initial neural paresis-causing lesion has occurred in the perinatal period, muscle contracture will later affect bone growth along with normal muscle lengthening (Hof, 2001). With today's therapeutic management, it is likely that such contracture is not adequately treated in paretic children as a large retrospective study in plantar flexor muscles recently showed that the range of ankle dorsiflexion decreases by 19 degrees during the first 18 years of life in children with infant paresis (Hägglund and Wagner, 2011). These disfigurements will become increasingly challenging, socially and psychologically, if appropriate preventative or curative treatment is not implemented.

## Spastic muscle overactivity

After damage to corticospinal pathways, lesion- and behaviour-induced adaptive changes take place within higher centres and the spinal cord (Gracies, 2005b). Intraspinal reorganization occurs as growth factors, adhesion and guidance molecules and other components fostering synapse neogenesis are produced by denervated ventral horns at spinal segments (Giger et al., 2010; Maier et al., 2008; Raineteau et al., 2002). Mature or maturing descending motor tracts (brainstem descending and contralesional corticospinal pathways) thus undergo intraspinal reconnections, through local cues guiding newly formed sprouts in the denervated spinal cord (Maier et al., 2008; Raineteau et al., 2002). Brainstem descending pathways (rubro-, tecto-, reticulo-, vestibulospinal) and contralesional corticospinal pathways are increasingly recruited at higher centres—potentially via frontal or transcallosal disinhibition after brain lesions—to take over some of the motor command execution (Ghosh et al., 2009; Giger et al., 2010;

Maier et al., 2008; Raineteau et al., 2002; Riddle and Baker, 2010). Most of these brainstem descending pathways tend to be permanently active at rest, thus creating the conditions for the emergence of permanent, dystonic muscle activity through their newly formed motoneuronal connections, as such ongoing descending activity impacts on a sensitized, hyperexcitable motor neuron ('denervation hypersensitivity', see below).

At each spinal level, local sprouting from neighbouring interneurons is also promoted, fostering the formation of new abnormal synapses between these interneurons and the somatic membrane of the deprived motor neurons. These new segmental or propriospinal synapses form a substratum for the emergence of motor neuron hyperexcitability and new abnormal or exaggerated reflex pathways (Gracies, 2005b). The superimposition of augmented descending and reflex inputs on hyperexcitable motor neurons leads to overall muscle overactivity, which adopts various forms.

## Spasticity

Spasticity has been the most commonly recognized manifestation among these gradually occurring reflex changes. Using a simplified definition as *an increase in the velocity-dependent stretch reflexes* (Gracies, 2005b), it is possible to observe spasticity at rest by excessive responses to muscle stretch or tendon taps. When compared to normal subjects, stretch-induced contraction at rest occurs at lower threshold and with increased amplitude in patients with deforming spastic paresis.

Thus, the optimal condition for detecting and evaluating spasticity is *the use of phasic stretch (i.e., the movement of stretch) at rest*. Spasticity does not constitute a highly disabling form of muscle overactivity, except in attempts at fast or ballistic active movements or when stretch-induced clonus is triggered and interferes with posture or movement in activities such as nursing or dressing.

## Spastic dystonia

From his animal studies using motor or premotor cortex ablations, Denny-Brown has coined the term spastic dystonia to describe the tonic, chronic muscle activity present at rest in the context of spasticity, a symptom confirmed by Laplane in humans affected by similar lesions (Denny-Brown, 1966; Gracies, 2005b; Laplane et al., 1977). Spastic dystonia represents spontaneous muscle overactivity at rest, without a specific triggering factor. A simple observation of patients with deforming spastic paresis at rest may often point to this type of muscle overactivity, as it enhances deformity of joint and body postures. Spastic dystonia thus represents an additional major cause of disfigurement and social disability, as it exacerbates the cosmetic consequences of soft tissue contracture.

Thus, the optimal condition for detecting and evaluating spastic dystonia is *natural observation at rest, without phasic or tonic stretch*. Simple experiments have demonstrated actual reduction of the degree of spastic dystonia with sustained stretch (Gracies and Simpson, 2004). The choice of the term *spastic* dystonia thus finds double justification: this form of dystonia is present in the context of spasticity and is itself stretch-sensitive.

## Spastic co-contraction

Spastic co-contraction is defined as an unwanted, excessive level of antagonistic muscle activity during voluntary agonist command, which is aggravated by stretch of the co-contracting muscle (Gracies, 2005b; Gracies et al., 1997). Spastic co-contraction is a descending phenomenon, most likely due to misdirection of the supraspinal drive during voluntary command (Gracies, 2005b; Gracies et al., 1997; Kukke and Sanger, 2011). It may be facilitated by increased recurrent inhibition, causing loss of reciprocal inhibition to antagonists during voluntary agonist command (Crone et al., 2003; Gracies, 2005b; Gracies et al., 2009; Vinti et al., 2012). Spastic co-contraction is aggravated as effort increases in intensity and duration (Gracies et al., 1997; Vinti et al., 2012).

Thus, the optimal condition for detecting and evaluating spastic co-contraction is *voluntary agonist command, regardless of any stretch imposed on muscles*. Spastic co-contraction likely represents the most disabling form of muscle overactivity in deforming spastic paresis, also in children with infant paresis, as it impedes force or movement generation, diminishes range of active motion and resists alternating movement (Damiano et al., 2000; Kukke and Sanger, 2011; Vinti et al., 2012).

## Other types of muscle overactivity

Other types of muscle overactivity comprise forms that may not be prominently stretch-sensitive.

These forms of overactivity include excessive extrasegmental co-contraction, termed 'synkinesis', 'overflow', 'associated reactions', or even 'athetosis' or 'chorea' depending among others on movement briskness or speed and on the author's discipline (Chui et al., 2010; Kukke and Sanger, 2011). Excessive extrasegmental co-contraction is an unwanted, abnormally high recruitment of muscles that are distant (at a different segmental level) from the agonist involved in the voluntary command (Gracies, 2005b). Extrasegmental co-contraction may become particularly prominent in children with infant paresis and constitute a separate source of 'dynamic deformity' and social and functional disability, which has been correlated with spasticity in one study (Chiu et al., 2010).

Excessive cutaneous or nociceptive responses represent another important form of muscle overactivity, which is often prominent and disabling in some forms of infant paresis or conditions such as spinal cord injury or multiple sclerosis. Finally, inappropriate motor recruitment during autonomic or reflex activities, such as breathing, coughing and yawning, is another characteristic feature in most forms of deforming spastic paresis (Gracies, 2005b).

## Clinical evaluation of deforming spastic paresis

The clinical assessment of *peripheral* paresis involves an ordinal evaluation of each muscle group as an agonist, i.e. *for its capacity to generate movement or agonist power*, using for example manual measurement with the Medical Research Council scale (John, 1984). This scale provides a number between 0 and 5 meant to represent the amount of command accessing the agonist. Such approach is not valid in deforming spastic paresis, as agonist weakness is impossible to assess manually because of the presence of co-contraction in the antagonist muscle (Crone et al., 2003; Gracies et al., 1997, 2009; Kukke and Sanger, 2011; Vinti et al., 2012).

In direct contrast, in deforming spastic paresis we recommend to assess each muscle group as an antagonist, i.e. *for its potential to oppose movement* (Gracies et al., 2010a). This strategy derives from Tardieu's concept that motor impairment in deforming spastic paresis owes more to resistance from hypoextensible soft tissue and excessively activated antagonistic muscles than to lessened

agonist command (Tardieu, 1966). We recommend to run a five-step assessment in which the first three steps (slow passive, fast passive and active movement against the muscle tested) measure the potential of muscles to oppose passive and active movements. Each step is quantified by estimating the joint angles at which resistance from the tested antagonist arrests each type of movement assessed (Gracies et al., 2010a). In this strategy, the zero is always defined as the angle of minimal stretch of the tested antagonist (Tardieu scale) (Gracies, 2001a; Gracies et al., 2010a,b; Patrick and Ada, 2006; Tardieu, 1966). The fourth step tests the ability to repeat active performance against the tested muscle. The final step evaluates limb function (Gracies et al., 2010a).

## Step 1: maximal range of passive motion ($X_{V1}$)

The clinician evaluates each muscle group using very slow and powerful stretch. This movement must be as slow as possible (V1, slow velocity), to minimize the probability of eliciting a stretch reflex, and as strong as possible for the clinician, to overcome most of the spastic dystonia and finally be arrested by a resistance that approximates the mere involvement of passive soft tissue. The maximal angle at which soft tissue resistance stops the movement (because of invincible resistance, patient discomfort or threat to soft tissue integrity as perceived by the clinician) is defined as the passive range of motion against the tested antagonist. In some cases (when testing large muscles in particular), severe spastic dystonia may not be fully overcome and thus may not be distinguished from soft tissue contracture. This may require a complementary evaluation, using focal motor anaesthetic block (Gracies and Simpson, 2003).

## Step 2: angle of catch ($X_{V3}$) and spasticity grade (Y)

Here the muscle group is evaluated using very fast stretch, at the fastest speed possible for the clinician (V3, fast velocity), to maximize the probability of eliciting a stretch reflex. It is of utmost importance that muscle rest be obtained prior to this fast stretch manoeuvre, using for example an inhibitory manoeuvre such as a brief sequence of fast passive repetitive movements in the direction opposite to that of the fast stretch manoeuvre (Gracies, 2001a; Gracies et al., 2010b). Two parameters are derived: the angle of catch or clonus ($X_{V3}$) represents the threshold to elicit the reflex, and the spasticity grade (Y) describes the type and the strength of the muscle reaction observed at $X_{V3}$ (Gracies, 2001a; Gracies et al., 2010a,b; Patrick and Ada, 2006).

## Step 3: active range of motion

The patient is now asked to reproduce the previously evaluated passive movements using active command against the tested antagonist, to reach as far as possible along the range until the active force produced by the agonist is matched by the combination of passive resistance and spastic co-contraction from the stretched antagonist. The maximal range of active motion—against the muscle tested—is obtained (Gracies et al., 2010a).

## Step 4: frequency of rapid alternating movements of maximal amplitude

The patient performs the same active movement over the maximal range as measured just before, then returns to the starting position and again, as many times as possible in a fixed amount of time (e.g., 15 seconds). The number of maximal amplitude movements performed indicates the ability of the subject to repeat fast active movements despite the likelihood of increased spastic co-contraction as fatigue acutely sets in during the series (Gracies et al., 2009; Vinti et al., 2012). The ability to repeat alternating movements is important for most everyday activities (walking, writing, bringing food to mouth, articulating language) and may in fact constitute the closest technical correlate to active limb function, among these four test manoeuvres.

## Step 5: limb function

### Upper limb

One may rate either objective patient performance as achieved before the rater, or the subjective perception of patient performance, by rater or

patient, based on interviews or questionnaires. To objectively rate patient performance, authors have often developed scores of motor impairment, which do not involve real-life tasks (Desrosiers, 1993; Fugl-Meyer et al., 1975; Heller et al., 1987; Lindmark and Hamrin, 1988; Lyle, 1981; Mathiowetz et al., 1985; Rapin et al., 1966). In children with infant paresis, analogous impairment tests include the Bruininks–Oseretsky Test of Motor Proficiency (Bruininks, 1978; Doll, 1946) and the Quality of Upper Extremity Skills Test (QUEST) (DeMatteo et al., 1992). Other scales, however, aim to directly assess real-life activities. In adults, these may be the Frenchay Arm Test, the Rivermead Motor Assessment, the Wolf Motor Function Test, the Jebsen–Taylor Hand Function Test or the Modified Frenchay Scale (Blanton and Wolf, 1999; Collen et al., 1990; Gracies et al., 2002; Jebsen et al., 1969; Lincoln and Leadbitter, 1979; Wade et al., 1983). In children with infant paresis, the Jebsen–Taylor Hand Function Test is also used and specific video-recorded tests have been developed such as the Melbourne Assessment (Johnson et al., 1994) and the Assisting Hand Assessment for unilateral deficiencies (Krumlinde-Sundholm and Eliasson, 2003).

Subjective patient perception on specific upper limb function in adult hemiparesis may be rated in four domains (limb positioning, hygiene, dressing, pain) in the Disability Assessment Scale (DAS), which has shown reliability and usefulness in adult therapeutic studies (Brashear et al., 2002). In children with infant paresis, the Canadian Occupational Performance Measure (COPM) is designed to assess outcomes in the areas of self-care, productivity and leisure, using a semi-structured interview, yielding two scores, for performance and satisfaction with performance (Law et al., 1990). In the Manual Ability Classification System, parents, teachers or the child itself are asked questions on the child's ability to handle objects in important daily activities: for example during play and leisure, eating and dressing (Eliasson et al., 2006).

Goal Attainment Scaling may be singled out as an attempt at assessing the result of a therapeutic intervention with respect to stated specific goals of the treatment, previously agreed upon between rater and patient, or rater and the patient's parents (Clark and Caudrey, 1983; Sakzewski et al., 2007). This measure may have good sensitivity to change in children with cerebral palsy (Sakzewski et al., 2007). However, it is often difficult to predict the most important effects that a therapeutic intervention will produce for a given patient; in addition, 'success' or 'failure' may itself be subjective as it may only depend on how high aims have been set for a given therapeutic intervention. Finally, such assessment is not able to characterize the functional level of a patient but simply whether an intervention has succeeded or not in modifying this level. Therefore, while Goal Attainment Scaling may be interesting as a complement to the functional assessments described above, it probably cannot replace these more systematic assessments.

## Lower limb

A major function of the lower limb is ambulation. To objectively rate lower limb function, walking tests are useful (10m walking test, 2-minute or 6-minute endurance tests), as walking speed has good ecological validity and correlates with most kinematics gait parameters (speed, step length) in hemiparesis (Moseley et al., 2004). In children with infant paresis, stride length, gait velocity and range of motion are related to the severity of the overall physical handicap. During a walking test, step length and cadence may be measured as well as the physiological cost index, which is the speed divided by the difference between the heart rates measured before and after the effort (Butler et al., 1984; Rose et al., 1985). Instrumental kinematic analysis may be proposed at the laboratory as a complement to these assessments, especially when surgery or another specific procedure is considered (Hutin et al., 2010; Skrotzky, 1983). Finally, a number of questionnaire-based subjective functional scales are available (e.g., the Functional Ambulation Classification or the SIP68 mobility subscale) to evaluate ambulation in daily life (Dobkin et al., 2010; Post et al., 1996). The Gross Motor Function Classification System (GMFCS) is a similar classification used for children with infant paresis, defining five levels of self-initiated ambulation capacities from level I (walks without limitations) to level V (transported in a manual wheelchair system) (Palisano et al., 2008). However, while appropriate to characterize the way patients rate their ambulation capacities, such scales may lack sensitivity to therapeutic interventions over short periods (Dobkin et al., 2010; Post et al., 1996).

# Management of deforming spastic paresis in children

## Treatment of the deformities due to soft tissue shortening: high-load and long-duration stretch

It is important to reiterate here that this treatment, while conceptually simple, is not adequately implemented in most centres today, particularly in children with infant paresis (cerebral palsy) who by the age of 7 years are already characterized by much less extensible muscles than age-matched typically developing children and in whom, as an example, the range of passive ankle dorsiflexion decreases by 19 degrees during the first 18 years of life (Alhusaini et al., 2010; Hägglund and Wagner, 2011). In fact, our personal observation when examining children with cerebral palsy, as they have grown up to be adults, is that their motor impairment owes more to resistance from soft tissue (mechanical) than to central command disorders (neurological), while the opposite is often true for patients with lesions acquired at an adult age.

In deforming spastic paresis, the intertwining between muscle contracture and stretch-sensitive muscle overactivity (Pollock and Davis, 1930; Ranson and Dixon, 1928; Tardieu et al., 1979) contributes to aggravating and consolidating asymmetrical shortening predominating on the more overactive agonist, with the emergence of increasingly fixed deformities (Gracies, 2005b). Here we are reviewing the large body of evidence for the beneficial effect of chronic stretch in deforming spastic paresis, to oppose soft tissue shortening and reduce stretch-sensitive muscle overactivity (Gracies, 2001b).

In animals, chronic stretch has been shown to promote muscle growth by increasing muscle mass, more so than muscle exercise, through genetic, ultrastructural, biochemical (protein content increase), histological changes (weight, length, number of sarcomeres in series, cross-sectional area of type I fibres) and angiogenesis (Carson and Booth, 1998; Cox et al., 2000; Egginton et al., 2001; Goldspink, 1999; Kelley, 1996). Short durations of daily intermittent stretch reversibly increase muscle mass even in muscles otherwise immobilized in short position (Bates, 1993; Carson et al., 1995; Sparrow, 1982; Williams, 1990). Brief muscle stretch also depresses subsequent stretch reflexes due to the slack in intrafusal fibres when muscle is back to its normal length, which reduces background spindle afferent discharge (Burke and Gandevia, 1995; Matthews, 1972; Proske et al., 1993).

## Use in children with spastic paresis

### Brief and sustained stretch: short-term beneficial impact on spastic overactivity and voluntary contractions

In healthy subjects a brief stretch prior to a maximal voluntary concentric contraction permits larger forces at contraction onset, in comparison with contractions starting from rest (Chapman et al., 1985). In adult subjects with deforming spastic paresis, passive joint movements reduce tone and stretch reflexes are depressed following muscle contraction in stretched position (Jahnke et al., 1989; Schmit et al., 2000; Wilson et al., 1999). In deforming spastic paresis, a single session of maintained stretch for 30 minutes to three hours reduces spasticity, especially when the stretch load imposed upon the spastic muscle is maximal (Gracies et al., 2000; Odeen and Knutsson, 1981; Tremblay et al., 1990). Brief muscle stretch also improves subsequent muscle contractions. In spastic paraparesis, spastic hip adductor co-contraction during efforts of hip abduction is thus reduced after a 30-minute stretch session (Odeen, 1981). Sustained stretch may also reduce corticospinal excitability and improve voluntary control of both the stretched muscle and its antagonist (Carey, 1990; Childers et al., 1999; Hummelsheim et al., 1994; Tremblay et al., 1990).

### Chronic stretch: daily stretch duration and optimal timing after injury—combination with treatment of overactivity

Chronic stretch prevents or treats contracture and reduces tone in adults and children with spastic paresis, all effects that correlate with both the daily duration of stretch and the number of days of stretch. The gain in range of motion has been shown to be proportional to the time spent in full range stretch (total end range time [TERT]), particularly in children with infant paresis (Flowers and LaStayo, 1994; McPherson et al., 1985; Tardieu et al., 1988; Zachazewski et al., 1982). Controlled studies testing casts or dynamic splints show that chronic stretch decreases spasticity and

spastic dystonia and increases range of motion more than traditional passive range of motion exercises (Brouwer et al., 2000; Harvey et al., 2009; Kaplan, 1962; Lin et al., 1999; McPherson, 1981; Otis et al., 1985). A single week of 24 hour/day casting may correct ankle plantar flexor contractures in adult patients with traumatic head injuries but stiffness and muscle overactivity return after removal of short duration immobilization (Ada and Canning, 1990, Dicman, 1959, Moseley, 1997, Tona and Schneck et al., 1993). In view of the very rapid muscle changes detectable after few hours of immobilization in short position (Gracies, 2005a), implementation of chronic stretch in vulnerable muscles may be beneficial almost immediately after CNS injury, even though controlled evidence for the benefits of ultra-early chronic stretch after CNS injury is lacking (Ada and Canning, 1990; Conine et al., 1990). Moreover, clinical studies in children with infant paresis confirm physiological experiments in animals indicating that overactivity and shortening are best treated simultaneously: a physical modality lengthening a muscle will have optimal results if combined with chemical or physical treatment relaxing the muscle (Eames et al., 1999; McLachlan, 1983).

## Practical stretch modalities

### Passive range of motion exercises

In this classic technique, the therapist manually stretches muscles at high load for periods of seconds to a few minutes (high-load brief stretch [HLBS]). While limiting loss of sarcomeres, muscle atrophy and modestly increasing range of motion in spastic paresis, this traditional modality is less effective than low-load prolonged stretch (LLPS) using casting or dynamic splinting in decreasing spastic hypertonia and increasing range of motion (Harvey et al., 2009; Light et al., 1984; Otis et al., 1985). In children with infant paresis, adding 30 minutes of electrical stimulation of an agonist to the passive stretch of the antagonist three times a week further improves the passive range of motion of the stretched antagonist (Khalili and Hajihassanie, 2008).

### Daily positioning

The literature shows different results depending on whether high-load or low-load stretch is used.

In subacute adult stroke patients, shoulder positioning in maximal external rotation (high load) for 30 minutes daily, using adjusted trays and soft strapping, reduces the rate of internal rotator contracture generation (Ada et al., 2005). In the spastic lower limb, low stretch loads applied for 30 minutes daily in spastic para- or tetraparesis (7.5 Nm for plantar flexors, 30 Nm for hamstrings) produce modest results after four weeks (Harvey et al., 2000, 2003). Caution must be exercised as compliance and results may be variable when stretch postures are prescribed to be manually applied by the ward staff (Turton and Britton, 2005).

## Self-stretch

Self-application of stretch postures has not been evaluated in controlled trials to our knowledge (Alkandari et al., 2012). Depending on the patient's physical and cognitive abilities and motivation and on the quality of the instructions received from the therapist or physician, the patient may apply this modality on him/herself, at least in distal muscles. This self-stretch management may have a number of advantages:

- A potentially longer duration of daily stretch per muscle, depending on the patient's self-discipline and availability
- A potentially higher load of stretch, depending on the patient's strength and endurance, in the healthy hemibody in particular
- Potential increased limb awareness, decreased disuse and overall increased responsibility and better 'ownership' of the patient regarding his/her own rehabilitation
- Cost-effectiveness in saving therapist time.

## Dynamic splints

Decisions to splint a spastic limb and as to which splint to use are often based more on personal experience than on hard controlled evidence (Lannin et al., 2007a). In neurorehabilitation, shortcomings of static splinting include aggravated disuse, lack of practicality with poor patient compliance, potential for pain, skin maceration and breakdown if the stretching force is excessive and for muscle atrophy if the stretching force is insufficient (Krajnik and Bridle, 1992). While first used in orthopaedic surgery to avoid complete immobilization while applying chronic stretch (Cannon and Strickland,

1985; Feldman, 1990), dynamic splinting has been increasingly used in adults and children with spastic paresis since the 1970s, particularly in the upper limb (Blair et al., 1995; Casey and Kratz, 1988; Scherling and Johnson, 1989). Among the many single-joint models designed, individually tailored Lycra™ splints and gloves have the advantage of stretching several joints at the same time, supinating and extending elbow, as well as extending wrist and fingers (Blair et al., 1995; Gracies et al., 2000). However, such splints may provide only low-load stretch and may be difficult to put on or off independently for patients (Milazzo and Gillen, 1998).

## Static splints

Despite the shortcomings reviewed above, static splints may provide chronic stretch while being easily removable by the patient, as opposed to casts. This allows monitoring of range of motion, skin and vascular condition, and preserving windows in the wearing schedule when passive and active movements are possible. However, as opposed to dynamic splints, static splints prevent normal limb use and reduce access to sensory input and self-management of the hand during the wearing time (Milazzo and Gillen, 1998). Thus, static splints tend to aggravate disuse, or learned non-use (Wolf et al., 1989).

The early concept of 'aggravated spasticity' through splinting at maximal range of motion (Bobath, 1979; Feldman, 1990) is now known to be incorrect, since the documented inhibitory effects of sustained and chronic stretch on spastic muscle overactivity (see above) (Childers et al., 1999; Hummelsheim et al., 1994). In addition, it has been shown that soft tissue stretch is more efficient when the stretch is performed at or close to full range (Flowers and LaStayo, 1994; Tardieu et al., 1988). However, these early 'antispastic' theories have exerted durable influence on the field and classical fabrication guidelines still often recommend that the joint be immobilized in its 'resting posture': e.g., forearm midway between pronation and supination, wrist at 10–30° of extension, metacarpophalangeal and interphalangeal joints flexed at 45° such as in the 'resting pan splint' and the 'submaximum range splint' (Feldman, 1990; McPherson et al., 1985; Milazzo and Gillen, 1998). Such systematic application of resting posture immobilization in spastic patients may also result from confusion between orthopaedic and neurological rehabilitation. In orthopaedic therapy, the preferred resting posture provides appropriate balance of soft tissue on either side of the joint. In deforming spastic paresis, immobilization may have to be deliberately 'imbalanced', i.e., producing high-load stretch of the more overactive muscle, which departs from the 'resting posture'. The good results obtained in open trials when using positions of maximal muscle stretch, or 'within 5 to 10 degrees of full range of motion' (Brennan, 1959; Kaplan, 1962; King, 1982; Lowe, 1995; Mills, 1984) have yet to be confirmed in controlled studies (Lannin et al., 2007a). Regarding the timing of use over the 24 hours, night-time use of static splints has often been viewed as preferable to wearing them during the waking day as the splints may aggravate learned non-use. However, controlled evidence is lacking that static splints applied for a few weeks meaningfully and durably reduce contracture in the muscles that were intended to be stretched (Lannin and Ada, 2011; Milazzo and Gillen, 1998). In children with cerebral palsy, while the literature is characterized by a relative paucity of controlled studies of stretching techniques, a long-term randomized trial of ankle splinting is currently under way (Maas et al., 2012).

## Casting and serial casting

A large variety of casts have been used to achieve steady stretch in the treatment of severe contractures in either lower or upper limbs, in both children or adults, including bivalve casts for intermittent use (Barnard et al., 1984; Booth et al., 1983; Cottalorda et al., 1997; Flett et al., 1999; Hylton and Kahn, 1973; King, 1982; Law et al., 1991; McNee et al., 2007; Sussman and Cusick, 1979; Verplancke et al., 2005; Westberry et al., 2006; Westin and Dye, 1983; Yasukawa, 1990; Zachazewski et al., 1982). Total contact casts apply constant pressure on the skin, which turns off thermal and rapidly adapting tactile receptors, reducing excitatory influence on motor neurons (Barnard et al., 1984; Feldman, 1990). In serial casting, each cast is left between 1 and 10 days, according to the severity of the contracture and the local status (circulation, sensation and motion) of the casted extremity. The gain in range of motion obtained after one cast is incorporated into a subsequent cast, commonly applied in submaximal range of motion, i.e., the maximum range minus 5 to 10 degrees (Feldman, 1990; Westberry et al., 2006). Serial casting thus allows progressive stretch with usually good compliance, particularly in children (Booth et al., 1983; Cottalorda et al., 1997; Feldman, 1990; Flett et al., 1999; Law et al., 1991; McNee et al., 2007; Verplancke et al., 2005; Westberry et al., 2006; Westin and Dye, 1983; Yasukawa, 1990). Serial casting has shown equal effectiveness with botulinum toxin injections in reducing calf tightness in ambulant children with cerebral palsy, although parents have consistently highlighted its inconvenience (Flett et al., 1999). Casts or splints with a flexor hinge allow incremental manual extension with a screwdriver, weekly for example, providing the same effect as serial casting without the need for cast removal (Feldman, 1990).

The optimal condition to apply casting is after focal treatment of muscle overactivity to minimize risks of soft tissue compromise (skin breakdown, oedema formation, circulatory impairment) and neurapraxia (Feldman, 1990; Westberry et al., 2006). Alertness and cognitive abilities are other important considerations. Unconsciousness, poor concentration, reduced memory or unilateral neglect represents unfavourable conditions as those patient may not be able to express pain or discomfort if a cast no longer fits (Ough et al., 1981). Previous unstable fracture, skin breakdown or inadequate circulation represent contra-indications to casting (Joachim-Grizaffi, 1998). Open-label studies suggest that casting may be less effective in teenagers than in younger children (Lannin et al., 2007b). Unfortunately, in children with infant paresis, cross-over trials of serial casting show modest results and parallel group randomized controlled trials are yet to include no-stretch comparison conditions (Lannin et al., 2007b; McNee et al., 2007).

## Stretch: a matter of load and duration

Despite some pessimistic reviews, positive results in the recent controlled literature in adults shed new light on the amount of stretch required to obtain meaningful soft tissue lengthening in deforming spastic paresis. In the calf muscles, while low-load stretch achieves only modest results, standing on the paretic leg for 30 minutes may provide a high-load stretch sufficient to achieve gradual calf muscle lengthening in adults with spastic paresis (Ben et al., 2005; Harvey et al., 2000, 2003; Katalinic et al., 2010). In the adult upper limb, 30 minutes per day in maximal external rotation reduces the development of internal rotator contracture while 30 minutes per day of shoulder extensor stretch at 90 degrees only (far from submaximal stretch load) does not (Ada et al., 2005).

# Treatment (or prevention) of paresis: motor training in children

The therapist involved with deforming spastic paresis should make every effort to improve the ability to voluntarily recruit selected muscles. The pathophysiological substrates of such improvement involve plasticity in the pathways of motor command preparation and execution. The therapist must thus capitalize on the innate capacity of the brain to change and adapt throughout the patient's life (Aisen et al., 2011). CNS plasticity may be *enhanced* by a number of interventions, including environmental enrichment, level of parental interaction, erythropoietin, chemical agents (antidepressants, vasoactive intestinal peptide, serotonin agents), transcranial magnetic stimulation, transcranial direct current stimulation, hypothermia, nutritional supplements and stem cells (Budhdeo and Rajapaksa, 2011; Holt and Mikati, 2011; Passemard et al., 2011). Once enhanced, plasticity may then be *guided* by two fundamental events: injury and training (Nudo, 2006).

## Injury-guided plasticity in children with infant paresis

In children with infant paresis, post-injury plasticity adopts particular features as the lesion occurs within an immature nervous system, more able than the adult brain to bypass the lesion in its development (Panigrahy et al., 2012). It is remarkable in that respect that there are no major differences between right and left infant hemiparetic patients overall, which is likely due to the greater plasticity of the immature brain (Khaw et al., 1994). Language functions, in particular, can be normal even in patients with extensive early left-hemispheric brain lesions, by language organization in the right hemisphere, which takes place in brain regions homotopic to the classical left-hemispheric language areas in normal subjects (Staudt, 2010). The corticospinal tract (CST) has a protracted postnatal development, and thus a protracted period of repair potential/vulnerability after perinatal

brain and spinal cord injury (Martin et al., 2011). Corticospinal motor projections have already reached their spinal target zones at the beginning of the third trimester of pregnancy, with initially bilateral projections from each hemisphere (Staudt, 2010). During normal development, the ipsilateral projections gradually withdraw, letting contralateral projections take charge of most of the motor command (Staudt, 2010). If, during this period, a unilateral brain lesion disrupts the corticospinal projections of one hemisphere, the ipsilateral projections from the contralesional hemisphere persist and allow that hemisphere to take over motor control over the paretic extremities, in addition to its contralateral side (Carr, 1996; Farmer et al., 1991). Depending on the time of the lesion, this may involve sprouting of the intact CST into the ipsilateral denervated half of the spinal cord (Vanek et al., 1998). The phenomenon of increase in ipsilateral command is also observed after bilateral cortical lesions (Maegaki et al., 1999). This mechanism of reorganization is available throughout the pre- and perinatal period, but its efficacy decreases with increasing age at the time of the insult (and perhaps with myelination), although it still persists in adults (see below) (Clowry, 2007; Staudt, 2010). As early injuries may thus interrupt, divert or reroute normal brain maturation, motor control at the spinal cord does not develop normally by lack of the normal influence of maturing descending corticospinal input and involve abnormal connections of remaining motor systems (Clowry, 2007; Staudt, 2010).

As for the somatosensory system, ascending thalamo-cortical somatosensory projections have not yet reached their cortical target zones at the beginning of the third trimester of pregnancy (Staudt, 2010). These projections can thus adjust to brain lesions acquired during this period and bypass periventricular white matter lesions to reach their original cortical target areas in the postcentral gyrus. Thus, somatosensory functions can be well preserved even in cases of large periventricular lesions (Staudt, 2010). In contrast, when the postcentral gyrus itself is affected, no signs for reorganization have been observed and somatosensory functions may be altered in these patients (Rose et al., 2011; Staudt, 2010). The motor signs in cerebral palsy may thus reflect both loss of CST connections and of sensorimotor thalamic pathways as well as development of abnormal connections of remaining motor systems to spinal motor circuits (Carr, 1996; Clowry, 2007;

Farmer et al., 1991; Maegaki et al., 1999; Martin et al., 2011; Rose et al., 2011; Staudt, 2010; Vanek et al., 1998).

## Behaviour-guided plasticity and motor training in infants at risk of cerebral palsy

First, there is a behaviour-induced potentially deleterious plasticity in the brain-damaged infant. If not treated (see below), an infant with cerebral damage will be characterized by a reduction of spontaneous movements and tone, potentially superimposed on impaired perception (Stigger et al., 2011). This is akin to a situation of 'sensorimotor restriction', which has been shown in newborn rodents to induce reduction in motor neuron sizes and branching, regardless of any preexisting brain damage (Stigger et al., 2011).

However, following Vojta's concept, a number of authors have advocated very early intensive training (within the first nine months of life, if possible) to take advantage of higher levels of behaviour-induced brain plasticity in that period (Banaszek, 2010; Cvjeticanin and Polovina, 1999; Hayasi and Arizono, 1999; Lesny et al., 1958; Vojta, 1973a). To perform such training appropriately, early diagnosis is critical (Amiel-Tison, 1968, 2002; Grenier, 1982; Grenier et al., 1995; Vojta, 1965). Apart from a specific infant-adapted neurological examination (Amiel-Tison, 1968, 2002; Grenier, 1982; Grenier et al., 1995; Vojta, 1965), it has been also suggested that palmar and fingerprints in the immediate postnatal period may help detect probability of brain damage and thus offer these children intensive motor training (Cvjeticanin and Polovina, 1999). Correlation between altered digitopalmar dermatoglyphics and severity of brain lesions has not been considered in other studies to our knowledge.

Training in toddlers has long been advocated by some groups, with techniques depending on the functional age, while some preferred softening up the term 'training'—and maybe the techniques involved—into 'education' (Barrett and Jones, 1967; Le Métayer, 1981; Monfraix and Tardieu, 1956; Vojta, 1973b). While a large number of reports exist and research with adequate methodology is applied increasingly often, these developments have not led to a substantial improvement in the scientific foundation of the interventions under study (Siebes et al., 2002). In Vojta's therapy, the early intensive training involves an extensive

family-oriented physiotherapy programme with isometric strengthening of muscles using tactile stimulation and exercises repeated several times a day to rebuild support, trunk erection and vertical mechanisms, improve automatic postural control and phase lower limb movement. Randomized controlled trials are yet to validate this therapy (Lesny et al., 1958; Vojta, 1973a). Single case studies, however, combined with high-sensitivity measures specific for children with infant paresis have made valuable contributions (Bodkin et al., 2003; Siebes et al., 2002). In particular, treadmill training and cycling induced by functional electrical stimulation for infants at high risk for neuromotor disabilities have been shown to be feasible (Bodkin et al., 2003; Trevis et al., 2012). Yet, few controlled studies have been carried out. A non-randomized study involved 10 infants with a gestational age of less than 33 weeks and a birth weight of less than 2000 g. The infants were first examined before 3 months of age (corrected for prematurity). The Vojta's method was applied in five infants vs five who did not undergo the programme. Four of the five who completed training could either stand still for five seconds or walk, 52 months after the beginning of the therapy programme. None of the five subjects with no training or insufficient training could accomplish this task 64 months following therapy initiation ($p = 0.03$). The authors concluded that a consistently applied physiotherapy programme resulted in better motor outcomes in this group of children at risk for developing 'spastic diplegic cerebral palsy' (Kanda et al., 2004).

An impressive attempt at studying the effects of very early training to reduce the incidence rate of cerebral palsy in children at risk has been published by a Chinese paediatric group from Beijing (Bao, 2005). The inclusion criterion for the study was based on an incidence rate of cerebral palsy 25 times higher in premature infants than in full-term infants in China: a total of 1053 premature infants (gestational age under 37 weeks, excluding those with congenital deformity and hereditary metabolic diseases) were classified into two groups depending on whether parents accepted and intended to actively participate in early intervention or not. There were 551 infants in the early intervention group and 502 in the routine care group. Intervention started less than a year after birth. In the intervention group, the premature infants received early intervention after discharge from hospital, in addition to routine care, once a month before corrected age of 6 months and once every two months after 6 months. The parents were instructed to stimulate the infant's cognition, language, emotion and communication ability, and the infants were given massage and subjected to exercise with active motor training. In the routine care group, infants received routine care only. The two groups turned out to be comparable for pregnancy complications, gestational age, birth weight, proportion of small for gestational age (SGA), proportion of single and multiple births, fetal stress, postnatal asphyxia, incidence of neonatal hypoxic ischaemic encephalopathy (HIE) and intracranial haemorrhage, Apgar Score and Neonatal Behavioural Neurological Assessment Score at 40 weeks of gestational age. At 1 year of age, the incidence of cerebral palsy was 0.9% (5/551; three mild and two severe cases) in the intervention group and 3.2% (16/502; seven moderate and nine severe cases) in the routine care group ($p < 0.01$). The authors concluded that early intervention can reduce the incidence of cerebral palsy of premature infants. Despite these compelling findings, this conclusion awaits confirmation from truly randomized studies (Bao, 2005). A recent Cochrane review concluded that in pre-term infants (<37 weeks), early intervention (within the first year of life) programmes have a positive influence on cognitive outcomes only, in the short-to-medium term (<5 years of age). However, heterogeneity was wide between the interventions considered (Spittle et al., 2007). Several recent controlled protocols did not have a no-training group or an intensive therapy group; otherwise, current research is often limited to pre–post designs (Hielkema et al., 2011; Law et al., 2011; Whittingham et al., 2011). To address this paucity in the literature and provide families of children at high risk for infant paresis with an evidence-based intervention to address behavioural and emotional problems as well as parenting challenges, randomized protocols are under way (Hielkema et al., 2010; Oberg et al., 2012; Wallender et al., 2010).

Among therapy techniques implemented in older children, already with a diagnosis of infant paresis (cerebral palsy), it is probably important to mention constraint-induced movement therapy, which may find in this population a more needed and appropriate indication than in patients with adult-acquired lesions. A randomized controlled clinical trial of constraint-induced therapy in which 18 children with diagnosed hemiparesis associated with cerebral palsy (7–96 months old) were randomly assigned to receive either constraint-induced therapy or conventional treatment showed that constraint-induced therapy produced major and sustained improvement in motoric function in the young children with hemiparesis in the study (Taub et al., 2004) This was corroborated in a non-randomized protocol, in children beyond 18 months of age, which evaluated an individually customized modified constraint-induced therapy vs conventional therapy. At 2 and 6 months, children who received constraint-induced therapy improved their ability to use their paretic hand (Assisting Hand Assessment) significantly more than the children in the control group (Eliasson et al., 2005).

## Perspectives: little fundamental difference between older children or adults with cerebral palsy and adults with adult-acquired lesions

As for the adult brain, a number of rehabilitation techniques are available in clinical practice to promote and guide brain plasticity with the aim to enhance motor function in children with deforming spastic paresis, as long as intensity of training, high number of repetition, focused attention and muscle activation are involved (see Chapters 1 and 11; Bayle and Gracies, 2012). Some of these techniques are now supported by the robust literature (chronic stretch, some motor training techniques, blocking agents), whereas others need further controlled clinical investigations to confirm or optimize their clinical benefit (e.g., non-invasive brain or peripheral stimulation) and to establish clinical relevance and long-term tolerance (e.g., chemicals used on a damaged brain). Novel management methods are also being proposed that rely on contracts between therapist and patient to foster patient sense of responsibility and self-discipline. They are called *Self-Rehabilitation Contracts*. These methods also require controlled evidence (Alkandari et al., 2012; Bayle and Gracies, 2012; Gracies, 2003).

## Conclusion

It may seem unfortunate that clinicians used to treating brain-damaged adults with deforming spastic paresis find that the population of grown-ups with cerebral palsy are the most difficult to improve. They may also observe that the hurdles to overcome in these adults with cerebral palsy have more to do with major soft tissue changes (akin to what is seen in a patient with an adult-acquired lesion who stopped rehabilitation for a couple of decades) than with major disturbances of neural command. When considering the literature on treatment of cerebral palsy, two unmet needs are obvious: (a) the lack of randomized controlled studies testing long-duration and high-load stretch in the more shortened muscles, as such interventions might have the potential to reshape muscles, prepare them for the growth spurts and a better function in adulthood, and (b) the lack of controlled randomized studies testing high-intensity training techniques in infants at high risk of cerebral palsy, as such interventions might have the potential to reshape motor circuits into better functioning units and thus reduce the level of handicap to be expected.

# References

Ada, L., Canning, C., 1990. Anticipating and avoiding muscle shortening. In: Ada, L., Canning, C. (Eds.), Key Issues in Neurological Physiotherapy. Butterworth-Heinmann, Oxford, pp. 219–236.

Ada, L., Goddard, E., McCully, J., Stavrinos, T., Bampton, J., 2005. Thirty minutes of positioning reduces the development of shoulder external rotation contracture after stroke: a randomized controlled trial. Arch. Phys. Med. Rehabil. 86, 230–234.

Aisen, M.L., Kerkovich, D., Mast, J., Mulroy, S., Wren, T.A., Kay, R.M., et al., 2011. Cerebral palsy: clinical care and neurological rehabilitation. Lancet Neurol. 10 (9), 844–852.

Alhusaini, A.A., Crosbie, J., Shepherd, R.B., Dean, C.M., Scheinberg, A., 2010. Mechanical properties of the plantarflexor musculotendinous unit during passive dorsiflexion in children with cerebral palsy compared with typically developing children. Dev. Med. Child Neurol. 52 (6), e101–e106.

Alkandari, S., Chahrour, R., Alkandari, M., Bayle, N., Tlili, L., Colas, C., et al., 2012. Effects of guided self-rehabilitation contracts together with repeated botulinum neurotoxin injections on walking speed in chronic hemiparesis. A prospective open-label study. Eur. J. Phys. Med. Rehabil. in press.

Amiel-Tison, C., 1968. Neurological evaluation of the maturity of newborn infants. Arch. Dis. Child. 43 (227), 89–93.

Amiel-Tison, C., 2002. Update of the Amiel-Tison neurologic assessment for the term neonate or at 40 weeks corrected age. Pediatr. Neurol. 27 (3), 196–212.

Banaszek, G., 2010. Vojta's method as the early neurodevelopmental diagnosis and therapy concept. Przegl. Lek. 67 (1), 67–76.

Bao, X.L., 2005. National Cooperative Research Group for Lowering Incidence of Cerebral Palsy of Premature Infants through Early Intervention. Lowering incidence of Cerebral Palsy of Premature Infants through Early Intervention. Zhonghua Er Ke Za Zhi 43 (4), 244–247.

Baptista, I.L., Leal, M.L., Artioli, G.G., Aoki, M.S., Fiamoncini, J., Turri, A.O., et al., 2010. Leucine attenuates skeletal muscle wasting via inhibition of ubiquitin ligases. Muscle Nerve 41, 800–808.

Barnard, P., Dill, H., Eldredge, P., Held, J.M., Judd, D.L., Nalette, E., 1984. Reduction of hypertonicity by early casting in a comatose head-injured individual. A case report. Phys. Ther. 64, 1540–1542.

Barrett, M.L., Jones, M.H., 1967. The 'sensory story'. A multi-sensory training procedure for toddlers. 1. Effect on motor function of hemiplegic hand in cerebral palsied children. Dev. Med. Child Neurol. 9 (4), 448–456.

Bates, G.P., 1993. The relationship between duration of stimulus per day and the extent of hypertrophy of slow-tonic skeletal muscle in the fowl, Gallus gallus. Comp. Biochem. Physiol. Comp. Physiol. 106, 755–758.

Bayle, N., Gracies, J.M., 2012. Management of deforming spastic paresis. In: Selzer, Textbook of Neural Repair and Rehabilitation. Cambridge University Press, in press.

Ben, M., Harvey, L., Denis, S., Glinsky, J., Goehl, G., Chee, S., et al., 2005. Does 12 weeks of regular standing prevent loss of ankle mobility and bone mineral density in people with recent spinal cord injuries? A randomized controlled trial. Aust. J. Physiother. 51, 251–256.

Blair, E., Ballantyne, J., Horsman, S., Chauvel, P., 1995. A study of a dynamic proximal stability splint in the management of children with cerebral palsy. Dev. Med. Child Neurol. 37, 544–554.

Blanton, S., Wolf, S.L., 1999. An application of upper-extremity constraint-induced movement therapy in a patient with subacute stroke. Phys. Ther. 79, 847–853.

Bobath, B., 1979. The application of physiological principles to stroke rehabilitation. Practitioner 223, 793–794.

Bodkin, A.W., Baxter, R.S., Heriza, C.B., 2003. Treadmill training for an infant born preterm with a grade III intraventricular hemorrhage. Phys. Ther. 83 (12), 1107–1118.

Booth, B.J., Doyle, M., Montgomery, J., 1983. Serial casting for the management of spasticity in the head-injured adult. Phys. Ther. 63, 1960–1966.

Brashear, A., Gordon, M.F., Elovic, E., 2002. Intramuscular injection of botulinum toxin for the treatment of wrist and finger spasticity after a stroke. N. Engl. J. Med. 347, 395–400.

Brennan, B.J., 1959. Response to stretch of hypertonic muscle groups in hemiplegia. Br. Med. J. 1, 1504–1507.

Brouwer, B., Davidson, L.K., Olney, S.J., 2000. Serial casting in idiopathic toe-walkers and children with spastic cerebral palsy. J. Pediatr. Orthop. 20, 221–225.

Bruininks, R.H., 1978. Bruininks–Oseretsky Test of Motor Proficiency–Owner's Manual. American Guidance Service, Circle Pines, MN.

Budhdeo, S., Rajapaksa, S., 2011. Functional recovery in cerebral palsy may be potentiated by administration of selective serotonin reuptake inhibitors. Med. Hypotheses 77 (3), 386–388.

Burke, D., Gandevia, S.C., 1995. The muscle spindle and its fusimotor control. In: Ferrell, W.R., Proske, U. (Eds.), Neural Control of Movement. Plenum Press, New York, pp. 19–25.

Butler, P., Engelbrecht, M., Major, R.E., Tait, J.H., Stallard, J., Patrick, J.H., 1984. Physiological cost index of walking for normal children and its use as an indicator of physical handicap. Dev. Med. Child Neurol. 26, 607–612.

Cannon, N.M., Strickland, J.W., 1985. Therapy following flexor tendon surgery. Hand Clin. 1, 147–165.

Carey, J.R., 1990. Manual stretch: effect on finger movement control and force control in stroke subjects with spastic extrinsic finger flexor muscles. Arch. Phys. Med. Rehabil. 71, 888–894.

Carr, L.J., 1996. Development and reorganization of descending motor pathways in children with hemiplegic cerebral palsy. Acta. Paediatr. Suppl. 416, 53–57.

Carson, J.A., Booth, F.W., 1998. Myogenin mRNA is elevated during rapid, slow, and maintenance phases of stretch-induced hypertrophy in chicken slow-tonic muscle. Pflugers Arch. 435, 850–858.

Carson, J.A., Alway, S.E., Yamaguchi, M., 1995. Time course of hypertrophic adaptations of the anterior latissimus dorsi muscle to stretch overload in aged Japanese quail. J. Gerontol. A. Biol. Sci. Med. Sci. 50, B391–B398.

Casey, C.A., Kratz, E.J., 1988. Soft splinting with neoprene: the thumb abduction supinator splint. Am. J. Occup. Ther. 42, 395–398.

Chapman, A.E., Caldwell, G.E., Selbie, W.S., 1985. Mechanical output following muscle stretch in forearm supination against inertial loads. J. Appl. Physiol. 59, 78–86.

Childers, M.K., Biswas, S.S., Petroski, G., Merveille, O., 1999. Inhibitory casting decreases a vibratory inhibition index of the H-reflex in the spastic upper limb. Arch. Phys. Med. Rehabil. 80, 714–716.

Chiu, H.C., Ada, L., Butler, J., Coulson, S., 2010. Characteristics of associated reactions in people with hemiplegic cerebral palsy. Physiother. Res. Int. [Epub ahead of print].

Clark, M.S., Caudrey, D.J., 1983. Evaluation of rehabilitation services: the use of goal attainment scaling. Int. Rehabil. Med. 5, 41–45.

Clowry, G.J., 2007. The dependence of spinal cord development on corticospinal input and its significance in understanding and treating spastic cerebral palsy. Neurosci. Biobehav. Rev. 31 (8), 1114–1124.

Collen, F.M., Wade, D.T., Bradshaw, C.M., 1990. Mobility after stroke: reliability of measures of impairment and disability. Int. Disabil. Stud. 12, 6–9.

Conine, T.A., Sullivan, T., Mackie, T., Goodman, M., 1990. Effect of serial casting for the prevention of equinus in patients with acute head injury. Arch. Phys. Med. Rehabil. 71, 310–312.

Cottalorda, J., Gautheron, V., Charmet, E., Chavrier, Y., 1997. Muscular lengthening of the triceps by successive casts in children with cerebral palsy. Rev. Chir. Orthop. Reparatrice Appar. Mot. 83, 368–371.

Cox, V.M., Williams, P.E., Wright, H., James, R.S., Gillott, K.L., Young, I.S., et al., 2000. Growth induced by incremental static stretch in adult rabbit latissimus dorsi muscle. Exp. Physiol. 85, 193–202.

Crone, C., Johnsen, L.L., Biering-Sorensen, F., Nielsen, J.B., 2003. Appearance of reciprocal facilitation of ankle extensors from ankle flexors in patients with stroke or spinal cord injury. Brain 126, 495–507.

Cvjeticanin, M., Polovina, A., 1999. Quantitative analysis of digitopalmar dermatoglyphics in male children with central nervous system lesion by quantification of clinical parameters

of locomotor disorder. Acta. Med. Croatica 53 (1), 5–10.

Damiano, D.L., Martellotta, T.L., Sullivan, D.J., Granata, K.P., Abel, M.F., 2000. Muscle force production and functional performance in spastic cerebral palsy: relationship of cocontraction. Arch. Phys. Med. Rehabil. 81 (7), 895–900.

DeMatteo, C., Law, M., Russell, D., Pollock, N., Rosenbaum, P., Walter, S., 1992. QUEST: Quality of Upper Extremity Skills Test. McMaster University, Neurodevelopmental Clinical Research Unit, Hamilton, ON.

Denny-Brown, D., 1966. The Cerebral Control of Movement. University Press, Liverpool, pp. 124–143.

Desrosiers, J., Hébert, R., Dutil, E., Bravo, G., 1993. Development and reliability of an upper extremity function test for the elderly: the Tempa. Can. J. Occup. Ther. 60, 9–16.

Dobkin, B.H., Plummer-d'Amato, P., Elashoff, R., Lee, J., SIRROWS Group, 2010. International randomized clinical trial, stroke inpatient rehabilitation with reinforcement of walking speed (SIRROWS), improves outcomes. Neurorehabil. Neural Repair 24, 235–242.

Doll, E.A., 1946. The Oseretsky Tests of Motor Proficiency. American Guidance Service, Circle Pines, MN.

Eames, N.W., Baker, R., Hill, N., Graham, K., Taylor, T., Cosgrove, A., 1999. The effect of botulinum toxin A on gastrocnemius length: magnitude and duration of response. Dev. Med. Child Neurol. 41, 226–232.

Egginton, S., Zhou, A., Brown, M.D., Hudlicka, O., 2001. Unorthodox angiogenesis in skeletal muscle. Cardiovasc Res. 49, 634–646.

Eliasson, A.C., Krumlinde-Sundholm, L., Shaw, K., Wang, C., 2005. Effects of constraint-induced movement therapy in young children with hemiplegic cerebral palsy: an adapted model. Dev. Med. Child Neur. 47 (4), 266–275.

Eliasson, A.C., Krumlinde-Sundholm, L., Rösblad, B., Beckung, E., Arner, M., Öhrvall, A.M., et al., 2006. The Manual Ability Classification System (MACS) for children with cerebral palsy: scale development and evidence of validity and reliability. Dev. Med. Child Neur. 48, 549–554.

Farmer, S.F., Harrison, L.M., Ingram, D.A., Stephens, J.A., 1991. Plasticity of central motor pathways in children with hemiplegic cerebral palsy. Neurology 41 (9), 1505–1510.

Feldman, P.A., 1990. Upper extremity casting and splinting. In: Glenn, Whyte, The Practical Management of Spasticity in Children and Adults. Lea & Febiger, Philadelphia–London, p. 149.

Flett, P.J., Stern, L.M., Waddy, H., Connell, T.M., Seeger, J.D., Gibson, S.K., 1999. Botulinum toxin A versus fixed cast stretching for dynamic calf tightness in cerebral palsy. J. Paediatr. Child Health 35, 71–77.

Flowers, K.R., LaStayo, P., 1994. Effect of total end range time on improving passive range of motion. J. Hand Ther. 7, 150–157.

Fugl-Meyer, A.R., Jaasko, L., Leyman, I., Olsson, S., Steglind, S., 1975. The post-stroke hemiplegic patient. A method for evaluation of physical performance. Scand. J. Rehab. Med. 7, 13–31.

Ghosh, A., Sydekum, E., Haiss, F., Peduzzi, S., Zörner, B., Schneider, R., et al., 2009. Functional and anatomical reorganization of the sensory-motor cortex after incomplete spinal cord injury in adult rats. J. Neurosci. 29, 12210–12219.

Giger, J.M., Bodell, P.W., Zeng, M., Baldwin, K.M., Haddad, F., 2009. Rapid muscle atrophy response to unloading: pretranslational processes involving MHC and actin. J. Appl. Physiol. 107, 1204–1212.

Giger, R.J., Hollis 2nd, E.R., Tuszynski, M.H., 2010. Guidance molecules in axon regeneration. Cold Spring Harb. Perspect Biol. 2 (7), a001867.

Goldspink, G., 1999. Changes in muscle mass and phenotype and the expression of autocrine and systemic growth factors by muscle in response to stretch and overload. J. Anat. 194, 323–334.

Gracies, J.M., 2001a. Evaluation de la spasticité–Apport de l'echelle de tardieu. Motricité Cérébrale 22, 1–16.

Gracies, J.M., 2001b. Pathophysiology of impairment in spasticity, and use of stretch as a treatment of spastic hypertonia. Phys. Med. Rehabil. Clin. N. Am. 12 (4), 747–768.

Gracies, J.M., 2003. Autoprise en charge du membre supérieur chez l'hémiplégique: expérience pilote d'un programme intensif d'étirements et de mouvements alternatifs rapides à domicile au long cours. Ann. Med. Phys. 46 (7), 429.

Gracies, J.M., 2005a. Pathophysiology of spastic paresis. I: paresis and soft tissue changes. Muscle Nerve 31, 535–551.

Gracies, J.M., 2005b. Pathophysiology of spastic paresis. II: Emergence of muscle overactivity. Muscle Nerve 31, 552–571.

Gracies, J.M., Simpson, D., 2003. Focal injection therapy. In: Hallett, M. (Ed.), The Handbook of Clinical Neurophysiology. Elsevier Science B.V., Philadelphia, pp. 651–695.

Gracies, J.M., Simpson, D.M., 2004. Spastic dystonia. In: Brin, M.F., Comella, C., Jankovic, J. (Eds.), Dystonia: Etiology, Classification, and Treatment. Lippincott Williams & Wilkins, Philadelphia, pp. 192–210.

Gracies, J.M., Wilson, L., Gandevia, S.C., Burke, D., 1997. Stretched position of spastic muscles aggravates their co-contraction in hemiplegic patients. Ann. Neurol. 42, 438–439.

Gracies, J.M., Marosszeky, J.E., Renton, R., Sandanam, J., Gandevia, S.C., Burke, D., 2000. Short-term effects of dynamic Lycra splints on upper limb in hemiplegic patients. Arch. Phys. Med. Rehabil. 81, 1547–1555.

Gracies, J.M., Hefter, H., Simpson, D., Moore, P., 2002. Botulinum toxin in spasticity. In: Moore, P., Naumann, M. (Eds.), Handbook of Botulinum Toxin Blackwell Science, New York, NY, pp. 221–274.

Gracies, J.M., Lugassy, M., Weisz, D.J., Vecchio, M., Flanagan, S., Simpson, D.M., 2009. Botulinum toxin dilution and endplate targeting in spasticity: a double-blind controlled study. Arch. Phys. Med. Rehab. 90, 9–16.

Gracies, J.M., Bayle, N., Vinti, M., Alkandari, S., Vu, P., Loche, C.M., et al., 2010a. Five-step clinical assessment in spastic paresis. Eur. J. Phys. Rehabil. Med. 46 (3), 411–421.

Gracies, J.M., Burke, K., Clegg, N.J., Browne, R., Rushing, C., Fehlings, D., et al., 2010b. Reliability of the Tardieu scale for assessing spasticity in children with cerebral palsy. Arch. Phys. Med. Rehabil. 91, 421–428.

Grenier, A., 1982. Early diagnosis of cerebral palsy … Why do it? Ann. Pediat. (Paris) 29 (7), 509–514.

Grenier, A., Hernandorena, X., Sainz, M., Contraires, B., Carré, M., Bouchet, E., 1995. Complementary neuromotor examination of infants at risk for sequelae. Why? How? Arch. Pediatr. 2 (10), 1007–1012.

Hägglund, G., Wagner, P., 2011. Spasticity of the gastrosoleus muscle is related to the development of reduced passive dorsiflexion of the ankle in children with cerebral palsy: a registry analysis of 2,796 examinations in 355 children. Acta Orthop. 82 (6), 744–748.

Harvey, L.A., Batty, J., Crosbie, J., Poulter, S., Herbert, R.D., 2000. A randomized trial assessing the effects of 4 weeks of daily stretching on ankle mobility in patients with spinal cord injuries. Arch. Phys. Med. Rehabil. 81, 1340–1347.

Harvey, L.A., Byak, A.J., Ostrovskaya, M., Glinsky, J., Katte, L., Herbert, R.D., 2003. Randomised trial of the effects of four weeks of daily stretch on extensibility of hamstring muscles in people with spinal cord injuries. Aust. J. Physiother. 49, 176–181.

Harvey, L.A., Herbert, R.D., Glinsky, J., Moseley, A.M., Bowden, J., 2009. Effects of 6 months of regular passive movements on ankle joint mobility in people with spinal cord injury: a randomized controlled trial. Spinal Cord 47 (1), 62–66.

Hayasi, M., Arizono, Y., 1999. Experience of very early Vojta therapy in two infants with severe perinatal hypoxic encephalopathy. No To Hattatsu 31 (6), 535–541.

Heller, A., Wade, D.T., Wood, V.A., Sunderland, A., Hewer, R.L., Ward, E., 1987. Arm function after stroke: measurement and recovery over the first three months. J. Neurol. Neurosurg. Psychiatry 50, 714–719.

Hielkema, T., Hamer, E.G., Reinders-Messelink, H.A., Maathuis, C.G., Bos, A.F., Dirks, T., et al., 2010. LEARN 2 MOVE 0–2 years: effects of a new intervention program in infants at very high risk for cerebral palsy; a randomized controlled trial. BMC Pediatr. 10, 76.

Hielkema, T., Blauw-Hospers, C.H., Dirks, T., Drijver-Messelink, M.,

Bos, A.F., Hadders-Algra, M., 2011. Does physiotherapeutic intervention affect motor outcome in high-risk infants? An approach combining a randomized controlled trial and process evaluation. Dev. Med. Child Neurol. 53 (3), e8–e15.

Hof, A.L., 2001. Changes in muscles and tendons due to neural motor disorders: implications for therapeutic intervention. Neural Plast. 8 (1–2), 71–81.

Holt, R.L., Mikati, M.A., 2011. Care for child development: basic science rationale and effects of interventions. Pediatr. Neurol. 44 (4), 239–253.

Hummelsheim, H., Munch, B., Butefisch, C., Neumann, S., 1994. Influence of sustained stretch on late muscular responses to magnetic brain stimulation in patients with upper motor neuron lesions. Scand. J. Rehabil. Med. 26, 3–9.

Hutin, E., Pradon, D., Barbier, F., Gracies, J.M., Bussel, B., Roche, N., 2010. Lower limb coordination in hemiparetic subjects: impact of botulinum toxin injections into rectus femoris. Neurorehabil. Neural Repair 24 (5), 442–449.

Hylton, N., Kahn, N., 1973. Casting used as an adjunct to N.D.T. Bobath Alumni Newsletter.

Jahnke, M.T., Proske, U., Struppler, A., 1989. Measurements of muscle stiffness, the electromyogram and activity in single muscle spindles of human flexor muscles following conditioning by passive stretch or contraction. Brain Res. 493, 103–112.

Jebsen, R.H., Taylor, N., Trieschmann, R.B., Trotter, M.J., Howard, L.A., 1969. An objective and standardized test of hand function. Arch. Phys. Med. Rehabil. 50, 311–319.

Joachim-Grizaffi, L., 1998. Casting applications. In: Gillen, G., Burkhardt, A. (Eds.), Stroke Rehabilitation. A Function-Based Algorithm. Mosby, St Louis, pp. 185–204.

John, J., 1984. Grading of muscle power: comparison of MRC and analog scales by physiotherapists. Medical Research Council. Int. J. Rehabil. Res. 7, 173–181.

Johnson, L.M., Randall, M.J., Reddihough, D.S., Oke, L.E., Byrt, T.A., Bach, T.M., 1994. Development of a clinical assessment of quality of movement for unilateral upper-limb

function. Dev. Med. Child Neurol. 36 (11), 965–973.

Kanda, T., Pidcock, F.S., Hayakawa, K., Yamori, Y., Shikata, Y., 2004. Motor outcome differences between two groups of children with spastic diplegia who received different intensities of early onset physiotherapy followed for 5 years. Brain Dev. 26 (2), 118–126.

Kaplan, N., 1962. Effect of splinting on reflex inhibition and sensorimotor stimulation treatment of spasticity. Arch. Phys. Med. Rehabil. 43, 565–569.

Katalinic, O.M., Harvey, L.A., Herbert, R.D., Moseley, A.M., Lannin, N.A., Schurr, K., 2010. Stretch for the treatment and prevention of contractures. Cochrane Database Syst. Rev. 8 (9), CD007455.

Kelley, G., 1996. Mechanical overload and skeletal muscle fiber hyperplasia: a meta-analysis. J. Appl. Physiol. 81, 1584–1588.

Khalili, M.A., Hajihassanie, A., 2008. Electrical simulation in addition to passive stretch has a small effect on spasticity and contracture in children with cerebral palsy: a randomised within-participant controlled trial. Aust. J. Physiother. 54 (3), 185–189.

Khaw, C.W., Tidemann, A.J., Stern, L.M., 1994. Study of hemiplegic cerebral palsy with a review of the literature. J. Paediatr. Child Health 30 (3), 224–229.

King, T.I., 1982. Plaster splinting as a means of reducing elbow flexor spasticity: a case study. Am. J. Occup. Ther. 36, 671–673.

Krajnik, S.R., Bridle, M.J., 1992. Hand splinting in quadriplegia: current practice. Am. J. Occup. Ther. 46, 149–156.

Krumlinde-Sundholm, L., Eliasson, A.-C., 2003. Development of the assisting hand assessment, a Rasch-built measure intended for children with unilateral upper limb impairments. Scand. J. Occup. Ther. 10, 16–26.

Kukke, S.N., Sanger, T.D., 2011. Contributors to excess antagonist activity during movement in children with secondary dystonia due to cerebral palsy. J. Neurophysiol. 105 (5), 2100–2107.

Lance, J.W., Feldman, R.G., Young, R.R., Koeller, C., 1980. Spasticity:

Disorder of Motor Control. Year Book Medical, Chicago, IL, pp. 185–204.

Lannin, N.A., Ada, L., 2011. Neurorehabilitation splinting: theory and principles of clinical use. NeuroRehabilitation 28 (1), 21–28.

Lannin, N.A., Cusick, A., McCluskey, A., Herbert, R.D., 2007a. Effects of splinting on wrist contracture after stroke: a randomized controlled trial. Stroke 38, 111–116.

Lannin, N.A., Novak, I., Cusick, A., 2007b. A systematic review of upper extremity casting for children and adults with central nervous system motor disorders. Clin. Rehabil. 21 (11), 963–976.

Laplane, D., Talairach, J., Meininger, V., Bancaud, J., Bouchareine, A., 1977. Motor consequences of motor area ablations in man. J. Neurol. Sci. 31 (1), 29–49.

Law, M., Baptiste, S., McColl, M., Opzoomer, A., Polatajko, H., Pollock, N., 1990. The Canadian occupational performance measure: an outcome measure for occupational therapy. Can. J. Occup. Ther. 57 (2), 82–87.

Law, M., Cadman, D., Rosenbaum, P., Walter, S., Russell, D., DeMatteo, C., 1991. Neurodevelopmental therapy and upper-extremity inhibitive casting for children with cerebral palsy. Dev. Med. Child Neurol. 33, 379–387.

Law, M.C., Darrah, J., Pollock, N., Wilson, B., Russell, D.J., Walter, S.D., et al., 2011. Focus on function: a cluster, randomized controlled trial comparing child–versus context-focused intervention for young children with cerebral palsy. Dev. Med. Child Neurol. 53 (7), 621–629.

Le Méayer, M., 1981. [Contribution to the investigation of neuro-motor patterns in the newborn and the infant: benefit for early therapeutic education (author's transl)]. Neuropsychiatr. Enfance. Adolesc. 29 (11–12), 587–600.

Lesny, I., Dittrich, J., Opatrny, E., Vojta, V., 1958. Therapeutic methods used at the Institute for the treatment of perinatal encephalopathy (cerebral palsy). Cesk Pediatr. 13 (5), 437–444.

Light, K.E., Nuzik, S., Personius, W., Barstrom, A., 1984. Low-load prolonged stretch vs. high-load brief stretch in treating knee contractures. Phys. Ther. 64, 330–333.

Lin, J.P., Brown, J.K., Walsh, E.G., 1999. Continuum of reflex excitability in hemiplegia: influence of muscle length and muscular transformation after heel-cord lengthening and immobilization on the pathophysiology of spasticity and clonus. Dev. Med. Child Neurol. 41, 534–548.

Lincoln, N.B., Leadbitter, D., 1979. Assessment of motor function in stroke. Physiotherapy 65, 48–51.

Lindmark, B., Hamrin, E., 1988. Evaluation of functional capacity after stroke as a basis for active intervention. Validation of a modified chart for motor capacity assessment. Scand. J. Rehabil. Med. 20, 111–115.

Lowe, C.T., 1995. Construction of hand splints. In: Trombly, C.A. (Ed.), Occupational Therapy for Physical Dysfunction, fourth ed. Williams & Wilkins, Baltimore, Md, pp. 583–597.

Lyle, R.C., 1981. A performance test for assessment of upper limb function in physical rehabilitation treatment and research. Intl. J. Rehabil. Res. 4, 483–492.

Maas, J.C., Dallmeijer, A.J., Huijing, P.A., Brunstrom-Hernandez, J.E., van Kampen, P.J., Jaspers, R.T., et al., 2012. Splint: the efficacy of orthotic management in rest to prevent equinus in children with cerebral palsy, a randomised controlled trial. BMC Pediatr. 12, 38.

Maegaki, Y., Maeoka, Y., Ishii, S., Eda, I., Ohtagaki, A., Kitahara, T., et al., 1999. Central motor reorganization in cerebral palsy patients with bilateral cerebral lesions. Pediatr. Res. 45, 559–567.

Maier, I.C., Baumann, K., Thallmair, M., Weinmann, O., Scholl, J., Schwab, M.E., 2008. Constraint induced movement therapy in the adult rat after unilateral corticospinal tract injury. J. Neurosci. 28, 9386–9403.

Martin, J.H., Chakrabarty, S., Friol, K.M., 2011. Harnessing activity-dependent plasticity to repair the damaged corticospinal tract in an animal model of cerebral palsy. Dev. Med. Child Neurol. 53 (Suppl. 4), 9–13.

Mathiowetz, V., Volland, G., Kashman, N., Weber, K., 1985. Adult norms for the box and block test of manual dexterity. Am. J. Occup. Ther. 39, 386–391.

Matthews, P.B.C., 1972. Mammalian Muscle Receptors and their Central Actions. Williams & Wilkins, London.

McLachlan, E.M., 1983. Modification of the atrophic effects of tenotomy on mouse soleus muscles by various hind limb nerve lesions and different levels of voluntary motor activity. Exp. Neurol. 81, 669–682.

McNee, A.E., Will, E., Lin, J.P., Eve, L.C., Gough, M., Morrissey, M.C., et al., 2007. The effect of serial casting on gait in children with cerebral palsy: preliminary results from a crossover trial. Gait Posture 25 (3), 463–468.

McPherson, J.J., 1981. Objective evaluation of a splint designed to reduce hypertonicity. Am. J. Occup. Ther. 35, 189–194.

McPherson, J.J., Becker, A.H., Franszczak, N., 1985. Dynamic splint to reduce the passive component of hypertonicity. Arch. Phys. Med. Rehabil. 66, 249–252.

Milazzo, S., Gillen, G., 1998. Splinting applications. In: Glen, G., Burkhardt, Stroke Rehabilitation. A Function-based Algorithm. Mosby, St Louis, pp. 161–184.

Mills, V.M., 1984. Electromyographic results of inhibitory splinting. Phys. Ther. 64, 190–193.

Monfraix, C., Tardieu, G., 1956. Concept of functional age; its application to the therapeutic training of cerebral motor handicaps. Rev. Prat. 6 (20), 2244–2252.

Moseley, A.M., 1997. The effect of casting combined with stretching on passive ankle dorsiflexion in adults with traumatic head injuries. Phys. Ther. 77, 240–247.

Moseley, A.M., Lanzarone, S., Bosman, J.M., van Loo, M.A., de Bie, R.A., Hassett, L., et al., 2004. Ecological validity of walking speed assessment after traumatic brain injury: a pilot study. J. Head Trauma Rehabil. 19 (4), 341–348.

Nudo, R.J., 2006. Plasticity. NeuroRx 3 (4), 420–427.

Oberg, G.K., Campbell, S.K., Girolami, G.L., Ustad, T., Jørgensen, L., Kaaresen, P.I., 2012. Study protocol: an early intervention program to improve motor outcome in preterm infants: a randomized controlled trial and a qualitative study of physiotherapy performance and

parental experiences. BMC Pediatr. 12, 15.

Odeen, I., 1981. Reduction of muscular hypertonus by long-term muscle stretch. Scand. J. Rehabil. Med. 13, 93–99.

Odeen, I., Knutsson, E., 1981. Evaluation of the effects of muscle stretch and weight load in patients with spastic paraplegia. Scand. J. Rehabil. Med. 13, 117–121.

Otis, J.C., Root, L., Kroll, M.A., 1985. Measurement of plantar flexor spasticity during treatment with tone-reducing casts. J. Pediatr. Orthop. 5, 682–686.

Ough, J.L., Garland, D.E., Jordan, C., Waters, R.L., 1981. Treatment of spastic joint contractures in mentally disabled adults. Orthop. Clin. North Am. 12, 143–151.

Palisano, R.J., Rosenbaum, P., Bartlett, D., Livingston, M.H., 2008. Content validity of the expanded and revised gross motor function classification system. Dev. Med. Child Neurol. 50 (10), 744–750.

Panigrahy, A., Wisnowski, J.L., Furtado, A., Lepore, N., Paquette, L., Bluml, S., 2012. Neuroimaging biomarkers of preterm brain injury: toward developing the preterm connectome. Pediatr. Radiol. 42 (Suppl 1), S33–S61.

Passemard, S., Sokolowska, P., Schwendimann, L., Gressens, P., 2011. VIP-induced neuroprotection of the developing brain. Curr. Pharm. Des. 17 (10), 1036–1039.

Patrick, E., Ada, L., 2006. The Tardieu Scale differentiates contracture from spasticity whereas the Ashworth Scale is confounded by it. Clin. Rehabil. 20, 173–182.

Pollock, L.J., Davis, L., 1930. Studies in decerebration. VI. The effect of deafferentation upon decerebrate rigidity. Am. J. Physiol. 98, 47–49.

Post, M.W., de Bruin, A., de Witte, L., Schrijvers, A., 1996. The SIP68: a measure of health-related functional status in rehabilitation medicine. Arch. Phys. Med. Rehabil. 77, 440–445.

Proske, U., Morgan, D.L., Gregory, E., 1993. Thixotropy in skeletal muscle and in muscle spindles: a review. Prog. Neurobiol. 41, 705–721.

Raineteau, O., Fouad, K., Bareyre, F.M., Schwab, M.E., 2002. Reorganization of descending motor tracts in the rat spinal cord. Eur. J. Neurosci. 16 (9), 1761–1771.

Hannan, L.M., Morrin, L.L.L., 2000. Elasticity and ductility of muscle in myostatic contracture caused by tetanus toxin. Am. J. Physiol. 86, 312–319.

Rapin, I., Tourk, L.M., Costa, L.D., 1966. Evaluation of the Purdue Pegboard as a screening test for brain damage. Dev. Med. Child Neurol. 8, 45–54.

Riddle, C.N., Baker, S.N., 2010. Convergence of pyramidal and medial brain stem descending pathways onto macaque cervical spinal interneurons. J. Neurophysiol. 103, 2821–2832.

Rose, J., Medeiros, J.M., Parker, R., 1985. Energy cost index as an estimate of energy expenditure of cerebral-palsied children during assisted ambulation. Dev. Med. Child Neurol. 27 (4), 485–490.

Rose, S., Guzzetta, A., Pannek, K., Boyd, R., 2011. MRI structural connectivity, disruption of primary sensorimotor pathways, and hand function in cerebral palsy. Brain Connect. 1 (4), 309–316.

Sakzewski, L., Boyd, R., Ziviani, J., 2007. Clinimetric properties of participation measures for 5- to 13-year-old children with cerebral palsy: a systematic review. Dev. Med. Child Neurol. 49 (3), 232–240.

Scherling, E., Johnson, H., 1989. A tone-reducing wrist-hand orthosis. Am. J. Occup. Ther. 43, 609–611.

Schmit, B.D., Dewald, J.P., Rymer, W.Z., 2000. Stretch reflex adaptation in elbow flexors during repeated passive movements in unilateral brain-injured patients. Arch. Phys. Med. Rehabil. 81, 269–278.

Siebes, R.C., Wijnroks, L., Vermeer, A., 2002. Qualitative analysis of therapeutic motor intervention programmes for children with cerebral palsy: an update. Dev. Med. Child Neurol. 44 (9), 593–603.

Skrotzky, K., 1983. Gait analysis in cerebral palsied and nonhandicapped children. Arch. Phys. Med. Rehab. 64 (7), 291–295.

Smith, L.R., Pontén, E., Hedström, Y., Ward, S.R., Chambers, H.G., Subramaniam, S., et al., 2009. Novel transcriptional profile in wrist muscles from cerebral palsy patients. BMC Med. Genomics 2, 44.

Sparrow, M.P., 1982. Regression of skeletal muscle of chicken wing after stretch-induced hypertrophy. Am. J. Physiol. 242, C333–C338.

Spittle, A.J., Orton, J., Doyle, L.W., Boyd, R., 2007. Early developmental intervention programs post hospital discharge to prevent motor and cognitive impairments in preterm infants. Cochrane Database Syst. Rev. (2)), CD005495.

Staudt, M., 2010. Reorganization after pre- and perinatal brain lesions. J. Anat. 217 (4), 469–474.

Stigger, F., do Nascimento, P.S., Dutra, M.F., Couto, G.K., Ilha, J., Achaval, M., et al., 2011. Treadmill training induces plasticity in spinal motoneurons and sciatic nerve after sensorimotor restriction during early postnatal period: new insights into the clinical approach for children with cerebral palsy. Int. J. Dev. Neurosci. 29 (8), 833–838.

Sussman, M.D., Cusick, B., 1979. Preliminary report: the role of short-leg, tone-reducing casts as an adjunct to physical therapy of patients with cerebral palsy. Johns Hopkins Med. J. 145, 112–114.

Tardieu, C., Tardieu, G., Colbeau-Justin, P., Huet de la Tour, E., Lespargot, A., 1979. Trophic muscle regulation in children with congenital cerebral lesions. J. Neurol. Sci. 42, 357–364.

Tardieu, C., Lespargot, A., Tabary, C., Bret, M.D., 1988. For how long must the soleus muscle be stretched each day to prevent contracture? Dev. Med. Child Neurol. 30, 3–10.

Tardieu, G., 1966. Evaluation et caractères distinctifs des diverses raideurs d'origine cérébrale. Chapitre VB1b, Les feuillets de l'infirmité motrice cérébrale, Association Nationale des IMC Ed., Paris,1–28.

Taub, E., Ramey, S.L., DeLuca, S., Echols, K., 2004. Efficacy of constraint-induced movement therapy for children with cerebral palsy with asymmetric motor impairment. Pediatrics 113 (2), 305–312.

Tona, J.L., Schneck, C.M., 1993. The efficacy of upper extremity inhibitive casting: a single-subject pilot study. Am. J. Occup. Ther. 47, 901–910.

Tremblay, F., Malouin, F., Richards, C.L., Dumas, F., 1990. Effects of prolonged muscle stretch on reflex and voluntary muscle activations

in children with spastic cerebral palsy. Scand. J. Rehabil. Med. 22, 171–180.

Trevisi, E., Gualdi, S., De Conti, C., Salghetti, A., Martinuzzi, A., Pedrocchi, A., et al., 2012. Cycling induced by functional electrical stimulation in children affected by cerebral palsy: case report. Eur. J. Phys. Rehabil. Med. 48 (1), 135–145.

Turton, A.J.T., Britton, E., 2005. A pilot randomized controlled trial of a daily muscle stretch regime to prevent contractures in the arm after stroke. Clin. Rehabil. 19, 600–612.

Vanek, P., Thallmair, M., Schwab, M.E., Kapfhammer, J.P., 1998. Increased lesion-induced sprouting of corticospinal fibres in the myelin-free rat spinal cord. Eur. J. Neurosci. 10 (1), 45–56.

Verplancke, D., Snape, S., Salisbury, C.F., Jones, P.W., Ward, A.B., 2005. A randomized controlled trial of botulinum toxin on lower limb spasticity following acute acquired severe brain injury. Clin. Rehabil. 19 (2), 117–125.

Vinti, M., Couillandre, A., Hausselle, J., Bayle, N., Primerano, A., Merlo, A., et al., 2012. Influence of effort intensity and gastrocnemius stretch on co-contraction and torque production in the healthy and paretic ankle. Clin. Neurophysiol. in press.

Vojta, V., 1965. Early diagnosis of a spastic infantile syndrome. Beitr. Orthop. Traumatol. 12 (9), 543–545.

Vojta, V., 1973a. Early management of children with cerebral palsy hazards. Analysis of final results. Monatsschr. Kinderheilkd. 121 (7), 271–273.

Vojta, V., 1973b. Early diagnosis and therapy of cerebral movement disorders in childhood. C. Reflexogenous locomotion–reflex creeping and reflex turning. C2. Its use in 207 risk children. Analysis of the final results. Z. Orthop. Ihre. Grenzgeb. 111 (3), 292–309.

Wade, D.T., Langton-Hewer, R., Wood, V.A., Skilbeck, C.E., Ismail, H.M., 1983. The hemiplegic arm after stroke: measurement and recovery. J. Neurol. Neurosurg. Psychiatry 46, 521–524.

Wallander, J.L., McClure, E., Biasini, F., Goudar, S.S., Pasha, O., Chomba, E., et al., 2010. Brain-hit investigators.

Brain research to ameliorate impaired neurodevelopment–home-based intervention trial (Brain-Hit). BMC Pediatr. 10, 27.

Westberry, D.E., Davids, J.R., Jacobs, J.M., Pugh, L.I., Tanner, S.L., 2006. Effectiveness of serial stretch casting for resistant or recurrent knee flexion contractures following hamstring lengthening in children with cerebral palsy. J. Pediatr. Orthop. 26 (1), 109–114.

Westin, G.W., Dye, S., 1983. Conservative management of cerebral palsy in the growing child. Foot Ankle 4, 160–163.

Whittingham, K., Wee, D., Boyd, R., 2011. Systematic review of the efficacy of parenting interventions for children with cerebral palsy. Child Care Health Dev. 37 (4), 475–483.

Williams, P.E., 1990. Use of intermittent stretch in the prevention of serial sarcomere loss in immobilised muscle. Ann. Rheum. Dis. 49, 316–317.

Wilson, L.R., Gracies, J.M., Burke, D., Gandevia, S.G., 1999. Evidence for fusimotor drive in stroke patients based on muscle spindle thixotropy. Neurosci. Lett. 264, 109–112.

Wolf, S.L., Lecraw, D.E., Barton, L.A., Jann, B.B., 1989. Forced use of hemiplegic upper extremities to reverse the effect of learned nonuse among chronic stroke and head-injured patients. Exp. Neurol. 104, 125–132.

Yasukawa, A., 1990. Upper extremity casting: adjunct treatment for a child with cerebral palsy hemiplegia. Am. J. Occup. Ther. 44, 840–846.

Zachazewski, J.E., Eberle, E.D., Jefferies, M., 1982. Effect of tone-inhibiting casts and orthoses on gait. A case report. Phys. Ther. 62, 453–455.

# Skeletal muscle changes due to cerebral palsy

Richard L. Lieber, Lucas R. Smith

## Review of skeletal muscle structure and function as related to cerebral palsy

### Basic principles of skeletal muscle contraction

The mechanical force required for voluntary motor activity is generated by skeletal muscles. This chapter provides an overview of how neurological signal is translated into the force and work that are required for motor movements.

Skeletal muscle activation requires numerous proteins and molecules working in concert. When a motor neuron fires, the neurotransmitter acetylcholine is released from the motor neuron into the synaptic cleft of the neuromuscular junction. Activated acetylcholine receptors on the muscle trigger an action potential that travels across and importantly through muscle cells via the T-tubule system (Block et al., 1988). Voltage-gated calcium channels permit calcium to enter the cell when the action potential passes. Located next to the voltage-gated calcium channels within the cell are ryanodine receptors on the sarcoplasmic reticulum that respond by producing a calcium-triggered calcium release from the sarcoplasmic reticulum store. Cytoplasmic calcium binds to the regulatory machinery on skeletal muscle myofilaments inducing a translocation of the troponin/tropomyosin complex to reveal the myosin binding site on actin (Zot and Potter, 1987), collectively termed the thin filament. Force is generated when myosin from the thick filament binds the thin filament and undergoes a power stroke to displace the filaments relative to each other, as first explained by the sliding filament theory (Huxley and Hanson, 1954; Huxley and Niedergerke, 1954).

A set of thick and thin filaments that interdigitate is referred to as a sarcomere and is the basic functional unit of muscle contraction. The sarcomere is bordered by Z-discs, connecting thin filaments from adjacent sarcomeres to create a myofibril from a series of sarcomeres. The myosin cross-bridge head is an ATPase, which requires ATP to release the thin filament and repeat the force generating cross-bridge cycle (Maruyama and Gergely, 1962). As calcium is pumped back into the sarcoplasmic reticulum, tropomyosin resumes its inhibitory position on the thin filament and muscle relaxation ensues. As muscle in patients with cerebral palsy has no genetic defect, these regulatory and force generating processes should remain intact. However it is possible that epigenetic modifications could impact the efficiency of translating motor neuron activity into muscle force.

The motor nerve has two important methods of controlling the amount of force a muscle produces. Temporal summation is achieved when action potentials are generated sequentially in less time than is required for the muscle to relax. The faster the frequency, the greater the calcium concentration within the cell and the more force generating myosin cross-bridges that will be formed until saturating calcium is achieved at around 100 Hz (frequency) (Blinks et al., 1978). Alternatively, spatial summation is the simultaneous firing of multiple motor neurons, which, in turn, activates more muscle fibres. The more fibres activated to promote cross-bridge cycling, the greater the magnitude of force.

The sliding filament theory leads to important functional implications that are inferred based on the length of a sarcomere and, thus, the amount of overlap between thick and thin filaments, referred to as the length–tension curve (Fig. 6.1) (Gordon et al., 1966). Typically divided up into three regions, the length–tension curve is based on the fact that the greater the overlap between thick and thin filaments, the greater the force a

sarcomere will generate. Thus, there is an optimal length when thin filaments directly overlap the thick filaments to produce a maximal force, termed the force plateau, which is achieved at 'optimal' sarcomere length. As the sarcomere is stretched, less overlap exists between filaments and thus less capacity for force generation in a region denoted the descending limb. If sarcomeres are shortened from the plateau, opposing thin filaments disrupt cross-bridge formation and any shortening beyond the length of thick filament is opposed mechanically. This region is referred to as the ascending limb. The sarcomere length–tension curve is vital to understanding muscle in cerebral palsy, as clinically the muscle is often referred to as short or stretched but precisely where the muscle operates on its length–tension curve relative to normal muscle is generally unknown.

These sarcomere lengths are all based on static, or isometric, muscle lengths. To understand the force a muscle generates one must know both its length and velocity as it relates to the force–velocity curve. When a muscle undergoes a shortening, or concentric, contraction the force produced is inversely proportional to the velocity of shortening (Huxley, 1969; Katz, 1939). This

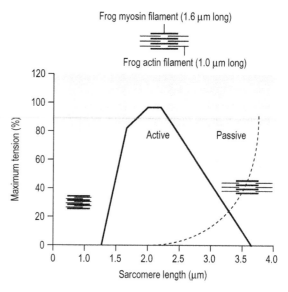

**Figure 6.1 •** The sarcomere length–tension curve for frog skeletal muscle obtained using sequential isometric contractions in single muscle fibres. The schematic arrangement of myofilaments in different regions of the length–tension curve is shown. The dotted line represents passive muscle tension.

is derived from the cross-bridge cycling rates, where, if filaments are sliding past each other, the cross-bridge has less chance to form. Alternatively, if muscle is activated while being lengthened (eccentric contraction), the force generated by muscle exceeds that produced isometrically. The large force generated in an eccentric contraction is largely independent of lengthening velocity, a property that is not fully understood (Harry et al., 1990). Muscle pathologies in cerebral palsy are not often viewed statically, so an understanding of how the forces are altered with motion will ultimately be critical to understanding the impairment.

Spatial summation indicates that the size of a muscle is a critical component of muscle activity. Further, the arrangement of muscle fibres, termed muscle architecture, is fundamental to determining function (Fig. 6.2). The ability to produce force is proportional to the number and size of fibres in a muscle: the muscle cross-sectional area (Gans and Bock, 1965). Many muscle fibres do not run the entire muscle length from origin to insertion parallel to the action of the muscle, but are instead at an angle, termed the pennation angle. The

pennation angle is used to correct the muscle cross-sectional area into physiological cross-sectional area, which is a strong predictor of force (Powell et al., 1984).

The other important architectural parameter is fibre length, normalized to sarcomere lengths. Normalized fibre length is related to the muscle excursion, the range of lengths in which the muscle can produce force (Wickiewicz et al., 1984; Winters et al., 2011). This is especially important when investigating muscle in cerebral palsy, as contracture development severely limits range of lengths over which a muscle can produce force. Furthermore, the length of fibres and sarcomeres changes as a muscle contracts, so it is important when comparing muscles to normalize fibre lengths. This can be done by using a reference sarcomere length; however, sarcomere length is much more difficult to measure in patients than fibre lengths. Muscle architectural measurements are essentially performed in order to estimate the number of sarcomeres in parallel (physiological cross-sectional area) and number of sarcomeres in series (normalized fibre length). Various muscles

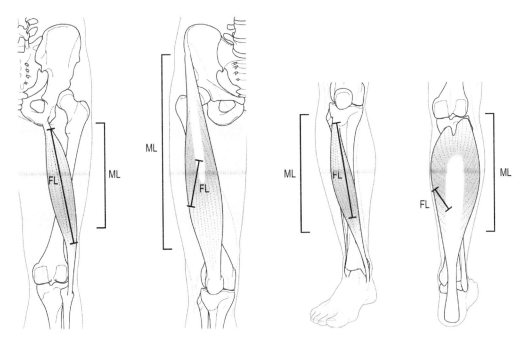

**Figure 6.2** • Schematic illustration of muscle architectural properties in the large muscle groups of the human lower limb. Functionally, quadriceps and plantarflexors are designed for force production based on their low fibre length/ muscle length ratios and large physiological cross-sectional areas. Conversely, hamstrings and dorsiflexors are designed for high excursion and velocity by nature of their high fibre length/muscle length ratios and relatively small physiological cross-sectional areas. ML, muscle length; FL, fibre length.

have specialized architectural properties based on functional requirements for either high force capacity or high excursion ability (Lieber and Friden, 2000). For example, the quadriceps muscles have relatively short fibres and high physiological cross-sectional areas and are ideal for high forces, whereas the hamstrings have comparatively long fibres and smaller physiological cross-sectional areas that are suited for high excursion (Fig. 6.2).

Our discussion of muscle so far has focused primarily on the muscle cells themselves; however, there are many other cell types present in skeletal muscle. There are, of course, fibroblasts and endothelial cells that provide the environment for muscle cells to function. Particularly in damaged or diseased muscle, there is an infiltration of many inflammatory cells that have the capacity to both impair or foster muscle regeneration (Tidball, 2005; Tidball and Villalta, 2010). The cells responsible for muscle regeneration are primarily the satellite cells, a muscle resident stem cell population named for their proximity just outside the muscle fibre but beneath the basal lamina (Fig. 6.3). Satellite cells have been shown to migrate to sites of muscle damage and divide into both a cell to replenish the satellite cell pool and a myoblast that differentiates and incorporates into an existing muscle fibre or fuses with other myoblasts to form a new myotube and eventually muscle fibre (Mauro, 1961; Yablonka-Reuveni, 2011). It is the overall interactions among these cell populations that create the pathologic state of muscle seen in muscle contractures of patients with cerebral palsy.

## Basic principles of passive mechanical properties of muscle

The material above describes how skeletal muscles produce force and perform work when activated by the nervous system. However, muscles are also capable of bearing considerable passive tension, without cross-bridge cycling, in response to stretch (Fig. 6.4). Thus, a passive length–tension curve is superimposed upon the active length–tension curve described above. Muscle passive tension limits range of motion in some joints, such as the hamstrings, which limit knee extension with the hip flexed. This is especially prevalent in patients with cerebral palsy as muscle passive tension results in debilitating joint contractures. The

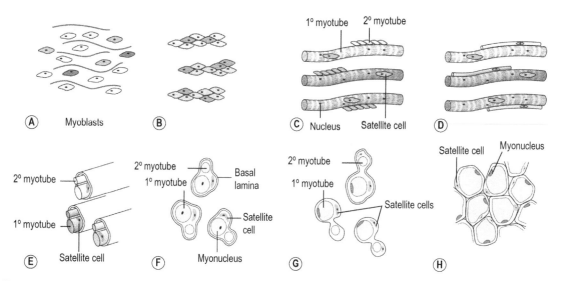

**Figure 6.3** • Schematic diagram of skeletal muscle development. **(A)** Primitive cells differentiate into myoblasts. **(B)** Myoblasts fuse together to form primary myotubes. **(C–F)** Later, secondary myotubes arise beneath the basal lamina of the primary myotubes. Fusion of myoblasts radially and longitudinally results in the formation of the muscle fibre beneath the basal lamina (shown in cross-section in E through H). In addition, some unfused myoblasts remain as satellite cells, which are maintained in the mature tissue. **(G)** As the muscle matures, primary and secondary myotubes separate, each with myonuclei and satellite cells, to become a mature fibre. **(H)** Finally, as the muscle fibres grow, they become arranged as tightly packed polygonal cells, characteristic of adult muscle.

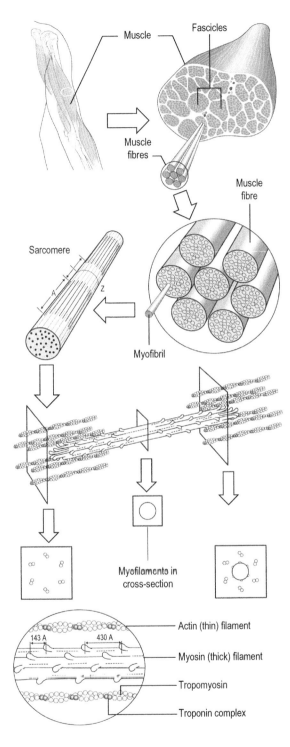

**Figure 6.4** • Structural hierarchy of skeletal muscle. Whole skeletal muscles (here a biceps muscle is shown) are composed of numerous fascicles of muscle fibres. Muscle fibres are composed of myofibrils arranged in parallel. Myofibrils are composed of sarcomeres arranged in series. Sarcomeres are composed of interdigitating actin and myosin filaments. Hexagonal array of interdigitating myosin and actin filaments which comprise the sarcomere. The myosin filament is composed of myosin molecules, and the actin filament is composed of actin monomers. Arranged at intervals along the actin filament are the regulatory proteins troponin and tropomyosin. Cross-sections through different portions of the sarcomere reveal the interdigitation of the filament systems. This type of sectioning experiment was used to define the mechanism of muscle contraction. (A-A band, I-I band, Z-Z band).

(Magid and Law, 1985). This suggested that, in frog muscle, collagen, intermediate filaments and cytoskeletal structures did not play a large role in bearing passive tension. It also mitigated the impact of other extracellular matrix components in contributing to passive tension of whole muscle.

Until the giant protein titin, the largest known protein, was discovered and shown to span half of the sarcomere from the Z-disc to the middle of the thick filament and provide a physical link between filaments (Horowits et al., 1986), it was unknown what could bear passive load within the sarcomere in the absence of cross-bridges. This made it a prime candidate for being responsible for the passive tension generated within the myofibril. Indeed experiments where titin was enzymatically removed resulted in fibres that were very compliant (Funatsu et al., 1990). Furthermore, it was demonstrated that titin had many splice variants with much of the variation in the length of the extensible PEVK (rich in proline, glutamate, valine and lysine) region. Studies showed that the size and corresponding length of a titin molecule was roughly related to the stiffness, with shorter isoforms being stiffer (Freiburg et al., 2000; Horowits, 1992). This presented strong evidence for titin bearing considerable muscle passive tension. It was thus possible the titin isoform was shifted to a smaller molecule in muscle of patients with cerebral palsy, contributing to the increased passive tension.

Later experiments showed that titin located in mammalian tissue such as rabbit did not bear as much of the passive load compared to frog

origin of this passive tension has been controversial and is not equal in all muscles. A seminal study in the field showed that, in frog muscle, most passive tension was borne within a single myofibril muscle (Prado et al., 2005). In this case the primary components responsible for load bearing were found to be extracellular. The extracellular matrix is a scaffold linking together muscle fibres on multiple levels. The endomysium surrounds individual fibres, the perimysium surrounds groups of fibres called fascicles, and the epimysium is a layer of connective tissue surrounding whole muscle. The extracellular matrix consists of many components, including collagens and proteoglycans. Collagen is the primary component of extracellular matrix in muscle thought to be responsible for much of the extracellular matrix stiffness (Borg and Caulfield, 1980; Duance et al., 1977; Gillies and Lieber, 2011). Changes to the extracellular matrix may be prevalent in cerebral palsy as the muscle is clinically often referred to as fibrotic (see below).

The passive tension in skeletal muscle is not purely a function of stretch (Fig. 6.5). Indeed, a stretched muscle will immediately resist stretch with a high force, followed by a period of relaxing stress to a lower steady state. This stress–relaxation principle makes muscle a viscoelastic material where the speed and time course of stretch are important components in determining passive tension (Magnusson, 1998; Meyer et al. 2011; Wang et al., 1993). These additional parameters have complicated models of passive tension in skeletal muscle (Best et al., 1994; Morgan et al.,

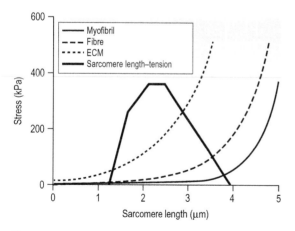

**Figure 6.5** • Passive stress of myofibril elements and ECM elements, and the average passive stress in the simulated fibre superimposed on the sarcomere length–tension diagram. Myofibril passive stress, ECM passive stress and the sarcomere length–tension relationship were estimated from the work by others.

1982). It is important to remember that passive muscle tension is not static in vivo just as one must consider the force–velocity curve when examining active tension. For example, during gait, as the quadriceps extends the knee, the force required to lengthen the hamstring is much greater than if the knee is very slowly extended. This property of passive tension is seen in cerebral palsy as the knee extension during a typical crouch gait is less than knee extension during passive stretching of the hamstring.

## Basic principles of plasticity in muscle

Skeletal muscle is a very adaptive tissue and subject to remodelling of the properties discussed previously, based on the pattern of use. Muscles that are subjected to high stress respond by undergoing muscle hypertrophy and increasing physiological cross-sectional area. Studies have shown that eccentric contractions, which produce the highest stresses, elicit the largest hypertrophy signal (Hather et al. 1991; Roig et al., 2009). It is possible for muscles to increase or decrease their physiological cross-sectional area by either changing the number of fibres or the size of present fibres. However, after development, muscle hypertrophy in mammalian muscle is accomplished primarily by fibre hypertrophy rather than the addition of new muscle fibres (Taylor and Wilkinson, 1986). Eccentric contractions of high stress are also capable of inducing muscle damage and injury. Repair of injured muscle often results in a fibrotic response (Kaariainen et al. 2000; Serrano and Munoz-Canoves, 2010). The tipping point between muscle contractions to maintain or increase mass and those that induce injury is critical. This is exaggerated in cerebral palsy where muscles have an altered capacity for growth and regeneration.

Conversely, muscles that are not subject to use undergo atrophy, as in the cases of limb immobilization, bed rest, or space flight (Lecker et al., 2004). Muscle atrophy is not just the opposite of hypertrophy, but an active process in which proteins are targeted for degradation in order to conserve the high-energy demand required for muscle upkeep. In order for muscle to effectively atrophy, proteins are 'marked' for degradation by ubiquitin, which is attached by a class of proteins

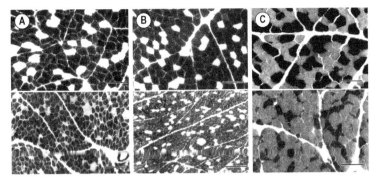

**Figure 6.6** • Light micrographs of the **(A)** vastus lateralis, **(B)** vastus medialis and **(C)** rectus femoris muscles. The top panel represents micrographs from normal muscle, and the bottom panel represents micrographs from immobilized muscles. All micrographs were taken at the same magnification. Fast fibres appear dark, and slow fibres appear light. Calibration bars = 100 μm. [Reprinted with permission from Lieber, R.L., Friden, J.O., Hargens, A.R., Danzin, L.A., Gershuni, D.H., 1998. Differential response of the dog quadriceps muscle to external skeletal fixation of the knee. Muscle Nerve 11, 193–201, with permission from John Wiley & Sons, Inc.]

termed ubiquitin ligases. Muscle that is actively undergoing atrophy has two ubiquitin ligases that are expressed to specifically mark contractile proteins for degradation (Bodine et al., 2001). The activation of muscle atrophy is often accompanied by muscle fibrosis as well, which occupies part of the space vacated by muscle fibres. Improper activation of the atrophy programme could compromise muscle in cerebral palsy.

Muscle plasticity is often referenced in relation to a change in fibre types. Muscle fibre types have important functional consequences for the muscle. Human muscle has primarily three fibre types, which are based largely on the myosin heavy chain isoform expressed. Type I, or slow, fibres have slower cross-bridge cycling rates and produce less force than other fibre types. However, type I fibres are highly oxidative and capable of repeated contractions with very little fatigue. Type IIa fibres have faster cross-bridge cycling rates and are capable of producing larger forces than type I fibres. They still maintain oxidative metabolism and are relatively fatigue resistant. Type IIx are the fastest and most powerful fibres in human muscle. However, they have very low oxidative capacity and rely upon glycolytic metabolism for energy demands and are thus very susceptible to fatigue. Each fibre from a motor unit consists primarily of the same fibre type. This allows a sequential activation where slow motor units dominate repetitive low force contractions and then fast fibres can be recruited for periodic high force contractions (Buller et al., 1960a, 1960b).

The proportion of fast and slow fibres varies across muscles, depending on their function (Fig. 6.6). With altered use it is possible to shift the proportion of fibre types within a muscle, with overactivity leading to a slower phenotype and decreased use leading to a faster phenotype. The potential magnitude of these changes in humans is controversial. However, as we have seen, the activation patterns in cerebral palsy are altered and indeed may represent a signal that is capable of inducing substantial fibre type plasticity in muscle of cerebral palsy patients.

Muscle is not only capable of adding sarcomeres in parallel with increased force but also of adding sarcomeres in series to create longer fibres and thus achieve greater excursion. Much of the research in this area was performed on cats, showing that when muscles are immobilized in a shortened position they reduce the number of sarcomeres in series and when they are placed at longer lengths they add sarcomeres in order to stay at the same point on the sarcomere length–tension curve (Tabary et al., 1972). This property of muscle is important during skeletal development as limbs extend the length of muscles, and also during surgical operations in which muscle length is altered (Boakes et al., 2007). We have seen, however, that changing muscle length with immobilization or surgery often is associated with other muscle plasticity adaptations that complicate models. Particularly, pathologic muscles may not demonstrate the ability to natively adapt the number of sarcomeres in order to maintain optimal sarcomere length.

Muscle in cerebral palsy is often referred to as 'shortened', bringing up the question as to whether this muscle is capable of plastically changing length and serial sarcomere number.

# Biomechanical and neurophysiological studies of limb mechanics in spasticity

## Reflex gain

Skeletal muscle in patients with cerebral palsy is often referred to as 'spastic muscle'. Spasticity is classically defined as a velocity-dependent resistance to stretch, with which there is an active response of muscle to resist stretch, or a catch (Lance, 1980). A spastic muscle may not have any actual muscle pathology, but instead be the result of hyperreflexia in the nervous system. It can be difficult to separate spasticity from intrinsic changes to the muscle itself. Previous studies have been conducted to delineate the passive, intrinsic and reflex-mediated increases in stiffness of spastic muscle in multiple sclerosis patients. While these patients did not have cerebral palsy, their results likely extend to cerebral palsy as well. The acquisition of these data can be complex, with the use of dynamometry, electromyography and nerve stimulation combined with signal processing methods to tease apart the intrinsic stiffness of the muscle from the overall muscle stiffness measured, which includes a reflex component (Fig. 6.7) (Lieber et al., 2004). An increase in reflex-mediated stiffness can be observed but interestingly, both studies also implicate the passive muscle stiffness as well (Mirbagheri et al., 2001; Sinkjaer and Magnussen, 1994). This increase in passive stiffness dominates particularly at the end of the range of motion where passive tension is highest. This indicates that the passive biomechanical properties of the muscle are being altered in cerebral palsy to increase joint stiffness, particularly in the case of fixed contracture where there is no reflex contribution, but joint motion is limited by increase in muscle stiffness. This is readily apparent in muscle lengthening surgeries of cerebral palsy patients, where the patient under general anaesthesia without reflex activity has a joint contracture that

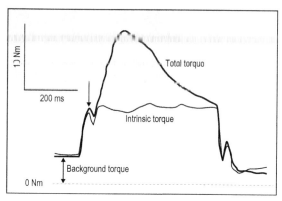

**Figure 6.7** • Example of a mechanical torque curve measured in a human subject during mechanical perturbation of the ankle and during electrical stimulation. In performing this experiment, plantarflexor muscles are first voluntarily activated to a preset level, in this case, about 5 Nm ('background torque'), and then the ankle is rapidly dorsiflexed at a known time (down arrow). This results in the 'total torque' trace, which is due to both intrinsic muscle properties as well as the reflex activation of the muscle due to the stretch reflex elicited (thick line). In a separate experiment, using neuromuscular electrical stimulation of the triceps via the tibial nerve, plantarflexion torque is again measured. But, this time, the torque recorded is only due to the intrinsic torque generated by muscle contraction, with (presumably) no neural component (thin line). Stiffness is calculated from these data in terms of torque/angle in units of Nm/degree. The zero torque level (0 Nm) is shown by the dotted line. Calibration bars are shown to the left of the figure. [Adapted with permission from Sinkjaer, T., Magnussen, I., 1994. Passive, intrinsic and reflex-mediated stiffness in the ankle extensors of hemiparetic patients. Brain 117, 355–363, with permission from Oxford University Press.]

is immediately relieved upon muscle or tendon lengthening.

## Intrinsic stiffness

Skeletal muscle is also known to undergo plastic changes in response to disease states, and here we examine the research on the plastic changes of muscle in response to cerebral palsy. Research in this field is slowed by the fact that there is no commonly accepted animal model of cerebral palsy, necessitating complex studies on human subjects (Foran et al., 2005). These studies examine the possible sources of increased intrinsic stiffness which is possible from multiple levels: decreased titin isoform size, increased muscle cell stiffness, increased extracellular matrix stiffness, changes in muscle architecture that increases muscle strain, or a combination of these factors (Fig. 6.8). Each of these factors may be altered in response to the primary pathologic neurological input to produce the increased intrinsic stiffness observed, or also from altered loading or treatment protocols that result. We must also consider that the muscle

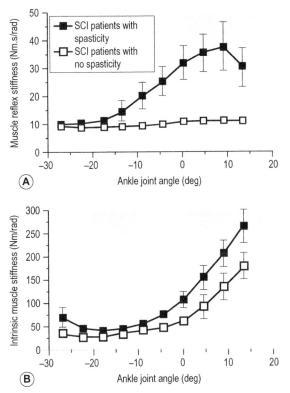

**Figure 6.8** • Joint dynamics measured in spinal cord-injured patients with spasticity (solid squares) compared to spinal cord-injured patients with no spasticity (open squares) using the 'parallel cascade' method. **(A)** Reflex stiffness. **(B)** Intrinsic stiffness. Note that both the intrinsic muscle stiffness and reflex gain are increased in spastic limbs, especially at dorsiflexed ankle positions. This is consistent with clinical experience where 'spasticity' increases with increasing muscle length. SCI, spinal cord injury [Adapted from Mirbagheri, M.M., Barbeau, H., Ladouceur, M., Kearney, R.E., 2001. Intrinsic and reflex stiffness in normal and spastic, spinal cord-injured subjects. Exp. Brain Res. 141 (4), 446–459, with kind permission from Springer Science + Business Media.]

is often in series with elastic tendons that may undergo plastic changes in cerebral palsy. Future studies are required to sort out the nature of this increased intrinsic stiffness.

There have been attempts to understand plastic changes in cerebral palsy from our knowledge of models on denervation, immobilization, increased use, or decreased use. Few abnormalities are found in the function of lower motor neurons in cerebral palsy aside from their altered input (Rose and McGill, 2005), suggesting a denervation model is insufficient. The loss of connections to lower motor neurons results in the negative features of upper motor neuron syndrome. However, much of the upper motor neuron signal is inhibitory and the loss of inhibition results in positive features of upper motor neuron syndrome. This does not allow for a neat fit into previously established muscle plasticity models, but instead a complex combination.

Although the upper motor neuron lesions in cerebral palsy are non-progressive, the secondary pathology often is progressive. The negative features of cerebral palsy result in muscle weakness and increased fatigability due to decreased drive to the lower motor neurons. Poor balance and other sensory deficits are also common negative features of cerebral palsy. The positive features of the upper motor neuron syndrome include hyperreflexia, clonus, co-contractions, and spasticity, which is most commonly referred to. The unique mix of positive and negative features often result in muscle contractures; however, the mechanism of this is not known (Kerr Graham and Selber, 2003). Muscle contractures result from a passive inextensibility of muscle that limits range of motion around a joint. Contractures represent a major form of disability in patients with cerebral palsy. Additionally, joint contractures have further downstream effects, creating bony torsion, joint instability and often degenerative arthritis. Contractures in muscle groups are commonly described by measuring the passive range of motion about a joint. Indirect studies performed on both passive and active joint mechanics present inconsistent evidence on fibre lengths (Smeulders et al., 2004; Tardieu et al., 1982a,b). To understand how these contractures develop, we must investigate the adaptations of skeletal muscle on multiple biological levels and further study how these muscle changes have tertiary results on tendon properties.

# Skeletal muscle in vivo morphology in cerebral palsy

## Fibre lengths in cerebral palsy

There is a general belief within the clinical community that muscle contractures are the result of shortened muscle. Studying this possibility in humans requires a non-invasive technique, yet MRI is difficult due to necessity of prolonged relaxation, exacerbated by spasticity and a primarily paediatric population as well as cost. This has led to many recent studies using ultrasound to measure fibre lengths in muscle from children with cerebral palsy. Ultrasound is best suited for superficial muscles that are known to undergo contracture in cerebral palsy and thus the gastrocnemius is studied almost exclusively (Fig. 6.9). Measurements are still complicated by splicing multiple fields, or projecting fascicles beyond the field. The earliest studies showed that fascicle lengths were not significantly different in cerebral palsy (Shortland et al., 2002). Later studies suggested that the fascicle lengths were shortened when not normalized to bone length (Mohagheghi et al., 2008). Subsequent studies have yielded mixed results based on muscle and normalization method (Mohagheghi

et al., 2007; Shortland et al., 2002), and a recent review is recommended for a detailed meta-analysis of literature data (Barrett and Lichtwark, 2010). We must, however, point out a major limitation of all ultrasound investigations, as excursion is proportional to normalized fibre length, and there is no internal muscle normalization available in any of these studies. This means that the muscle length is dependent on the position of the joint and provides another complicating factor in these studies. Ultrasound studies would yield the same fibre length on a shorter fibre stretched to a given joint position as a muscle with longer fibres, assuming tendon length was equivalent. Conversely, it is possible to measure a shorter fascicle length at the same joint position when the muscle sarcomeres are just shortened due to tendon elongation. These discrepancies cannot be resolved by normalizing to bone length or tendon length. A fuller understanding requires the knowledge of sarcomere lengths and a much more invasive procedure.

## Intraoperative sarcomere length in cerebral palsy

Knowing that fibre shortening could be the result of shortening the sarcomeres within a muscle, it is the relative number of sarcomeres in series that provides knowledge of muscle excursion which impacts the function in patients with cerebral palsy. Ideally, image technologies would exist that allow a direct measure of the number of sarcomeres in series of these patients, but none is currently available. However, animal studies have shown that within a muscle the sarcomere length is relatively constant along the length of the muscle, excluding the sarcomeres at the muscle–tendon junction (Huxley and Peachey, 1961; Paolini et al., 1976). This facilitates studying sarcomeres at a single region of muscle using a method such as laser diffraction. Laser diffraction takes advantage of the fact that skeletal muscle is striated, or striped, creating a visual diffraction pattern based on the distance between stripes, which is the sarcomere length (Cleworth and Edman, 1969).

A series of studies has actually employed this technique intraoperatively to investigate muscles in cerebral palsy. The initial study measured sarcomere lengths in wrist flexors of patients with cerebral palsy, and unexpectedly found a dramatically *increased* sarcomere length even though the muscles

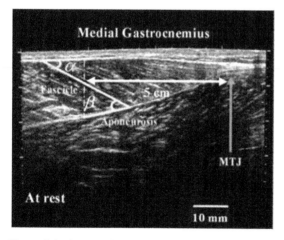

**Figure 6.9** • Longitudinal ultrasonic images of the medial gastrocnemius muscle at rest. The skin is on the top of the image, and the left side corresponds to proximal. The myotendinous junction (MTJ) is defined by the vertical arrow. α and β are the posterior and anterior pennation angles, respectively. (Please refer to colour plate section)

were *shortened* (Fig. 6.10) (Lieber and Friden, 2002). This was counterintuitive to see long sarcomeres in a supposedly shortened muscle. However, it suggests that there may be a great reduction in sarcomeres in series, so much so that the remaining sarcomeres are stretched to excessively long lengths, creating a very short normalized fibre length. To further accentuate the importance of this increased strain on the sarcomeres, a follow-up study showed that, for wrist flexor contractures, the measured sarcomere length in wrist flexors correlated with disability in terms of wrist extension angle, while wrist extensor sarcomere lengths did not (Lieber and Friden, 2002; Ponten et al., 2005). While this supported the shorter normalized fibre length hypothesis, further studies raised new questions. For example, in vivo real-time measurements of sarcomere length allowed sarcomere length measurement during joint rotation. When the wrists of these patients were moved, the change in sarcomere length was the same in both the patients with cerebral palsy and controls. This suggested that muscles in cerebral palsy had the same number of sarcomeres even when stretched. This implies that another mechanism of adaptation is possible with tendon shortening, muscle pennation angle changes, or moment arms increasing (Lieber and Friden, 2002).

To investigate sarcomere length changes further in the spastic wrist flexors, a study examined the muscle force as muscle length was altered during tendon transfer surgery. If sarcomere lengths were overstretched on the descending limb of the length–tension curve, the maximum force would be expected to occur at a flexed position and full extension would predict very little active tension and high passive forces. However, the study revealed the muscles seemed to operate roughly on the plateau of the length–tension curve (Smeulders et al., 2004). Of course, this study did not directly measure sarcomere and did not compare how the length–tension properties would compare to a control population due to the surgical requirement. Importantly, many of the patients also did not have fixed contractures, but dynamic contractures that were relieved under anaesthesia.

There has also been a recent study in vivo of sarcomere length of hamstring muscle in patients with cerebral palsy. In this case, a muscle biopsy was taken using specialized clamps to ensure the muscle fibres biopsied were held at constant length after excision and throughout a fixation process (Ward et al., 2009). Again, sarcomere lengths

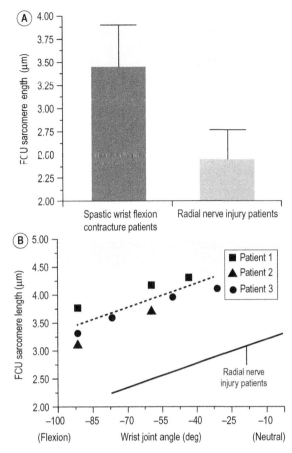

**Figure 6.10 • (A)** Sarcomere length measured from the flexor carpi ulnaris (FCU) muscle of a patient with spastic wrist flexion contracture and a patient with a radial nerve injury that denervates wrist extensors but leaves the FCU intact. This allows us to use the FCU from radial nerve patients as 'control' data. Note that the sarcomeres are abnormally long in muscle from these patients, in spite of the fact that their muscles are abnormally short. Data represents mean ± SEM for each group. (Data replotted from Lieber and Frieden, 2002.) **(B)** Sarcomere length measured from the FCU muscle during surgery for the spastic wrist joint contracture. Sarcomere length is measured in the muscle as the wrist joint is rotated. Each symbol type represents data from a single patient. Note that the linear regression relationship (dotted line) from the three contracture patients parallels the normal sarcomere length–joint angle relationship for the FCU obtained from radial nerve injury patients (solid line). This is an indirect method to show that fibre length is the same in both patient populations. [Adapted with permission from Lieber, R.L., Friden, J., 2002. Spasticity causes a fundamental rearrangement of muscle-joint interaction. Muscle Nerve 25, 265–270. Reprinted with permission of John Wiley & Sons, Inc.]

observed were much longer that those expected from a control population (Smith et al., 2011). While this may suggest normalized fibre shortening, all that it conclusively shows is that muscle in cerebral palsy is under increased strain. Currently there are no studies that investigate normalized fibre length directly by measuring both sarcomere length and fibre length concurrently to predict how muscle excursion may be limited in patients with cerebral palsy. Aside from muscle excursion, the increased sarcomere strain observed does imply these muscles are operating on the descending limb of their length–tension curves, which has important consequences for explaining loss in muscle strength.

## Estimates of in vivo tension in cerebral palsy

Fibre length in relation to excursion plays an important role in cerebral palsy muscle, but so does physiological cross-sectional area, which relates to muscle strength. A multitude of studies performed have shown that patients with cerebral palsy have reduced voluntary force producing capabilities with functional consequences (MacPhail and Kramer, 1995; Ross and Engsberg, 2007). Unlike fibre length, studies investigating physiological cross-sectional area have consistently shown a decrease. MRI studies on hemiplegic patients allow well-controlled comparisons of muscle area (Elder et al., 2003), with a definitive decrease in muscle area (Fig. 6.11). It should be acknowledged

that muscle area in this study did not correct for pennation angle and is thus not precisely a physiological cross-sectional area. The investigation goes on to report that specific tension, i.e., the amount of force a muscle produces per area, is also decreased in cerebral palsy. While this could be the result of compromised muscle integrity as the authors suggest, it may also be due to a decrease in pennation angle or comparisons at sarcomere lengths on the descending limb of the length–tension curve.

As ultrasound has proven to be the most widely used muscle imaging modality in patients with cerebral palsy, further studies have sought to use it in examination of muscle area. Studies have examined muscle thickness using ultrasound as a correlate to muscle area in supporting the findings of decreased area (Moreau et al., 2009, 2010). This was shown in vastus lateralis as well as the more typically involved rectus femoris. While pennation angle was measured, no correction was made for physiological cross-sectional area. A subsequent study did calculate physiological cross-sectional area and demonstrate its decrease in patients with cerebral palsy (Barber et al., 2011). Although these ultrasound studies on muscle area do not measure active tension to calculate a specific tension, their correlation with functional status in patients emphasizes the importance of muscle area (Bandholm et al. 2009; Mohagheghi et al., 2007; Moreau et al., 2009). Methods of increasing muscle area may thus have therapeutic effects on patients with cerebral palsy.

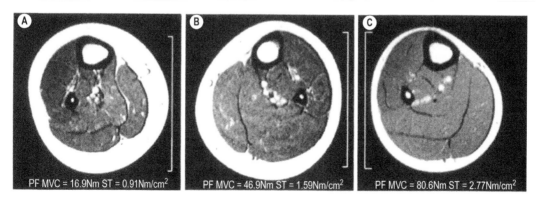

PF MVC = 16.9Nm ST = 0.91Nm/cm$^2$    PF MVC = 46.9Nm ST = 1.59Nm/cm$^2$    PF MVC = 80.6Nm ST = 2.77Nm/cm$^2$

**Figure 6.11** • MRI images obtained from both legs from a child with hemiplegia: **(A)** hemiplegic affected leg, **(B)** hemiplegic control leg and **(C)** one leg of a control child, matched by age weight and height. Plantarflexion (PF) maximal voluntary contraction (MVC) is reported for each limb, along with specific tension (ST). Calibration bar = 8 cm. Nm, Newton meters.

# Skeletal muscle tissue properties in cerebral palsy

## Histology

Muscle imaging modalities are able to measure muscle properties non-invasively, but investigating muscle at the cell level requires acquisition of muscle biopsies, complicated again by the lack of an animal model for cerebral palsy (Foran et al., 2005). The most basic form of analysis of muscle tissue is histological examination. Typically, skeletal muscle has tightly packed polygonal fibres and this contractile material represents the vast majority of muscle area. However, muscle from patients with spasticity undergo many histological changes, including increased variability in fibre size, increased number of abnormally shaped fibres and increased extracellular matrix space (Fig. 6.12) (Booth et al., 2001; Castle et al., 1979; Dietz et al., 1986; Ito et al., 1996; Romanini et al., 1989). Similar changes in muscle histology are also seen in various muscle diseases, including Duchenne muscular dystrophy. While the functional consequence of these histological changes can be difficult to predict, it provides strong evidence that muscle in cerebral palsy is indeed pathologic.

Another aspect of muscle that can be examined using a histological staining method is the distribution of fibre type. Staining for oxidative processes or myosin heavy chain isoform can distinguish fibre types, although fibre type distributions may also be determined by myosin heavy chain content (Fry et al., 1994). The negative features of upper motor neuron syndrome would predict decreased use and a faster phenotype, while the positive features such as spasticity would predict increased use and shifting to a slower phenotype. Several studies have reported an increased percentage of slow fibres (Dietz et al., 1986; Ito et al., 1996; Marbini et al., 2002) in patients with upper motor neuron syndrome, while others have reported a shift to a faster distribution of fibres (Ponten and Stal, 2007, 2008; Sjostrom et al., 1980). Still more studies have shown no fibre type change at all (Castle et al., 1979; Romanini et al., 1989), demonstrating there is no consistent model of activity that encapsulates cerebral palsy muscle. This emphasizes the complexity of the neuronal signal and could be different between upper and lower extremities in cerebral palsy or even from muscle to muscle.

Additional studies have made use of immuno-histochemical techniques to study specific proteins within cerebral palsy muscle. Knowing the aetiology is neurological in origin, one study investigated the neuromuscular junction. Typically, the neuro-muscular junction is defined by acetylcholine esterase, a prominent protein involved in breaking down acetylcholine to terminate synaptic transmission and allow reuptake by the presynaptic nerve. In biopsies of paraspinal muscles of cerebral palsy patients undergoing spinal fusion, acetylcholine receptors were regularly found outside of the neuromuscular junction (Theroux et al., 2002). This suggests a disorganization of the neuromuscular junction in cerebral palsy and the possibility the muscle is attempting to recruit new muscle fibres and increase contractile activity.

Using similar immunohistological techniques investigators have also probed fibrillar collagen content within cerebral palsy muscle (Booth et al., 2001). The histological evidence supported the notion that muscle in cerebral palsy is fibrotic by

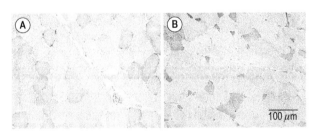

**Figure 6.12 •** Muscle fibre morphology is abnormal in spastic muscle. Light micrograph of a muscle obtained from a 19-year-old hemiplegic boy. **(A)** Non-spastic extensor carpi radialis brevis muscle. Histochemical stain of the NADH oxidative enzyme that labels fibre type I and type IIA dark, and type IIB lighter. **(B)** Spastic flexor carpi ulnaris muscle. Note the spastic muscle demonstrates greater fibre size variability. (Please refer to colour plate section). [Micrographs courtesy of Dr Eva Pontén, Karolinska Institute, Stockholm, Sweden.]

demonstrating increases in collagen intensity with the endomysium as the primary area of collagen accumulation. A more recent investigation also qualitatively showed an increase in both fibrillar collagen type I as well as an increase in laminin, a major component of the basal lamina (Smith et al., 2011). Both studies also used hydroxyproline to quantify the overall collagen content and show that it is increased in cerebral palsy. Emphasizing the role of fibrosis, collagen content had a significant correlation with GMFCS (Booth et al., 2001). The role of this increased collagen and extracellular matrix of cerebral palsy muscle is unknown. It could inhibit muscle regenerative capacity or may also be a contributor to the increased passive tension observed in these muscles.

## Mechanics of muscles and muscle fibres

Previous studies showed that muscle organization could be responsible for increased stiffness of muscle in contracture, but an intrinsic change in muscle stiffness is also possible. While measuring passive stiffness of isolated whole muscle is not possible in human subjects, muscle fibres can be isolated from muscle biopsies and mechanical measurements performed. An early study tested fibres from a variety of muscles biopsies acquired during surgery in patients with cerebral palsy and controls. By measuring sarcomere length and passive force across a series of stretches the investigators were able to determine that fibres in cerebral palsy were approximately twice as stiff as controls (Friden and Lieber, 2003). It should be noted that these forces were measured after allowing two minutes for the fibre to stress relax to a static force and disregarded the viscous component of these fibres. These results also corresponded to a lower resting sarcomere length in cerebral palsy muscle. Studies in stroke victims also found increased fibre stiffness in patients with spasticity, but only within type IIx fibres (Olsson et al., 2006). These data suggest that intrinsic changes to the fibres themselves contribute to muscle contracture. A similar study was conducted subsequently, but tested a larger sample size of muscle fibres from the same hamstring muscles to compare cerebral palsy to controls (Smith et al., 2011). As opposed to the previous study, this time no difference in stiffness was observed between cerebral palsy single fibres compared to controls.

These differences could result from differences in experimental design, but while the first study suggests fibre stiffness contributes to contracture (Friden and Lieber, 2003), the second study shows that this is not a necessary adaptation that leads to changed muscle stiffness in cerebral palsy (Smith et al., 2011).

The most likely candidate for any increase in fibre stiffness would come from the giant molecular titin, which provides a physical link between thick and thin filaments. Shorter titin molecules in cerebral palsy would predict both the stiffness increase and decrease in resting sarcomere length observed in the previous study (Friden and Lieber, 2003). However, when titin size was measured in either individual fibres or muscle biopsies, there was no significant difference between cerebral palsy and control muscle in lower extremity muscles (Smith et al., 2011). Nonetheless there are other components of titin that are also capable of altering its stiffness other than molecular size, such as phosphorylation state (Kruger et al., 2009). Still, if muscle stiffness is changing, the components outside of the fibre may play a role as well.

Outside of the muscle fibre, the extracellular matrix may also contribute to passive stiffness. One method of examining the extracellular matrix is to mechanically test bundles of fibres that include the constituent extracellular matrix and subtract the fibre stiffness tested from the same biopsy. This method shows that bundles are stiffer than fibres in both control and cerebral palsy, emphasizing the role of extracellular matrix in passive mechanical properties. Surprisingly, the study revealed that bundles from cerebral palsy biopsies were much more compliant than control. While these bundles were more compliant, they still showed a greater area fraction of extracellular matrix in corroboration with previous studies. This confounding result suggests that even with stiffer fibres and more extracellular matrix present, the extracellular matrix is organized in a way that confers much less mechanical stiffness to the tissue (Lieber et al., 2003). It also opposes the hypothesis that stiffness is due to an intrinsic change of muscle properties. Again, the subsequent study looking specifically at hamstring muscle showed the opposite result. Here, bundles again became stiffer than fibres, but only at longer sarcomere lengths, where it is thought the extracellular matrix contributes more to passive tension. Stiffness was increased in cerebral palsy muscle compared to controls, making the extrapolation of these tissue level results to the

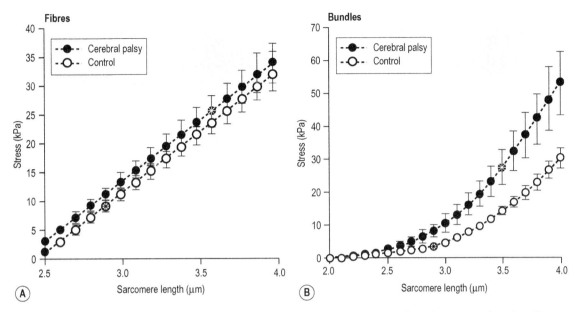

**Figure 6.13** • Passive tension as a function of sarcomere length for fibres and bundles, after stress relaxation. Plots represent the average of the fits from each individual sample ± SEM. The stress vs sarcomere length fit was **(A)** linear for fibres and **(B)** quadratic for bundles. Gracilis fibres show no difference between CP and control. CP gracilis bundles show a significant increase in stress at high sarcomere lengths compared to control. (*) In symbol designates the approximate sarcomere length at 90° of hip and knee flexion.

joint level more applicable. This study showed that the increased stiffness of bundles was similar to the increased collagen content, suggesting collagen as the source of extracellular matrix stiffening and the consequence of muscle fibrosis (Smith et al., 2011).

While we have primarily examined muscle properties independently, it is also possible to combine them to predict overall muscle tension in vivo. Specifically, when muscle bundle mechanical properties were combined with sarcomere length measurements in a similar patient population, it was possible to predict in vivo muscle tension (Fig. 6.13) (Smith et al., 2011). While the muscle tissue itself can account for up to a twofold increase in stiffness, if we compare stiffness at sarcomere lengths found in vivo at the same joint position, the results predict a sixfold increase in stiffness. This demonstrates the importance of combining our knowledge of muscle tissue property changes with in vivo structural studies in cerebral palsy.

## Muscle gene expression

Microarray technology permits the simultaneous collection of gene expression data on thousands of genes (Fig. 6.14). This allows an unbiased means of investigating tissue to determine which cellular mechanisms may be interacting to create the pathologic condition. The muscle parameters measured by studies discussed most likely have their roots in transcriptional changes in the muscle. (It is important to remember in the context of these studies that expression levels do not necessarily correlate with protein levels.) A recent study compared wrist flexor and extensor muscles from patients with cerebral palsy to controls undergoing wrist fracture surgery. Importantly, muscles from patients with cerebral palsy clustered independently of controls, showing a robust distinction between the muscle transcriptional profile in cerebral palsy and controls (Smith et al., 2009).

Cerebral palsy biopsies showed 205 genes that were significantly altered, covering a range of cellular processes. Placing gene expression in the context of physiological pathways, the results demonstrated that spastic muscle in cerebral palsy adapts transcriptionally by altering extracellular matrix, fibre type and myogenic potential. Extracellular matrix adaptations occur primarily in the basal lamina, although there is increase in fibrillar collagen components as well. Fibre type is

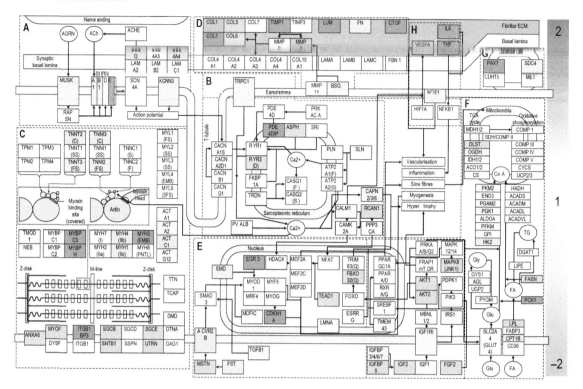

**Figure 6.14** • Linked map of functional muscle gene networks. Colour is determined by the expression ratio (CP/typically developing). Grey expression represents transcripts not present on the chip or below present threshold. Green connectors represent activation and red connectors represent inhibition in the direction of the arrow. Pathways represented are: A, neuromuscular junction; B, excitation contraction coupling; C, muscle contraction; D, extracellular matrix; E, muscle signalling; F, inflammation; G energy metabolism; H, satellite cells. (Please refer to colour plate section)

shifted to fast isoforms compared to normal muscle, as evidenced by contractile gene isoforms and decrease in oxidative metabolic gene transcription. Interestingly, there were also many signs of muscle immaturity such as a large increase in embryonic myosin heavy chain. Paradoxically, the muscles showed evidence of both competing pathways of fibre hypertrophy with an increase in the anabolic IGF1 gene in parallel with an increase in myostatin, a gene responsible for stopping muscle growth. As the first transcriptional profile performed on spastic muscle of patients with cerebral palsy, these adaptations were not characteristic of those observed in other disease states—emphasizing the unique muscle pathology in cerebral palsy (Smith et al., 2009).

A follow-up microarray experiment was conducted on muscle hamstring biopsies (Smith et al., 2012a). This was a more robust study,

using 40 microarrays and a well-controlled patient population. Again, patients with cerebral palsy had a unique transcriptional profile evidenced by clustering algorithms. However, with the increased statistical power, 1398 genes were significantly altered, necessitating the use of more global analysis. Ontology analysis revealed several categories of genes that were altered in cerebral palsy, and was expanded to also investigate pathways, transcription factors and microRNA. Additional markers of muscle immaturity were also observed to be up-regulated in cerebral palsy, supporting the notion that the muscle is not allowed to develop properly under the altered neurological input. Many of the up-regulated transcripts were found within the extracellular matrix, further emphasizing the role of fibrosis. Contrasting the results of the upper extremity, however, there was evidence of a fast-to-slow fibre type transition. This contrast was also observed in myostatin signalling, which was down-regulated in the hamstrings, implying a signal for muscle hypertrophy. In fact, surprisingly, there was little overlap between specific transcripts of the upper and lower extremity changes beyond the increases in extracellular matrix genes (Smith et al., 2009).

Measuring these transcriptional changes in the same hamstring biopsies as mechanical measurements allowed investigation of some functional consequences of these alterations (Smith et al., 2011, 2012a). Most demonstratively, the genes that had a significant correlation with bundle stiffness were part of the extracellular matrix. This again highlights the functional consequences of fibrosis in muscle from cerebral palsy patients. However these transcriptional studies are not capable of determining which cells within muscle are responsible for altered expression. More specific analysis would be required to enable therapies to target the cell populations responsible.

## Stem cell populations in cerebral palsy muscle

Knowing the changes in cell populations present in muscle contracture would enable deeper understanding of experiments performed on muscle in cerebral palsy. Flow cytometry has long been used in blood and liquid tissue to quantify cell populations, but recently has been applied to enzymatically digested muscle tissue, enabling analysis of mononuclear cells (Montarras et al. 2005). Despite being unable to isolate mature muscle fibres, this method can identify and purify mononuclear cell populations to investigate their role in muscle tissue. Mononuclear cells within muscle, including fibroblasts, macrophages, endothelial cells (Fig. 6.15), and others may be quantified with proper labelling. Knowledge of the cells present in muscle tissue may provide insights as to the tissue components that contribute to contracture development; for example, is the fibrosis observed the result of more fibroblasts present in the muscle? Recent articles on mouse muscle demonstrate that, resident within muscle, is a novel cell population capable of differentiating into fibroblasts, adipocytes, or even assisting muscle regeneration (Joe et al., 2010; Uezumi et al., 2010). It is also possible to investigate

the population of resident satellite cells within a muscle directly responsible for muscle regeneration and growth. The only flow cytometry studies conducted on human muscle show that satellite cell population increases with eccentric exercise (McKay et al., 2010).

Preliminary data have been collected on hamstring biopsies from patients with cerebral palsy using flow cytometry (Smith et al., 2012b). After mononuclear cells were isolated using enzymatic digestion and filtration, cells were labelled with various fluorescent antibodies. The antibodies used were a combination of NCAM and PAX7 for satellite cell determination (McKay et al., 2010), CD45 for hematopoietic cells (Tchilian et al., 2001), CD34 for hematopoietic plus endothelial cells (Elknerová et al., 2007), ER-TR7 for fibroblast determination (Strutz et al., 1995), and PDGFRα for fibro/adipogenic progenitor cells (Uezumi et al., 2010). Initial results showed that NCAM and PAX7 co-localized, enabling the use of NCAM only in further experiments, which was also demonstrated in other studies (McKay et al., 2010). The surprising initial results have also shown an approximately twofold decrease in the satellite cell population in biopsies from patients with cerebral palsy (Smith et al., 2012b). Other

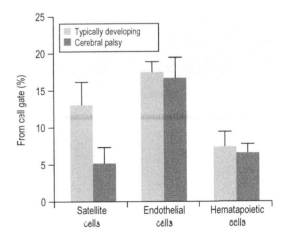

**Figure 6.15 •** Cell distributions from muscle biopsies of patients with cerebral palsy or typically developing. Cell types represented are satellite cells, endothelial cells and hematopoietic cells. There are significantly fewer satellite cells in muscle biopsies from patients with cerebral palsy, implicating reduced muscle repair and growth potential.

populations did not change or were not efficiently labelled, but this provides a cellular explanation for the inhibited growth potential seen in cerebral palsy muscle. This brings up the potential of cellular therapies for treatment of muscle contracture. Further studies are required to better understand the nature of muscle adaptations in cerebral palsy at the cellular level and to direct the next generation of therapies for muscle contracture treatment and prevention.

# References

Bandholm, T., Magnusson, P., Jensen, B.R., Sonne-Holm, S., 2009. Dorsiflexor muscle-group thickness in children with cerebral palsy: relation to cross-sectional area. NeuroRehabilitation 24 (4), 299–306.

Barber, L., Hastings-Ison, T., Baker, R., Barrett, R., Lichtwark, G., 2011. Medial gastrocnemius muscle volume and fascicle length in children aged 2 to 5 years with cerebral palsy. Dev. Med. Child Neurol. 53 (6), 543–548.

Barrett, R.S., Lichtwark, G.A., 2010. Gross muscle morphology and structure in spastic cerebral palsy: a systematic review. Dev. Med. Child Neurol. 52 (9), 794–804.

Best, T.M., McElhaney, J., Garrett Jr., W.E., Myers, B.S., 1994. Characterization of the passive responses of live skeletal muscle using the quasi-linear theory of viscoelasticity. J. Biomech. 27 (4), 413–419.

Blinks, J.R., Rudel, R., Taylor, S.R., 1978. Calcium transients in isolated amphibian skeletal muscle fibres: detection with aequorin. J. Physiol. 277, 291–323.

Block, B.A., Imagawa, T., Campbell, K.P., Franzini-Armstrong, C., 1988. Structural evidence for direct interaction between the molecular components of the transverse tubule/sarcoplasmic reticulum junction in skeletal muscle. J. Cell Biol. 107 (6 Pt 2), 2587–2600.

Boakes, J.L., Foran, J., Ward, S.R., Lieber, R.L., 2007. Muscle adaptation by serial sarcomere addition 1 year after femoral lengthening. Clin. Orthop. Relat. Res. 456, 250–253.

Bodine, S.C., Latres, E., Baumhueter, S., Lai, V.K., Nunez, L., Clarke, B.A., et al., 2001. Identification of ubiquitin ligases required for skeletal muscle atrophy. Science 294 (5547), 1704–1708.

Booth, C.M., Cortina-Borja, M.J., Theologis, T.N., 2001. Collagen accumulation in muscles of children with cerebral palsy and correlation with severity of spasticity. Dev. Med. Child Neurol. 43 (5), 314–320.

Borg, T.K., Caulfield, J.B., 1980. Morphology of connective tissue in skeletal muscle. Tissue Cell 12 (1), 197–207.

Buller, A.J., Eccles, J.C., Eccles, R.M., 1960a. Differentiation of fast and slow muscles in the cat hind limb. J. Physiol. 150, 399–416.

Buller, A.J., Eccles, J.C., Eccles, R.M., 1960b. Interactions between motoneurones and muscles in respect of the characteristic speeds of their responses. J. Physiol. 150, 417–439.

Castle, M.E., Reyman, T.A., Schneider, M., 1979. Pathology of spastic muscle in cerebral palsy. Clin. Orthop. Relat. Res. 142, 223–232.

Cleworth, D., Edman, K.A., 1969. Laser diffraction studies on single skeletal muscle fibres. Science 163 (864), 296–298.

Dietz, V., Ketelsen, U.P., Berger, W., Quintern, J., 1986. Motor unit involvement in spastic paresis. Relationship between leg muscle activation and histochemistry. J. Neurol. Sci. 75 (1), 89–103.

Duance, V.C., Restall, D.J., Beard, H., Bourne, F.J., Bailey, A.J., 1977. The location of three collagen types in skeletal muscle. FEBS Lett. 79 (2), 248–252.

Elder, G.C., Kirk, J., Stewart, G., Cook, K., Weir, D., Marshall, A., et al., 2003. Contributing factors to muscle weakness in children with cerebral palsy. Dev. Med. Child Neurol. 45 (8), 542–550.

Elknerová, K., Lacinová, Z., Soucek, J., Marinov, I., Stöckbauer, P., 2007. Growth inhibitory effect of the antibody to hematopoietic stem cell antigen CD34 in leukemic cell lines. Neoplasma 54 (4), 311–320.

Foran, J.R., Steinman, S., Barash, I., Chambers, H.G., Lieber, R.L., 2005. Structural and mechanical alterations in spastic skeletal muscle. Dev. Med. Child Neurol. 47 (10), 713–717.

Freiburg, A., Trombitas, K., Hell, W., Cazorla, O., Fougerousse, F., Centner, T., et al., 2000. Series of exon-skipping events in the elastic spring region of titin as the structural basis for myofibrillar elastic diversity. Circ. Res. 86 (11), 1114–1121.

Friden, J., Lieber, R.L., 2003. Spastic muscle cells are shorter and stiffer than normal cells. Muscle Nerve 27 (2), 157–164.

Fry, A.C., Allemeier, C.A., Staron, R.S., 1994. Correlation between percentage fibre type area and myosin heavy chain content in human skeletal muscle. Eur. J. Appl. Physiol. Occup. Physiol. 68 (3), 246–251.

Funatsu, T., Higuchi, H., Ishiwata, S., 1990. Elastic filaments in skeletal muscle revealed by selective removal of thin filaments with plasma gelsolin. J. Cell Biol. 110 (1), 53–62.

Gans, C., Bock, W.J., 1965. The functional significance of muscle architecture—a theoretical analysis. Ergeb. Anat. Entwicklungsgesch 38, 115–142.

Gillies, A.R., Lieber, R.L., 2011. Structure and function of the skeletal muscle extracellular matrix. Muscle Nerve 44 (3), 318–331.

Gordon, A.M., Huxley, A.F., Julian, F.J., 1966. The variation in isometric tension with sarcomere length in vertebrate muscle fibres. J. Physiol. 184 (1), 170–192.

Harry, J.D., Ward, A.W., Heglund, N.C., Morgan, D.L., McMahon, T.A., 1990. Cross-bridge cycling theories cannot explain high-speed lengthening behavior in frog muscle. Biophys. J. 57 (2), 201–208.

Hather, B.M., Tesch, P.A., Buchanan, P., Dudley, G.A., 1991. Influence of eccentric actions on skeletal muscle adaptations to resistance training. Acta Physiol. Scand. 143 (2), 177–185.

Horowits, R., 1992. Passive force generation and titin isoforms in mammalian skeletal muscle. Biophys. J. 61 (2), 392–398.

Horowits, R., Kempner, E.S., Bisher, M.E., Podolsky, R.J., 1986. A physiological role for titin and nebulin in skeletal muscle. Nature 323 (6084), 160–164.

Huxley, H., Hanson, J., 1954. Changes in the cross-striations of muscle during contraction and stretch and their structural interpretation. Nature 173 (4412), 973–976.

Huxley, H.E., 1969. The mechanism of muscular contraction. Science 164 (886), 1356–1365.

Huxley, A.F., Niedergerke, R., 1954. Structural changes in muscle during contraction; interference microscopy of living muscle fibres. Nature 173 (4412), 971–973.

Huxley, A.F., Peachey, L.D., 1961. The maximum length for contraction in vertebrate striated muscle. J. Physiol. 156, 150–165.

Ito, J., Araki, A., Tanaka, H., Tasaki, T., Cho, K., Yamazaki, R., 1996. Muscle histopathology in spastic cerebral palsy. Brain Dev. 18 (4), 299–303.

Joe, A.W., Yi, L., Natarajan, A., Le Grand, F., So, L., Wang, J., et al., 2010. Muscle injury activates resident fibro/adipogenic progenitors that facilitate myogenesis. Nat. Cell Biol. 12 (2), 153–163.

Kaariainen, M., Jarvinen, T., Jarvinen, M., Rantanen, J., Kalimo, H., 2000. Relation between myofibres and connective tissue during muscle injury repair. Scand. J. Med. Sci. Sports 10 (6), 332–337.

Katz, B., 1939. The relation between force and speed in muscular contraction. J. Physiol. 96 (1), 45–64.

Kerr Graham, H., Selber, P., 2003. Musculoskeletal aspects of cerebral palsy. J. Bone Joint Surg. Br. 85 (2), 157–166.

Kruger, M., Kotter, S., Grutzner, A., Lang, P., Andresen, C., Redfield, M.M., et al., 2009. Protein kinase G modulates human myocardial passive stiffness by phosphorylation of the titin springs. Circ. Res. 104 (1), 87–94.

Lance, J.W. (Ed.), 1980. Symposium Synopsis. Ed Spasticity: Disordered Motor Control. Year Book; Chicago.

Lecker, S.H., Jagoe, R.T., Gilbert, A., Gomes, M., Baracos, V., Bailey, J., et al., 2004. Multiple types of skeletal muscle atrophy involve a common program of changes in gene expression. FASEB J. 18 (1), 39–51.

Lieber, R.L., Friden, J., 2000. Functional and clinical significance of skeletal muscle architecture. Muscle Nerve 23 (11), 1647–1666.

Lieber, R.L., Friden, J., 2002. Spasticity causes a fundamental rearrangement of muscle–joint interaction. Muscle Nerve 25 (2), 265–270.

Lieber, R.L., Runesson, E., Einarsson, F., Friden, J., 2003. Inferior mechanical properties of spastic muscle bundles due to hypertrophic but compromised extracellular matrix material. Muscle Nerve 28 (4), 464–471.

Lieber, R.L., Steinman, S., Barash, I.A., Chambers, H., 2004. Structural and functional changes in spastic skeletal muscle. Muscle Nerve 29 (5), 615–627.

MacPhail, H.E., Kramer, J.F., 1995. Effect of isokinetic strength-training on functional ability and walking efficiency in adolescents with cerebral palsy. Dev. Med. Child Neurol. 37 (9), 763–775.

Magid, A., Law, D.J., 1985. Myofibrils bear most of the resting tension in frog skeletal muscle. Science 230 (4731), 1280–1282.

Magnusson, S.P., 1998. Passive properties of human skeletal muscle during stretch maneuvers. A review. Scand. J. Med. Sci. Sports 8 (2), 65–77.

Marbini, A., Ferrari, A., Cioni, G., Bellanova, M.F., Fusco, C., Gemignani, F., 2002. Immunohistochemical study of muscle biopsy in children with cerebral palsy. Brain Dev. 24 (2), 63–66.

Maruyama, K., Gergely, J., 1962. Interaction of actomyosin with adenosine triphosphate at low ionic strength. I. Dissociation of actomyosin during the clear phase. J. Biol. Chem. 237, 1095–1099.

Mauro, A., 1961. Satellite cell of skeletal muscle fibres. J. Biophys. Biochem. Cytol. 9, 493–495.

McKay, B.R., Toth, K.G., Tarnopolsky, M.A., Parise, G., 2010. Satellite cell number and cell cycle kinetics in response to acute myotrauma in humans: immunohistochemistry versus flow cytometry. J. Physiol. 588 (Pt 17), 3307–3320.

Meyer, G.A., McCulloch, A.D., Lieber, R.L., 2011. A nonlinear model of passive muscle viscosity. J. Biomech. Eng. 133 (9), 091007.

Mirbagheri, M.M., Barbeau, H., Ladouceur, M., Kearney, R.E., 2001. Intrinsic and reflex stiffness in normal and spastic, spinal cord injured subjects. Exp. Brain Res. 141 (4), 446–459.

Mohagheghi, A.A., Khan, T., Meadows, T.H., Giannikas, K., Baltzopoulos, V., Maganaris, C.N., 2007. Differences in gastrocnemius muscle architecture between the paretic and non-paretic legs in children with hemiplegic cerebral palsy. Clin. Biomech. (Bristol, Avon) 22 (6), 718–724.

Mohagheghi, A.A., Khan, T., Meadows, T.H., Giannikas, K., Baltzopoulos, V., Maganaris, C.N., 2008. In vivo gastrocnemius muscle fascicle length in children with and without diplegic cerebral palsy. Dev. Med. Child Neurol. 50 (1), 44–50.

Montarras, D., Morgan, J., Collins, C., Relaix, F., Zaffran, S., Cumano, A., et al., 2005. Direct isolation of satellite cells for skeletal muscle regeneration. Science 309 (5743), 2064–2067.

Moreau, N.G., Teefey, S.A., Damiano, D.L., 2009. In vivo muscle architecture and size of the rectus femoris and vastus lateralis in children and adolescents with cerebral palsy. Dev. Med. Child Neurol. 51 (10), 800–806.

Moreau, N.G., Simpson, K.N., Teefey, S.A., Damiano, D.L., 2010. Muscle architecture predicts maximum strength and is related to activity levels in cerebral palsy. Phys. Ther. 90 (11), 1619–1630.

Morgan, D.L., Mochon, S., Julian, F.J., 1982. A quantitative model of intersarcomere dynamics during fixed-end contractions of single frog muscle fibres. Biophys. J. 39 (2), 189–196.

Olsson, M.C., Kruger, M., Meyer, L.H., Ahnlund, L., Gransberg, L., Linke, W.A., et al., 2006. Fibre type-specific increase in passive muscle tension in spinal cord-injured subjects with spasticity. J. Physiol. 577 (Pt 1), 339–352.

Paolini, P.J., Sabbadini, R., Roos, K.P., Baskin, R.J., 1976. Sarcomere length dispersion in single skeletal muscle fibres and fibre bundles. Biophys. J. 14 (9), 010-030.

Ponten, E., Friden, J., Thornell, L.E., Lieber, R.L., 2005. Spastic wrist flexors are more severely affected than wrist extensors in children with cerebral palsy. Dev. Med. Child Neurol. 47 (6), 384–389.

Ponten, E., Lindstrom, M., Kadi, F., 2008. Higher amount of MyHC IIX in a wrist flexor in tetraplegic compared to hemiplegic cerebral palsy. J. Neurol. Sci. 266 (1-2), 51–56.

Ponten, E.M., Stal, P.S., 2007. Decreased capillarization and a shift to fast myosin heavy chain IIx in the biceps brachii muscle from young adults with spastic paresis. J. Neurol. Sci. 253 (1-2), 25–33.

Powell, P.L., Roy, R.R., Kanim, P., Bello, M.A., Edgerton, V.R., 1984. Predictability of skeletal muscle tension from architectural determinations in guinea pig hindlimbs. J. Appl. Physiol. 57 (6), 1715–1721.

Prado, L.G., Makarenko, I., Andresen, C., Kruger, M., Opitz, C.A., Linke, W.A., 2005. Isoform diversity of giant proteins in relation to passive and active contractile properties of rabbit skeletal muscles. J. Gen. Physiol. 126 (5), 461–480.

Roig, M., O'Brien, K., Kirk, G., Murray, R., McKinnon, P., Shadgan, B., et al., 2009. The effects of eccentric versus concentric resistance training on muscle strength and mass in healthy adults: a systematic review with meta-analysis. Br. J. Sports Med. 43 (8), 556–568.

Romanini, L., Villani, C., Meloni, C., Calvisi, V., 1989. Histological and morphological aspects of muscle in infantile cerebral palsy. Ital. J. Orthop. Traumatol. 15 (1), 87–93.

Rose, J., McGill, K.C., 2005. Neuromuscular activation and motor-unit firing characteristics in cerebral palsy. Dev. Med. Child Neurol. 47 (5), 329–336.

Ross, S.A., Engsberg, J.R., 2007. Relationships between spasticity, strength, gait, and the GMFM-66 in persons with spastic diplegia cerebral palsy. Arch. Phys. Med. Rehabil. 88 (9), 1114–1120.

Serrano, A.L., Munoz-Canoves, P., 2010. Regulation and dysregulation of fibrosis in skeletal muscle. Exp. Cell Res. 316 (18), 3050–3058.

Shortland, A.P., Harris, C.A., Gough, M., Robinson, R.O., 2002. Architecture of the medial gastrocnemius in children with spastic diplegia. Dev. Med. Child Neurol. 44 (3), 158–163.

Sinkjaer, T., Magnussen, I., 1994. Passive, intrinsic and reflex-mediated stiffness in the ankle extensors of hemiparetic patients. Brain 117 (Pt 2), 355–363.

Sjostrom, M., Fugl-Meyer, A.R., Nordin, G., Wahlby, L., 1980. Post-stroke hemiplegia; crural muscle strength and structure. Scand. J. Rehabil. Med. Suppl. 7, 53–67.

Smeulders, M.J., Kreulen, M., Hage, J.J., Huijing, P.A., van der Horst, C.M., 2004. Overstretching of sarcomeres may not cause cerebral palsy muscle contracture. J. Orthop. Res. 22 (6), 1331–1335.

Smith, L.R., Ponten, E., Hedstrom, Y., Ward, S.R., Chambers, H.G., Subramaniam, S., et al., 2009. Novel transcriptional profile in wrist muscles from cerebral palsy patients. BMC Med. Genomics 2, 44.

Smith, L.R., Lee, K.S., Ward, S.R., Chambers, H.G., Lieber, R.L., 2011. Hamstring contractures in children with spastic cerebral palsy result from a stiffer extracellular matrix and increased in vivo sarcomere length. J. Physiol. 589 (Pt 10), 2625–2639.

Smith, L.R., Chambers, H.G., Subramaniam, S., Lieber, R.L., 2012a. Transcriptional abnormalities of hamstring muscle contractures in children with cerebral palsy. PLoS One 7 (8), e40686. (Epub 2012 Aug 16).

Smith, L.R., Chambers, H.G., Lieber, R.L., December 5, 2012b. Reduced satellite cell population may lead to contractures in children with cerebral palsy. Dev. Med. Child Neurol. doi: 10.1111/dmcn.12027 [Epub ahead of print](in press).

Strutz, F., Okada, H., Lo, C.W., Danoff, T., Carone, R.L., Tomaszewski, J.E., et al., 1995. Identification and characterization of a fibroblast marker: FSP1. J. Cell Biol. 130 (2), 393–405.

Tabary, J.C., Tabary, C., Tardieu, C., Tardieu, G., Goldspink, G., 1972. Physiological and structural changes in the cat's soleus muscle due to immobilization at different lengths by plaster casts. J. Physiol. 224 (1), 231 244.

Tardieu, C., Huet de la Tour, E., Bret, M.D., Tardieu, G., 1982a. Muscle hypoextensibility in children with cerebral palsy: I. Clinical and experimental observations. Arch. Phys. Med. Rehabil. 63 (3), 97–102.

Tardieu, G., Tardieu, C., Colbeau-Justin, P., Lespargot, A., 1982b. Muscle hypoextensibility in children with cerebral palsy: II. Therapeutic implications. Arch. Phys. Med. Rehabil. 63 (3), 103–107.

Taylor, N.A., Wilkinson, J.G., 1986. Exercise-induced skeletal muscle growth. Hypertrophy or hyperplasia? Sports Med. 3 (3), 190–200.

Tchilian, E.Z., Wallace, D.L., Wells, R.S., Flower, D.R., Morgan, G., Beverley, P.C., 2001. A deletion in the gene encoding the CD45 antigen in a patient with SCID. J. Immunol. 166 (2), 1308–1313.

Theroux, M.C., Akins, R.E., Barone, C., Boyce, B., Miller, F., Dabney, K.W., 2002. Neuromuscular junctions in cerebral palsy: presence of extrajunctional acetylcholine receptors. Anesthesiology 96 (2), 330–335.

Tidball, J.G., 2005. Inflammatory processes in muscle injury and repair. Am. J. Physiol. Regul., Integr. Comp. Physiol. 288 (2), R345–R353.

Tidball, J.G., Villalta, S.A., 2010. Regulatory interactions between muscle and the immune system during muscle regeneration. Am. J. Physiol. Regul., Integr. Comp. Physiol. 298 (5), R1173–R1187.

Uezumi, A., Fukada, S., Yamamoto, N., Takeda, S., Tsuchida, K., 2010. Mesenchymal progenitors distinct from satellite cells contribute to ectopic fat cell formation in skeletal muscle. Nat. Cell Biol. 12 (2), 143–152.

Wang, K., McCarter, R., Wright, J., Beverly, J., Ramirez-Mitchell, R., 1993. Viscoelasticity of the sarcomere matrix of skeletal muscles. The titin–myosin composite filament is a dual-stage molecular spring. Biophys. J. 64 (4), 1161–1177.

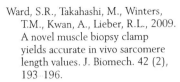

Ward, S.R., Takahashi, M., Winters, T.M., Kwan, A., Lieber, R.L., 2009. A novel muscle biopsy clamp yields accurate in vivo sarcomere length values. J. Biomech. 42 (2), 193–196.

Wickiewicz, T.L., Roy, R.R., Powell, P.L., Perrine, J.J., Edgerton, V.R., 1984. Muscle architecture and force–velocity relationships in humans. J. Appl. Physiol. 57 (2), 435–443.

Winters, T.M., Takahashi, M., Lieber, R.L., Ward, S.R., 2011. Whole muscle length–tension relationships are accurately modeled as scaled sarcomeres in rabbit hindlimb muscles. J. Biomech. 44 (1), 109–115.

Yablonka-Reuveni, Z., 2011. The skeletal muscle satellite cell: still young and fascinating at 50. J. Histochem. Cytochem. 59 (12), 1041–1059.

Zot, A.S., Potter, J.D., 1987. Structural aspects of troponin–tropomyosin regulation of skeletal muscle contraction. Annu. Rev. Biophys. Biophys. Chem. 16, 535–559.

# Early muscle development in children with cerebral palsy: the consequences for further muscle growth, muscle function, and long-term mobility

7

Martin Gough, Adam P. Shortland

## CHAPTER CONTENTS

How might a non-progressive central nervous system lesion lead to progressive musculoskeletal deformity and impairment of function? How early does muscle deformity occur in children with cerebral palsy (CP)? Is it possible that intervention in infancy and early childhood may alter the development of muscle deformity? Although we lack empirical evidence, our growing understanding of normal skeletal muscle development and growth suggests that muscle deformity in CP may be related to an impairment of growth and to subsequent adaptation to altered use. To explore this concept and its implications, it may be helpful to first review normal skeletal muscle structure and function and the alterations described in muscle in CP, and then discuss normal skeletal muscle development and growth. We can then consider how early muscle development may be altered in children with CP, how skeletal muscles may respond to subsequent use in children with CP, and the implications this may have for intervention. Muscle structure and function, and the alterations

noted in children with CP, have been discussed in detail in Chapter 6, and the development of the corticospinal tract and spinal cord networks have been discussed in Chapter 2. They are discussed briefly again below to facilitate discussion of the questions raised above.

## Skeletal muscle structure and function

Skeletal muscle contraction occurs through the interaction of two proteins, actin and myosin. These proteins form filaments that overlap in the sarcomere, the basic functional unit of the muscle cell. In the presence of calcium, actin binds to myosin and the resulting configurational change in myosin results in a relative change in the position of the actin and myosin filaments. A range of structural proteins are needed to facilitate and stabilize this interaction. Other intracellular proteins form supportive structures called costameres which transmit the force generated by the interaction of the actin and myosin filaments through the cell membrane. The costameres link the sarcomeres to the basal lamina, which is in turn linked to a continuous three-dimensional network of connective tissue surrounding fibres, fascicles and whole muscles which is connected to internal and external tendons and to the surrounding fascia (for a review see Purslow, 2002).

Human muscles may be classified depending on the predominant type of myosin heavy chain (MHC) isoform present into slow (MHCIβ) and fast (MHCIIa, MHCIIx) muscles, although rather than having discrete muscle fibre types each muscle fibre may contain a range of different MHC isoforms (Pette and Staron, 2000). Thyroid hormone up-regulates the genes expressing fast MHC isoforms, whereas nerve activity-dependent transcription of the genes expressing MHCIβ is necessary for the development and maintenance of slow fibres (Schiaffino et al., 2007). The MHC isoform expressed by a muscle cell varies depending on how the muscle is used: there is a shift towards a slower MHC isoform with more frequent and tonic muscle activation, whereas with reduced or phasic activity there is a shift towards a faster MHC isoform (Pette and Staron, 2000; Schiaffino et al., 2007).

Energy is needed within the muscle cell for actin/myosin interaction, for rapid storage of calcium in the sarcoplasmic reticulum after contraction, and for intracellular protein synthesis and degradation. This energy is provided predominantly by intracellular organelles called mitochondria. A 'slow-twitch' muscle fibre produces force slowly and relaxes slowly, but can maintain force production

for prolonged periods because of its use of oxidative metabolism. A 'fast-twitch' muscle fibre produces force rapidly and relaxes rapidly but may not be able to sustain this force as the energy demands involved may outstrip the oxidative capacity of the fibre.

Skeletal muscle is a highly adaptable tissue, and is able to respond to altered demand by changes in the expression of genes within the cell nucleus. Factors influencing muscle gene expression include the pattern of neuronal activation, the energy substrates available and the presence of local hormones and growth factors (Fig. 7.1). Signalling pathways allow a balance between active muscle protein synthesis and active protein degradation, which in turn determines the size and function of the muscle cell (Gundersen, 2011). Innervation, growth factors and nutrition appear to promote protein synthesis, while denervation, immobilization, systemic inflammation and starvation result in active protein degradation and muscle atrophy (Gundersen, 2011) (Fig. 7.2). Growth factors may have different actions on different components of the muscle: myostatin, which inhibits muscle fibre growth, is important

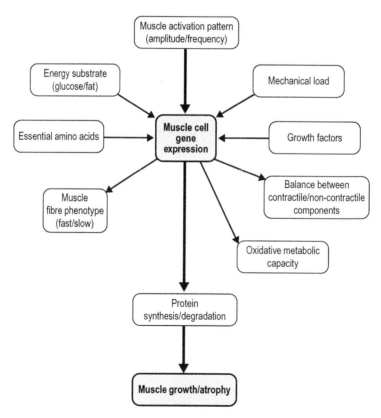

**Figure 7.1** • Factors influencing muscle growth.

in muscle repair and appears to promote growth of the connective tissue matrix (Zhu et al., 2007). Insulin-like growth factor 1 (IGF-1) is released by the muscle when active and promotes protein synthesis within the muscle fibre through pathways involving mammalian target of rapamycin (mTOR) (Clemmons, 2009; Otto and Patel, 2010). Protein synthesis in muscle may also be stimulated directly by ingested essential amino acids, particularly leucine, acting through mTOR (Drummond et al., 2009). This action of ingested amino acids may, however, be inhibited during periods of starvation or stress (Fujita et al., 2007).

The mitochondrial content of the sarcomere, and the ability of the sarcomere to use energy substrates such as glucose or fat, appears to be influenced by pathways within the cell that are sensitive to neuronal activation such as those involving the calcineurin-NFAT (nuclear activated factor of T cells) system (Schiaffino et al., 2007; Westerblad et al., 2010). Calcineurin-NFAT also appears to be important in determining the type of MHC expressed, which will influence the contraction speed of the muscle (Pette and Staron, 2000; Schiaffino et al., 2007). Skeletal muscle responds to both increased use and decreased use: cast immobilization, for instance, will lead to a reduction in muscle fibre protein synthesis and a shift towards protein degradation within the muscle fibre. This is an active process that involves the tagging of muscle fibres by ubiquitin prior to proteolysis and in which myostatin appears to be involved (Gundersen, 2011). Cast immobilization of the quadriceps in the human results in a reduction in protein synthesis within 48 hours (Urso et al., 2006) and also in a reduction of the normal protein synthesis response of muscle to ingested amino acids (Glover et al., 2008).

A muscle fibre thus consists of a composite and complex network with a close balance and interaction between contractile and non-contractile elements which is influenced by a number of factors, including innervation, the mechanical load imposed, and the presence of local or systemic growth factors. Of these factors, the most important factor appears to be the pattern of neuronal activation and the ionic changes and mechanical stresses associated with contraction. A focal impairment of muscle growth with replacement of the muscle fibres by fat and fibrous tissue was noted in neonatal mouse models of brachial plexus palsy following neurotomy (Kim et al., 2010; Nikolau et al., 2011) or denervation using botulinum toxin A (Kim et al., 2009). Neuromuscular electrical stimulation has been shown to lessen reductions in muscle volume, and to moderate the increase in fat content and the reduction in muscle oxidative capacity after chronic spinal cord injury in humans (Biering-Sorenson et al., 2009).

Muscle protein synthesis is suppressed during periods of active contraction, but there appears to be a subsequent increase in protein synthesis

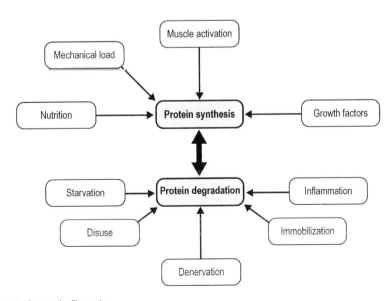

**Figure 7.2** • Control of muscle fibre size.

(Atherton and Rennie, 2009). Stretch without contraction in the human gastrocnemius does not appear to lead to protein synthesis (Fowles et al., 2000), and cultured muscle cells show a prolonged inhibition of protein synthesis after mechanical stretch without activation (Atherton et al., 2009). Rather than resulting in muscle growth, repeated passive stretch instead appears to promote expression of the atrophy pathway in the rat soleus (Gomes et al., 2006). Van Dyke et al. (2012) recently showed that passive stretch of the adult rat soleus following tenotomy did not alter the rate of sarcomere loss in comparison to unstretched tenotomized muscle: sarcomere loss was reduced but not prevented when stretch was combined with electrical stimulation of the muscle.

Each skeletal muscle fibre is innervated by an alpha-motor neuron (αMN): the αMN and its associated muscle fibres form a motor unit (MU). There is a close relationship between the size of a MU, the size of the αMN, and the force produced by the MU. Small MUs have a small number of slow fibres innervated by a small αMN, and large MUs have a large number of fast fibres innervated by a large αMN. These MUs are distributed throughout the muscle and allow the graded development of the force of contraction (Henneman and Olson, 1965); small motor units are activated initially, and as the force required increases, larger motor units are recruited and the rate of contraction of individual motor units is increased. This allows smaller fibres with greater endurance to be used more often, and reserves the energy-expensive large MUs for movements where speed and force of contraction are important. Muscles are composed of multiple motor units distributed over large volumes of the muscle: the combination of a mechanically robust connective tissue framework and a distributed MU network allows the smooth transmission of lateral and axial forces.

Most skeletal muscles are pennate, with muscle fibres arranged at an angle to the tendon. This leads to a small loss of force for an individual muscle fibre but this is offset by the increased force available due to the greater number of fibres which can be accommodated per unit muscle volume. The force produced by a muscle is related to the physiological cross-sectional area. The speed of contraction and range of contraction of a muscle are influenced by muscle fibre length, with longer fibres (with more sarcomeres in series) having a faster rate of contraction and greater range, and

shorter muscles (with more sarcomeres in parallel) producing more force over a shorter range. The force generated is influenced by the physiological cross-sectional area (PCSA) of the muscle, which represents the sum of the cross-sectional areas of the individual muscle fibres. Muscle fibres rarely lie in the long axis of the muscle, so the anatomical cross-sectional area and the PCSA are not the same. Muscle fibre type, muscle architecture and MU composition thus combine to define the response of a muscle to activation.

# Skeletal muscle changes in children with CP

There is, as yet, limited information on skeletal muscle changes in children with CP. Muscle biopsy studies in this group have noted marked fibre size variability and predominance of either fast or slow fibres: this may reflect the heterogeneous functional level of the children involved and variation in the muscles assessed. In a recent systematic review, Barrett and Lichtwark (2010) noted that the most consistent morphological and structural change evident in the muscles of children with spastic CP was reduced size, as indicated by reduced muscle volume, reduced cross-sectional area and reduced muscle thickness. There have been conflicting reports on muscle fibre length changes, with some groups reporting no alteration in muscle fibre lengths and other groups reporting reduced muscle fibre lengths. Most of the studies on muscle fibre lengths involved the gastrocnemius muscle: recently, Moreau et al. (2009) described muscle fibre shortness in the rectus femoris and unchanged muscle fibre lengths in the vastus lateralis, suggesting that rather than a uniform change, the alteration seen in muscle in children with CP may reflect a combination of influences, including the nature of the central lesion, the level of function of the child, the morphology of individual muscles, and possibly the effect of previous intervention. Lieber et al. (2004) have assessed the morphology of the flexor carpi ulnaris in children undergoing surgery and noted increased sarcomere lengths and increased stiffness of muscle fibres: whether these changes are primary or secondary is unclear. In a recent study, this group assessed biopsies from the semitendinosus and gracilis muscles in 17 cases with CP and 14 controls (Smith et al., 2011). They found markedly reduced muscle fibre diameter and reduced muscle cross-sectional area. Sarcomere lengths appeared to be increased at rest compared to controls: this was more marked with increasing deformity and with greater limitation of function. The involved muscles were also stiffer due to increased collagen content.

Muscle function appears to be altered in children with CP. Stackhouse et al. (2005) investigated the quadriceps femoris and triceps surae muscles in children with CP: they found that children with CP had reduced muscle strength due to impaired activation of the muscles and to co-contraction of antagonist muscles. Voluntary activation of the quadriceps was reduced by 33% and 45% in triceps surae in the CP group in comparison to controls, suggesting a limitation in the extent to which muscle fibres could be activated in response to increasing demand in children with CP. There may also be limitation in rate-coding, which is the ability of a muscle to increase the strength of contraction by increasing the frequency of contraction. Rose and McGill (2005) looked at voluntary activation of the gastrocnemius and tibialis anterior in children with CP. They found a similar activation rate to controls at lower frequencies of activation but noted that the children with CP were unable to increase the frequency of activation of smaller MUs, and as noted by Stackhouse et al., (2005), were unable to recruit larger (higher threshold) MUs. The speed of contraction and the speed of relaxation may also be altered: Downing et al. (2009) looked at the rate at which a moment could be generated and relaxed across the lower limb joints of ambulant children with CP. They found that children with CP took 89% longer to generate a peak moment and 71% longer to reduce the moment in comparison to controls: this was particularly marked in the distal muscles of the lower limb and was felt by the authors to be of sufficient severity to adversely affect ambulation. This may be related to altered or prolonged activation of the αMN by the spinal cord networks or to changes of oxidative metabolic capacity or calcium control within the muscle cell, as noted by Smith et al. (2009).

The changes seen in gross muscle function and morphology in CP are mirrored by changes in gene activation and expression within the sarcomere. Smith et al. (2009) looked at the pattern of gene expression in the flexor carpi ulnaris of children with CP and noted a shift towards a faster muscle phenotype with expression of MHCs not usually seen in children. These included the fetal and

perinatal isoform and even MHCIIb, which is normally not expressed in humans, despite up-regulation of the pathway for slow oxidative fibre-type determination. They also noted increased levels of parvalbumin, a calcium-binding protein which would affect the relaxation rate. They noted that their findings did not fit a simple model of increased use or disuse of muscle. Ponten et al. (2008) looked at MHC expression in the flexor carpi ulnaris in children with CP with different levels of functional involvement: she found a shift towards greater expression of MHCI in children with greater levels of function and of MHCII isoforms in children with reduced upper limb function.

The timing of onset of muscle deformity in children with CP is not clear. A reduction in medial gastrocnemius volume, PCSA and fascicle length has been noted in children with spastic CP aged between 2 and 5 years associated with a reduction in passive dorsiflexion (Barber et al., 2011), suggesting that muscle changes may occur at an earlier age than is generally considered. Before discussing how this may occur, it may be helpful to briefly review our understanding of normal skeletal muscle development and growth.

# Normal skeletal muscle development and growth

Primary myotubes are formed in the human embryo at around eight post-conception weeks (PCW) following migration of myoblasts into the developing limb bud (Ijkema-Paassen and Gramsbergen, 2005). Activation of muscle fibres by αMNs occurs soon after formation of the myotubes, and muscle contraction is seen between eight and ten PCW (Prechtl, 1993). This muscle contraction occurs before ingrowth of the corticospinal tract (CST), and appears to represent the activity of intrinsic spinal cord networks capable of ordered discharge without corticospinal or afferent input (Vinay et al., 2002). The afferent (sensory) axons from skeletal muscle appear to reach the spinal cord grey matter by 7.5 PCW and make dense connections (which are later refined) to innervate motor neurons by 8.5–9 PCW, going on to establish the monosynaptic reflex pathway by 14 PCW (for a review, see Clowry, 2007). Muscle fibres in the adult human are each innervated by a single axon but initially each muscle fibre is innervated by a number of αMNs: this is termed polyneuronal innervation. Regression of polyneuronal innervation occurs in the rat soleus prior to the onset of locomotion (Ijkema-Paassen and Gramsbergen, 2005), but there is limited evidence about the timing of neuronal regression and the development of mononeuronal activation in the human. Gramsbergen et al. (1997) studied the innervation of human psoas fibres and found that mononeuronal activation occurs by 12 weeks postnatally.

Development of motor function appears to be greatly dependent on the ingrowth of the CST to the spinal cord (see Fig. 7.3). The CST appears to have a number of functions including control of afferent inputs, control of spinal reflexes, direct and indirect excitation of motor neurons, and inhibition of motor neurons, together with trophic effects on spinal networks during development (Lemon and Griffiths, 2005). CST axons invade the human spinal cord from 17 to 29PCW and innervate the ventral horn from 31 to 35PCW, influencing the development of the cord networks, in particular the development of inhibitory interneurons (Clowry, 2007). Martin et al. (2005) identified three CST developmental stages: namely, growth of axons to the cord; refinement of grey matter termination; and development of motor control. He suggested that refinement and elimination of cord synapses

occur between 1 and 2 years of age in humans and may be related to activity-dependent competition between developing CST terminals and other spinal neural systems. As the corticospinal system and cord networks develop, the motor cortex can activate cord circuits and αMNs with lower levels of input through the use of postsynaptic facilitation, increased neurotransmitter expression, and an increase in CST axon branches (Chakrabarty and Martin, 2010). Regression of polyneuronal innervation of muscle appears to occur after the onset of CST innervation (Clowry, 2007) and is likely to be influenced by the effect of the CST on cord networks.

The refinement of spinal cord networks appears to be important for αMN function. Eken et al. (2008) studied MU activity in rat soleus muscles and found that the mean duration of muscle activity increased from 3.4 seconds at seven days to 62 seconds in adults, with most of this increase occurring after the age of three weeks. They suggested that postnatal development of tonic firing in soleus MUs depends on concurrent appearance of monoamine-dependent plateau potentials in αMNs due to interaction between the developing CST and intrinsic cord networks. The neuromuscular junction also undergoes development during this period. In the rat

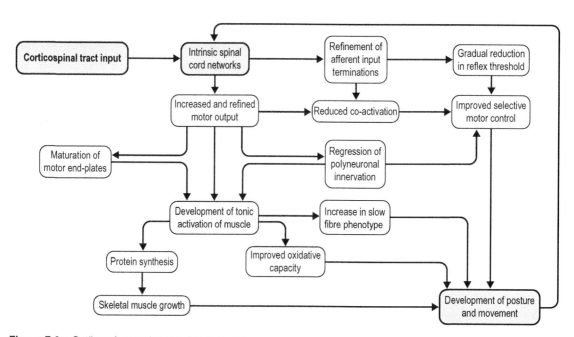

**Figure 7.3** • Outline of normal motor development.

neuromuscular junction, a gradual change from immature, low-threshold calcium channels associated with the acetylcholine receptor to faster, higher threshold channels in the mature muscle has been noted (Navarrete and Vrbova, 1993). These immature channels may be re-expressed following denervation (Hughes et al., 2006). The refinement of intrinsic cord networks due to interaction with the CST thus appears to allow amplification of the CST input, development of tonic activation of muscle, maturation of the neuromuscular junction, regression of polyneuronal innervation and the refinement of afferent input (Chakrabarty and Martin, 2010; Clowry, 2007; Eken et al., 2008; Martin, 2005).

Primary myotubes express embryonic MHC and the form of MHC seen in adult slow muscle, MHCIβ (Biressi et al., 2007). Secondary myotubes, formed by a subsequent wave of migrating myoblasts, express embryonic and perinatal MHC isoforms. Although MHC expression in primary myotubes appears independent of innervation, the development of subsequent muscle fibres and their expression of MHC isoforms appears to be closely related to their pattern of innervation (Ijkema-Paassen and Gramsbergen, 2005). There is limited data on MHC expression in the human fetus. Schloon et al. (1979) noted a predominance (95%) of fast fibres before 34 weeks' gestation, with an increase in the percentage of slow fibres to 40% at term, but the histochemical classification used would have included developmental MHC isoforms (embryonic and perinatal) as well as MHCII muscle fibres. Studies in mice (Agbulut et al., 2003) suggest a sequential expression of MHC isoforms due to down-regulation of developmental (embryonic and perinatal) isoforms, and up-regulation and stabilization of the adult MHC isoforms, with MHCIIa and MHCIIx expressed postnatally.

Muscle fibre growth and the development of the connective tissue network of muscle appears to be marked in the antenatal and perinatal period. In the human, the muscle fibres in sartorius appear to double in diameter between midgestation and term (Moore et al., 1971) and an accelerated growth in overall muscle fibre diameter in humans has been noted between 35 weeks' gestation and term (Schloon et al., 1979). This early marked growth of muscle fibres appears to be dependent on an adequate supply of protein in the form of amino acids: this has been noted to be most marked in pigs in late gestation and in the perinatal period

(Brameld et al., 1998). Muscle protein synthesis in neonatal pigs is associated with an increased sensitivity to growth hormones, insulin and amino acids: this increased sensitivity appears to decrease with age (Suryawan et al., 2007) and in the neonatal pig is associated with a marked increase in individual mitochondrial activity associated with an increase in mitochondrial number (Schmidt and Herpin, 1997). The importance of early nutrition in muscle growth is also suggested by studies on the effect of the timing of nutritional restriction in animal studies. In rats, under-nutrition prior to weaning has been shown to cause permanent stunting of muscle growth. In contrast, the effect of under-nutrition subsequent to weaning can generally be reversed (Bedi et al., 1982). Skeletal muscle is likely to be an expensive tissue in terms of protein requirements, and muscle growth may be selectively limited in the antenatal or perinatal period if nutrition is impaired. A relative inhibition of fetal skeletal muscle growth has been noted in a sheep model of late placental insufficiency/ intrauterine growth retardation, suggesting that skeletal muscle growth may be preferentially down-regulated if early nutrition is compromised (Thorn et al., 2009).

Because of the pennate nature of skeletal muscle, skeletal muscle growth involves changes in muscle fibre diameter and in muscle fibre length. Oertel et al. (1988) studied postmortem sections of the human vastus lateralis and deltoid and noted an increase in mean fibre diameter from 10–12 μm shortly after birth to 40–60 μm between the ages of 15 and 20 years. Lexell et al. (1992) noted that the mean fibre diameter of the human vastus lateralis in postmortem specimens increases more than twofold between the ages of 5 and 20 years, and found that this was closely associated with a similar increase noted in muscle cross-sectional area. They noted an increase in the percentage of fast muscle fibres in the vastus lateralis from 35% at age 5 years to 50% at age 20 years: this was thought to represent a transition of muscle fibres from a slow to a fast phenotype. Increases in the amplitude of activation of muscle fibres may contribute to the increasing percentage of fast muscle phenotypes and the development of large MUs with growth, as although fast MHC isoforms are present at birth their subsequent expression depends on neurological innervation and hormonal factors (Agbulut et al., 2003). Longitudinal growth of the mouse gastrocnemius muscle belly occurs predominantly through muscle fibre hypertrophy rather than by increased muscle fibre length (White et al., 2010), but the situation in humans appears more complex. Binzoni et al. (2001) noted an increase in the pennation angle of the human medial gastrocnemius during growth which they felt reflected muscle fibre hypertrophy. Benard et al. (2011) used ultrasound to study the growth of the medial gastrocnemius in children aged between 5 and 12 years. They found that muscle fibre length and diameter increase with growth, but, because of the pennate nature of the gastrocnemius, longitudinal muscle fibre growth accounts for only 20% of the longitudinal growth of the medial gastrocnemius muscle belly: the remaining 80% was related to the increase in diameter of the muscle fibres. The contribution of muscle fibre growth in length and in diameter to longitudinal growth and increased volume of the muscle belly is likely to vary depending on the morphology of the muscle.

Growth and development of muscle fibres is accompanied by development and organization of the connective tissue framework within the muscle, which results in an organized arrangement of muscle fibres within the muscle. Myostatin appears to be suppressed during perinatal and early postnatal muscle growth in rats, possibly to enhance development of the contractile component of muscle (Nishimura et al., 2007). Muscle fibre development and growth, the metabolic capacity of the muscle fibre and the development of the connective tissue network of muscle appear to reflect the interplay of a number of factors, including neuronal, nutritional and hormonal factors and the initial and subsequent pattern of muscle use. The mouse models of neonatal brachial plexus palsy noted above (Kim et al., 2009, 2010; Nikolau et al., 2011) suggest that the pattern of neuronal activation of muscle may be particularly important in postnatal muscle fibre growth and the development of the muscle phenotype.

Muscle development and growth do not occur in isolation. The development of motor control appears to be facilitated by interaction of the musculoskeletal and corticospinal systems (Vinay et al., 2002). Forssberg (1985) reviewed human locomotor patterns in newborns (<2 months old), during supported locomotion (6–12 months old) and during early independent walking (10–18 months old) and noted co-contraction of agonists and antagonists. He suggested that innate pattern

generators in the spinal cord produce the infant stepping, and also generate the basic locomotor rhythm in adults, but that neural circuits specific for humans transform the original, non-plantigrade motor activity to a plantigrade motor pattern. Sutherland et al. (1988) noted differences in the activation patterns of tibialis anterior (prolonged activity in stance), vastus medialis (prolonged activity in swing) and in the gastrocnemius and soleus (prolonged activity beginning near the middle of swing) in children 1–2 years old. These patterns gradually changed until by the age of 4 years a more mature pattern was seen in the majority of the muscles assessed. These changes appear to be associated with an improvement in the ability of the child to filter afferent input and to develop reciprocal inhibition. O'Sullivan et al. (1991) noted a gradual increase in the stimulus needed to invoke a monosynaptic reflex in typically developing children, increasing from a low level at birth to an adult level by the age of 6 years. The increase in threshold was associated with a reduction in activation of other muscles, including antagonists in the reflex response.

Although we think of the development of motor control in terms of efferent output from the CNS, afferent input from muscles and afferent input generated by movement are also important: the development of a cortical motor map in the cat, for example, appears to depend on activity and motor experience (Martin et al., 2005). The refinement of the CST terminations and connections in the spinal cord, and of afferent fibres from muscle, appears to be driven by movement: blocking limb use in the cat between 3 and 7 weeks postnatally with the use of botulinum toxin resulted in a persistent abnormal morphology of CST axon terminals and a persistent prehension deficit (Martin et al., 2004). This may be related to competition between the CST, muscle afferent fibres and other inputs for cord synapses as suggested by Clowry et al. (2006) who noted similar findings in rats following the use of botulinum toxin in the second postnatal week to cause temporary limb paresis. These findings suggest close interaction between muscle development and function and continued motor development, with skeletal muscle acting as an important component of a feedback loop.

Acquisition of the ability to stand, and subsequently take steps, requires appropriate motor control but also requires the presence of lower limb extensor muscles capable of producing sufficient force and with sufficient metabolic capacity to sustain generation of this force. An impairment of muscle development will result in an impaired capacity for movement and function, which may exacerbate any limitation in motor control. As will be discussed in the next section, there are a number of possible ways in which muscle development and growth may be altered in children with CP.

## Possible mechanisms leading to altered muscle development and growth in CP

Although we lack information about early development of skeletal muscle in children with CP, altered interaction of the neuronal, nutritional and endocrine factors noted above could influence muscle development in a manner consistent with the subsequent alteration in muscle morphology and function described earlier. The reduced input of the CST to the developing spinal cord networks, and the resulting impaired development of these networks as discussed in Chapter 1, are likely to be particularly important factors

influencing subsequent muscle function and motor development (see Fig. 7.4). Persistence of polyneuronal innervation of muscle fibres and an inability to maximally activate muscle fibres because of incomplete development of spinal cord networks could result in a reduced ability to develop and activate individual MUs and impaired development of motor end-plates. The adverse effect of this on the development of motor control could be exacerbated by impaired or failed refinement of afferent input terminations and by impaired presynaptic inhibition because of reduced CST input: this could lead to a continued heightened motor response to afferent input with persistent antagonist activation. Spasticity, the velocity-dependent resistance of a muscle to stretch, is likely to be related to an impaired refinement of afferent input terminations to the cord and a persistently reduced ability to filter this increased input: this would suggest an associative rather than a causative role for spasticity in the impairment of muscle growth in CP.

Impaired development of the intrinsic cord networks because of impaired CST input is also likely to result in impaired development of tonic activation of muscle which appears to be needed, as discussed above, to promote the development and

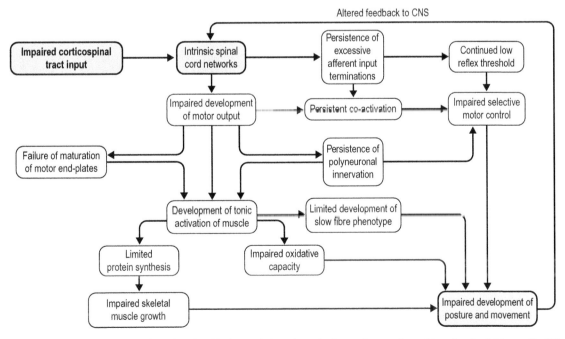

**Figure 7.4 •** Possible mechanisms involved in the early impairment of muscle growth and function in children with CP.

growth of slow muscle fibres which are essential to the development of posture and ambulation. As discussed earlier, a reduction in muscle fibres diameter will affect muscle belly length because of the pennate nature of skeletal muscle: a reduced rate of muscle fibres hypertrophy with growth may thus present clinically as progressive shortness of the muscle belly. This may be associated with an alteration in tendon length and may explain the findings of Fry et al. (2004) of a relative increase in tendon length and a reduction in muscle belly length in children with CP. These changes in muscle morphology may not be noted on clinical examination, which is generally focused on the measurement of passive range of joints. It is likely that our clinical measurements are insensitive to changes in the morphology of the musculature of very young children with CP, perhaps due to the compliance of musculotendinous units as a whole at this age, and this may colour our understanding of the development of muscle deformity. An early impairment of muscle growth and development would explain the findings of Barber et al. (2011), noted above, of reduced gastrocnemius muscle size and volume in children at the age of two years. The metabolic capacity of muscle will also be influenced by an altered innervation pattern: reduced muscle activation is likely to result in reduced muscle oxidative capacity through pathways discussed above, such as those involving calcineurin-NFAT (Schiaffino et al., 2007; Westerblad et al., 2010). This could reduce muscle endurance, which would in turn affect muscle function. Conversely, the quadriceps in ambulant children with CP has been found to be less fatiguable than in control children (Stackhouse et al., 2005): this may represent a response to increased use.

The neonatal mouse brachial plexus models noted above (Kim et al., 2009, 2010; Nikolau et al., 2011) suggest that a reduction of muscle activation may result in impaired muscle growth, replacement of muscle by fat and fibrous tissue, and the development of fixed deformity. A deficit in muscle growth and development due to reduced activation may be exacerbated by other factors. Children born preterm may have impaired muscle growth because of nutritional causes (Hay and Thureen, 2010; Yao and Chang, 1993), and as noted above impaired early nutrition may result in a preferential down-regulation of muscle growth (Thorn et al., 2009). The increased sensitivity of skeletal muscle to growth stimuli in the perinatal period has been discussed above: the combination of impaired muscle activation and potentially impaired nutrition may result in reduced sensitivity to, or failure of, the accelerated muscle development which occurs in the last trimester and in infancy. The presence of sepsis or inflammation in the perinatal period may alter the balance between growth of contractile and non-contractile material within the muscle through enhancement of the action of myostatin (Kollias and McDermott, 2008; Menconi et al., 2010; Nishimura et al., 2007; Zhu et al., 2007): the use of steroids during this period may further impair muscle growth (Menconi et al., 2010).

It may not be possible, even with subsequent appropriate innervation and nutrition, for muscle growth and function to subsequently reach normal levels. If impaired innervation of the muscle persists, there is likely to be a continued significant impairment of muscle growth and function as in the mouse models noted above. The impairment of muscle growth and function seen in children with CP may reflect the underlying neurological phenotype: children in Gross Motor Function Classification System (GMFCS) level II, for instance, may have enough small MUs developed to allow sufficient development of slow muscle fibres to enable independent ambulation but insufficient subsequent development of large MUs to allow normal levels of activity with growth, whereas children at GMFCS level III may have impaired development of slow muscle, in terms of both muscle volume and oxidative capacity, to an extent which prevents the acquisition of independent ambulation. The lack of development of slow muscle fibres in children at GMFCS level V may contribute significantly to their motor impairment. The relationship between early impairment of muscle growth in children with CP and their ultimate level on the GMFCS has not been fully delineated, although there is some evidence that muscle size and GMFCS levels are associated in cross-sectional studies (Ohata et al., 2008).

Muscles in children with CP appear to be smaller than those in their typically developing peers (Barrett and Lichtwark, 2011) even from an early age (Barber et al., 2011): in addition, they appear to have delayed activation and relaxation to an extent which would interfere with normal gait (Downing et al., 2009) and to have difficulty in recruiting available muscle fibres that will further limit their ability to generate force. This combination of reduced muscle size, reduced and poorly modulated muscle activation, persistent co-contraction, and a reduction in muscle fascicle length and diameter may be the factors underlying the development of an equinus gait pattern in children with CP, in which muscle activation appears to be reduced and poorly modulated rather than increased (Berger, 1998; Berger et al., 1982). While an equinus gait may reduce the demands on the ankle plantarflexor muscles, it is likely to result in increased eccentric loading of these muscles: this is supported by the findings of Gagliano et al. (2009), who noted altered expression of the genes responsible for collagen turnover in the tendons of children with CP that suggested an adaptation to higher levels of stress.

Increased loading of a small and weak muscle, particularly eccentric loading, may lead to injury and subsequent enhancement of the connective tissue network of muscle and possible suppression of muscle fibre growth through the action of myostatin (Zhu et al., 2007). This would explain the increased sarcomere lengths noted at rest in the semitendinosus in children with CP in the presence of increased connective tissue (Smith et al., 2011). Muscle injury due to altered loading may also lead to fibrosis and replacement of muscle fibres by fat (Serrano and Munoz-Canoves, 2010), which could exacerbate altered muscle morphology due to the underlying neurological injury. Fibrosis and fatty change in the muscles of ambulant children may be related to overuse and chronic injury, while muscle changes in non-ambulant children may be related to impaired early muscle development because of reduced innervation. Overuse in the muscles of ambulant children would be likely to result in injury and atrophy of some muscle fibres and hypertrophy of other fibres, as was noted in the biopsy studies reviewed by Barrett and Lichtwark (2010).

The reduced muscle size, variable muscle fibre size, increased intermuscular fat (Johnson et al., 2009) and connective tissue noted in the skeletal muscles of children with CP may thus be related to an early impairment of muscle growth and development due to a combination of neurological, nutritional and endocrine factors with subsequent altered adaptation to use. The interaction of these factors is likely to be influenced by the underlying muscle morphology and phenotype and by the pattern of muscle use. It may also potentially be influenced by intervention: this will be discussed in the next section.

# Implications for early intervention

Early intervention to skeletal muscles in children is frequently performed with the aim of maintaining or improving musculotendinous unit length, with passive joint range being used as a surrogate measure. The current model of the development of deformity in skeletal muscle in children with CP includes the concept of impaired muscle growth, but this is generally considered to be due to increased resistance of a muscle to stretch due to the presence of spasticity. Non-operative intervention to lengthen muscle generally involves the use of muscle stretch, either applied for a short period or over a prolonged period, with the aim of preventing muscle deformity and facilitating muscle growth by the addition of sarcomeres to muscle fibres. The perceived involvement of spasticity is addressed by denervation of muscle using botulinum toxin, with the aim of improving the capacity of a muscle to respond to passive stretch and in this way to facilitate muscle growth and function. Consensus statements have recommended the use of continuous passive stretch for children with CP from the age of six months (Gericke, 2006) and the use of repeat intramuscular botulinum toxin injection from the age of two years Heinen et al., 2010.

Passive muscle stretch, namely stretch imposed on a muscle rather than intrinsic to muscle contraction, has not however been shown to correct deformity or promote muscle growth whether used as part of a therapy programme (Butler and Darrah, 2001; Pin et al., 2006), through the use of orthoses (Morris, 2002) or through serial casting (Blackmore et al., 2007). A recent Cochrane review (Katalinic et al., 2010) concluded that in people with neurological conditions, there was moderate to high-quality evidence to indicate that passive stretch does not have clinically important immediate, short-term or long-term effects on joint mobility. This is likely to reflect the limited role of passive stretch on muscle growth as discussed above. Even if stretch of muscle did promote sarcomerogenesis, this would have a limited benefit in terms of muscle belly length because of the limited contribution of muscle fibre length to musculotendinous unit length (Benard et al., 2011). The moderate short-term alteration in musculotendinous unit length following botulinum toxin injection appears to be related to reduced muscle activity because of denervation; whether this mild short-term benefit offsets the potential associated impairment of muscle growth is open to question (Gough et al., 2005).

The combination of botulinum toxin and muscle immobilization or passive stretch may not have a positive effect on muscle growth but may have a negative effect. The importance of innervation in muscle growth and maintenance of function, and the adverse effect of immobilization on muscle growth, have been discussed above. Botulinum toxin use in adult animal muscles has been reported to cause marked atrophy (Gough, 2009; Gough et al., 2005). An adverse effect of an intervention on growing muscle may result in a permanent deficit in muscle size or volume: the use of botulinum toxin in 29-day-old rats resulted in marked atrophy and an impairment of muscle growth that did not respond to subsequent exercise (Velders et al., 2008). There are as yet no studies assessing the long-term outcome of botulinum toxin use on muscle growth and function in children with CP. Tedroff et al. (2009) reviewed the outcome in children with CP treated with botulinum toxin for spasticity or limitation of joint motion and noted a progressive reduction in joint passive ranges, following an initial improvement. They concluded that botulinum toxin was not effective in preventing muscle deformity and suggested that it may instead promote the development of deformity. Schroeder et al. (2010) have recently written to express concern about the use of botulinum toxin in children because of the finding of long-standing muscle atrophy and denervation in adult muscles injected with botulinum toxin (Schroeder et al., 2009).

As discussed earlier, contractile activity leads to an alteration in mitochondrial gene expression and an increase in mitochondrial number (Bigard et al., 2000; Hood, 2001). Because of this, skeletal muscle immobilization and denervation have the potential not only to adversely affect muscle growth but also to affect muscle development in terms of metabolic capacity and resistance to fatigue. Contractile activity, working through the calcineurin-NFAT pathway, appears to promote the expression of genes involved in lipid and glucose metabolism which influence muscle metabolic pathways and the metabolic substrates used for energy production (Long et al., 2007). This is particularly important when the importance of muscle in terms of lipid and carbohydrate metabolism, and as an end-organ

of insulin action, is considered: early alteration in the development of muscle metabolic pathways may have long-term implications with a potential increase in the risk of development of type 2 diabetes, cardiovascular disease, or obesity (Barnes and Ozanne, 2011; Bauman, 2009).

A reduction in innervation through the use of botulinum toxin is also likely to adversely affect development of the motor end-plate, where expression of immature calcium channels has been noted following denervation (Hughes et al., 2006). This may be particularly important in children with CP, where the neuromuscular junction has been shown to be disorganized with an association between the dysmorphic changes seen and the severity of the motor deficit (Theroux et al., 2005). A reduction in innervation may also delay or prevent the change from polyneuronal innervation to mononeuronal innervation, which is highly dependent on innervation (Brown et al., 1982). This could have implications for the development of selective motor control.

It is important to remember that skeletal muscle is not just a highly plastic organ which provides the force needed for movement: it is also an essential link in the feedback loop which allows structural development of central nervous system networks and topography which is essential for motor development. This has been discussed earlier in relation to spinal cord networks, where refinement of the terminals of the afferent fibres from skeletal muscle which is related to movement may contribute to the reduction in the threshold for stretch reflex and the reduction in co-contraction of antagonist and agonist muscles seen with typical motor development (Gibson and Clowry, 1999). Skeletal muscle activity also appears to contribute, however, to development of sensory and motor representation in the cerebral cortex (Chakrabarty and Martin, 2000, Martin et al., 2004, 2005). In the adult animal, a reduction of limb use through immobilization may adversely affect both the cortical sensory map (Coq and Xervi, 1999) and the cortical motor map (Liepert et al., 1995).

Skeletal muscle immobilization or denervation in infancy may have similar adverse effects. Hoon et al. (2009) used diffusion tensor imaging to assess the corticospinal tract and posterior thalamocortical radiation of children with CP born preterm, and described abnormalities of both pathways. They noted, however, that the alteration in the posterior thalamocortical radiation was correlated more closely with reduced contralateral touch threshold, proprioception and motor severity than was the case with the changes in the corticospinal tract. Marin-Padilla (1997) discussed the input deprivation and output isolation of the grey matter in children with CP resulting from axonal lesions in the white matter, which in turn resulted in altered differentiation and maturation in the cortex. The pre-existing motor and sensory deficits in children with CP may potentially be exacerbated by early intervention aimed primarily but unsuccessfully at promoting musculotendinous unit length through a combination of passive stretch, immobilization and denervation of muscle.

On a more positive note, the plasticity of developing muscle and the role of muscle use and movement in CNS development raise exciting potential prospects for intervention. An early focus on enhancing muscle growth and function may benefit both muscle growth and metabolic capacity, and in this way reduce the incidence of musculoskeletal deformity and improve muscle endurance and function. It may also provide a portal through which the development of the central nervous system may be influenced. Early intervention also allows the prospect of ameliorating or preventing the subsequent adaptive changes in muscle due to reduced use and altered loading, and in this way promoting muscle growth and optimizing the outcome of future intervention such as muscle strengthening or surgery to lengthen the musculotendinous unit.

Early intervention programmes in preterm infants have not been shown to improve subsequent motor outcome but evidence in this area is limited (for a review, see Orton et al., 2009). Hadders-Algra (2011) has suggested that early promotion of self-produced motor activity in infants at risk of developmental disorders may improve motor outcome. This may be particularly important in children with CP where the importance of muscle growth and development and its relevance to motor development does not appear to have been emphasized previously. The key to early muscle growth and development appears to be promotion of muscle use and muscle contraction: an early intervention programme for children with CP which specifically focuses on encouraging and facilitating muscle use would have the potential to benefit subsequent muscle growth and motor development. This issue is discussed in Chapter 1. Methods of training that target active stretching

of muscles as part of a task-specific training and exercise programme are described in Chapter 11. Implementation of such a programme would require early identification of children at risk of development of CP and early referral for physiotherapy: it may also require the development of a more specific and individually tailored physiotherapeutic approach designed to maximize muscle use in infants and in this way enhance muscle growth and function.

As yet, it is difficult to be other than speculative about other potential options for early intervention. The present focus on reducing inflammation and infection in the perinatal period, and on optimizing nutrition in the postnatal period, also has the potential as noted above to benefit muscle growth and to promote the development of the contractile component of muscle rather than the connective tissue framework. We do not as yet have a way of supporting or enhancing the input of the corticospinal tract to the developing spinal cord networks and in this way enhancing muscle growth and development: intervention such as transcortical magnetic stimulation may have a role in the future but this would require considerable further investigation. In a similar manner, a greater understanding of the role of local and systemic growth factors may allow manipulation of muscle growth and development in the early postnatal period and in infancy. Given the many factors involved in muscle growth, an approach which combines facilitation and encouragement of muscle use, optimization of muscle innervation patterns and nutritional support, together with the use of muscle growth factors, may be the most effective approach. This is however speculative: in the meantime early promotion and encouragement of muscle use, together with caution about the early use of muscle immobilization, passive stretching and denervation, is recommended for infants and young children with CP.

## Conclusion

The development of muscle deformity in children with CP appears to reflect an impairment of muscle growth due to a number of interacting factors. The predominant factor appears to be reduced or impaired development of muscle innervation which is likely to be related to the impaired development of spinal cord intrinsic networks, as well as afferent and efferent connections, due to a reduction in input from the corticospinal tract. The changes noted in the muscles of older children with CP appear to be related to a combination of impaired growth and altered adaptation, which it may be possible to prevent or at least ameliorate. The present early management of muscle deformity, which includes acute or prolonged muscle stretch and muscle denervation, does not appear to address the factors causing impairment of muscle growth and may contribute further to impaired growth and subsequent altered development of muscle. It may also impair subsequent CNS development which is influenced by muscle activation and movement. A shift in focus to the early promotion of muscle use may be a more effective approach.

Early intervention to muscle in CP has the potential to enhance muscle growth with a consequent potential benefit in motor development and in long-term mobility and metabolic function, but exploration and development of this concept will require research and close communication and interaction between clinicians and basic scientists. In the meantime, the evidence available would suggest a focus on the promotion of early muscle use and the avoidance of disuse through the development of specific physiotherapy programmes together with early identification and referral of children at risk of CP. Skeletal muscle in children with CP remains plastic: the challenge we face is to consider how we may use this adaptability to enhance muscle growth and function and in this way prevent or reduce deformity and enhance the present and future function of the child with CP.

# References

Agbulut, O., Noirez, P., Beaumont, F., Butler-Browne, G., 2003. Myosin heavy chain isoforms in postnatal muscle development of mice. Biol. Cell 95, 399–406.

Atherton, P.J., Rennie, M.J., 2009. It's no go for protein when it's all go. J. Physiol. 587 (7), 1373–1374.

Atherton, P.J., Szewczyk, N.J., Selby, A., Rankin, D., Hillier, K., Smith, K., et al., 2009. Cyclic stretch reduces myofibrillar protein synthesis despite increases in FAK and anabolic signalling in L6 cells. J. Physiol. 587 (14), 3719–3727.

Barber, L., Hastings-Ison, T., Baker, R., Barrett, R., Lichtwark, G., 2011. Medial gastrocnemius volume and fascicle length in children aged 2 to 5 years with cerebral palsy. Dev. Med. Child. Neurol. 53, 543–548.

Barnes, S.K., Ozanne, S.E., 2011. Pathways linking the early environment to long-term health and lifespan. Prog. Biophys. Mol. Biol. 106, 323–336.

Barrett, R.S., Lichtwark, G.A., 2010. Gross muscle morphology and structure in spastic cerebral palsy: a systematic review. Dev. Med. Child Neurol. 52, 794–804.

Bauman, W.A., 2009. The potential metabolic consequences of cerebral palsy: inferences from the general population and persons with spinal cord injury. Dev. Med. Child Neurol. 51 (Suppl. 4), 64–78.

Bedi, K.S., Birzgalis, A.R., Mahon, M., Smart, J.L., Wareham, A.C., 1982. Early life undernutrition in rats. Br. J. Nutr. 47, 417–431.

Benard, M.R., Harlaar, J., Becher, J.G., Huijing, P.A., Jaspers, R.T., 2011. Effects of growth on geometry of gastrocnemius muscle in children: a three-dimensional ultrasound analysis. J. Anat. 219, 388–402.

Berger, W., 1998. Characteristics of locomotor control in children with cerebral palsy. Neurosci. Biobehav. Rev. 22, 579–582.

Berger, W., Quintern, J., Dietz, V., 1982. Pathophysiology of gait in children with cerebral palsy. Electroenceph. Clin Neurophysiol. 53, 538–548.

Biering-Sorensen, B., Kristensen, I.B., Kjaer, M., Biering-Sorensen, F., 2009. Muscle after spinal cord injury. Muscle Nerve 40, 499–519.

Bigard, X., Sanchez, H., Zoll, J., 2000. Calcineurin co-regulates contractile and metabolic components of slow muscle phenotype. J. Biol. Chem. 275, 19653–19660.

Binzoni, T., Bianchi, S., Hanquinet, S., Kaelin, A., Sayegh, Y., Dumont, M., et al., 2001. Human gastrocnemius medialis pennation angle as a function of age: from newborn to the elderly. J. Physiol. Anthropol. 20, 293–298.

Biressi, S., Molinaro, M., Cossu, G., 2007. Cellular heterogeneity during vertebrate skeletal muscle development. Dev. Biol. 308, 281–293.

Blackmore, A.M., Boettcher-Hunt, E., Jordan, M., Chan, M.D., 2007. A systematic review of the effects of casting on equinus in children with cerebral palsy. Dev. Med. Child Neurol. 49, 781–790.

Brameld, J.M., Buttery, P.J., Dawson, J.M., Harper, J.M.M., 1998. Nutritional and hormonal control of skeletal-muscle cell growth and differentiation. Proc. Nutr. Soc. 57, 207–217.

Brown, M.C., Hopkins, W.G., Keynes, R.J., 1982. Short and long-term effects of paralysis on the motor innervation of two different neonatal mouse muscles. J. Physiol. 329, 439–450.

Butler, C., Darrah, J., 2001. Effects of neurodevelopmental treatment (NDT) for cerebral palsy: an AACPDM evidence report. Dev. Med. Child Neurol. 43, 778–790.

Chakrabarty, S., Martin, J.H., 2000. Postnatal development of the motor representation in primary motor cortex. J. Neurophysiol. 84, 2582–2594.

Chakrabarty, S., Martin, J.H., 2010. Postnatal development of a segmental switch enables corticospinal tract transmission to spinal forelimb motor circuits. J. Neurosci. 30, 2277–2288.

Clemmons, D.R., 2009. Role of IGF-I in skeletal muscle mass maintenance. Trends Endocrinol. Metabol. 20, 349–356.

Clowry, G., 2007. The dependence of spinal cord development on corticospinal input and its significance in understanding and treating spastic cerebral palsy. Neurosci. Behav. Rev. 31, 1114–1124.

Clowry, G.J., Walker, L., Davies, P., 2006. The effects of botulinum toxin induced muscle paresis during a critical period upon muscle and spinal cord development in the rat. Exp. Neurol. 202, 456–469.

Coq, J.O., Xervi, C., 1999. Tactile impoverishment and sensorimotor restriction deteriorate the forepaw cutaneous map in the primary somatosensory cortex of adult rats. Exp. Brain. Res. 129, 518–531.

Downing, A.L., Ganley, K.J., Fay, D.R., Abbas, J.J., 2009. Temporal characteristics of lower extremity moment generation in children with cerebral palsy. Muscle Nerve 39, 800–809.

Drummond, M.J., Dreyer, H.C., Fry, C.S., Glynn, E.L., Rasmussen, B.B., 2009. Nutritional and contractile regulation of human skeletal muscle protein synthesis and mTORC1 signaling. J. Appl. Physiol. 106, 1374–1384.

Eken, T., Elder, G.C.B., Lamo, T., 2008. Development of tonic firing behaviour in rat soleus muscle. J. Neurophysiol. 99, 1899–1905.

Forssberg, H., 1985. Ontogeny of human locomotor control I: infant stepping, supported locomotion and transition to independent locomotion. Exp. Brain Res. 57, 480–493.

Fowles, J.R., MacDougall, J.D., Tarnopolsky, M.A., Sale, D.G., Roy, B.D., Yarasheski, K.E., 2000. The effects of acute passive stretch on muscle protein synthesis in humans. Can. J. Appl. Physiol. 25, 165–180.

Fry, N.R., Gough, M., Shortland, A.P., 2004. Three-dimensional realisation of muscle morphology and architecture using ultrasound. Gait Posture 20, 177–182.

Fujita, S., Dreyer, H.C., Drummond, M.J., Glynn, E.L., Cadenas, J.G., Yoshizawa, F., et al., 2007. Nutrient signaling in the regulation of human muscle protein synthesis. J. Physiol. 582 (2), 813–823.

Gagliano, N., Pelillo, F., Chiriva-Internati, M., Picciolini, O., Costa, F., Schutt, R.C., et al., 2009. Expression profiling of genes involved in collagen turnover in tendons from cerebral palsy patients. Conn. Tiss. Res. 50, 203–208.

Gericke, T., 2006. Postural management for children with cerebral palsy: consensus statement. Dev. Med. Child Neurol. 48, 244.

Gibson, C.L., Clowry, G.J., 1999. Retraction of muscle afferents from the rat ventral horn during development. NeuroReport 10, 231–235.

Glover, E.I., Phillips, S.M., Oates, B.R., Tang, J.E., Tarnopolsky, M.A., Selby, A., et al., 2008. Immobilization induces anabolic resistance in human myofibrillar protein synthesis with low and high dose amino acid infusion. J. Physiol. 586 (24), 6049–6061.

Gomes, A.R., Soares, A.G., Peviani, S., Nascimento, R.B., Moriscot, A.S., Salvini, T.F., 2006. The effect of 30 minutes of passive stretch on the myogenic differentiation, myostatin, and atrogin-1 gene expressions. Arch. Phys. Med. Rehabil. 87, 241–246.

Gough, M., 2009. Does botulinum toxin prevent or promote deformity in children with cerebral palsy? Dev. Med. Child. Neurol. 51, 89–90. (Commentary).

Gough, M., Fairhurst, C., Shortland, A.P., 2005. Botulinum toxin and cerebral palsy: time for reflection? Dev. Med. Child Neurol. 47, 709–712. (Review).

Gramsbergen, A., Ijkema-Paasen, J., Nikkels, P.G.J., Hadders-Algra, M., 1997. Regression of polyneuronal innervation in the human psoas muscle. Early Hum. Dev. 49, 49–61.

Gundersen, K., 2011. Excitation-transcription coupling in skeletal muscle: the molecular pathways of exercise. Biol. Rev. Camb. Philos. Soc. 86, 564–600.

Hadders-Algra, M., 2011. Challenges and limitations in early intervention. Dev. Med. Child Neurol. 53 (Suppl. 4), 52–55.

Hay, W.W., Thureen, P., 2010. Protein for preterm infants: how much is needed? How much is enough? How much is too much? Pediatr. Neonatol. 51, 198–207.

Heinen, F., Desloovere, K., Schroeder, A.S., et al., 2010. The updated European Consensus 2009 on the use of Botulinum toxin for children with cerebral palsy. Eur. J. Paediatr. Neurol. 14, 45–66.

Henneman, E., Olson, C.B., 1965. Relations between structure and function in the design of skeletal muscles. J. Neurophysiol., 581–598.

Hood, D.A., 2001. Invited review: contractile activity-induced mitochondrial biogenesis in skeletal muscle. J. Appl. Physiol. 90, 1137–1157.

Hoon, A.H., Stashinko, E.E., Nagae, L.M., et al., 2009. Sensory and motor deficits in children with cerebral palsy born preterm correlate with diffusion tensor imaging abnormalities in thalamocortical pathways. Dev. Med. Child. Neurol. 51, 697–704.

Hughes, B.W., Kusner, L.L., Kaminski, H.J., 2006. Molecular architecture of the neuromuscular junction. Muscle Nerve 33, 445–461.

Ijkema-Paassen, I., Gramsbergen, A., 2005. Development of postural muscles and their innervation. Neural Plast. 12, 141–151.

Johnson, D.L., Miller, F., Subramanian, P., Modlesky, C.M., 2009. Adipose tissue infiltration of skeletal muscle in children with cerebral palsy. J. Pediatr. 154, 715–720.

Katalinic, O.M., Harvey, L.A., Herbert, R.D., Moseley, A.M., Lannin, N.A., Schurr, K., 2010. Stretch for the treatment and prevention of contractures (Review). Cochrane Database Syst. Rev. (9).

Kim, H.M., Galatz, L.M., Das, R., Patel, N., Thomopoulos, S., 2009. Recovery potential after postnatal shoulder paralysis: an animal model of neonatal brachial plexus palsy. J. Bone Joint Surg. Am. 91, 879–891.

Kim, H.M., Galatz, L.M., Das, R., Patel, N., Thomopoulos, S., 2010. Musculoskeletal deformities secondary to neurotomy of the superior trunk of the brachial plexus in neonatal mice. J. Orthop. Res. 28, 1391–1398.

Kollias, H.D., McDermott, J.C., 2008. Transforming growth factor-β and myostatin signaling in skeletal muscle. J. Appl. Physiol. 104, 579–587.

Leon, R.N., Griffiths, J., 2005. Comparing the function of the corticospinal system in different species: organizational differences for motor specialization? Muscle Nerve 32, 261–279.

Lexell, J., Sjostrom, M., Nordlund, A.-S., Taylor, C.C., 1992. Growth and development of human muscle: a quantitative morphological study of whole vastus lateralis from childhood to adult age. Muscle Nerve 15, 404–409.

Lieber, R.L., Steinman, S., Barash, I.A., Chambers, H., 2004. Structural and functional changes in spastic skeletal muscle. Muscle Nerve 29, 615–627.

Liepert, J., Tegenthoff, M., Malin, J.P., 1995. Changes of cortical motor area size during immobilization. Electroenceph. Clin. Neurol. 97, 382–386.

Long, Y.C., Glund, S., Garcia-Roves, P.M., Zierath, J.R., 2007. Calcineurin regulates skeletal muscle metabolism via coordinated changes in gene expression. J. Biol. Chem. 282, 1607–1614.

Marin-Padilla, M., 1997. Developmental neuropathology and impact of perinatal brain damage. II: white matter lesions of the neocortex. J. Neuropathol. Exp. Neurol. 56, 219–235.

Martin, J.H., 2005. The corticospinal system: from development to motor control. Neuroscientist 11, 161–173.

Martin, J.H., Choy, M., Pullman, S., Meng, Z., 2004. Corticospinal system development depends on motor experience. J. Neurosci. 24, 2122–2132.

Martin, J.H., Engber, D., Meng, Z., 2005. Effect of forelimb use on postnatal development of the forelimb motor representation in primary motor cortex of the cat. J. Neurophysiol. 93, 2822–2831.

Menconi, M.J., Arany, Z.P., Alamdari, N., Aversa, Z., Gonnella, P., O'Neal, P., et al., 2010. Sepsis and glucocorticoids downregulate the expression of the nuclear cofactor PGC-1beta in skeletal muscle. Am.

J. Physiol. Endocrinol. Metab. 299, E533–E543.

Moore, M.J., Rubino, J.J., Holden, M., Adams, R.D., 1971. Biometric analyses of normal skeletal muscle. Acta Neuropath. 19, 51–69.

Moreau, N.G., Teefey, S.A., Damiano, D.L., 2009. In vivo muscle architecture and size of the rectus femoris and vastus lateralis in children and adolescents with cerebral palsy. Dev. Med.. Child Neurol. 51, 800–806.

Morris, C., 2002. A review of the efficacy of lower-limb orthoses used for cerebral palsy. Dev. Med. Child Neurol. 44, 205–211.

Navarrete, R., Vrbova, G., 1993. Activity-dependent interactions between motoneurons and muscles: their role in the development of the motor unit. Prog. Neurobiol. 41, 93–124.

Nikolaou, S., Peterson, E., Kim, A., Wylie, C., Cornwall, R., 2011. Impaired growth of denervated muscle contributes to contracture formation following neonatal brachial plexus injury. J. Bone Joint Surg. Am. 93, 461–470.

Nishimura, T., Oyama, K., Kishioka, Y., Wakamatsu, J., Hattori, A., 2007. Spatiotemporal expression of decorin and myostatin during rat skeletal muscle development. Biochem. Biophys. Res. Comm. 361, 896–902.

Oertel, G., 1988. Morphometric analysis of normal skeletal muscles in infancy, childhood and adolescence: an autopsy study. J. Neurol. Sci. 88, 303–313.

Ohata, K., Tsuboyama, T., Haruta, T., Ichihashi, N., Kato, T., Nakamura, T., 2008. Relation between muscle thickness, spasticity, and activity limitations in children and adolescents with cerebral palsy. Dev. Med. Child. Neurol. 50, 152–156.

Orton, J., Spittle, S., Doyle, L., Anderson, P., Boyd, R., 2009. Do early intervention programmes improve cognitive and motor outcomes for preterm infants after discharge? A systemic review. Dev. Med. Child. Neurol. 51, 851–859.

Otto, A., Patel, K., 2010. Signalling and the control of skeletal muscle size. Exp. Cell Res. 316, 3059–3066.

O'Sullivan, M.C., Eyre, J.A., Miller, S., 1991. Radiation of phasic stretch reflex in biceps brachii to muscles

of the arm in man and its restriction during dvelopment. J. Physiol. 439, 529–543.

Pette, D., Staron, R.S., 2000. Myosin isoforms, muscle fibre types, and transitions. Microsc. Res. Tech. 50, 500–509.

Pin, T., Dyke, P., Chan, M., 2006. The effectiveness of passive stretching in children with cerebral palsy. Dev. Med. Child Neurol. 48, 855–862.

Ponten, E., Lindstrom, M., Kadi, F., 2008. Higher amount of MyHC IIX in a wrist flexor in tetraplegic compared to hemiplegic cerebral palsy. J. Neurol. Sci. 266, 51–56.

Prechtl, H.F.R., 1993. Principles of early motor development in the human. In: Kalverboer, A.F., Hopkins, B., Gueze, R. (Eds.), Motor Development in Early and Later Childhood: Longitudinal Approaches. Cambridge University Press, pp. 35–50.

Purslow, P.P., 2002. The structure and functional significance of variations in the connective tissue within muscle. Comp. Biochem. Physiol. Part A 133, 947–966.

Rose, J., McGill, K.C., 2005. Neuromuscular activation and motor-unit firing characteristics in cerebral palsy. Dev. Med. Child Neurol. 47, 329–336.

Schiaffino, S., Sandri, M., Murgia, M., 2007. Activity-dependent signaling pathways controlling muscle diversity and plasticity. Physiology 22, 269–278.

Schloon, H., Schlottmann, J., Lenard, H.G., Goebel, H.H., 1979. The development of skeletal muscles in premature infants I: fibre size and histochemical differentiation. Eur. J. Pediatr. 131, 49–60.

Schmidt, I., Herpin, P., 1997. Postnatal changes in mitochondrial protein mass and respiration in skeletal muscle from the newborn pig. Comp. Biochem. Physiol. 118B, 639–647.

Schroeder, A.S., Ertl-Wagner, B., Britsch, S., et al., 2009. Muscle biopsy substantiates long-term MRI alterations one year after a single dose of botulinum toxin injected into the lateral gastrocnemius muscle of healthy volunteers. Mov. Disord. 24, 1494–1503.

Schroeder, A.S., Koerte, I., Berweck, S., Ertl-Wagner, B., Heinen, F., 2010.

How doctors think – and treat with botulinum toxin. Dev. Med. Child Neurol. 52, 875–876. (letter).

Serrano, A.L., Munoz-Canoves, P., 2010. Regulation and dysregulation of fibrosis in skeletal muscle. Exp. Cell Res. 316, 3050–3058.

Smith, L.R., Pontén, E., Hedström, Y., Ward, S.R., Chambers, H.G., Subramaniam, S., et al., 2009. Novel transcriptional profile in wrist muscles from cerebral palsy patients. BMC Med. Genomics 2, 44.

Smith, L.R., Lee, K.S., Ward, S.R., Chambers, H.G., Lieber, R.L., 2011. Hamstring contractures in children with spastic cerebral palsy result from a stiffer ECM and increased in vivo sarcomere length. J. Physiol. 589, 2625–2639.

Stackhouse, S.K., Binder-Macleod, S.A., Lee, S.C.K., 2005. Voluntary muscle activation, contractile properties, and fatigability in children with and without cerebral palsy. Muscle Nerve 31, 594–601.

Suryawan, A., Orellana, R.A., Nguyen, H.V., Jeyapalan, A.S., Fleming, J.R., Davis, T.A., 2007. Activation by insulin and amino acids of signaling components leading to translation initiation in skeletal muscle of neonatal pigs is developmentally regulated. Am. J. Physiol. Endocrinol. Metab. 293, E1597–E1605.

Sutherland, D.H., Olshen, R.A., Biden, E.N., Wyatt, M.P., 1988. The development of mature walking. Clinics in Developmental Medicine No. 104/105. MacKeith Press, Oxford, pp. 154–162.

Tedroff, K., Granath, F., Forssberg, H., Haglund-Akerling, Y., 2009. Long-term effects of botulinum toxin A in children with cerebral palsy. Dev. Med. Child Neurol. 51, 120–127.

Theroux, M.C., Oberman, K.G., Lahaye, J., et al., 2005. Dysmorphic neuromuscular junctions associated with motor ability in cerebral palsy. Muscle Nerve 32, 626–632.

Thorn, S.R., Regnault, T.R.H., Brown, L.D., Rozance, P.J., Keng, J., Roper, M., et al., 2009. Intrauterine growth restriction increases fetal gluconeogenic capacity and reduces messenger ribonucleic acid translation initiation and nutrient sensing in fetal liver and skeletal muscle. Endocrinologica 150, 3021–3030.

Urso, M.L., Scrimgeour, A.G., Chen, Y.W., Thompson, P.D., Clarkson, P.M., 2006. Analysis of human skeletal muscle after 48 h immobilization reveals alteration in mRNA and protein for extracellular matrix components. J. Appl. Physiol. 101, 1136–1148.

Van Dyke, J., Bain, J.L.W., Riley, D.A., 2012. Preserving sarcomere number after tenotomy requires stretch and contraction. Muscle Nerve 45, 367–375.

Velders, M., Legerlotz, K., Falconer, S., et al., 2008. Effect of botulinum toxin A-induced paralysis and exercise training on mechanosensing and signalling gene expression in juvenile rat gastrocnemius muscle. Exp. Physiol. 93, 1273–1283.

Vinay, L., Brocard, F., Clarac, F., Norreel, J.C., Pearlstein, E., Pflieger, J.F., 2002. Development of posture and locomotion: an interplay of endogenously generated activities and neurotrophic actions of descending pathways. Brain Res. Rev. 40, 118–129.

Westerblad, H., Bruton, J.D., Katz, A., 2010. Skeletal muscle: energy metabolism, fibre types, fatigue and adaptability. Experim. Cell Res. 316, 3093–3099.

White, R.B., Bierinx, A.-S., Gnocchi, V.F., Zammit, P.S., 2010. Dynamics of muscle fibre growth during postnatal mouse development. BMC Dev. Biol. 10, 21.

Yao, K.T., Chang, M.-H., 1993. Growth and body composition of preterm, small-for-gestational age infants at a postmenstrual age of 37–40 weeks. Early Hum. Dev. 33, 117–131.

Zhu, J., Li, Y., Shen, W., Qiao, C., Ambrosio, F., Lavasani, M., et al., 2007. Relationships between transforming growth factor-beta1, myostatin and decorin: implications for skeletal muscle fibrosis. J. Biol. Chem. 282, 25852–25863.

# PART 4

## Early and Active Intervention to Optimize Growth, Development and Functional Motor Performance

# Early diagnosis and prognosis in cerebral palsy

8

Giovanni Cioni, Vittorio Belmonti, Christa Einspieler

The quality of care for the infants born with an extremely low birth weight, or with other conditions of high neurological risk, has achieved extraordinary progress in the last decades. Survival and quality of life have considerably increased for these children, but they still remain at risk for neurological damage, caused by perinatal infections, hypoxic-ischaemic damage, haemorrhagic insult, or by a combination of these factors. Negative outcome includes cerebral palsy (CP), intellectual disability, perceptual and sensory disorders, behavioural disorders and other.

The incidence of CP in particular has been considered the marker of the quality of neonatal care and utilized as an outcome measure in many studies, although cognitive and behavioural problems are by far more common. Those more subtle disorders, which are important for participation and quality of life of the children, are difficult to diagnose in the first weeks or months of life. Conversely, it is largely agreed that an early diagnosis of CP should be possible, or better, should be necessary even in the neonatal period, for a number of reasons.

Although all infants discharged by a neonatal intensive care unit (NICU) and potentially at risk for a neurodevelopmental disorder should enter a follow-up programme, children diagnosed as carrying a risk of CP require medical and social resources that are limited in several countries. Furthermore, an early diagnosis of CP is necessary in order to start early intervention, to tailor it according to the infant's needs, to modify positively the natural history of her/his condition, and to evaluate the results of the intervention. Randomization of the subjects for early interventional trials, based on neuroprotective drugs, environmental changes, etc., requires detailed prognostic data.

Finally, another major reason for all the efforts made on early diagnosis of CP deals with information in regard to the parents, who obviously ask about the neurodevelopmental outcome of their infants, and their questions are: 'will he/she be able to walk?' or 'to take and use an object?'

Although prognostic hints for a CP diagnosis are needed in the neonatal period, many textbooks and manuals still postpone the possibility of a diagnosis of CP to the end of a so-called 'silent period', lasting some weeks or even, for mild forms of CP, some months after term age.

The possibility that neonatal neuroimaging can enable recognition of brain pathology that may lead to a diagnosis of CP is today largely accepted in terms of the type and timing of the brain lesions typical of the different forms of CP (Krägeloh-Mann, 2004), although it is questioned by some authors (O'Shea et al., 1998). A recent paper by de Vries et al. (2011) has unravelled the 'myth' that CP cannot be predicted by neonatal neuroimaging, when this technique is correctly applied. The authors show evidence from a number of papers that the non-ambulatory most severe CP can be predicted in the majority of the cases by a combination of sequential brain US and by MRI carried out at term age. Additional useful indices can be obtained by assessing the myelination of the PLIC (posterior limb of internal capsule) and diffusion-weighted imaging techniques. Moreover, there are interesting research directions that may further improve, by sophisticated MRI techniques, the prognostic value of neonatal neuroimaging in the less severe forms of CP.

However, brain MRI in most centres requires the transfer of the infant from the NICU. In addition, the equipment is extremely expensive and therefore not affordable for all centers and countries.

It has also to be remarked that even the most advanced neuroimaging techniques can only show structural changes of the brain and does not provide information on the functional status of the nervous system. For this and other reasons, a clinical assessment is always necessary.

# Techniques for the clinical assessment of the neonatal nervous system

Neonatal neurological examination is generally carried out through traditional neurological methods, largely based on muscle tone and neonatal reflexes. However, it is now widely recognized that the human nervous system can express many complex and rapidly changing functions from as early as the first weeks of gestation. Fetuses and newborns are complex organisms producing a great deal of endogenously generated behaviours.

Some of the standard neurological examination methods, though standing as milestones of modern infant neurology, are still influenced by considerations drawn from adult neurology and experiments on animal models. For instance, Saint-Anne Dargassies (1977) developed a pioneering examination protocol based on the evaluation of active and passive tone. Other methods were then proposed in the following decades, including items for muscle tone, postural-motor milestones and, in some cases, behavioural aspects.

The neurological examination protocol proposed in the same period by Prechtl (1977) (not to be confused with the method the same author has later proposed), has been standardized and validated only for the examination of infants at term. It includes the extremely important concept of behavioural states, but many of its items are still based on muscle tone and responses integrated at a low level in the CNS. Moreover, it is rather time-consuming and cannot be applied to preterm infants.

The Neonatal Behavioural Assessment Scale (NBAS) is a technique developed by Brazelton (Brazelton and Nugent, 1995) for examining the behaviour of term infants during the first couple of months of age. Its conceptual basis is founded on the assumption that the newborn has active and specific responses to environmental stimulations, rather than passive behaviour. On the basis of NBAS, Als (1984) standardized a behavioural scale for preterm infants, the Assessment of Preterm Infant Behaviour (APIB), thought to be employed in neonatal intensive care units also for providing and monitoring individualized intervention programmes. These techniques are time-consuming and not easily applicable in clinical settings. Moreover, a high intra-individual day-to-day variability in the responses has been shown for the same test (Sameroff, 1978). Their main applications are in research and early intervention protocols.

Currently, the most recently updated and extensively validated method for the neurological examination of preterm and full-term newborn infants is the Hammersmith Neonatal Neurological Examination (HNNE), first published by Dubowitz and Dubowitz (1981) and updated by Dubowitz et al. (1999). These authors adapted tests drawn from the previous works of Prechtl, Saint-Anne Dargassies and Brazelton, into a simplified and user-friendly pro forma, also including items based on the concepts of Prechtl and co-workers on spontaneous motor activity (see below). The items are organized in six sections: posture and tone; tone patterns; reflexes; movements; abnormal signs; and behaviour. Typical normal and abnormal patterns are extensively described in the manual (Dubowitz et al., 1999) and have proven easily recognizable and clinically useful for diagnosis and prognosis. For research purposes, an optimality score for full-term and preterm newborn infants was also calculated (Mercuri et al., 2003).

On the basis of the neonatal examination, the same authors also developed a protocol for use after the neonatal period in infants up to 24 months of age: the Hammersmith Infant Neurological Examination (HINE) (Dubowitz et al., 1999), divided into three sections: one, non-age-dependent neurological items; a second providing a summary of motor milestones; and a third made of three simple behavioural items. Its prognostic value as to motor outcome has been found high both in preterm infants born before 31 weeks of gestation (Frisone et al., 2002) and in term infants with hypoxic-ischemic encephalopathy (Haataja et al., 2001).

Although both HNNE and HINE have been tested in several clinical and research settings, they also present some limitations. Most items are still correlated with muscle tone and reflexes and the distinction between normal and abnormal patterns may turn out, to some extent, rigid and schematic, hardly comprising the whole complexity of the infant's repertoire. Moreover, while several studies have reported statistically significant correlations between clinical findings, and mid- and long-term outcome, some others have reported a relevant number of false-positive and false-negative results, especially among preterm infants (see Volpe, 2008, for a review of follow-up studies).

# Prechtl's method on the qualitative assessment of general movements

The basic requirements for an ideal method of neurological assessment for newborn infants were outlined by Heinz Prechtl as follows: it had to be non-invasive, non-time-consuming, and highly sensitive to variations of the age-specific functional repertoire (Prechtl, 1990). None of the traditional protocols of neonatal neurological assessment completely matched these criteria. The observation and categorization of all spontaneous movements in the first months of life led Prechtl and his co-workers to the identification of several normal and abnormal motor patterns. Among others, the so-called 'general movements' (GMs) were identified as on-going global movements involving all body parts and appeared particularly suitable for assessment (Prechtl, 1990, 2001). This gave birth to Prechtl's Method on the Qualitative Assessment of General Movements in Preterm, Term and Young Infants (see the published handbook: Einspieler et al., 2004).

Though based on global and qualitative judgement, GM assessment has proven a very sound method. Its validity and reliability have been extensively evaluated in a number of studies, mainly dealing with the prediction of CP (Cioni et al., 2000; Ferrari et al., 2002; Prechtl, 1997), but also with that of minor neurological disorders (Bruggink et al., 2008; Einspieler et al., 2007; Groen et al. 2005), Rett syndrome (Einspieler et al., 2005a,b), cognitive development (Bruggink et al., 2010) and autistic spectrum disorders (Phagava et al., 2008).

Normal GMs involve the whole body in a complex sequence of arm, leg, neck and trunk movements. They wax and wane in intensity, force and speed, and have a gradual beginning and end. Rotations along the axis of the limbs and slight changes in the direction of movement make them fluent and elegant and create the impression of complexity and variability. GMs appear as early as nine to 12 weeks postmenstrual age (PMA) and continue after birth without substantially changing their form until 46 to 49 weeks PMA, irrespective of when birth occurs. At 46 to 49 weeks PMA, a major change in form sets in, being fulfilled around 3 months post-term, when the so-called fidgety movements (FMs) appear (Hadders-Algra and Prechtl, 1992; Prechtl, 1990). From 5 to 6 months post-term, GMs fade out, while new, voluntary motor patterns emerge.

Though complex and variable by definition, GMs can be classified into a limited number of recognizable patterns, related to PMA and either normal or abnormal. Normal GMs are briefly reported in Table 8.1.

As already stated, in the FMs period various other motor patterns gradually emerge and mingle with GMs, thus building up the so-called 'associated motor repertoire', whose richness and age-adequacy have been related to the optimality

**Table 8.1  Description of normal and abnormal general movement patterns**

**Normal GMs**

*From 9 to 49 weeks PMA*

| | |
|---|---|
| Fetal and preterm general movements (GMs) | Similar to writhing movements (see below), but wider and jerkier, especially in the lower limbs |
| Writhing movements (WMs) | Variable amplitude, slow-to-moderate speed, typically ellipsoid limb trajectories lying close to the sagittal plane with superimposed rotations. Mostly expressed around term age (40 weeks PMA) |

*From 46 up to 64 weeks PMA*

| | |
|---|---|
| Fidgety movements (FMs) | Smaller than WMs, moderate average speed with variable acceleration in all directions, migrating through all body parts as an on-going flow of movement. Continual in the awake infant, except during fussing, crying and focused attention. Peak of expression around 3 months post-term (52 weeks PMA) |

**Abnormal GMs**

*Preterm and WMs period*

| | |
|---|---|
| Poor repertoire (PR) | Monotonous sequences, few movement components, repetitive and not so complex as in normal WMs. Fluency may be reduced too, but is usually more spared than complexity and variability |
| Cramped-synchronized (CS) | No complexity, no fluency, no variability: all limb and trunk muscles contract and relax almost simultaneously |
| Chaotic (Ch) | Large amplitude, high jerk and chaotic order without any fluency or smoothness. Rare, often evolving into CS |
| Hypokinesia | No or very few GMs are detectable during several hours (infrequent pattern, mostly seen in the first days after the onset of a severe hypoxic-ischaemic encephalopathy) |

*FMs period*

| | |
|---|---|
| Absent FMs (F−) | FMs are never observed in the whole period |
| Abnormal FMs (AF) | Fidgety-like movements, but amplitude, average speed and jerkiness are exaggerated |

of later motor co-ordination (Bruggink et al., 2008) and cognitive functions (Bruggink et al., 2010).

GMs of infants with cerebral impairment lack complexity, fluency and/or variability. Abnormal GM patterns can be sorted into two groups depending on whether they are observed before or after the onset of FMs, i.e., in the preterm/ writhing movement period or in the FMs period. The description of these patterns is also reported in Table 8.1.

The global visual perception of movement quality (Gestalt perception) has proven a powerful and reliable instrument to recognize normal and abnormal GMs, but only if scorers are properly trained and the technique is carefully applied. A thorough description of the standardized assessment procedure can be found in the GMs handbook (Einspieler et al., 2004). Notably, the standard GM assessment is performed off-line on selected video recordings, but it has also proven reliable (especially in the FMs period) when performed live, as part of the routine neurological examination. The methodology of Prechtl's GM assessment has evolved to today's standardized and highly reliable form through several years. Concerns about its possible biases (e.g., because of poor validation in non-European countries) may still arise (see, for instance, Darsaklis et al., 2011), but they can be overestimated if earlier studies are considered together with newer ones, or if results obtained in different clinical populations (e.g. high-risk and low-risk babies) are mixed-up. Recently, the most predictive features of GMs have been definitely pointed out and their clinical role extensively reviewed, as summarized in the following paragraphs, especially in relation to prediction of CP.

## Absent fidgety movements at 3–5 months is the most sensitive sign for CP prediction

In 1997, Heinz Prechtl and associates carried out the most important study to date on the predictive value of GM assessment, indicating it to be a reliable and valid tool for distinguishing between infants who are at significant risk of developing CP and infants who are not (Prechtl et al., 1997). The findings were based on a longitudinal study on 130 infants who represented the whole spectrum of perinatal brain ultrasound findings. Central to the study were the age-specific FMs, i.e., normal FMs observed at least once between 3 and 5 months post-term age. Ninety-six per cent of the infants with normal FMs ($n = 70$) had a normal neurological outcome. Abnormal quality or total absence of FMs were followed by neurological abnormalities (most of them CP) in 95% of the 60 infants. Specificity and sensitivity of the assessment of FMs (96% and 95%, respectively) were higher than those of cranial ultrasound (83% and 80%, respectively). Since then, various groups have emphasized the significance of FMs for the early prediction of CP. Burger and Louw (2009) reviewed 15 studies on the predictive value of FMs and reported a sensitivity >91% and a specificity >81%. So far, the largest sample recruited in a longitudinal study has been of 903 children, which yielded a sensitivity of 98% and a specificity of 94% (Romeo et al., 2009).

As already mentioned, GM assessment is based on global and qualitative judgement, but has proven highly reliable and consistent, both

inter- and intra-subjectively, especially in the FMs period. Its high level of objectivity has been documented by an inter-scorer agreement ranging from 89% to 93%, and by an average kappa of 0.88, both obtained in a total of 15 studies (Einspieler and Prechtl, 2005; Fjørtoft et al., 2009). Such high values can be achieved after a few days of extensive training (Valentin et al., 2005). A high intra-individual consistency of GM quality was demonstrated by kappa values from 0.90 to 0.96 (Mutlu et al., 2008). Due to the utmost importance of FMs for prognosis, recent research has struggled to provide automated and objective methods for their identification. A computer-based video analysis technique has been recently developed by Adde et al. (2009, 2010), yielding a sensitivity of 85% and a specificity of 88% for CP prediction.

The mere absence of FMs, however, has never been found specific for a particular CP subtype, nor it can predict CP severity. This fact indicates that several neural structures, at least the corticospinal fibres, the basal ganglia and the cerebellum, need to be intact to generate normal FMs. The latter are thought to be a necessary step for an optimal calibration of the sensory-motor system (Prechtl et al., 1997). Interestingly enough, normal FMs are also absent in infants with some genetic disorders. FMs are thus very sensitive for prognosis, while other motor features, combined with the absence of FMs, have proven useful to predict CP type and severity.

## Cramped-synchronized general movements at preterm and term age are a very specific predictive sign for spastic CP

Fetal, preterm and writhing GMs display three patterns of abnormality, among them the so-called cramped-synchronized (CS) GMs. CS GMs appear very rigid and abrupt; all limb and trunk muscles appear to contract almost simultaneously and relax almost simultaneously (Ferrari et al., 1990). If normal GMs are characterized by fluency, complexity and variability, CS GMs lack all these three main features. Observing this pattern consistently over several weeks is highly predictive (98%) for the eventual development of spastic CP (Table 8.2 and Figure 8.1) (Prechtl, 1997). The sooner CS GMs evolve and the longer they last, the

**Table 8.2 Developmental trajectories with a high predictive power for normal development and the development of CP.**

| GMs during preterm age | Writing GMs (at term) | Fidgety GMs (3-5 months) | Neurological outcome | Reference |
|---|---|---|---|---|
| Poor repertoire or normal GMs | Poor repertoire or normal GMs | Normal fidgety movements | Normal | Cioni et al. (1997a, 1997b); Einspieler et al. (2004, 2005a); Ferrari et al. (1990); Hadders-Algra (2004); Prechtl (1990, 1997, 2001); Prechtl et al. (1997) |
| Poor repertoire or cramped-synchronized GMs | Cramped-synchronized GMs | Absence of fidgety movements; abnormal findings in neurological examination | Bilateral spastic CP | Adde et al. (2010); Bruggink et al. (2009); Burger and Louw (2009); Cioni et al. (1997a, 1997b); Einspieler et al. (2004, 2005a); Ferrari et al. (1990, 2002, 2011); Hadders-Algra (2004); Hamer et al. (2011); Prechtl (1990, 2001); Prechtl et al. (1997); Romeo et al. (2009); Snider et al. (2008); Spittle et al. (2008, 2009, 2010) |
| Poor repertoire or cramped-synchronized GMs | Poor repertoire or cramped-synchronized GMs | Absence of fidgety movements and asymmetrical segmental movements; normal or abnormal findings in neurological examination | Unilateral spastic CP | Cioni et al. (2000); Einspieler (2008); Einspieler et al. (2004); Guzzetta et al. (2003, 2010); Romeo et al (2009) |
| Poor repertoire GMs | Poor repertoire GMs, circular arm movements and finger spreading | Absence of fidgety movements, absence of foot-to-foot contact, circular arm movements and finger spreading | Dyskinetic CP | Einspieler et al. (2002, 2004) |

[From Einspieler C, Marschik PB, Prechtl HFR. 2011. Early markers for cerebral palsy. In: Panteliades, C.P. (Ed.), Cerebral Palsy. A Multidisciplinary Approach. Dustri-Verlag, Munich–Orlando.]

more severe the future motor impairment will be (Ferrari et al., 2002). Conversely, a transient CS feature (i.e., observed on one of several longitudinal observations of the same infant), usually does not predict CP (Figure 8.2). Moreover, CS GMs are not very sensitive (may not be present or they may be inconsistent in CP) and do not usually occur in children with non-spastic CP.

## The asymmetry of selective distal movements at 3 months predicts unilateral CP

Children with spastic CP show abnormal GMs during their first weeks of life and have no FMs at 3 to 5 months post-term age, which is also true for unilateral

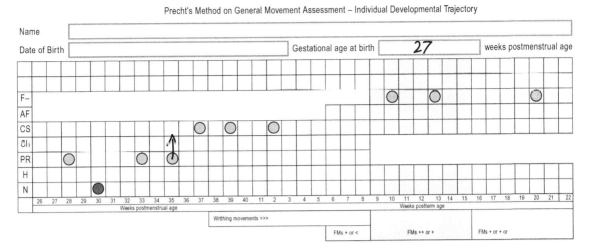

N, normal age-specific GMs; **FMs**, fidgety movements; **H**, hypokinesis (no GMs during the recording); **PR**, poor repertoire of GMs; **Ch**, chaotic GMs; **CS**, cramped-synchronized GMs; **AF**, abnormal fidgety movements; **F−**, absent fidgety movements

**Figure 8.1** • Individual developmental trajectory of an infant born preterm, small for gestational age (SGA), whose outcome was a spastic diplegia. He showed initially PR GMs, transiently improving towards normal GMs, and then worsening until the development of a predominant CS pattern, followed by an absence of FMs.

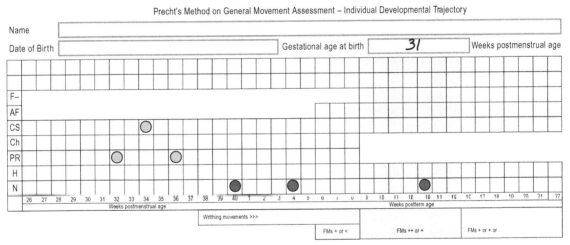

N, normal age-specific GMs; **FMs**, fidgety movements; **H**, hypokinesis (no GMs during the recording); **PR**, poor repertoire of GMs; **Ch**, chaotic GMs; **CS**, cramped-synchronized GMs; **AF**, abnormal fidgety movements; **F−**, absent fidgety movements

**Figure 8.2** • Individual developmental trajectory of an infant born preterm with normal outcome. He showed PR GMs, evolving towards a transient CS pattern, then again to PR GMs, followed by normal writhing and fidgety movements

forms of CP. Incidentally, this finding denies the presence of a 'silent period' in children with unilateral CP (Cioni et al., 2000; Guzzetta et al., 2003). At about 2 to 4 months post-term, the first asymmetries can also be observed (Table 8.2): the so-called 'segmental movements' (i.e., isolated finger and toe movements that are part of the spontaneous motor repertoire) are reduced or even absent in the side contralateral to the lesion, regardless of head position (Cioni et al., 2000; Guzzetta et al., 2003, 2010). Of note is that at this age neurological examination may still yield normal results (see below).

# GM features that can predict dyskinetic CP

Until the second month post-term, infants who will later become dyskinetic show a so-called 'poor repertoire' (PR) pattern of GMs (Einspieler et al., 2002). A monotonous sequence of movement components and a lack of complexity characterize PR GMs (Ferrari et al. 1990). Apart from the PR pattern, which is by no means specific, these infants have been found to move their arms repeatedly and stereotypically in circles and to spread their fingers in an exaggerated manner (Einspieler et al., 2002). Characteristically, these abnormal circular arm movements are present at least until the age of 5 months post-term. They are uni- or bilateral, monotonous, slow forward rotations originating in the shoulder. From 3 to 5 months, FMs and limb movements towards the midline (particularly foot-to-foot contact) are absent (Table 8.2).

# Motor optimality scores and the prediction of CP severity

A semi-quantitative assessment of GM quality can be achieved by applying Prechtl's optimality concept (Prechtl, 1990). A score for optimal or non-optimal performance is given to every movement criterion, such as amplitude, speed, movement character, sequence, range in space, onset and offset of GMs. Two different optimality scoring lists have been reported: the first one for preterm and term age (Ferrari et al., 1990); and the second one covering the whole motor behaviour, not only GMs, of 3 to 5-month-old infants (Einspieler et al., 2004; Fjørtoft et al., 2009). In fact, as previously mentioned, the motor repertoire of infants aged 3 to 5 months consists not only of FMs but also of other motor patterns, e.g., kicking, swiping and wiggling-oscillating arm movements, movements towards the midline, leg lifts, arching and axial rolling (Einspieler, 2008). The motor optimality score at 3 to 5 months is thus the sum of five components: (1) the presence and quality of FMs; (2) the presence and normality of other movement patterns; (3) the presence and normality of postural patterns; (4) the age-adequacy of the concurrent motor repertoire; and (5) the quality of the concurrent motor repertoire. The presence and quality of FMs is always the most important feature and is weighted more than the other components.

GM optimality scores can be used for statistical calculations and comparisons with other measures, especially in research settings. Optimality scoring should never be carried out prior to or together with the global assessment of GMs by means of Gestalt observation, as the latter is easily disrupted by detailed analysis.

A recent study by Bruggink et al. (2009) investigated the predictive value of the motor optimality score at 3 to 5 months in relation to the level of self-mobility of CP children at school age. In this study, the abnormal quality of the concurrent motor repertoire was separately classified as monotonous, jerky and/or cramped. Of the 347 prospectively enrolled participants, 37 developed CP and were classified according to the GMFCS (Palisano et al., 1997). The higher the motor optimality score, the better was the GMFCS level. The positive and the negative predictive values of the optimality score (cutoff = 9) for the outcome (either levels I–II or levels III–V) were both around 70%. The various single features of the motor repertoire included (1) a cramped movement character, (2) a reduced age-adequate motor repertoire, (3) monotonous kicking, and, obviously, (4) the absence of FMs, and were all associated with lower levels of self-mobility.

# Integrating GM assessment with traditional neurological examination and neuroimaging techniques

GM assessment may be carried out as an isolated means of observation (for research purposes, serial checks, or when the infant cannot be otherwise evaluated), but is more often part of a comprehensive assessment protocol. As indicated in the introduction of this chapter, irrespective of their clinical properties, the traditional neurological examination and the assessment of GMs have different conceptual backgrounds. The former invariably consists of a list of individual items, each of which is separately scored and aims to evaluate a particular 'function' or structure of the nervous system. Most of the items are usually based on muscle tone, reflex reactions, postural patterns, single 'bad signs' and motor milestones. By contrast, GM assessment is a global, simultaneous appreciation of movement quality, which cannot be further distinguished into any individual 'components', at least not during the same session (detailed analysis and the assessment of isolated distal movements must take place after the GM pattern has been determined). GMs are more related to the general well-being of the central nervous system than any other single behavioural feature, and have been recognized as the most prominent and consistent age-specific motor behaviour shown by young infants (Prechtl, 1990, 1997). On the other hand, they still provide little information on the anatomical structures involved in pathological processes. In summary, while traditional neurological items can be seen in tighter relationship with brain *impairment* (what the child cannot do), GMs are more sensitive to the age-specific brain *function* (Palmer, 2004).

The integration of GM assessment with traditional neurological examination is particularly useful for distinguishing unilateral from bilateral CP. In an Italy-wide multicentre study (Romeo et al., 2009), 13 of 903 preterm infants were eventually diagnosed with unilateral CP. Eleven of them had shown no FMs, which is remarkable since nine of them had had only a persistent flare on the brain ultrasound with no signs of unilateral damage. Surprisingly, the HINE scores of all but one infant were within the normal range. By contrast, most of the infants who later developed bilateral CP had abnormal HINE scores. These results also lead to the important conclusion that a 3- to 4-month-old infant with a normal neurological score but an absence of FMs and asymmetric segmental movements is at a high risk of developing unilateral CP (Einspieler, 2008).

Another important tool for the early diagnosis of brain impairment is neonatal MRI. So far, only few studies have addressed the relationship between specific MRI findings and GM patterns. In very preterm infants, both white matter lesions (Spittle et al., 2009) and a reduced cerebellar diameter, but not grey matter abnormalities, were associated with absent FMs (Spittle et al., 2010). In infants born at term, however, the severity of the injury to the central grey matter and basal ganglia correlated

with a lack of FMs (Ferrari et al., 2011). In the latter study, CS GMs were highly specific for CP (100%), while MRI was by far more sensitive (100%). This high sensitivity of MRI abnormalities may sometimes be misleading for diagnosis, for instance in the case of tiny focal lesions: about half of neonatal cerebral infarctions are known not to develop into CP (Wu et al., 2005). Definite GM abnormalities (especially absent FMs and CS GMs), have on the contrary a very high positive predictive value, which means that CP will very likely follow. Again, the integration of different approaches, born with different purposes and from distant professional areas, is the best way of obtaining comprehensive information on the child's actual well-being and future development.

## Conclusion

The methodological breakthrough of the GM assessment, which is non-intrusive, easy to acquire and cost-effective, lies in its predictive value for the development of neurological deficits, in particular CP, at a much earlier age than before. Recognition of abnormal GMs can help to improve earlier detection of CP if this technique can be successfully incorporated into follow-up programmes and developmental surveillance (Palmer, 2004), combining it with neuroimaging (especially MRI) and neurological assessment. The great advantage of detecting an increased risk of CP at such an early stage consists in the possibility of intervention long before the emergence of pathological and adaptive features. The consistent presence of cramped-synchronized GMs, and even more so the absence of FMs, puts an infant at such a high risk of CP that early physiotherapeutic intervention is justified. It is no less important to identify infants who, despite an increased risk based on their clinical history, have normal GMs and can thus be expected to have a normal neurological outcome. In addition, the design of randomized control studies to test the effectiveness of early physical or other interventions for those infants who had neonatal adverse events and are at risk for neurodevelopmental disorders requires precise criteria for case selection and group allocation. The evaluation of GMs can be an important tool for these studies.

# References

Adde, L., Helbostad, J.L., Jensenius, A.R., Taraldsen, G., Støen, R., 2009. Using computer-based video analysis in the study of fidgety movements. Early Hum. Dev. 85, 541–547.

Adde, L., Helbostad, J.L., Jensenius, A.R., Taraldsen, G., Grunewaldt, K.H., Støen, R., 2010. Early prediction of cerebral palsy by computer-based video analysis of general movements: a feasibility study. Dev. Med. Child Neurol. 53, 773–778.

Als, H., 1984. Newborn behavioral assessment. In: Burns, W.J., Lavigne, J.V. (Eds.), Progress in Pediatric Psychology. Grune & Stratton, New York, pp. 1–46.

Brazelton, T.B., Nugent, J.K., 1995. Neonatal Behavioral Assessment, third ed. Mac Keith Press, London.

Bruggink, J.L., Einspieler, C., Butcher, P.R., Van Braeckel, K.N., Prechtl, H.F.R., Bos, A.F., 2008. The quality of the early motor repertoire in preterm infants predicts minor neurologic dysfunction at school age. J. Pediatr. 153, 32–39.

Bruggink, J.L., Cioni, G., Einspieler, C., Maathuis, C.G., Pascale, R., Bos, A.F., 2009. Early motor repertoire is related to level of self-mobility in children with cerebral palsy at school age. Dev. Med. Child Neurol. 51, 878–885.

Bruggink, J.L., Van Braeckel, K.N., Bos, A.F., 2010. The early motor repertoire of children born preterm is associated with intelligence at school age. Pediatrics 125 (6), e1356–e1363.

Burger, M., Louw, Q.A., 2009. The predictive validity of general movements—A systematic review. Eur. J. Paediatr. Neurol. 13, 408–420.

Cioni, G., Ferrari, F., Einspieler, C., Paolicelli, P.B., Barbani, M.T., Prechtl, H.F.R., 1997a. Comparison between observation of spontaneous movements and neurological examination in preterm infants. J. Pediatr. 130, 704–711.

Cioni, G., Prechtl, H.F.R., Ferrari, F., Paolicelli, P.B., Einspieler, C., Roversi, M.F., 1997b. Which better predicts later outcome in full term infants: quality of general movements or neurological examination? Early Hum. Dev. 50, 71–85.

Cioni, G., Bos, A.F., Einspieler, C., et al., 2000. Early neurological signs in preterm infants with unilateral intraparenchymal echodensity. Neuropediatrics 31, 240–251.

Darsaklis, V., Snider, L.M., Majnemer, A., Mazer, B., 2011. Predictive validity of Prechtl's Method on the Qualitative Assessment of General Movements: a systematic review of the evidence. Dev. Med. Child Neurol. 53, 896–906.

de Vries, L.S., van Haastert, I.C., Benders, M.J., Groenendaal, F., 2011. Myth: cerebral palsy cannot be predicted by neonatal brain imaging. Semin. Fetal Neonat. Med. 16, 279–287.

Dubowitz, L.M.S., 1981. The neurological assessment of the preterm and full-term newborn infant. Clinics in developmental medicine, No. 79. London. Heinemann.

Dubowitz, L.M.S., Dubowitz, V., Mercuri, E., 1999. The Neurological Assessment of the Preterm and Fullterm Newborn Infant, second ed. Mac Keith Press, London. (distributed by Cambridge University Press)

Einspieler, C., 2008. Early markers for unilateral spastic cerebral palsy in premature infants. Nature Clin. Pract. Neurol. 4, 186–187.

Einspieler, C., Prechtl, H.F., 2005. Prechtl's assessment of general movements: a diagnostic tool for the functional assessment of the young nervous system. Ment. Retard. Dev. Disabil. Res. Rev. 11, 61–67.

Einspieler, C., Cioni, G., Paolicelli, P.B., et al., 2002. The early markers for later dyskinetic cerebral palsy are different from those for spastic cerebral palsy. Neuropediatrics 33, 73–78.

Einspieler, C., Prechtl, H.F., Bos, A.F., Ferrari, F., Cioni, G., 2004. Prechtl's Method on the Qualitative Assessment of General Movements in Preterm, Term and Young Infants. (incl. CD-ROM). Mac Keith Press, London (distributed by Cambridge University Press).

Einspieler, C., Kerr, A., Prechtl, H.F.R., 2005a. Abnormal general movements in girls with Rett disorder: the first four months of life. Brain Dev. 27, 8–13.

Einspieler, C., Kerr, A.M., Prechtl, H.F.R., 2005b. Is the early development of girls with Rett disorder really normal? Pediatr. Res. 57, 696–700.

Einspieler, C., Marschik, P.B., Milioti, S., Nakajima, Y., Bos, A.F., Prechtl, H.F.R., 2007. Are abnormal fidgety movements an early marker for complex minor neurological dysfunction at puberty? Early Hum. Dev. 83, 521–525.

Einspieler, C., Marschik, P.B., Prechtl, H.F.R., 2011. Early markers for cerebral palsy. In: Panteliades, C.P. (Ed.), Cerebral Palsy. A Multidisciplinary Approach. Dustri-Verlag, Munich–Orlando.

Ferrari, F., Cioni, G., Prechtl, H.F.R., 1990. Qualitative changes of general movements in preterm infants with brain lesions. Early Hum. Dev. 23, 193–233.

Ferrari, F., Cioni, G., Einspieler, C., Roversi, M.F., Bos, A.F., Paolicelli, P.B., 2002. Cramped synchronised general movements in preterm infants as an early marker for cerebral palsy. Arch. Pediatr. Adolesc. Med. 156, 460–467.

Ferrari, F., Todeschini, A., Guidotti, I., et al., 2011. General movements in full-term infants with perinatal asphyxia are related to basal ganglia and thalamic lesions. J. Pediatr. 158, 904–911.

Fjørtoft, T., Einspieler, C., Adde, L., Strand, L.I., 2009. Inter-observer reliability of the 'Assessment of Motor Repertoire—3 to 5 Months' based on video recordings of infants. Early Hum. Dev. 85, 297–302.

Frisone, M.F., Mercuri, E., Laroche, S., Foglia, C., Maalouf, E.F., Haataja, L., et al., 2002. Prognostic value of the neurologic optimality score at 9 and 18 months in preterm infants born before 31 weeks' gestation. J. Pediatr. 140, 57–60.

Groen, S.E., de Blécourt, A.C., Postema, K., Hadders-Algra, M., 2005. General movements in early infancy predict neuromotor development at 9 to 12 years of age. Dev. Med. Child Neurol. 47, 731–738.

Guzzetta, A., Mercuri, E., Rapisardi, G., et al., 2003. General movements detect early signs of hemiplegia in term infants with neonatal cerebral infarction. Neuropediatrics 34, 61–66.

Guzzetta, A., Pizzardi, A., Belmonti, V., Boldrini, A., Carotenuto, M., D'Acunto, G., et al., 2010. Hand movements at 3 months predict later hemiplegia in term infants with neonatal cerebral infarction. Dev. Med. Child Neurol. 52, 767–772.

Haataja, L., Mercuri, E., Guzzetta, A., Rutherford, M., Counsel, l.S., Frisone, F.M., et al., 2001. Neurologic examination in infants with hypoxic-ischemic encephalopathy at age 9 to 14 months: use of optimality scores and correlation with magnetic resonance imaging findings. J. Pediatr. 138, 332–337.

Hadders-Algra, M., 2004. General movements: a window for early identification of children at high risk for developmental disorders. J. Pediatr. (Suppl. 145), S12–S18.

Hadders-Algra, M., Prechtl, H.F.R., 1992. Developmental course of general movements in early infancy. I. Descriptive analysis of change in form. Early Hum. Dev. 28, 201–213.

Hamer, E.G., Bos, A.F., Hadders-Algra, M., 2011. Assessment of specific characteristics of abnormal general movements: does it enhance the prediction of cerebral palsy? Dev. Med. Child Neurol. 53, 751–756.

Krageloh-Mann, I., 2004. Imaging of early brain injury and cortical plasticity. Exp. Neurol. 190 (Suppl. 1), S84–S90. (Review).

Mercuri, E., Guzzetta, A., Laroche, S., Ricci, D., van Haastert, I., Simpson, A., et al., 2003. Neurologic examination of preterm infants at term age: comparison with term infants. J. Pediatr. 142, 647–655.

Mutlu, A., Einspieler, C., Marschik, P.B., Livanelioglu, A., 2008. Intra-individual consistency in the quality of neonatal general movements. Neonatology 93, 213–216.

O'Shea, T.M., Klinepeter, K.L., Dillard, R.G., 1998. Prenatal events and the risk of cerebral palsy in very low birth weight infants. Am. J. Epidemiol. 147, 362–369.

Palisano, R.J., Rosenbaum, P.L., Walter, S., Russell, D.J., Wood, E.P., Galuppi, B.E., 1997. Development and reliability of a system to classify gross motor function in children with cerebral palsy. Dev. Med. Child Neurol. 39, 214–223.

Palmer, F.B., 2004. Strategies for the early diagnosis of cerebral palsy. J. Pediatr. 145, S8–S11.

Phagava, H., Muratori, F., Einspieler, C., et al., 2008. General movements in infants with autism spectrum disorders. Georgian Med. News 156, 100–105.

Prechtl, H.F., 1990. Qualitative changes of spontaneous movements in fetus and preterm infant are a marker of neurological dysfunction. Early Hum. Dev. 23, 151–158.

Prechtl, H.F.R., 1997. State of the art of a new functional assessment of the young nervous system. An early predictor of cerebral palsy. Early Hum. Dev. 50, 1–11.

Prechtl, H.F.R., 2001. General movement assessment as a method of developmental neurology: new paradigms and their consequences. The 1999 Ronnie Mac Keith Lecture. Dev. Med. Child Neurol. 43, 836–842.

Prechtl, H.F., Einspieler, C., Cioni, G., Bos, A.F., Ferrari, F., Sontheimer, D., 1997. An early marker for neurological deficits after perinatal brain lesions. Lancet 349, 1361–1363.

Romeo, D.M., Guzzetta, A., Scoto, M., et al., 2009. Early neurologic assessment in preterm infants: integration of traditional neurological examination and observation of general movements. Eur. J. Paediatr. Neurol. 12, 183–189.

Saint-Anne Dargassies, S., 1977. Neurological Development in the Full-Term and Premature Neonate. Excerpta Medica, New York.

Sameroff, A.J., 1978. Summary and conclusions: the future of newborn assessment. In: Sameroff, A.J. (Ed.), Organization and Stability of Newborn Behavior. Monographs of the Society for Research in Child Development, (5–6): 43 pp. 102–117.

Snider, L.M., Majnemer, A., Mazer, B., Campbell, S., Bos, A.F., 2008. A comparison of the general movements assessment with traditional approaches to newborn and infant assessment: concurrent validity. Early Hum. Dev. 84, 297–303.

Spittle, A.J., Doyle, L.W., Boyd, R.N., 2008. A systematic review of the clinimetric properties of neuromotor assessments for preterm infants during the first year of life. Dev. Med. Child Neurol. 50, 254–266.

Spittle, A.J., Boyd, R.N., Inder, T.E., Doyle, L.W., 2009. Predicting motor development in very preterm infants at 12 months' corrected age: the role of qualitative magnetic resonance imaging and general movement assessment. Pediatrics 123, 512–517.

Spittle, A.J., Doyle, L.W., Anderson, P.J., et al., 2010. Reduced cerebellar diameter in very preterm infants with abnormal general movements. Early Hum. Dev. 86, 1–5.

Valentin, T., Uhl, K., Einspieler, C., 2005. The effectiveness of training in Prechtl's method on the qualitative assessment of general movements. Early Hum. Dev. 81, 623–627.

Volpe, J.J., 2008. Neurology of the Newborn, fifth ed. W.B. Saunders, Philadelphia, PA.

Wu, Y.W., Lynch, J.K., Nelson, K.B., 2005. Perinatal arterial stroke: understanding mechanisms and outcomes. Semin. Neurol. 25, 424–434.

# Effects of motor activity on brain and muscle development in cerebral palsy

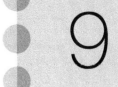

Diane L. Damiano

## CHAPTER CONTENTS

Brain and muscle plasticity in response to brain injury and specific types of physiotherapy have been demonstrated in cerebral palsy (CP) (Cope et al., 2010; McNee et al., 2009). Despite this exciting evidence, physiotherapists who provide early intervention services for infants with cerebral palsy and their families face a quandary. After several decades and multiple studies, the consensus among systematic reviews on physiotherapy for infants with or at high risk for cerebral palsy is that early intervention aiming to improve motor outcomes regardless of type has not been shown to produce positive mean group changes that are more than what would be expected due to maturation (Hadders-Algra, 2011). Comparisons with control groups receiving no or another intervention have similar results of no group differences in motor development.

Some of the interventions appear to improve cognitive outcomes in infants (Blauw-Hospers et al., 2007; Orton et al., 2009), facilitate bonding (Kaaresen et al., 2008) or reduce parental stress (Badr et al., 2006), which are clearly important. However, these positive changes provide an interesting contrast to the consistent absence of statistically and/or clinically significant improvements in motor development. The consensus from all of these studies is perhaps even more baffling today as evidence is rapidly accumulating on the remarkable potential for the brain to recover from injury that is purported to be even greater in a more immature nervous system (Villablanca and Hovda, 2000). In fact, it seems almost inconceivable that early intervention strategies not only show no appreciable benefit on motor functioning but also fail to show a dramatic effect. Newer innovative treatment strategies have emerged that are based on sound developmental principles such as coping and caring for children with special needs (COPCA) (Blauw-Hospers et al., 2007) or context-based approaches (Law et al., 2011), yet evidence of superiority still remains elusive for these, as shown by results from well-controlled randomized controlled trials (RCTs) (Hielkema et al., 2011; Law et al., 2011). How can we forge a path forward based on these disappointing results that fly in the face of what we know are tremendous possibilities for brain plasticity and recovery of function?

This chapter will explore possible explanations for this apparent 'disconnect', focusing primarily on the amount, type and timing of interventions that have been provided to infants and families and on study design issues and challenges. Intervention features will be evaluated in light of the current evidence that supports the fundamental role of motor activity in promoting brain and muscle development and plasticity throughout the lifespan. Central to these discussions are current assumptions and knowledge on the uniqueness of the infant with regard to these processes and the associated implications for therapeutic strategies.

# Infancy is a unique period of neural development and plasticity

Although developmental changes occur in the brain throughout the lifespan, the processes that occur in infancy are dramatic and unique in many ways. During infancy there is an overabundance of neural pathways that are established and then pruned through programmed cell death (apoptosis) as well as experience-dependent enhancement or attenuation of synaptic connections within and across brain regions (Johnston, 2009). A brain injury disrupts normal developmental processes in ways that we are only recently beginning to understand. We now know that the brains of children with CP reorganize substantially in response to injury, as seen in infants with hemiplegia who may retain a higher percentage of bilateral corticospinal projections or whose brain may reorganize so that the dominant hemisphere provides ipsilateral input to the non-dominant extremity (Staudt, 2010). While these processes may restore some degree of functionality to the affected extremity, this is accomplished by the formation or strengthening of pathways between remaining brain regions, rather than by direct repair of the damaged areas. Substitution of function may also occur that could be at the expense of recovery or development in another skill or domain. These imperfect repair processes may also impose distinct limits on rehabilitation potential, at least given the current state of medical care and science. In children with congenital hemiplegia, the pattern of reorganization is intricately related to dexterity of the paretic hand, with those who demonstrate shared representation of the paretic and non-paretic hand in the intact hemisphere having the worst prognosis (Vandermeeren et al., 2009). In some cases where the damage occurs prior to or in a critical period of the development of a specific functional capability, that function may never develop (Rittenhouse et al., 1999).

It has been well-argued that 'developing brain' is not a term that should be reserved just for the first few years of life (Kolb and Gibb, 2011). The brain is always developing, with no age limit on plasticity (Thickbroom and Mastaglia, 2009), but has different capabilities and vulnerabilities that depend on its current stage of development and thus may have divergent responses to the same insult at different time periods. An example is the differential effect of a traumatic brain injury in early versus late adolescence, in that motor outcomes are typically worse in the earlier years but frontal lobe outcomes are better compared with later adolescence where the pattern is often reversed (Kolb and Gibb, 2011). Anderson et al. (2011) describe a 'recovery continuum' for infants with early brain insults, with the opposing processes of heightened vulnerability versus plasticity in the immature brain at the two extremes of the outcome spectrum representing poor or excellent outcomes, respectively. They state that where a given child falls on that continuum depends on injury factors, e.g., the location, extent and timing of injury and environmental factors, e.g., parenting, socio-economic status and interventions; each of these factors may act independently or synergistically. Even though cerebral palsy is not a genetically transmitted disorder (although several genetic disorders have been uncovered that had been errantly diagnosed as CP), individual genetic factors may be largely responsible for modulating responses to environmental stress, injury and recovery and further contribute to variability in prognosis and response to treatment. A fascinating study on adaptive plasticity of the motor cortex in 16 pairs of identical monozygotic vs dizygotic twins demonstrated a strong 'heritability estimate', concluding that 'genetic factors may contribute significantly to inter-individual variability in plasticity paradigms', which may have implications for motor learning and rehabilitation potential (Missitzi et al., 2011). It has also been shown that maladaptive plastic changes are 'plastic' themselves, which provides even greater optimism for promoting and refining brain repair and reorganization over a more prolonged time period (Martin, 2012).

# Interaction of brain and muscle injury and plasticity

Injury to the brain leads to alterations at all levels of the central nervous system as well as the peripheral nervous system with the converse also being true. For example, diffuse muscle atrophy can occur in the affected extremities after a middle cerebral artery infarct, or there can be a dramatic loss of cortical representation of an amputated limb. Movement is produced through the interplay of the central and peripheral nervous systems and therefore can be impaired by a disruption at any level with widespread secondary effects. In cerebral palsy the initial injury is, of course, in the central nervous system, which leads to deficits in motor function in specific body parts depending on the location and extent of the injury, often with a predictable bias towards preservation of some movements or patterns of movement over others. Further confounding the picture, the amount of voluntary motor activity in an affected body part is often less than that in an unaffected body part, which then leads to a competitive disadvantage for that body part at the joint level, the level of the neuromuscular junction and at the level of synapses in the brain. Muscle atrophy and increased intrinsic stiffness, joint contractures and bony deformities may all develop as a result of these movement biases. Current treatments in CP such as strength training, botulinum toxin injections or orthopaedic surgery have some measurable effects in alleviating some of the secondary musculoskeletal consequences in the short term, but since the brain injury is still present, the abnormal influences persist and continue to exert effects peripherally. These, in turn, may have further central effects, an iterative process that causes a 'static' injury to worsen over time, with additional confounding negative influences from other processes such as physical growth and ageing. Until recently, trying to manage the secondary peripheral effects was deemed to be the most, if not the only, effective management strategy. This approach has at best been marginally successful in maintaining or positively influencing the level of functional mobility for individuals with CP and has largely failed to successfully prevent the precipitous decline in function in older individuals (Ando and Ueda, 2000; Bottos and Gericke, 2003).

Due to recent advances in neuroscience, our therapeutic approaches are beginning to be directed at the primary site of injury. The realization of the vast capacity of the brain to remodel and to some extent recover has dramatically shifted our focus on trying to better understand and therapeutically manipulate this process. The goal of what we need to try to accomplish was beautifully stated by Martin (2012) and highlights the formidable challenge ahead: 'We must repair the damaged motor systems, so the brain reconnects with motor neurons. These connections must be sufficiently strong and precise to enable robust and proper voluntary muscle recruitment.' This underscores why it is so important that muscles are sufficiently developed and structurally intact to both help drive and respond to these central nervous system changes.

## Muscle plasticity in infants with cerebral palsy

Muscles are now known to be one of the most malleable ('plastic') tissues in the body and respond very dramatically to increases or decreases in mechanical loading and activation throughout their lifespan (Narici and Maganaris, 2007). Muscle fibres respond to external stimuli or lack thereof by either a change in size or protein isoform content. Infants are believed to have nearly all of their adult muscle fibres present at birth, but have little antigravity muscle control, unlike many animals who walk independently shortly after birth. Dynamic systems theory, espoused by Thelen and Ulrich (1991), challenged the primacy of the neuromaturational explanation of motor development and explored biomechanical factors underlying this process. They postulated that the rate-limiting steps for the emergence of independent walking in infants were the development of postural control and adequate extensor muscle strength. Compelling indirect evidence for the critical importance of strength development in infancy can be seen through cross-cultural differences in infant handling and positioning practices. Clearly, those cultural practices that stimulate more antigravity movements or weight-bearing activities lead to systematically earlier skill acquisition. An example of how infant handling can influence motor development is the recent change in the USA in the recommended safe sleeping position for infants from prone to supine. This has had an appreciable adverse effect on the development of extensor strength and related milestone achievement, leading to public service announcements to encourage more 'tummy time' during play activities to ensure that children have sufficient opportunities to acquire adequate strength.

Synapse formation at the neuromuscular junction in infancy mirrors the process that is occurring in the brain. In older children and adults, each muscle fibre is innervated by a single alpha motor neuron. However, during development many of the fibres are innervated by multiple axons. As in the brain, synapse elimination is an activity-dependent event with competition across axons (Lieber, 2010). Scientific data on the development of muscle strength and fibre type differentiation in infants is surprisingly lacking and is mainly inferred from invasive studies in young and older animals and in adult humans. Schiaffino et al. (2007) demonstrated remarkable plasticity in terms of fibre size (activity-dependent increases or decreases) and fibre type transformation in mature animal muscles from slow to fast isoforms in response to denervation and electrical stimulation. They further demonstrated the far greater capacity of immature versus mature muscle to remodel in response to external stimuli. There appears to be a set amount and intensity of physical activity that maintains muscle mass within a range that is commensurate with daily activity requirements. If activity levels drop or increase substantially, muscle adaptations are evident. The optimal amount of activity to maintain muscle integrity is difficult to estimate and in our increasingly sedentary society, 'average' activity amounts may be too low of a standard (Booth and Laye, 2010). Movement is ubiquitous and pervasive during fetal and child development and has been shown to be reduced in amount and amplitude in infants with motor disabilities as compared to those with typical development (Bell et al., 2010; Spittle et al., 2008; Vaal et al., 2000). How to provide them sufficient opportunities for self-initiated movement when movement production is the major deficit is a major challenge for physiotherapists and families.

Intense and repetitive activation of muscles not only stimulates their own growth but also stimulates the release of neural and other growth factors that can enhance cognitive functioning and promote physical growth (Bell et al., 2010). These findings have major implications for children with cerebral palsy who typically move less and often have prolonged delays or difficulties in the acquisition of upright motor skills. Many children with CP also have restricted growth that correlates with their degree of involvement, which could reasonably be assumed to be mediated in part by their restricted muscle activity, although that has not been tested empirically.

Alterations in spastic muscle extend far beyond changes in size and likely originate in infancy, although no longitudinal investigation of muscle changes during development in CP has been reported. Reported differences in CP include counter-intuitively longer sarcomere resting length in contracted muscles, marked disruptions in the extracellular matrix with excessive collagen content, and fat infiltration in muscle tissue, among others (Barrett and Lichtwark, 2010; Grant-Beuttler et al., 2000; Johnson et al., 2009; Lieber et al., 2004; Marbini et al., 2002; Theroux et al., 2005). The extent to which any of these structural changes can be modified is unknown, although recent evidence on changes in muscle volume after strength training has been reported (McNee et al., 2009). Activity enhancement should be the primary goal of early motor intervention for both the brain and the muscles, but how to best accomplish this in each child, when the best time to do this is and how much should be done are major unanswered questions (Damiano, 2006). Critical stages in brain and muscle development and the points at which the various maladaptive changes are likely to be irreversible also need to be determined.

## Efficacy and effectiveness of early intervention: study design considerations

A standard population-based approach to early intervention that produces large and lasting treatment effects on motor development has not yet been identified, and in a diverse population such as CP this may not even be possible. Randomized controlled trials are the optimal source of evidence regarding treatment efficacy when there is a well-defined and homogeneous sample of participants, each of whom would be anticipated to respond similarly to the same intervention when the intervention is also clearly defined and administered in the same way to all subjects, and when the groups created by randomization have a similar investment in and perception of personal benefit (or not) as a result of their participation. Individual variability in baseline characteristics that are not considered in the randomization process and which affect the subsequent response to intervention is the nemesis of RCTs. Early intervention studies typically include a heterogeneous sample of infants that may share some characteristics, e.g., low birth weight, extreme prematurity, delayed motor milestones, or abnormal movement characteristics, but individual subjects could have very diverse aetiologies, brain injuries, and personal and environmental histories. Since the CP diagnosis is often delayed, many studies include a large percentage of subjects who do not even go on to develop CP. Determining the prognosis in early infancy for developing CP in the first place, and then estimating the subsequent degree of motor severity, has improved with early infant motor assessments that may better predict motor prognosis (Campbell et al., 2006; Einspieler and Prechtl, 2005) and imaging advances. However, this remains an imprecise science and, even when children appear very similar there can be tremendous individual variability in outcomes.

Future RCTs in this population could be improved by including more homogeneous samples and by focusing on a specific training component (rather than comparing intervention programmes, each with multiple elements) shown in preliminary studies to have a powerful effect on motor function. An excellent example is the myriad of RCTs examining intense upper limb training in patients with hemiplegia which have been able to demonstrate efficacy (Hoare et al., 2007). However, long-standing convictions that only evidence from RCTs merit consideration are unfounded and many are now urging researchers to look beyond RCTs and consider other potentially more appropriate designs for examining treatment effectiveness in this population. While extensive individual variability is difficult to control or account for in RCTs, other study designs are being recommended for and applied to early intervention studies that exploit the sources of variability in patient characteristics and processes of care. Comparative effectiveness, also referred to as practice-based evidence, research designs aim to identify associations of specific characteristics with outcomes but require datasets that are large enough to include all the variables presumed to substantially influence the target outcome (Horn, 2010). One recent example of the type of information that can be gleaned from these types of designs is by Hielkema et al. (2011) who explored the sources of variability in outcomes in their non-conclusive RCT comparing an innovative treatment (COPCA) and traditional physiotherapy (Bobath therapy). They dissected the components of the

two interventions and related each to outcomes. In the COPCA programme, parents were coached on how to facilitate motor development in their child, whereas the traditional therapy approach provided instructions to parents on how to perform specific techniques, with the former associated with better outcomes and the latter with worse outcomes. The authors suggested that the first approach was more empowering to the parents and enabled them to interact more effectively to promote their child's mobility on a daily basis in the context of everyday activities. Strategies that challenged the child to produce self-initiated movements were associated with better outcomes, whereas more passive positioning or sensory stimulation techniques were associated with worse outcomes. No association was found between efforts to improve movement quality and outcomes. Analytic methods that can decompose intervention programmes into active, ineffective and potentially detrimental elements are incredibly informative processes that can be directly and rapidly translated into clinical practice, and these need to be a far higher research priority in this population.

It is interesting to now revisit the much-cited RCT published by Palmer et al. (1988) comparing two groups of infants, one which participated in an infant stimulation programme for six months followed by physical therapy for the next six months compared to a group that had physical therapy (Bobath therapy) the entire 12 months. Their results showed that the physical therapy alone group (i.e., group 2) did not have superior motor outcomes and were actually worse at both assessment points, sparked considerable controversy at the time, with many in the therapy community expressing scepticism about these results and suggesting other possible explanations for their findings. However, closer examination of the intervention descriptions is quite illuminating and may make these results far less surprising given what we now know. The specific focus of the physical therapy programme was facilitation of the righting and equilibrium responses once considered to underlie the development of motor milestones. In contrast, the infant stimulation group followed an established programme of developmentally appropriate and progressively challenging activities to stimulate all aspects of development, and specifically did not include any activities that targeted righting or equilibrium responses. The therapy involved considerable handling and manipulating of the infant to stimulate a response, similar to traditional Bobath or neurodevelopmental therapy (NDT) methods, rather than encouraging greater self-exploration of their environment as was the goal in the infant stimulation programme. These results are virtually identical to the associations of these two same strategies with worse and better outcomes, respectively, found in the study by Hielkema et al. (2011).

## Types and amounts of interventions that have been delivered

Despite the multiple clinical studies and in several cases high-quality RCTs on early intervention approaches, consistent patterns or a consensus on which, if any, are the most effective or efficacious have not emerged. Potential explanations, beyond the individual variability in response that can be obscured by mean group analyses, may include the fact that many interventions are based on an overarching treatment philosophy that is applied individually at the discretion of the clinician, rather than being a well-defined set of exercises that is administered in a standardized manner across subjects. NDT is one such philosophy that has dominated the field for several decades and has been the most well-studied. Many therapists worldwide have been trained in this method, which even offers a specialized 'Baby course'. However, the consensus from reviews of the many studies that included NDT as the experimental or traditional physiotherapy (control group) method was that it does not confer any benefits compared to alternatives and fails to alter motor prognosis (Butler and Darrah, 2001). NDT has evolved considerably over the years, incorporating other contemporary approaches to the point where the basic tenets are hardly recognizable (Mayston, 2008), so more recent studies on NDT may not be evaluating the same intervention as in previous studies. In addition to NDT, several other approaches to improve motor outcomes have been reported. Spittle et al. (2007), in their review of early intervention studies in premature infants, identified six different treatment categories across 16 studies as well as differences in who the intervention was directed to: the child, the caregiver or the interaction between them.

These ranged from educating parents on motor development, providing direct 'stimulation' in therapy, or fostering interactions through helping parents better decipher their child's behavioural cues. Again, no consistent positive effect on motor outcomes from any approach was identified.

Dosage questions are also intricately linked to the effectiveness of an intervention. If a treatment is not found to be effective, the argument can reasonably be posed that the treatment may not have been delivered often enough or well enough for an adequate duration. However, the counter-argument can be made that if a treatment has not been shown to be at least marginally effective in a smaller dose, more of the same will also fail to be effective. Most early intervention programmes have been conducted for at most a few hours per week, which is a very small percentage of the total time the infant is awake and trying to move. Therefore, lack of efficacy due to inadequate dosing may be one explanation. Alternatively, focusing on the infant's family and environment would seem to be the optimal way to provide sufficient movement and developmental experiences on a daily basis to measurably enhance skill development and neuroplasticity. However, the results of two recent RCTs on family and context-based approaches were similarly unimpressive (Hielkema et al., 2011; Law et al., 2011). So where do we go from here?

## The future of physiotherapy for infants with CP

The basic science argues that we should not yet resign ourselves to the current status quo. Given the growing body of compelling evidence for the activity dependence of both brain and muscle development, and the increasing recognition that infants as well as older children with CP are far too sedentary and that when they do move, some of their self-selected movement choices may lead to maladaptive changes (e.g., overuse of the non-paretic side), a strong rationale exists for continued investigation of activity-based therapies to promote neural recovery. The brain injury in CP creates abnormally strong or inappropriate 'competitions' between activity patterns of muscles about a joint or between limbs and ultimately between synapses in both the central and peripheral nervous systems, with those that are stronger being reinforced and those that are weaker or non-existent being overtaken or eliminated. Apparently, much is to be learned from the increasing evidence supporting constraint-induced movement therapy (CIMT) which directly addresses the distorted competition between limbs by limiting the movement of the more functional limb and promoting skilled activity in the more impaired limb. This approach has also been shown to have a positive effect on cortical reorganization in older children with CP that correlates with motor skill improvement (Cope et al., 2010). Bimanual training, focusing on greater participation of the impaired limb in bimanual activities, has also demonstrated effectiveness even though the shift in the relative use of the two limbs is not as great (Hung et al., 2011). Whether the two approaches have different effects on cortical reorganization has not been investigated, but given that CIMT provides a more dramatic reversal of the competitive situation and that bimanual training recreates a more typical developmental scenario, differences could be quite informative. Since the corticospinal tract is so active in infancy, some caution may be advisable if the unilateral focus were too extreme, because it may be possible to disrupt the development of the more functional limb. Altering the competitive advantage across limbs seems fairly straightforward to accomplish for infants with unilateral deficits, but it is far more challenging to determine whether this would even be feasible or effective for children who have bilateral involvement. The implications in terms of motor learning or brain plasticity of being able to perform a task well on one limb (hemiplegia) versus not being able to do it well on either limb (diplegia) are intriguing but are as yet unknown.

CIMT also incorporates repetitive practice of functionally relevant tasks that is consistent with task-oriented interventions shown to be successful in adults with central nervous system injuries and in infants with Down syndrome (Rensink et al., 2009; Ulrich et al., 2001). The meaningfulness or 'salience' of a task and the level of cognitive engagement required also enhance the potential neuroplastic effects, and these principles could be applied to patients with both unilateral and bilateral involvement. Two recent RCTs in infants born less than 33 weeks premature used task-oriented methods to progressively train greater reaching-to-toy movements with the hands, and also the feet, and were successful in increasing the number and duration of these behaviours compared to a control social stimulation group (Heathcock and Galloway, 2009; Heathcock et al., 2005). However, these infants practiced a task they were already able to do. The dilemma with many infants with CP is that they may not be able to initiate a specific movement to be able to practice it at all or correctly. As a result, these children often develop adaptive strategies to accomplish a specific functional goal in the short term that ultimately limits movement efficiency and flexibility in the long term. In the absence of intervention, this less than optimal strategy is then reinforced through repetition. Facilitating and handling techniques were used with infants for many years to help simulate more desirable movement patterns, but these techniques may have actually restricted learning in that they also compensated for rather than addressed the deficits that prevented the child from doing the task him or herself and did not allow the child to develop accurate intrinsic feedback.

Motor-powered devices and/or harnessed support systems that encourage, facilitate or assist movement are increasingly prevalent in rehabilitation. The most common systems involve body weight supported step training. The previous example of a lower extremity study in infants that trained a 'reaching' task with the feet required considerable cognitive engagement (Heathcock and Galloway, 2009). However, efficacy and superiority of more cyclical and less cognitively engaging tasks such as walking on a treadmill have not been conclusively demonstrated in adults (Duncan et al., 2011) or children with cerebral palsy (Damiano and DeJong, 2009). This should perhaps not be so surprising because as noted in dynamical systems theory, step generation is only one component of independent walking with antigravity strength, trunk and limb control and balance even more crucial. These two may be hampered in their development by existing harness or exoskeleton systems that limit loading and provide support rather than challenge trunk control.

Newer support systems are needed, such as the ZeroG system (Hidler et al., 2011), which provides a consistent amount of support within a wide range of movement excursion that still requires control of all parts of the body, most notably the trunk. For typically developing infants, much of their motor experience is centred around attempting to transition between movements and/or recovering their balance when leaning or falling outside their limits of stability. Safe, effective strategies and devices to mimic these experiences in infants with restricted movement capabilities are needed and are beginning to be developed (Hadders-Algra, 2008; Stergiou et al., 2006). Variability in the speed and type of motion facilitated is limited in many robotic or motor-driven devices such as treadmills or robotic gait-devices, although variability is a key component of adaptive motor control and one that is often lacking in children with brain injuries (Prosser et al., 2012; Ragonesi and Galloway, 2012). One cautionary note is that external devices may pose the danger of 'over-assisting' movement to the same or even greater extent than physical handling. These should be used only as much or as long as needed and no more and should promote and respond to, rather than guide or control, movement intention.

All of these strategies involve some level of direct intervention or manipulation to alter the environment, the task requirements, or the resources the infant is able to utilize to produce the desired movement. These appear to be in opposition to other therapeutic approaches prevalent today that focus mainly on empowering and supporting parents to provide any needed care or 'therapy' for their infants. However, to direct neuroplastic changes, a combination of approaches may be necessary to promote very specific movement experiences for those children who may not be able to experience them otherwise. If the use of these types of devices is shown to be superior in producing functional and neuroplastic changes, the next stage in their technical development should be to make these safe and available for everyday use.

## Summary and conclusions

For years, there has been much appropriate clinical sensitivity about not trying to make children with CP 'normal', because that has not yet been thought possible. But what if it were possible? The evidence of rapid and often dramatic motor recovery in children post-hemispherectomy, with those who are younger tending to have better outcomes (de Bode et al. 2005), provides considerable cause for optimism for children with CP. Based on recent research in multiple neurologic disorders, several neurorehabilitation principles have been emerging that are, perhaps not surprisingly, nearly identical with the principles underlying the process of motor skill learning in infants, i.e., movement must be self-initiated, meaningful, and repeated often but in a variable manner (see Chapters 1 and 11). The major challenge for physiotherapy for infants with CP is to devise training strategies or devices that would enable them to perform movements that are difficult or even impossible for them to do with their existing resources or in their current environments, and then to effectively motivate them to practice these *often*, in a varied manner that allows errors as well as successes. Examples are aquatic environments or 'smart' harnesses or robotic devices that sense intention or eliminate the weight of the limb— all of which are aimed to make movement easier. These strategies are likely to be the most effective for brain and muscle development soon after injury or just as a movement or its precursors begins to emerge. While many consider it highly improbable that any means of promoting motor activity alone will be able to completely 'cure' the brain injury in CP, activity-based therapies will likely lead to some degree of recovery as well as play a fundamental role in helping direct more effective repair processes stimulated by drugs or other molecular-based approaches (Sadowsky and McDonald, 2009). The state of the science suggests that effectiveness of early intervention should be the rule rather than the exception, and that the challenge is now up to those working in field of paediatrics to determine how best to enable these infants to 'move' from brain injury to maximal recovery.

## References

Anderson, V., Spencer-Smith, M., Wood, A., 2011. Do children really recover better? Neurobehavioural plasticity after early brain insult. Brain 134 (Pt 8), 2197–2221.

Ando, N., Ueda, S., 2000. Functional deterioration in adults with cerebral palsy. Clin. Rehabil. 14 (3), 300–306.

Badr, L.K., Garg, M., Kamath, M., 2006. Intervention for infants with brain injury: results of a randomized controlled study. Infant. Behav. Dev. 29 (1), 80–90.

Barrett, R.S., Lichtwark, G.A., 2010. Gross muscle morphology and structure in spastic cerebral palsy: a systematic review. Dev. Med. Child Neurol. 52, 794–804.

Bell, K.L., Boyd, R.N., Tweedy, S.M., Weir, K.A., Stevenson, R.D., Davies, P.S., 2010. A prospective, longitudinal study of growth, nutrition and sedentary behaviour in young children with cerebral palsy. BMC Public Health 10, 179.

Blauw-Hospers, C.H., de Graaf-Peters, V.B., Dirks, T., Bos, A.F., Hadders-Algra, M., 2007. Does early intervention in infants at high risk for a developmental motor disorder improve motor and cognitive development? Neurosci. Biobehav. Rev. 31 (8), 1201–1212.

Booth, F.W., Laye, M.J., 2010. The future: genes, physical activity and health. Acta Physiol. (Oxf) 199 (4), 549–556.

Bottos, M., Gericke, C., 2003. Ambulatory capacity in cerebral palsy: prognostic criteria and consequences for intervention. Dev. Med. Child Neurol. 45 (11), 786–790.

Butler, C., Darrah, J., 2001. Effects of neurodevelopmental treatment (NDT) for cerebral palsy: an AACPDM evidence report. Dev. Med. Child Neurol. 43 (11), 778–790.

Campbell, S.K., Levy, P., Zawacki, L., Liao, P.J., 2006. Population-based age standards for interpreting results on the test of motor infant performance. Pediatr. Phys. Ther. 18 (2), 119–125.

Cope, S.M., Liu, X.C., Verber, M.D., Cayo, C., Rao, S., Tassone, J.C., 2010. Upper limb function and brain reorganization after constraint-induced movement therapy in children with hemiplegia. Dev. Neurorehabil. 13 (1), 19–30.

Damiano, D.L., 2006. Activity, activity, activity: rethinking our physical therapy approach to cerebral palsy. Phys. Ther. 86, 1534–1540.

Damiano, D.L., DeJong, S.L., 2009. A systematic review of the effectiveness of treadmill training and body weight support in pediatric rehabilitation. J. Neurol. Phys. Ther. 33 (1), 27–44.

deBode, S., Firestine, A., Mathern, G.W, Dobkin, B., 2005. Residual motor control and cortical representations of function following hemispherectomy: effects of etiology. J. Child Neurol. 20 (1), 64–75.

Duncan, P.W., Sullivan, K.J., Behrman, A.L., Azen, S.P., Wu, S.S., Nadeau, S.E., et al., 2011. LEAPS Investigative Team. Body-weight-supported treadmill rehabilitation after stroke. N. Engl. J. Med. 364 (21), 2026–2036.

Einspieler, C., Prechtl, H.F., 2005. Prechtl's assessment of general movements: a diagnostic tool for the functional assessment of the young nervous system. Ment. Retard. Dev. Disabil. Res. Rev. 11, 61–67.

Grant-Beuttler, M., Palisano, R.J., Miller, D.P., Reddien Wagner, B., Heriza, C.B., Shewokis, P.A., 2000. Gastrocnemius-soleus muscle tendon unit changes over the first 12 weeks of adjusted age in infants born preterm. Phys. Ther. 89, 136–148.

Hadders-Algra, M., 2008. Reduced variability in motor behaviour: an indicator of impaired cerebral connectivity? Early Hum. Dev. 84 (12), 787–789.

Hadders-Algra, M., 2011. Challenges and limitations in early intervention. Dev. Med. Child Neurol. 53 (Suppl. 4), 52–55.

Heathcock, J.C., Galloway, J.C., 2009. Exploring objects with feet advances movement in infants born preterm: a randomized controlled trial. Phys. Ther. 89, 1027–1038.

Heathcock, J.C., Bhat, A.N., Lobo, M.A., Galloway, J.C., 2005. The relative kicking frequency of infants born full-term and preterm during learning and short-term and long-term memory periods of the mobile paradigm. Phys. Ther. 85, 8–18.

Hidler, J., Brennan, D., Black, I., Nichols, D., Brady, K., Nef, T., 2011. ZeroG: overground gait and balance training system. J. Rehabil. Res. Dev. 48 (4), 287–298.

Hielkema, T., Blauw-Hospers, C.H., Dirks, T., Drijver-Messelink, M., Bos, A.F., Hadders-Algra, M., 2011. Does physiotherapeutic intervention affect motor outcome in high-risk infants? An approach combining a randomized controlled trial and process evaluation. Dev. Med. Child Neurol. 53 (3), e8–15.

Hoare, B.J., Wasiak, J., Imms, C., Carey, L., 2007. Constraint-induced movement therapy in the treatment of the upper limb in children with hemiplegic cerebral palsy. Cochrane Database Syst. Rev. 18 (2), CD004149.

Horn, S.D., 2010. Invited commentary. Phys. Ther. 90 (11), 1673–1675.

Hung, Y.C., Casertano, L., Hillman, A., Gordon, A.M., 2011. The effect of intensive bimanual training on coordination of the hands in children

with congenital hemiplegia. Res. Dev. Disabil. 32 (6), 2724–2731.

Johnson, D.L., Miller, F., Subramanian, P., Modlesky, C.M., 2009. Adipose tissue infiltration of skeletal muscle in children with cerebral palsy. J. Pediatr. 154, 715–720.

Johnston, M.V., 2009. Plasticity in the developing brain: implications for rehabilitation. Dev. Disabil. Res. Rev. 15 (2), 94–101.

Kaaresen, P.I., Rønning, J.A., Tunby, J., Nordhov, S.M., Ulvund, S.E., Dahl, L.B., 2008. A randomized controlled trial of an early intervention program in low birth weight children: outcome at 2 years. Early Hum. Dev. 84 (3), 201–209.

Kolb, B., Gibb, R., 2011. Brain plasticity and behaviour in the developing brain. J. Can. Acad. Child Adolesc. Psychiatry 20 (4), 265–276.

Law, M.C., Darrah, J., Pollock, N., Wilson, B., Russell, D.J., Walter, S.D., et al., 2011. Focus on function: a cluster, randomized controlled trial comparing child- versus context-focused intervention for young children with cerebral palsy. Dev. Med. Child Neurol. 53 (7), 621–629.

Lieber, R.L., 2010. Skeletal Muscle Structure, Function and Plasticity, third ed. Lippincott Williams & Wilkins, Philadelphia, PA, pp. 8–11.

Lieber, R.L., Steinman, S., Barash, I.A., Chambers, H., 2004. Structural and functional changes in spastic skeletal muscle. Muscle Nerve 29, 615–627.

Marbini, A., Ferrari, A., Cioni, G., Bellanova, M.F., Fusco, C., Gemignani, F., 2002. Immunohistochemical study of muscle biopsy in children with cerebral palsy. Brain Dev. 24, 63–66.

Martin, J.H., 2012. Systems neurobiology of restorative neurology and future directions for repair of the damaged motor systems. Clin. Neurol. Neurosurg. 114 (5), 515–523. (Epub ahead of print).

Mayston, M., 2008. Bobath concept: Bobath@50: mid-life crisis–what of the future? Physiother. Res. Int. 13 (3), 131–136.

McNee, A.E., Gough, M., Morrissey, M.C., Shortland, A.P., 2009. Increases in muscle volume after plantarflexor strength training in children with spastic cerebral palsy. Dev. Med. Child Neurol. 51 (6), 429–435.

Missitzi, J., Gentner, R., Geladas, N., Politis, P., Karandreas, N., Classen, J., et al. 2011. Plasticity in human motor cortex is in part genetically determined. J. Physiol. 589, 297–306.

Narici, M.V., Maganaris, C.N., 2007. Plasticity of the muscle tendon complex with disuse and aging. Exerc. Sport Sci. Rev. 35 (3), 126–134.

Orton, J., Spittle, A., Doyle, L., Anderson, P., Boyd, R., 2009. Do early intervention programmes improve cognitive and motor outcomes for preterm infants after discharge? A systematic review. Dev. Med. Child Neurol. 51 (11), 851–859.

Palmer, F.B., Shapiro, B.K., Wachtel, R.C., Allen, M.C., Hiller, J.E., Harryman, S.E., et al., 1988. The effects of physical therapy on cerebral palsy. A controlled trial in infants with spastic diplegia. N. Engl. J. Med. 318 (13), 803–808.

Prosser, L.A., Ohlrigh, L.B., Curatalo, L.A., Alter, K.E., Damiano, D.L., 2012. Feasibility and preliminary effectiveness of a novel mobility training intervention in infants and toddlers with cerebral palsy. Dev. Neurorehabil. 15 (4), 259–266.

Ragonesi, C.B., Galloway, J.C., 2012. Short-term, early intensive power mobility training: case report of an infant at risk for cerebral palsy. Pediatr. Phys. Ther. 24 (2), 141–148.

Rensink, M., Schuurmans, M., Lindeman, E., Hafsteinsdóttir, T., 2009. Task-oriented training in rehabilitation after stroke:

systematic review. J. Adv. Nurs. 65 (4), 737–754.

Rittenhouse, C.D., Shouval, H.Z., Paradiso, M.A., Bear, M.F., 1999. Monocular deprivation induces homosynaptic long-term depression in visual cortex. Nature 28, 347–350.

Sadowsky, C.L., McDonald, J.W., 2009. Activity-based restorative therapies: concepts and applications in spinal cord injury-related neurorehabilitation. Dev. Disabil. Res. Rev. 15 (2), 112–116.

Schiaffino, S., Sandri, M., Murgia, M., 2007. Activity-dependent signaling pathways controlling muscle diversity and plasticity. Physiologica 22, 269–278.

Spittle, A.J., Orton, J., Doyle, L.W., Boyd, R., 2007. Early developmental intervention programs post hospital discharge to prevent motor and cognitive impairments in preterm infants. Cochrane Database Syst. Rev. 18 (2), CD005495.

Spittle, A.J., Brown, N.C., Doyle, L.W., Boyd, R.N., Hunt, R.W., Bear, M., et al., 2008. Quality of general movements is related to white matter pathology in very preterm infants. Pediatrics 121, e1184–e1189.

Staudt, M., 2010. Reorganization after pre- and perinatal brain lesions. J. Anat. 217 (4), 469–474.

Stergiou, N., Harbourne, R., Cavanaugh, J., 2006. Optimal movement variability: a new theoretical perspective for neurologic physical therapy. J. Neurol. Phys. Ther. 30 (3), 120–129.

Thelen, E., Ulrich, B.D., 1991. Hidden skills: a dynamic systems analysis of treadmill stepping during the first year. Monogr. Soc. Res. Child Dev. 56, 1–98. discussion 9–104.

Theroux, M.C., Oberman, K.G., Lahaye, J., Boyce, B.A., Duhadaway, D., Miller, F., et al., 2005. Dysmorphic neuromuscular junctions associated with motor ability in cerebral palsy. Muscle Nerve 2005 (32), 626–632.

Thickbroom, G.W., Mastaglia, F.L., 2009. Plasticity in neurological disorders and challenges for noninvasive brain stimulation (NBS). J. Neuroeng. Rehabil. 6, 4.

Ulrich, D.A., Ulrich, B.D., Angulo-Kinzler, R.M., Yun, J., 2001. Treadmill training of infants with Down syndrome: evidence-based developmental outcomes. Pediatrics 108, E84.

Vaal, J., van Soest, A.J., Hopkins, B., Sie, L.T., van der Knaap, M.S., 2000. Development of spontaneous leg movements in infants with and without periventricular leukomalacia. Exp. Brain Res. 135, 94–105.

Vandermeeren, Y., Davare, M., Duque, J., Olivier, E., 2009. Reorganization of cortical hand representation in congenital hemiplegia. Eur. J. Neurosci. 29 (4), 845–854.

Villablanca, J.R., Hovda, D.A., 2000. Developmental neuroplasticity in a model of cerebral hemispherectomy and stroke. Neuroscience 95 (3), 625–637.

# The consequences of independent locomotion for brain and psychological development

David I. Anderson, Joseph J. Campos, Monica Rivera, Audun Dahl, Ichiro Uchiyama, and Marianne Barbu-Roth

## CHAPTER CONTENTS

> As we look along the scale of life, whether in time or in order of organization, muscle is there before nerve, and nerve is there before mind, 'recognizable mind.' It would seem to be the motor act under 'urge to live' which has been the cradle of mind. The motor act, mechanically integrating the individual, would seem to have started mind on its road to recognizability.
>
> Sherrington, 1951, p. 161

Clinicians and researchers who specialize in motor development and motor rehabilitation are intimately familiar with the constraints our bodies and physical abilities place on potential interactions with the world. Each new skill or change in body function is celebrated as an important step along the path toward functional independence. The changes build on each other in a predictable and logical sequence. Clinicians and researchers are far less familiar, however, with the notion that these same bodies and physical abilities constrain the way we perceive and think. Moreover, many are surprised to learn that self-generated movement, along with its perceptual consequences, is a primary driving force behind brain and behavioural development. This notion has serious implications for children with physical disabilities that impede skillful interaction with the physical and social environment, particularly if there are critical periods in brain development.

The field of developmental paediatrics has long held a bias against motoric processes affecting psychological development (Young, 1977). Related to this bias is the established paradigm for analysing children with developmental disabilities a paradigm wherein causal analysis begins with the brain and stops at the musculature, failing to consider how the process in fact continues and loops back from movement to brain. This chapter challenges these biases and presents evidence from a multitude of carefully crafted experiments documenting that motoric developments bring about profound psychological reorganizations in an array of crucial psychological domains. We maintain that these motorically paced reorganizations are not well known, or at all, by segments of the paediatric community; and we propose implications for understanding cerebral palsy (CP) and similar motoric disabilities, the functional deficits in whom are thus too often not appreciated.

This chapter concentrates on the effects of self-produced locomotion on changes in spatial-cognitive functioning and the implications these effects have for children with physical disabilities like CP. Successful independent mobility is an excellent example of the more general effects that motor activity can have on psychological development. We believe that the early promotion of functional mobility is crucial in maximizing children's potential for independent living. Our contribution is in showing that independent mobility has consequences that extend far beyond independence in everyday activities. Mobility generates and maintains psychological changes that are crucial for adapting to a complex world (Campos et al., 2000). This idea, which is an illustration of the well-accepted notion that animals play an active role in their own development, is not new. However, its translation to the clinical setting has lagged behind the experimental discoveries (Campos et al., 1982), despite the fact that many children with disabilities could profit from the knowledge at hand.

# Brief historical perspective on motor activity and psychological functioning

Movement is indeed the mother of all cognition

Sheets-Johnstone, 1999, p. xxi

Modern philosophers and scientists have speculated about movement's role in perception and cognition since the 1700s, when Bishop Berkeley published *An Essay Towards a New Theory of Vision*. Berkeley argued that because visual stimuli were impoverished and ambiguous, motor experience was necessary to make sense of the visual world. His ideas inspired a number of different motor theories of perception that were popular at various times during the 20th century (for a review, see Weimer, 1977). The 1950s were a particularly generative period for theorizing about the role of motor activity in psychological functioning. Sherrington (1951) highlighted that the brain evolved to control movement and so movement must be fundamental to thinking. Sperry (1952) argued that the entire output of our thinking consists of little more than patterns of movement and Piaget (1952, 1954) stressed that the origins of intelligence were in an infant's sensorimotor interactions with the

world. Like Berkeley, Piaget believed that motor experience was necessary to structure patterns of sensory stimuli that were initially meaningless. The theorizing in the 1950s set the stage for a wave of important animal experiments in the late 1950s and 1960s. Those experiments showed convincingly that the normal development of visual–motor co-ordination was dependent on self-produced movement.

Held and Hein's (1963) kitten experiment is the best-known illustration of the early plasticity of the perceptual systems and the critical link between movement experience and perceptual development. Kittens were raised in the dark and then exposed to a patterned environment in an active or passive locomotion condition. All kittens moved along the inside perimeter of a black and white striped cylinder. However, the passive kittens rode in a gondola that was yoked to the movements of the active kitten via a horizontal rod and tether. After training, only the active kittens showed spatially adaptive behaviour by avoiding a drop-off and extending their forelimbs in preparation for contact with a surface. In a clever confirmation and extension of the original findings, Hein et al. (1970) covered one of the kitten's eyes with a patch as it moved actively in the cylinder. The kittens behaved adaptively in response to the drop-off and surface only when tested with the active eye but not the passive eye, highlighting the specificity of the effects of locomotor experience on visual–spatial development.

# The neglect of motor activity's role in psychological functioning

Though widely cited in the psychological literature, Held and Hein's work did not stimulate a wave of research on the motor contributions to perceptual and psychological development that might have been expected. On the contrary, the role of motoric factors in psychological development is still downplayed by the scientific community, despite an impressive body of empirical evidence suggesting that motor activity makes a central contribution to psychological function (Campos et al., 2000; Rakison and Woodward, 2008). Bertenthal and Campos (1990) listed three reasons why the study of the functional consequences of motor development had received little attention until then. The first was the apparent failure to confirm Gesell's (1928) proposal that precocious motor development in infancy predicts IQ in later childhood. The second was the lack of methods available until recently to adequately measure motor processes, and the third was the tendency to explain developmental changes on the basis of innate predetermined mechanisms (e.g., Diamond, 1990), a bias that continues to exist in many circles (e.g., Spelke and Kinzler, 2009).

The limitations of quasi-experimental designs have further encouraged researchers to downplay the role of motor factors in psychological development because these designs cannot rule out maturation as an explanation for differences in psychological performance between groups that differ in motor competence. In fact, researchers consider the study of functional consequences of the causal link between motor development and cognitive (as well as social and emotional) development to be a methodological Gordian Knot. (In Greek mythology, the Gordian Knot was an intricate knot that resisted all attempts to untie it until Alexander the Great cut it with his sword. The Gordian Knot is often used as a metaphor for an intractable problem.) Haith and Benson (1998) commented: 'It is not possible in any single study to control all key variables and potential confounds, including age of locomotor onset, age at spatial-cognitive testing, duration of locomotor experience, manipulation of type of locomotor experience, and level of locomotor skill. Researchers will need to account for these and other variables through multiple studies that converge on similar outcomes (p. 217).' In subsequent sections we will show how our laboratory has addressed this challenge.

Methodological issues are only part of the problem; the neglect of motor contributions to psychological development seems to be symptomatic of a broader neglect of the importance of motor processes in mainstream psychological phenomenon. In discussing the neglect, David Rosenbaum has gone as far as to dub motor control the *Cinderella of psychology* (Rosenbaum, 2005). Rosenbaum cites psychology's intellectual roots in philosophy, where the contents of the mind have always held centre stage, as a primary reason for the tendency to overlook motor contributions to mental life. However, it is clear that the bias from philosophy cannot fully explain the neglect, given that many philosophers, including Berkeley, have shown a keen interest in the motor contributions to mind.

# A resurgence of interest in motor contributions to mind

In the words of the Bob Dylan, evidence suggests that 'the times they are a-changin.' Several trends have coalesced over the last few years to make the relation between motor activity and psychological function a legitimate and increasingly popular topic of investigation. The first trend has been the resurgence of interest in motor development, spurred largely by the popularity of the dynamic systems and the ecological approaches to the study of perception and action (Gibson and Pick, 2000; Thelen and Smith, 1994, 2006). Secondly, these approaches have also increased acceptance among psychologists of the idea that cognition is embodied; in other words, that our bodies and their potential for action provide the substrate for all psychological activity (Casasanto, 2011; Clark, 1997; Thelen, 2000; Varela et al., 1992; Wilson, 2002). Thirdly, researchers in the field of neuroscience, which has always had an interest in motor control, have discovered close anatomical linkages in brain areas known to be involved in cognitive and motor functions (e.g., Diamond, 2000). The linkage between the basal ganglia and the dorsolateral prefrontal cortex has been known for some time; however, Diamond (2000) has more recently argued that the connections between the cerebellum and the dorsolateral prefrontal cortex suggest that the cerebellum might also play an important role in cognitive functions. This suggestion is particularly relevant to cognitive deficits seen in children with CP because children with bilateral spastic CP are hypothesized to have disruptions to white matter tracts that connect the prefrontal and posterior brain regions, the basal ganglia, and related dopaminergic pathways, in addition to the disruptions to motor tracts (Bottcher, 2010; Christ et al., 2003).

Some research suggests that the efficiency with which information is processed from the somatosensory system might also contribute to cognition. A study by Craft et al. (1995) showed that children with spastic diplegic CP who underwent selective dorsal rhizotomy to minimize overactive reflex activation in lower limb muscles showed dramatic improvements in attentional control and cognitive performance relative to controls who did not undergo the procedure. More recently, Dalvand et al. (2012) have supported this idea by arguing that the significant relation between motor and intellectual function seen in children with CP can be at least partially explained by a lack of mobility and consequently a lack of sensory stimulation to the brain regions involved in the control of motor and cognitive functions.

The fourth trend relates to the most recent discoveries about brain plasticity. The role that experience plays in shaping the brain has garnered wide attention and at the same time has contributed to greater acceptance of the idea that motor activity influences brain development (Doidge, 2007; Gomes da Silva et al., 2012). Researchers are now more willing to accept a role for experience in developmental changes that were once considered genetically/maturationally determined. The fifth trend is the renewed interest shown in predicting academic performance from early measures of motor and cognitive function (Piek et al., 2008). Finally, the widespread problems of depression and obesity have popularized research into exercise/physical activity as non-pharmacological interventions (Ratey, 2007) and indirectly popularized examination of the broader link between motor activity and psychological function. Several studies have shown that exercise and physical activity induce the production of neurotransmitters and neurotrophins that are critical to learning, memory, and higher-order thinking (Erickson et al., 2012).

In summary, the relation between motor activity and psychological function has long been a topic of interest in modern scientific inquiry. Surprisingly, the role of movement in psychological development has not attracted the attention one would expect given movement's centrality in everyday life. Recent trends suggest the situation is changing. In the following sections, we highlight research on the relation between mobility and psychological development that is attracting attention thanks to the resurgence of interest more generally in the relationship between motor activity and psychological function. We focus on the implications this body of work has for optimizing psychological competence in children with disabilities such as in CP, in the final section of the chapter.

# Independent mobility and psychological development in the human infant

Clinicians and researchers in the motor domain are well aware of the contribution earlier motor skills make to the development of later motor skills. Agency, the ability to act instrumentally to realize one's goals or intentions, influences all aspects of development (Bidell and Fischer, 1997). Each new motor accomplishment heralds an increasing degree of independence and provides a foundation from which to launch the acquisition of new skills. Skill development occurs in a predictable sequence, such that each new skill builds logically on previous ones. For example, the onset of reliable head control and then sitting lead to step-function improvements in reaching, grasping, and manipulation (Rochat, 1992; Thelen and Spencer, 1998), and experience with belly crawling facilitates the development of proficiency in hands-and-knees crawling (Adolph et al., 1998).

Many clinicians are unaware, however, that motor development contributes to developmental changes beyond the motor domain. Piaget (1952, 1954) built an entire theory of cognitive development on this premise, arguing that sensorimotor interactions with the world provide the building blocks for intellectual functioning. Piaget believed that sensory information is structured initially by the patterning of motor activity. Moreover, observing the consequences of movement permits the discovery of novel solutions to old problems and reveals new problems as the solutions to familiar goals are blocked by unexpected obstacles. An explosion of new goals, new choices, and potential interactions with the world confront infants as they become increasingly agentic. Agency recruits experience, which in turn builds agency. The two are interwoven throughout development in an intimate dance that permits an ever-increasing degree of autonomy and mastery over the environment. Although Piaget's work has fallen out of favour, contemporary theorists have increasingly emphasized the importance of self-generated exploration as a driving force behind developmental change (Bidell and Fischer, 1997; Edelman, 1987; Gibson, 1988; Thelen and Smith, 1994).

The link between independent mobility and psychological development is one of the best illustrations of the contributions that motor activity makes to psychological development. It is now clear that locomotor experience plays a central role in infant psychological development (Campos et al., 2000). Major changes in visual–motor co-ordination, visual–spatial understanding, problem solving, memory, emotion and social interaction occur after the onset of prone locomotion. The onset of prone locomotion has been associated more broadly with a reorganization in brain functioning (Bell and Fox, 1997). Thus, prone locomotion (typically in the form of hands-and-knees crawling) appears to catalyse a psychological revolution in the latter half of life's first year, facilitating changes in an incredibly diverse set of skills that underlie adaptive behaviour. In this section, we will focus on changes in three areas—*visual proprioception*, *spatial search*, and *spatial coding*—to highlight how researchers have uncovered the relation between independent mobility and psychological development. These three areas were chosen because they index *spatial cognition*, a psychological skill that has attracted increasing attention in its own right because it provides a broad foundation for a host of higher-order intellectual skills that permit us to function in an increasingly technological society (Mix et al., 2010; Newcombe and Frick, 2010).

## Visual proprioception: what is it and why is it important?

James Gibson (1966, 1979) famously pointed out that vision is possible because of the structuring of ambient light reflected from the various surfaces that comprise the environment. Each surface has many tiny surfaces (patches or texture elements) that reflect bundles of narrow cones of light differently, depending on their orientation relative to the light source, their orientation relative to their neighbours, and their chemical composition. These bundles of reflected light form a densely structured optic array that is unique from any given point of observation. Consequently, when the head moves, whether through head turning, whole body postural sway, or locomotion, the surrounding optic array changes; it deforms or flows in a manner that co-varies precisely with the speed and direction of self-movement. *Visual proprioception*, then, is the optically produced awareness of self-motion that stems from the co-variation between self-motion and the optic flow field (Gibson, 1966, 1979; Lee, 1978, 1980). Optic flow is a rich source of information for the control of self-motion and its imposition on stationary observers can elicit very powerful postural and emotional reactions. Anyone who has felt their stomach drop while sitting or standing stationary in a simulated space flight or

rollercoaster ride at an amusement park can attest to the powerful effect of optic flow.

Visual proprioception is a widely under-appreciated psychological phenomenon, despite its obvious importance for the control of the postures and movements that are fundamental to the expression of all skilled activity (Anderson et al., 2004). The perception and control of self-motion is not only vitally important for motor skill development but also sensitivity to self-motion appears to play a central role in the development of the *self*—the sense of oneself as a unique entity, distinct from the external surround. The ability to perceive self-motion as distinct from motion of the surround provides the foundation from which the infant begins to differentiate herself from the environment (Neisser, 1988). This notion is particularly relevant to the current discussion, because recent research has shown that an infant's ability to differentiate self-propelled from externally caused motion improves after the onset of crawling (Cicchino and Rakison, 2008). In addition, as we will see later, the ability to differentiate self-movement from externally generated movement has been implicated in a limited sense of agency experienced by children with CP (Ritterband-Rosenbaum et al., 2012).

### The development of visual proprioception

Although the ability to perceive and utilize optic flow has been examined relative to multiple aspects of behaviour (Gilmore et al., 2007; Warren and Wertheim, 1990), the primary focus here is on the development of visual proprioceptive control of head, trunk, and whole-body stability in sitting and standing. The developmental work on the visual proprioceptive control of balance has largely been conducted using the moving room paradigm, or a variant of the paradigm, originally designed by David Lee and colleagues (e.g., Lishman and Lee, 1973). The moving room is a large enclosure that can be moved back and forth relative to a stationary observer (see Fig. 10.1). Responsiveness to optic flow is assessed by measuring the infant's postural sway in relation to movement of the walls.

When looking in the direction of locomotion, the eyes are exposed to different geometrical patterns of optic flow; global optic flow in the entire field of view, radial optic flow (like a starburst pattern) in the central field of view, and lamellar optic

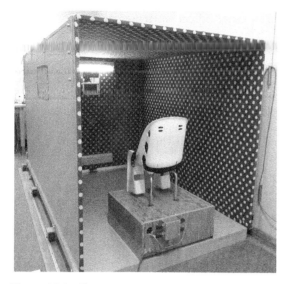

**Figure 10.1** • The moving room. The infant experiences global optic flow when all the walls are moved together, radial optic flow when only the front wall is moved, and lamellar optic flow when only the side walls and ceiling are moved.

flow (like the lines of longitude on a globe) in the periphery of the field (see Fig. 10.2). Stoffregen (1985) has observed that adults show greater postural responsiveness to lamellar optic flow in the periphery (generated by moving only the side walls of the room) than radial optic flow in the centre of the field of view (generated by moving only the front wall). Anyone who has experienced a false perception of self-motion when a train adjacent to the one in which you are sitting starts moving can appreciate the power of peripheral lamellar optic flow in conveying information about self-motion.

## Responsiveness to global optic flow

When infants are exposed to global optic flow (whole room motion) in a moving room the *magnitude* of their postural compensation shows an interesting trajectory—it peaks during the early acquisition of a new posture and then diminishes as the posture comes under greater control only to peak again during the early acquisition of the next posture. For example, Butterworth and Pope (1981) have shown that infants as young as 2 months of age, when seated and provided with support for the trunk, will show postural compensation of the head when the whole room is moved toward them, with the magnitude of

head sway decreasing with age and experience in controlling the head. Similarly, Butterworth and Hicks (1977) have observed that seated infants sway less in response to whole room movement as they gain increasing experience with the standing posture. However, the onset of standing and the onset of walking seem to be times when the infant is particularly responsive to global optic flow. The coupling between whole room motion and postural sway peaks between 9 and 10 months of age, at about the age where infants are just beginning to learn how to stand without support (though, curiously, also at the time they are mastering crawling) (Bertenthal et al., 1997; Delorme et al., 1989). Peaks in responsiveness to whole room movement that coincide with the onset of sitting, the onset of standing, and the onset of walking have been noted (Foster et al., 1996). Other research groups (Lee and Aronson, 1974; Schmuckler and Gibson, 1989; Stoffregen et al., 1987) have reported that the magnitude of the balance disturbance caused by the moving room is much higher in inexperienced walkers than experienced walkers. Newly walking infants are often literally 'bowled over' by the imposed global optic flow.

## Responsiveness to peripheral lamellar optic flow (PLOF)

The development of responsiveness to PLOF provides an example of the role of experience in *functionalizing* visual information for the control of posture. Utilizing the moving room paradigm, it was found that 5-month-old infants were essentially unresponsive to PLOF when exposed to side-wall movement in a moving room (Bertenthal and Bai, 1989). The same lack of responsiveness was reported in 7 month olds (Higgins et al., 1996). In contrast, both studies noted major changes in responsiveness between 7 and 9 months of age, changes that the authors speculated were related to experience with independent mobility. The link between mobility experience and responsiveness to PLOF was subsequently affirmed in a second experiment (Higgins et al., 1996). Eight-month-old infants who were proficient at crawling on hands and knees or moving about in wheeled walkers showed significantly higher postural responsiveness to side-wall motion in the moving room than same-aged infants who were not yet locomoting independently.

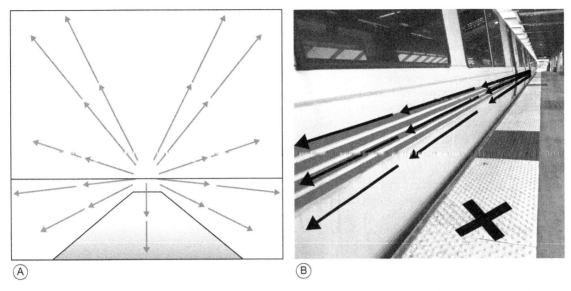

**Figure 10.2 • (A)** A pilot's view of global optic flow experienced during landing an aircraft. The flow emanates from the location to which the pilot is heading. It has a radial structure in the centre of the field of view and an increasingly lamellar structure in the periphery. **(B)** Lamellar optic flow experienced when a train passes a passenger standing on the platform.

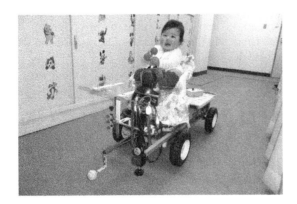

**Figure 10.3 •** The powered mobility device (PMD) used by Uchiyama et al. (2008).

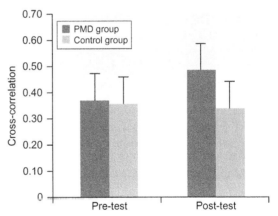

**Figure 10.4 •** Changes in the coupling between side-wall movement in the moving room and postural sway before and after training in a powered mobility device in the Uchiyama et al. (2008) study.

These findings have recently been confirmed and extended using a randomized controlled trial (RCT) (Uchiyama et al., 2008). In the RCT, prelocomotor infants were taught to drive a baby go-cart (powered mobility device [PMD]) by pulling on a joystick mounted at the front of the device (Fig. 10.3). Infants were tested for responsiveness to PLOF before and after 15 days of training. A control group received the same pre- and post-testing, but no training. The findings were remarkably clear—the PMD infants' responsiveness to side-wall motion in the moving room increased significantly as a function of their training, whereas the control group showed no changes in visual–postural coupling at all (Fig. 10.4). Equally importantly, the PMD-trained infants, as well as hands-and-knees crawlers and infants with 'artificial' walker experience who were tested in a preliminary study showed heightened emotional reactions to the imposed optic flow (Uchiyama et al., 2008). The latter findings are important because they suggest that the postural compensation induced by the imposed peripheral optic flow was more meaningful to the infants with locomotor experience than those without locomotor experience. Presumably, the meaningfulness came from the threat to stability that was associated with the imposition of the newly functionalized peripheral optic flow in the locomotor infants but not the prelocomotor infants.

Another interesting finding was the increase in positive emotion (smiling) associated with learning to control the PMD (Uchiyama et al., 2008). The increase in smiling coincided with dramatic increases in the amount of pulling engaged in by the infant, implying that once the joystick had become functionalized as a means to an end (i.e., the infant understood that pulling the joystick caused the PMD to move forward), the infant had a heightened sense of agency—a heightened sense of control of the self relative to the environment.

The consequences of PMD training for prelocomotor infants have been replicated and extended (Dahl et al., 2013). In addition to showing heightened responsiveness to PLOF, PMD-trained infants also displayed greater cardiac indications of wariness of heights when lowered to the deep side of a visual cliff (see Fig. 10.5). This finding is significant for researchers interested in the psychological consequences of motor activity because wariness of heights was one of the first psychological outcomes linked to experience with independent mobility (see Campos, 1976). In other words, the contemporary work on mobility and

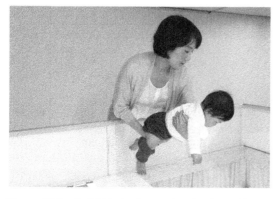

**Figure 10.5 •** A child being lowered to the deep side of the visual cliff in the Dahl et al. (2013) study.

psychological development had its origins in the serendipitous and surprising discovery that infants did not display wariness of heights until they had acquired experience with independent locomotion.

Despite the clear role that locomotor experience has been shown to play in facilitating the use of peripheral optic flow for balance, there is evidence for a precocious competence in the neonate for responding to lamellar optic flow (e.g., Barbu-Roth et al., 2009; Jouen, 1988, 1990; Jouen et al., 2000). For example, Jouen et al. (2000) reported that neonates (3 days old), who were reclined in a specially designed infant seat between two television monitors, showed head retraction to a continuously moving optical pattern. This precocious sensitivity highlights a consistent finding in perceptual development—infants can detect information well before that information is useful for guiding action (Goldfield, 1995). Following Haith (1993), we have referred to perceptual, cognitive, and emotional biases and precocities as *partial accomplishments*. These biases are the rudimentary primitives from which functional skills are constructed. Consequently, locomotor experience appears to play a pivotal role in *functionalizing* these primitives for utilization in the control of skilled behaviour.

## How does mobility experience contribute to changes in visual proprioception?

Though visual proprioception will obviously improve as the visual system's ability to pick up information improves via accommodation, convergence, decreasing thresholds for motion detection, oculomotor co-ordination, and widening of the field of view, locomotion presses the infant to differentiate global, radial, and lamellar optic flow. The press can be understood with respect to the demands placed on the visual system during locomotion. Gibson (1979) has noted that vision serves three important functions in mobility: (1) detecting that the surface supports locomotion; (2) steering through apertures and around obstacles; and (3) maintaining postural stability. Essentially, the individual must concurrently process information about self-motion and attend to the layout of surfaces and objects during locomotion. The newly locomoting infant is pressed to differentiate spatially delimited patterns of optical flow so that the various demands on the visual system can be accomplished successfully and efficiently (Gibson and Schmuckler, 1989). Relegating the control of postural stability to the peripheral field of view frees the central field of view to accomplish the task of surface scanning and steering and to focus on other features of the environment that might be important to secondary tasks that are nested into the primary task of locomotion: noting landmarks, for example.

The overall process by which visual proprioception becomes more finely tuned involves the *education of attention* (Gibson, 1979) to specific patterns of information that are potentially usable for postural control, differentiation of spatially delimited regions of optic flow, and precise mapping, via self-produced experience, of specific patterns of optic flow onto specific neuromuscular control strategies. With experience, functionalization leads to increasing specificity in behaviour over time, which then increases the effectiveness, efficiency, and adaptability of behaviour to the task and to the environment in which it occurs. Because visual proprioception plays such an integral role in balance and because balance is so essential to the development of all skilled interaction with the environment, deficits in visual proprioception can seriously compromise children's skill development. Moreover, given the contribution that visual proprioception makes to the development of a concept of the self and given how important self-awareness is to having a sense of agency, deficits in visual proprioception have serious implications for the child's development of a sense of agency.

## The development of spatial understanding

Locomotion is more than simply organizing a pattern of movement to make forward progression. Functional locomotion requires that the individual has an intimate understanding of the spatial layout and his or her relation to it. In the previous section we noted that visual proprioception provides infants with one of the earliest means to differentiate themselves from the environment because specific patterns of optic flow are associated with their own movements versus movements of objects and surfaces. Improvements in visual proprioception refine the infant's perception of orientation relative to the external surrounds and consequently feed into a deeper appreciation of external space. Optic flow will ultimately be used to gauge heading direction (Banton and Bertenthal, 1997; Gilmore and Rettke, 2003) and judge speed and distance after the onset of independent locomotion (Campos et al., 2000). However, functional locomotion also relies on navigation and memory. Maintaining an orientation to the external layout, knowing where we are going and where we have been, remembering landmarks, and recalling where objects are located or hidden once we have moved are all features of *spatial cognition* (Clearfield, 2004; McKenzie, 1987). The functional independence that comes with locomotion would be very limited indeed without spatial-cognitive skills.

In this section, we describe research on the development of two spatial-cognitive skills that have been linked to mobility experience: manual search for hidden objects and position constancy. The former refers to an ability to find hidden objects from a stationary position, whereas the latter refers to an ability to find objects and places following self-displacement. We then discuss the processes by which locomotor experience may contribute to changes in these important skills.

### Manual search for hidden objects

One of the most puzzling spatial-cognitive phenomena in infancy is the difficulty that infants have in searching correctly for an object hidden in one of two locations. Although infants between 8 and 9 months of age are able to successfully retrieve an object hidden within reach at one location, they often do not succeed when the object is hidden under one of two adjacent locations, even when the locations are perceptually distinct (Bremner, 1978; Piaget, 1954). More curiously, infants at this age will often fail to retrieve a hidden object after it has been moved to a new location, even though they have successfully retrieved it from the old location and they saw it being moved to the new location. Infants will surprisingly perseverate at searching in the old location. The perseverative search is referred to as the *A-not-B error*. The longer the delay imposed in searching for the object when it is hidden in a new place, the poorer the infant's performance (Diamond, 1990).

The A-not-B error gained widespread attention thanks to Piaget (1954), who used it to highlight the importance of action in the child's intellectual development. Piaget (1954) believed that infants made the error, in part, because they coded the positions of objects egocentrically (relative to their own body) rather than allocentrically (relative to each other or to stable environmental features). Contemporary explanations suggest that many factors play a role in the error (Munakata, 1998; Smith et al., 1999). Regardless of the explanation, it is now clear that locomotor experience is related to the infant's overcoming of the error (see Smith et al., 1999).

A number of researchers, including Piaget (1954), have speculated about a link between skill in spatial search and locomotor experience (Acredolo, 1978, 1985; Bremner, 1985; Bremner and Bryant, 1977; Campos et al., 1978). However, Horobin and Acredolo (1986) were the first to test the link. Their results showed clearly that 31–41-week-old infants with greater amounts of locomotor experience were more likely to search successfully at the B location on a series of progressively challenging hiding tasks. These findings were replicated and extended using a similarly challenging series of spatial search tasks (Kermoian and Campos, 1988). The tasks ranged from retrieving an object partially hidden under a single location to the A-not-B task with a seven-second delay between hiding and search. The infants in the study were all 8.5 months of age, but differed in the amount of experience each had with independent mobility; one group was prelocomotor, a second group was prelocomotor but had experience moving in an infant walker, and a third group had experience with hands-and-knees crawling. The results showed clearly that infants with hands-and-knees crawling experience or walker experience significantly outperformed prelocomotor infants on the spatial search tasks. Moreover, search performance improved with greater amounts of locomotor experience. For example, 76% of hands-and-knees crawling and walker infants with nine or more weeks of locomotor experience successfully searched in the B location on the A-not-B test with a three-second delay compared to only 13% of prelocomotor infants.

Of special relevance to the purpose of this chapter are the findings from a third experiment. Infants who were the same age as those tested in experiments 1 and 2 and who had between one and nine weeks of *belly crawling* experience performed like prelocomotor infants on the spatial search tasks. Moreover, no relation between the amount of belly crawling experience and spatial search

performance was found. The differences in spatial search performance between infants with hands-and-knees crawling or walker experience and those with belly crawling experience was attributed to the effort involved in crawling on the belly. Belly crawlers were thought to devote so much effort and attention to organizing prone progression that they were unable to devote attention to processing the perceptual consequences associated with moving through the world. We will discuss the implications of this idea for the motorically disabled child at the end of this section.

These findings have been replicated and extended (Tao and Dong, 1997), using cross-sectional and longitudinal investigations, and taking advantage of ecologically and culturally mediated delays in the onset of independent mobility in urban Chinese infants. Specifically, infants in Beijing who were delayed in locomotion by two to four months relative to North American norms initially performed poorly on the A-not-B test, then improved dramatically as a function of locomotor experience, regardless of the age of onset of locomotion.

Even more pertinent to the current chapter, aspects of these findings have been confirmed in a longitudinal study of seven infants with spina bifida who were delayed in the onset of locomotion relative to typically developing infants (Campos et al., 2009). The infants were tested on a two-position hiding task in which a toy was hidden only in one location, with a second hiding location serving as a distractor. The infant's ability to follow the gaze and point of an experimenter toward an object that was outside their field of view was also tested. Note that an ability to follow the point and gaze, also referred to as *referential gestural communication*, has also been linked to experience with locomotion. The infants were tested monthly after they were recruited into the study until two months after the delayed onset of independent locomotion, which occurred at 10.5 months of age in four of the infants and 8.5, 11.5, and 13.5 months of age in the other three infants. The results revealed dramatic improvement on the task following the onset of locomotion. Infants searched successfully for the hidden object on only 14% of trials while they were prelocomotor, but improved to 64% correct search following delayed onset of locomotion (Fig. 10.6). Similarly, in the referential gestural communication task, the infants were much more likely to look in the correct direction

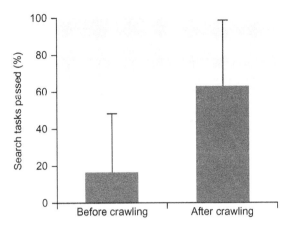

**Figure 10.6** • Changes in spatial search performance following the delayed onset of locomotion in infants with spina bifida in the Campos et al. (2009) study.

of the experimenter's gaze and point and less likely to look at the experimenter, following the delayed onset of locomotion.

## How does locomotor experience contribute to the development of spatial search?

Surprisingly, the processes by which locomotor experience contribute to improvements in spatial search are not well understood, despite the significant degree of attention that has been devoted to understanding the A-not-B error. The need to explain the spatial component of manual search for hidden objects, i.e., where is the object located, as well as the temporal component, i.e., improved tolerance of increasing delays between hiding and search, has added to the challenge of developing viable explanations. We have noted previously (Campos et al., 2000) that at least four different factors seem to underlie changes in search performance: (1) shifts from egocentric to allocentric coding strategies; (2) new attentional strategies and improved discrimination of task-relevant information; (3) improvements in means–ends behaviours and greater tolerance of delays in goal attainment, possibly related to changes in working memory; and (4) refined understanding of others' intentions.

### A shift in coding strategies

The idea that changes in spatial search performance reflect shifts from egocentric to allocentric coding strategies was first proposed by Piaget (1954).

He reasoned that prelocomotor infants could rely on egocentric coding strategies because they interacted with their environment from a stationary position. Thus an object on the left would always be found on the left and an object on the right would always be found on the right. The infant can remember where objects are located on the basis of movements towards those objects, using what has been referred to as *response learning* (Clearfield, 2004). However, egocentric coding strategies are unreliable once the infant starts to locomote because the mobile infant's relation to the environment constantly changes. Allocentric coding strategies, where the locations of objects are coded relative to other objects and places, are much more reliable when one's own relation to the environment constantly changes. We will take this issue up again in the subsequent section on spatial coding.

It is relevant to note that a form of response learning has been implicated in the A-not-B error by those who have taken an embodied cognition approach to explaining the phenomenon (Clearfield et al., 2006; Smith et al., 1999; Thelen et al., 2001). These researchers have argued that the postural set adopted by the infant, as well as the kinematic characteristics of the reaches made during search, contribute significantly to perseveration at the A location. However, it is interesting to note that where postural set has been implicated as a factor in perseverative search (e.g., Smith et al., 1999), others have noted that the infant's spatial relation to the task may be a more important factor (Lew et al., 2007). Regardless of how an infant's tendency to behave egocentrically contributes to performance on the A-not-B error, it is important to note that a shift from egocentric to allocentric responding cannot explain how locomotor experience contributes to improved success on search tasks that do not involve moving an object from one hiding location to another (e.g., Campos et al., 2009).

### New attentional strategies

Locomotor infants are commonly observed to be more attentive and less distractible during spatial search tasks (Campos et al., 2000). Visual attention was first proposed as a mediator between locomotor experience and success on spatial search tasks by Acredolo and colleagues (Acredolo, 1985; Acredolo et al., 1984; Horobin and Acredolo, 1986). Infants who kept an eye on the hiding location were more likely to retrieve the object successfully. Keeping an eye on objects may be a particularly helpful way for a locomotor infant to retrieve those objects after they have moved. Moreover, keeping an eye on objects may also refine an infant's ability to discriminate perceptually relevant information about the self and the environment, through the process of education of attention, which facilitates knowing where one is going and where one has been. Improved spatial discrimination of relevant task features has been proposed as one means by which locomotor experience might contribute to improved performance on the A-not-B task (Smith et al., 1999).

## Improvements in means–ends behaviours and working memory

The explanations for the A-not-B error described thus far have focused on the spatial component of the task. Improvements in means–ends behaviours (e.g., Diamond, 1991) and greater tolerance for delays between initiating a behaviour and completing it have been proposed to account for the temporal component of the error: the finding that errors increase as the delay between hiding and search increases. The logic is that locomotor goals require more time to complete than discrete actions such as reaching, and so the infant must keep the locomotor goal in mind for a longer period of time, taxing working memory. In addition, the means by which locomotor goals are accomplished, through a repeating sequence of intra- and interlimb co-ordination, are more complex than the means involved in organizing discrete movements. Thus, locomotion provides infants with new problems to solve, potentially leading to refinements in problem solving that carry over to other tasks and contexts, and locomotion taxes working memory because it forces the infant to tolerate longer delays in goal attainment. Both factors could explain the locomotor infant's ability to tolerate longer delays between hiding and search on the A-not-B task.

A recent study linking locomotor experience to greater flexibility in memory retrieval is particularly relevant to the locomotor infant's ability to tolerate longer delays in the A-not-B task. Herbert et al. (2007) tested 9-month-old infants, with and without crawling experience, on a deferred imitation task. An experimenter demonstrated an action on a toy and the infants were tested 24 hours later to see if they would perform the same action. Crawlers and pre-crawlers imitated the action when they were given the same toy in the same context in which they were tested (laboratory or home); however, crawlers were significantly more likely than pre-crawlers to imitate the action when the toy and the testing context were different. The authors argued that locomotor experience promotes flexibility in memory retrieval because the locomotor infant has abundant opportunities to deploy their memories in novel situations. Given that locomotion has been linked to long-term memory, it is not unreasonable to think that locomotion might also contribute to changes in working memory, with such changes subsequently contributing to greater tolerance of delays in hide-and-seek tasks. Reported correlations between motor ability and working memory in school-aged children (Piek et al., 2008) add further support to the idea that locomotor experience might contribute to working memory development.

## Improved understanding of others' intentions

Improvement in understanding others' intentions is the final process by which locomotion could contribute to success on spatial search tasks. We have already noted that locomotor infants are more attentive and less distractible during search tasks. However, they also appear to search for communicative signals from the experimenter. This search is likely related to their ability to follow the referential gestural communication of an experimenter (e.g., Campos et al., 2009) and increased distal communication with the parent after the onset of locomotion (Campos et al., 2000). The importance of social communication in the A-not-B error has recently been highlighted by an experiment showing that perseverative search errors are considerably reduced when communication between the experimenter and infant is minimized (Topál et al., 2008). The burgeoning literature on the link between action production and action understanding (e.g., Sommerville and Woodward, 2010) is also relevant to the potential mediating role of understanding others' intentions in locomotor infants' ability to solve spatial search problems. This literature suggests that an infant's understanding of other people's actions as being goal-directed is a function of their own action experience. Consequently, experience with self-generated actions should contribute to understanding the intentions of others.

## Position constancy

Position constancy refers to an ability to find an object or location despite a shift in one's spatial relation to that object or location. It presupposes basic skill in spatial search, because without such skill position constancy would be impossible. Position constancy is of great importance to neurologists, who find different neurological mechanisms underlying different strategies to attain position constancy, and to developmentalists, who see in position constancy a window into the development of spatial cognition. The ability to relocate objects and places following self-displacement is a necessity for mobile organisms. An animal that cannot relocate places where food is stored, where shelter is available, or where predators lurk, will likely have a short lifespan, indeed. Position constancy is essential to navigation, a much broader component of spatial cognition and one to which we will return at the end of the chapter. Neurologists are particularly interested in the brain processes that support navigation and they have provided convincing evidence that experience with navigation contributes to structural changes in the brain. For example, London taxi drivers, who are held to some of the most rigorous standards in the world relative to knowing their city, have greater grey matter volume in the mid-posterior hippocampi, a brain structure well-known to be involved in navigation. Moreover, greater driving experience is associated with greater posterior hippocampal grey matter volume (Maguire et al., 2000, 2006). So, the need to know a complex environment places highly specific demands on the brain structures that support navigation and leads to measurable changes in those structures.

### Attentiveness to far space may contribute to position constancy

Greater attentiveness to far space may be one of the precursors to position constancy in the locomotor infant. Locomotor infants will attend to far space during the course of locomotion to a destination, but locomotor infants also show a general attentiveness to far space relative to prelocomotor infants. Gustafson (1984) reported that prelocomotor infants were far less likely to attend to objects, people, and room features in far space when placed on the floor than when placed in an upright position in an infant walker. In addition,

the extent to which prelocomotor infants attended to far space while in the walker was no different to the extent that hands-and-knees crawlers attended to far space. Freedman (1992) reported similar findings. Infants with locomotor experience, whether via a walker or hands-and-knees crawling, deployed their attention to far space differently than prelocomotors. The locomotor infants looked at specific objects in the room when attending to far space, whereas the prelocomotor infants tended to look at nothing in particular. In addition, the locomotor infants looked toward far space more often while manipulating toys in near space than the prelocomotors. Parental reports provide additional evidence that infants shift their attention to far space more often after the onset of independent locomotion. An interview study showed that parents of locomotor infants were much more likely to report that their infants attended to distal events than were parents of prelocomotor infants (Campos et al., 1992).

Refinements in visual proprioception after the onset of independent locomotion should also contribute to the infant's ability to keep track of her orientation to the environment because optic flow patterns contain information about heading direction in addition to information about speed of locomotion and postural stability (Gilmore and Rettke, 2003). However, infants must also learn to detect and utilize other sources of information about the self and the environment to navigate successfully. In the previous section, a shift from egocentric to allocentric coding strategies was proposed as an explanation for improvements in performance on the A-not-B task. The same shift, though in a more advanced form, can account for improvements in spatial coding.

### Strategies underlying position constancy

Two types of egocentric, or self-referenced, strategies are available to the infant during locomotion: *response learning* and *dead reckoning* (Clearfield, 2004). Response learning, which has already been implicated in A-not-B performance, involves remembering a sequence of movements, such as turn left, then right and then left again, to get to a destination. It works well when the infant always starts in the same position relative to the target, but it fails when the infant's relation to the environment changes. For example, it could not be used to return from the target location to the start position. Dead reckoning is a more complicated self-referenced strategy. It involves continuously updating position by keeping track of the distance and direction of movements. Dead reckoning skills are not likely to emerge until after the child has had considerable experience with locomotion (Acredolo, 1978) and, even then, such skills are only likely to be used for short distances.

Two types of allocentric, or environment-referenced (ER), strategies are also available to the infant during locomotion: *cue learning*, where an association is learned between a location and a stable landmark, and *place learning*, where a location is specified by noting its spatial relation (direction and distance) between two or more stable landmarks (Clearfield, 2004). The landmarks are used to triangulate the position of the location. Clearly, then, place learning is more complicated than cue learning.

Even though infants are capable of using ER spatial coding strategies to some degree before the onset of independent locomotion, several authors have proposed, or implied, that locomotor experience should facilitate the use of such strategies (e.g., Acredolo, 1978, 1995; Bremner, 1993; Bremner and Bryant, 1977; Lepecq, 1990; Piaget, 1954). Campos et al. (2000) have noted that precocious ER strategies are likely to be used under the following conditions: (1) landmarks are very close to the searched-for object or location; (2) the landmarks are salient; (3) infants are tested in a familiar environment; and (4) no training trials are used during the initial localization of the target to prevent the development of response learning. Locomotion appears to create contexts in which ER strategies must be utilized in increasingly complex ways.

## Locomotion and the development of ER strategies

One of the first studies linking locomotor experience to increased use of ER strategies was conducted by Enderby (1984), who tested three groups of 36-week-old infants in a paradigm developed by Acredolo (1978). One group of infants was prelocomotor, another had at least three weeks of locomotor experience, and the third was prelocomotor but had at least 40 hours of walker experience. The infants were tested in a curtained enclosure that had a window on either side of the infant. One window was marked with salient landmarks consisting of flashing lights, bright stripes, and a blue star on the wall next to

the window. The infants first learned to anticipate the appearance of an experimenter at one of the windows five seconds after a buzzer sounded. The test trials began after the infant had correctly anticipated the appearance of the experimenter on four out of five trials. Immediately after the criterion had been reached, the infant was translated forward a short distance and rotated 180 degrees to face the other side of the enclosure. The buzzer was sounded, though the experimenter did not appear at the window, and the infant's initial direction of looking was recorded.

The locomotor infants in Enderby's study showed significantly better position constancy than the prelocomotor infants. Locomotor infants correctly anticipated the window at which the experimenter should have appeared on 40% of the test trials, whereas prelocomotor infants correctly anticipated on only 15% of test trials. Infants with walker experience correctly anticipated the experimenter's appearance on 35% of trials. These findings were replicated by Bertenthal et al. (1984), though correct anticipation on the test trials was significantly higher in all groups: 74% of trials for locomotor infants, 56% of trials for prelocomotor infants, and 95% of trials for infants with walker experience. The authors reported a longitudinal case study of an infant with an orthopaedic handicap who performed poorly on the test trials until a heavy cast was removed from the leg and the infant achieved a relatively late onset of independent locomotion. Taken together, the findings from these three studies provide strong evidence that locomotor experience plays a role in the development and deployment of more sophisticated ER strategies in the localization of places.

Bai and Bertenthal (1992) adapted a paradigm developed by Bremner (1978) to further examine the link between locomotor experience and ER localization strategies. Three groups of 33-week-old infants were tested. One group was prelocomotor, one group had 2.7 weeks of belly crawling experience, and one group had 7.2 weeks of hands-and-knees crawling experience. The task was a hide-and-seek task in which an object was hidden under one of two different coloured cups that were placed side by side in front of the infant. Prior to searching for the object, the infant was rotated 180 degrees around the other side of the table on which the cups were placed or the table was rotated 180 degrees. The position of the cups relative to the infant changed as a consequence of both types of rotation. The data from the first trial showed a particularly strong effect of locomotor experience. Infants with hands-and-knees crawling experience successfully retrieved the object on 72% of trials following rotation to the other side of the table compared to a 25% success rate for the prelocomotors. As in Kermoian and Campos's (1988) spatial search experiment, the belly crawlers in Bai and Bertenthal's study performed liked prelocomotors, searching successfully on only 30% of trials. Notably, the groups did not differ on their search performance when the table was rotated, probably because this type of displacement is rarely experienced by any infant, regardless of locomotor experience.

A completely different paradigm was developed by Clearfield (2004) to study the link between locomotor experience and the use of ER strategies in 8-, 11-, and 14-month-old infants. The 8-month-old infants were novice crawlers, the 11-month-old infants were experienced crawlers, and the 14-month-old infants were novice walkers. The paradigm was an adaptation of the classic Morris water maze task used to study spatial memory in rats. Infants were first taught to locate the position of their mother who stood on the outside of a 2 ft high and 10 ft in diameter octagonal enclosure. The infant was carried to the mother and then turned away from the mother and placed in front of another wall of the enclosure. The infants' task was to find their way back to the mother. In the test trials, the mother ducked behind the barrier when the infant was turned away from her. Several distal landmarks were available immediately beyond the enclosure to help code the mother's position, including four video cameras, a bright orange flag that hung from one of the cameras, and a cluster of three shiny lights.

The results of Clearfield's (2004) first experiment showed a clear effect of locomotor experience on search performance. All infants with less than six weeks of locomotor experience, whether crawling or walking, were unable to find the mother on the test trials. In contrast, a step-function improvement in successful search was seen in infants with more than six weeks of locomotor experience. Interestingly, the novice walkers did not seem to profit from their previous crawling experience when attempting to locate the mothers from their new walking posture. Novice and expert crawlers and walkers were tested with

a direct landmark in a second experiment. The landmark was a large quilting ring covered with fluorescent green fabric with brightly coloured bugs on it and glittery stars. The landmark was on a curtain immediately behind the mother and just above her head. Again, a clear effect of locomotor experience was found. Novice crawlers and walkers with less than six weeks of locomotor experience could not find their mother, whereas those with more than six weeks of locomotor experience were much more successful.

### How does locomotor experience contribute to the development of position constancy?

The explanation for the role of locomotor experience in the development of position constancy is straightforward. As noted in the introduction to this section, egocentric coding strategies are much less effective once one becomes mobile. With locomotion, an object that once was in front of the infant can now be adjacent to, or even behind the child. If the locomotion also involves a rotational component, an object to the left can wind up on the right; an object to the right can subsequently be on the left. Because locomotor experience complicates a simple egocentric search strategy, the newly locomotor infant experiences a pressure to use a search strategy that links the position of an object to stable environmental landmarks, rather than to her body. For this reason infants with locomotor experience are more likely to invoke an allocentric, landmark-based, coding strategy in spatial search, and the use of landmarks will make position constancy more likely. Note that the use of landmark-based coding strategies represents a much deeper appreciation of external space and the relations among the features that occupy external space. That appreciation must feed into higher intellectual processes involved with imagining, thinking, planning, problem solving, and remembering.

## Mobility and psychological development: implications for infants with disabilities

It is now clear that independent mobility makes a pivotal contribution to psychological development. The previous sections have provided a sampling of the evidence linking locomotor experience to one aspect of psychological development, spatial-cognitive development, and discussed the processes by which locomotion might contribute to specific psychological changes. A better understanding of the processes by which locomotion facilitates psychological change can provide insights into alternative developmental pathways that therapists might exploit to promote psychological change when independent locomotion might be severely delayed or impossible to acquire. The consequences of independent mobility are, however, much broader than those that have been outlined so far. In the final section of this chapter, we focus on the implications that the link between locomotor experience and psychological development has for children with motor disabilities that impede independent mobility. We have already noted that infants who are delayed in the onset of locomotion for neurological or orthopaedic reasons have also been shown to be delayed in the development of spatial-cognitive skills. In addition, we have noted that infants who engage in effortful forms of locomotion, like belly crawling, do not appear to profit, in terms of psychological consequences, from their locomotor experience. We suspect that at least some of the cognitive deficits that have been noted in older children and adults with motor disabilities might be attributable to a lack of locomotor experience or delays in locomotor experience, particularly if those delays straddle critical periods in the development of the psychological skills in question.

## Spatial-cognitive deficits in individuals with motoric disabilities

The idea that motoric limitations might contribute to limitations in perceptual and spatial-cognitive functioning in some children with motoric disabilities is not new (e.g., Abercrombie, 1964, 1968; Kershner, 1974). Limited evidence currently exists, however, to support the idea, particularly as it pertains to children with CP and, as noted much earlier, the current model in developmental paediatrics does not stress the importance of psychological development in children with disabilities. A major problem with accepting a role for motoric factors in the psychological development of children with physical disabilities has been the difficulty associated with separating the role of brain damage from that of activity

limitation in any psychological deficits that are discovered. Brain damage is often the cause of the primary motor impairments seen in children with physical disabilities (clearly so in the case of CP) and that same damage is obviously implicated in any co-occurring spatial-cognitive deficits.

Despite this problem, there seems to be growing sympathy for a potential role for motoric limitations in the psychological delays and deficits seen in children with CP. This sympathy is associated with the new consensus that CP is much more than a disruption in posture and movement. CP is now defined as a multifaceted condition, with disturbances in sensory-motor coupling, perception, cognition, executive functioning, communication, and behaviour, along with the associated problems of epilepsy and secondary musculoskeletal deficits, accompanying the primary motor limitations (Bax et al., 2005). Although it is well established that 23–44% of children with CP possess intellectual deficits (Odding et al., 2006), the addition of *alternative disturbances* into the definition has sparked greater interest in those deficits.

## Specific psychological issues seen in children with CP

Some excellent reviews of the psychological problems experienced by children with CP have recently been published (Bax et al., 2005; Bjorgaas et al., 2012; Bottcher, 2010; Parkes et al., 2008; Pirilä and van der Meere, 2010; Straub and Obrzut, 2009). These reviews have highlighted that some of the most commonly impaired skills (i.e., in visual perception in spatial cognition, in memory, and in attention) are the same skills that have been linked to experience with self-produced locomotion in typically developing infants. Specific components of these skills emerge during early infancy, show dramatic spurts following the onset of independent locomotion, and continue to develop well into the school years. An intriguing aspect of the psychological deficits observed in children with CP is that similar deficits are found in children with other motor disabilities such as myelomeningocele (MMC). For example, cognitive attentional problems like orienting to and disengaging from stimuli are found in CP and MMC (Dennis et al., 2005; Schatz et al., 2001) and visual attention, visual mapping, and mathematical reasoning are spatial-cognitive abilities with known dysfunction in both populations (Dennis et al., 2006; Pirilä and van der Meere, 2010; Straub and Obrzut, 2009; Taylor et al., 2010). As MMC involves entirely separate CNS disruption than that seen in CP, it is difficult to see how the deficits could result entirely from damage to specifically localized brain regions, as is commonly assumed by many who have uncovered these deficits (Bottcher, 2010 provides an excellent discussion of this assumption).

While cortical damage clearly does play a role in the psychological deficits experienced by children with CP, there is growing recognition that diminished early and ongoing spatial exploratory experiences may also play a role. For example, as noted earlier in the chapter, Dalvand et al. (2012) have argued that the significant relation between motor and intellectual function observed in children with CP can be partially explained by a lack of mobility-generated sensory data to the brain regions involved in the control of motor and cognitive functions. Similarly, Ploughman (2008) has argued that the reduction in physical activity associated with motor disability has a detrimental effect on learning and memory. While we must be cognizant of the contributions that brain areas once thought to play an exclusive role in motor control are now recognized to play in cognitive function, it is time to seriously consider the idea that impoverished motor activity might play an independent role in some of the psychological deficits seen in children with physical disabilities. In addition, it is time to consider the highly likely possibility that impoverished motor activity exacerbates some of the psychological deficits attributable to motor-independent brain damage. With that idea in mind, in the final section of the chapter, we will highlight some of the growing evidence that supports the importance of spatial exploratory experiences in the development of a spatial skill that has enormous implications for functional independence in children with physical disabilities—navigation. Moreover, navigation has major implications for participation and socialization in the wider world. Such participation is dramatically curtailed when individuals have difficulties finding their way from place to place.

## The role of limited exploratory experience and agency in navigation deficits

One of the first studies to examine the effects of limited exploration on the development of navigation skills was conducted by Simms (1987). Earlier in the chapter we discussed the shift from egocentric to ER (landmark)-based coding that accompanies the shift to independent locomotion in typically developing children. The development of spatial coding does not end, however, once the child has acquired the ability to use landmarks. Rather, it continues to develop as children learn routes to target locations and ultimately learn to integrate routes and landmarks into an overall representation of the environment (Piaget and Inhelder, 1948; Siegel and White, 1975). In Simms's (1987) study, nine young adults with spina bifida and nine able-bodied controls had to learn routes while being driven through a traffic-free road system and a busy village. Compared to the able-bodied controls, the young people with spina bifida took significantly longer to learn a route, noticed fewer landmarks, were less able to mark routes on a map, and produced poorer hand-drawn maps. Notably, the participants' level of mobility was linked to spatial skill, with walkers performing better than wheelchair users.

Nigel Foreman has been one of the most vocal proponents of the idea that motoric limitations can have a negative impact on spatial-cognitive skills such as those involved in locomotion. For example, with colleagues he studied spatial awareness in 10 children with physical disabilities that restricted independent mobility (Foreman et al., 1989). Compared with age-matched classmates, the children with disabilities were significantly poorer at drawing maps of their classrooms, placing objects on classroom maps, and pointing toward distant landmarks on the school campus. Importantly, the children with disabilities showed deficiencies in spatial awareness, regardless of whether or not they had brain damage. Foreman argued that the deficiencies probably resulted from the lack of active decision making associated with the children frequently receiving assistance to move from place to place.

Subsequent studies provided evidence to support Foreman's assertion about the importance of agency in the development of spatial awareness. In two experiments, 4- to 6-year-old children were tested on their ability to retrieve objects that were strategically positioned within a large room (Foreman et al., 1990). The children were first familiarized with the object positions in one of four locomotor conditions: (1) independently walking between positions; (2) walking but being led by an experimenter; (3) passively transported in a wheelchair; or (4) passively transported in a wheelchair while directing the experimenter where to go. The results showed that children who walked independently or directed the experimenter while being pushed in the wheelchair performed most successfully on the task. Thus, agency, regardless of how it was exercised, was the crucial determinant of spatial search performance following navigation through the room. A considerable body of research with typically developing children now shows that active locomotion facilitates spatial search performance (Yan et al., 1998)

A further study suggested that a critical period may exist in the development of some types of spatial competence (Stanton et al., 2002). Thirty-four physically disabled teenagers (with a mean age of 14.1 years) who were all capable of independent locomotion were compared to 24 age-matched able-bodied teenagers in their ability to learn a route in a computer-simulated maze. Though both groups were able to learn the route, the physically disabled teenagers had more difficulties than their able-bodied peers choosing correct short-cuts, indicating that they had not learned the spatial layout of the maze as thoroughly. Moreover, the performance of disabled participants whose mobility was impaired earlier in development was poorer than that of teenagers whose mobility became impaired later in childhood. Stanton et al. (2002) argued that early impairments to locomotion had a more deleterious and longer lasting effect on spatial learning because children missed a window of opportunity for learning about important spatial relations. This hypothesis deserves much closer scrutiny because it clearly has enormous implications for when interventions to improve locomotion and spatial competence should be started. How the timing of experience influences the extent to which the consequences of self-produced activity have enduring effects represents one of the largest gaps in our understanding of the relation between motor activity and psychological development.

Building on earlier work, Wiedenbauer and Jansen-Osmann (2006) recently confirmed that children with physical disabilities have difficulties acquiring spatial knowledge related to navigation. Eighteen children with spina bifida and 18 healthy controls, matched in terms of age (mean = 11.5 years), sex, and verbal IQ, were compared on their ability to learn a route through a maze in a virtual environment. A joystick enabled the participants to 'walk' through the maze. The results were very clear: children with spina bifida took significantly longer to learn the route and once the route had been learned made more errors on a test trial in which landmarks had been removed from the maze. However, even though the children with spina bifida recalled fewer landmarks and identified fewer landmarks at their correct location than the healthy controls, these differences were not significant.

Wiedenbauer and Jansen-Osmann (2006) highlighted the specificity in the spatial deficits seen in children with spina bifida. Route learning, a behavioural-based measure of spatial understanding, was compromised, whereas memory for landmarks was not. The performance on the test trial without landmarks suggested that the children with spina bifida were dependent on the landmarks for navigation, while their healthy peers seemed to utilize a more refined understanding of the spatial configuration of the entire environment. In other words, children with spina bifida used landmark-based spatial coding strategies that were more consistent with those employed by younger children. Consistent with Stanton et al. (2002), the authors argued that the deficits in spatial knowledge seen in the children with spina bifida were likely the result of restricted early spatial experiences resulting from the children's physical disabilities.

Similar conclusions about the importance of early spatial experiences for the development of navigation skills in children with CP were reached by Pavlova et al. (2007). Fourteen adolescents (13–16 years of age), who were born prematurely and had periventricular leukomalacia (PVL) with leg-dominated bilateral spastic CP, were compared to eight same-aged children who were born prematurely but with no brain damage, and eight same-aged children who were born at term and also had no brain damage, on the labyrinth test from the Wechsler Intelligence Scale for Children. The participants had to find their way out of the centre of a two-dimension maze presented on a piece of paper. The adolescents with PVL performed much more poorly on the labyrinth task than the two control groups but no more poorly on a visual attention task or tasks designed to measure perceptual organization (picture completion, event arrangement, block design, and object assembly). These findings further underscore the specificity of the effects of physical disability on spatial competence.

Moreover, Pavlova et al. (2007) found a significant relation between performance on the labyrinth test and the severity of functional motor impairment of the lower extremities but not the upper extremities. The relation was not, however, a function of brain damage to the same areas subserving lower limb control and navigation skill. When motor disability and the extent of right frontal PVL were entered into a step-wise multiple regression analysis, motor disability was entered first and explained a significant percentage of the variance (49%) in navigation skill. The extent of right frontal PVL was entered second and explained a further 25% of variance. Thus, the severity of motor disability and the severity of brain damage made independent contributions to task performance. Again, consistent with previous researchers, the authors concluded that the normal development of skill in visual navigation was prevented by the diminished active spatial exploration associated with impaired lower limb function.

## A final note on agency

Two recent studies provide further evidence that spatial understanding in children with CP might be compromised by a limited sense of agency. Ritterband-Rosenbaum et al. (2011) showed that children with spastic CP had significantly larger problems than healthy children in determining whether an observed movement was caused by themselves or a computer. The task required participants to use a stylus to make aiming movements on a digitizer pad. The participant's arm was blocked from view by a horizontal board, so that the only feedback they received on their movement was from the movement trace displayed on a monitor in front of them. A computer program randomly displaced the traces by 10 or 15 degrees and the participants were required to specify at the end of each trial whether they or the computer had made the movement. The sense of agency disappears when there is a discrepancy between the intended and actual sensory consequences associated with an action.

Ritterband-Rosenbaum et al.'s (2011) findings were confirmed in a follow-up study on two groups of children with CP (Ritterband-Rosenbaum et al., 2012). One group ($n = 20$, mean age = 11.1 years) was given 20 weeks of training on a web-based training program for CP children (Move It to Improve It), designed to improve cognitive,

perceptual, and motor abilities (Bilde et al., 2011), whereas the other group ($n = 20$, mean age = 12.0 years) continued with their regular daily routine. The training led to significant improvements in the children's ability to determine whether the movements they observed on the monitor had been made by themselves or the computer. The authors attributed the improvements in performance to a heightened sense of agency that resulted from a strengthening of sensory–motor interactions during the training. These findings are important for at least two reasons: first, they highlight the deficits in agency experienced by children with CP, and second, they show that novel interventions are already available to help improve the child's sense of agency. Presumably, the benefits of these interventions generalize beyond the items that are targeted for training and the contexts in which training occurs, though this is clearly an issue for future research to confirm.

# Conclusions and future directions

Humans play an active role in their own development, such that the quality of interactions with the environment will have a profound impact on developmental outcomes. This notion is particularly apparent in the remarkably broad range of psychological changes that follow the onset of independent mobility. It is now patently clear that locomotion serves to orchestrate many of these changes. What, then, are the implications for children with motoric disabilities like CP? Evidence is mounting that children with CP suffer a range of psychological problems in addition to their obvious motor limitations. To what extent these problems are consequences of motor limitations or exacerbated by such limitations is unclear at this point. However, it is noteworthy that many of the psychological skills that improve dramatically after the onset of independent mobility in typically developing infants are the same skills that prove to be problematic in children with CP. This intriguing link between the facilitation of psychological skills seen after the onset of locomotion in typically developing infants and the depression of such skills in children with impaired mobility deserves much closer scrutiny.

Further attention is warranted on the ecology within which the young child with CP acquires locomotion (see Chapter 9). Even though the majority of children with CP will develop some form of independent mobility, locomotion is often much more effortful than it is for typically developing children, making it much more difficult to profit from the experiences associated with locomotion. Moreover, the contexts in which locomotion is acquired are quite different for the child with CP than for the typically developing child. A child ambulating with the physical therapist in the gym is not required to *pay attention* to the environment in the same way as a typically developing child because the environment is typically kept stationary and free of hazards. In addition, attentional focus is often directed on the extremities or on posture ('keep your back straight', or 'heel first') rather than on environmental features. Therefore, children with disabilities often lack an essential aspect of natural mobility when they are learning to ambulate, circumstances that encourage the processing of self-motion relative to environmental features. Therapists must keep in mind when they are designing interventions to promote independent mobility that functional locomotion taxes perceptual, spatial-cognitive, attentional, and working memory skills. Ironically, many of these skills are consequences of locomotion itself. Effective interventions should provide systematically increasing challenges to information processing and planning during locomotion in addition to working on the neural and musculoskeletal structures that support balance and forward progression. This idea is taken up again in Chapter 10, where suggestions are given for how to improve the ecological validity of treadmill training interventions for infants with disabilities.

The therapist should also pay close attention to the social context in which motor skills are acquired and the facilitatory effect that motor development has on social and emotional development. Social interaction is often the goal of locomotion; whether crawling or walking toward a caregiver, or to show their new toy to a friend, the end results of locomotor efforts are socially mediated. Socio-emotional development is an area that we have neglected entirely in this chapter, yet a comprehensive European survey of 8- to 12-year-old children ($n = 818$) with CP reported that the most frequent problems found in the sample were peer relationships, hyperactivity, and emotional issues (Parkes et al., 2008). Lack of mobility and disordered movement, particularly where speech and communication are involved, can have a profound effect on the opportunities that are available for developing social skills. Moreover, considerable evidence with typically developing infants has linked socio-emotional development to experience with self-produced locomotion (Campos et al., 2000). Recent work in our laboratory has also linked the onset of walking to a major spurt in productive and receptive language (Walle and Campos, unpublished), suggesting that upright locomotion creates social contexts that promote language development. This finding has major implications for children with CP whose speech and locomotion are compromised.

Finally, the wise therapist will be cognizant of the presence of alternative developmental pathways during ontogenesis. Alternative pathways have been implicated in the apparently normal development of Piagetian sensorimotor skills thought to require manual and locomotor exploration in children whose mothers had taken thalidomide. These infants were able to acquire functionally equivalent skills by using their feet, heads, mouths, and orthopaedic appliances to acquire the motoric experiences they otherwise lacked (Decarie, 1969; Kopp and Shaperman, 1973). Thus, children who are unable to locomote, or who can only locomote with great effort, might be able to acquire certain psychological skills via non-locomotor means. This finding does not downplay the importance of locomotion in psychological development, because locomotion is still the most common means by which many psychological skills are dramatically reorganized, thus providing one more reason to develop effective training and exercise programmes for young infants with disabilities. The finding does highlight, however, that crawling or walking per se are not the driving forces behind psychological change. Rather, it is the experiences that stem from independent mobility and agency that have the catalysing effect on psychological development. As noted already, innovative efforts are already underway to explore ways in which non-locomotor interventions can be used to facilitate psychological development in children with physical disabilities (see also Akhutina et al., 2003). We applaud these efforts and hope they continue. We also call on researchers to take up the challenge of identifying how motoric limitations might influence psychological development during infancy and beyond and to address whether critical periods exist in the development of the psychological skills in question. Tremendous scope exists in this area for making a major contribution to our understanding of child development and for changing the face of clinical practice.

# References

Abercrombie, M.L.J. 1964. Perceptual and Visuomotor Disorders in Cerebral Palsy: A Review of the Literature. Spastics Society/ Heinemann, London.

Abercrombie, M.L.J., 1968. Some notes of spatial disability: movement intelligence quotient and attentiveness. Dev. Med. Child Neurol. 10, 206–213.

Acredolo, C., 1995. Intuition and gist. Special issue: a symposium on fuzzy-trace theory. Learn. Individ. Differ. 7 (2), 83–86.

Acredolo, L.P., 1978. Development of spatial orientation in infancy. Dev. Psychol. 14 (3), 224–234.

Acredolo, L.P., 1985. Coordinating perspectives on infant spatial orientation. In: Cohen, R. (Ed.), The Development of Spatial Cognition. LEA, Hillsdale, NJ, pp. 115–140.

Acredolo, L.P., Adams, A., Goodwyn, S.W., 1984. The role of self-produced movement and visual tracking in infant spatial orientation. J. Exp. Child Psychol. 38 (2), 312–327.

Adolph, K.E., Vereijken, B., Denny, M.A., 1998. Learning to crawl. Child Dev. 69 (5), 1299–1312.

Akhutina, T., Foreman, N., Krichevets, A., Matikka, L., Narhi, V., Pylaeva, N., et al., 2003. Improving spatial functioning in children with cerebral palsy using computerized and traditional game tasks. Disabil. Rehabil. 25 (24), 1361–1371.

Anderson, D.I., Campos, J.J., Barbu-Roth, M.A., 2004. A developmental perspective on visual proprioception. In: Bremner, G., Slater, A. (Eds.), Theories of Infant Development. Blackwell Publishing Ltd., Malden, MA, pp. 30–69.

Bai, D.L., Bertenthal, B.I., 1992. Locomotor status and the development of spatial search skills. Child Dev. 63, 215–226.

Banton, T., Bertenthal, B.I., 1997. Multiple developmental pathways for motion processing. Optom. Vis. Sci. 74, 751–760.

Barbu-Roth, M., Anderson, D.I., Despre, A., Provasi, J., Cabrol, D., Campos, J.J., 2009. Neonatal stepping in relation to terrestrial optic flow. Child Dev. 80 (1), 8–14.

Bax, M., Goldstein, M., Rosenbaum, P., Leviton, A., Paneth, N., 2005. Proposed definition and classification of cerebral palsy, April 2005: introduction. Dev. Med. Child. Neurol. 47, 571–576.

Bell, M.A., Fox, N.A., 1997. Individual differences in object permanence performance at 8 months: locomotor experience and brain electrical activity. Dev. Psychobiol. 31, 287–297.

Bertenthal, B.I., Bai, D.L., 1989. Infants' sensitivity to optic flow for controlling posture. Dev. Psychol. 25, 936–945.

Bertenthal, B.I., Campos, J.J., 1990. A systems approach to the organizing effects of self-produced locomotion during infancy In: Rovee-Collier, C. Lipsitt, L. (Eds.), Advances in Infancy Research, Vol. 6. Ablex, Norwood, NJ, pp. 1–60.

Bertenthal, B.I., Campos, J.J., Barrett, K., 1984. Self-produced locomotion: an organizer of emotional, cognitive, and social development in infancy. In: Emde, R., Harmon, R. (Eds.), Continuities and Discontinuities in Development. Plenum Press, New York, pp. 175–210.

Bertenthal, B.I., Rose, J.L., Bai, D.L., 1997. Perception–action coupling in the development of visual control of posture. J. Exp. Psychol. Hum. Percept. Perform. 23, 1631–1643.

Bidell, T.R., Fischer, K.W., 1997. Between nature and nurture: the role of human agency in the epigenesist of intelligence. In: Sternberg, R.J., Grigorenko, E. (Eds.), Intelligence, Heredity, and Environment. Cambridge University Press, Cambridge.

Bilde, P.E., Kliim-Due, M., Rasmussen, B., Petersen, L.Z., Petersen, T.H., Nielsen, J.B., 2011. Individualized, home-based interactive training of cerebral palsy children delivered through the Internet. BMC Neurol., 11.

Bjorgaas, H.M., Hysing, M., Elgen, I., 2012. Psychiatric disorders among children with cerebral palsy at school starting age. Res. Dev. Disabil. 33, 1287–1293.

Bottcher, L., 2010. Children with spastic cerebral palsy, their cognitive functioning and social participation: a review. Child Neuropsychol. 16, 209–228.

Bremner, J.G., 1978. Egocentric versus allocentric spatial coding in 9-month-old infants: factors influencing the choice of code. Dev. Psychol. 14, 346–355.

Bremner, J.G., 1985. Object tracking and search in infancy: a review of data and a theoretical evaluation. Dev. Rev. 5 (4), 371–396.

Bremner, J.G., 1993. Motor abilities as causal agents in infant cognitive development. In: Savelsbergh, G.J.P. (Ed.), The Development of Coordination in Infancy. Elsevier Science Publishers B. V., Amsterdam, Netherlands, pp. 47–77.

Bremner, J.G., Bryant, P.E., 1977. Place versus response as the basis of spatial errors made by young infants. J. Exp. Child Psychol. 23, 162–171.

Butterworth, G., Hicks, L., 1977. Visual proprioception and postural stability in infancy: a developmental study. Perception 6 (3), 255–262.

Butterworth, G., Pope, M., 1981. Origine et fonction de la proprioception visuelle chez l'enfant. In: de Schonen, S. (Ed.), Le Développement Dans La Première Année. Presses Universitaires de France, Paris, pp. 107–128.

Campos, J.J., 1976. Heart rate: a sensitive tool for the study of emotional development in the infant.

In: Lipsitt, L. (Ed.), Developmental Psychobiology: The Significance of Infancy. Lawrence Erlbaum Associates, Hillsdale, NY, pp. 1–31.

Campos, J.J., Hiatt, S., Ramsay, D., Henderson, C., Svejda, M., 1978. The emergence of fear on the visual cliff. In: Lewis, M., Rosenblum, L. (Eds.), The Origins of Affect. Plenum Press, New York, pp. 149–182.

Campos, J.J., Svejda, M.J., Campos, R.G., Bertenthal, B., 1982. The emergence of self-produced locomotion: its importance for psychological development in infancy. In: Bricker, D.O. (Ed.), Intervention with At-Risk and Handicapped Infants: From Research to Application. University Park Press, Baltimore, pp. 195–216.

Campos, J.J., Bertenthal, B.I., Kermoian, R., 1992. Early experience and emotional development: the emergence of wariness of heights. Psychol. Sci. 3, 61–64.

Campos, J.J., Anderson, D.I., Barbu-Roth, M.A., Hubbard, E.M., Hertenstein, M.J., Witherington, D., 2000. Travel broadens the mind. Infancy 1, 149–219.

Campos, J.J., Anderson, D.I., Telzrow, R., 2009. Locomotor experience influences the spatial cognitive development of infants with spina bifida. Zeitschrift für Entwicklungspsychologie und Pädagogische Psychologie 41 (4), 181–188.

Casasanto, D., 2011. Different bodies, different minds: the body specificity of language and thought. Curr. Dir. Psychol. Sci. 20 (6), 378–383.

Christ, S.E., White, D.A., Brunstrom, J.E., Abrams, R.A., 2003. Inhibitory control following perinatal brain injury. Neuropsychology 17 (1), 171–178.

Cicchino, J.B., Rakison, D.H., 2008. Producing and processing self-propelled motion in infancy. Dev. Psychol. 44 (5), 1232–1241.

Clark, A., 1997. Being There: Putting Brain, Body, and World Together Again. MIT Press, Cambridge, MA.

Clearfield, M., 2004. The role of crawling and walking experience in infant spatial memory. J. Exp. Child Psychol. 89, 214–241.

Clearfield, M.W., Deidrich, F.J., Smith, L.B., Thelen, E., 2006. Young infants reach correctly in A-not-B tasks: on

the development of stability and preservation. Infant Behav. Dev. 29, 135–144.

Craft, S., Park, T.S., White, D.A., Schatz, J., Noetzel, M., Arnold, S., 1995. Changes in cognitive performance in children with spastic diplegic cerebral palsy following selective dorsal rhizotomy. Pediatr. Neurosurg. 23, 68–75.

Dahl, A., Campos, J.J.,Anderson, D.I., Uchiyama, I., Witherington, D.C., Ueno, M., et al., 2013. The epigenesis of wariness of heights. (Psychol. Sci.).

Dalvand, H., Dehghan, L., Hadian, M.R., Feizy, A., Hosseini, S.A., 2012. Relationship between gross motor and intellectual function in children with cerebral palsy: a cross-sectional study. Arch. Phys. Med. Rehabil. 93, 480–484.

Decarie, T., 1969. A study of the mental and emotional development of the thalidomide child In: Foss, B. (Ed.), Determinants of Infant Behaviour, 4. Methven & Co. Ltd., London.

Delorme, A., Frigon, J., Lagacé, C., 1989. Infants' reactions to visual movement of the environment. Perception 18, 667–673.

Dennis, M., Edelstein, K., Copeland, K., Frederick, J., Francis, D.J., Hetherington, R., et al., 2005. Covert orienting to exogenous and endogenous cues in children with spina bifida. Neuropsychologia 43, 976–987.

Dennis, M., Landry, S.H., Barnes, M., Fletcher, J.M., 2006. A model of neurocognitive function in spina bifida over the lifespan. J. Int. Neuropsychol. Soc. 12, 285–296.

Diamond, A., 1990. The development and neural bases of memory functions as indexed by the AB and delayed responses tasks in human infants and infant monkeys. In: Diamond, A. (Ed.), The Development and Neural Bases of Higher Cognitive Functions. The New York Academy of Science, New York, pp. 267–309.

Diamond, A., 1991. Neuropsychological insights into the meaning of object concept development. In: Carey, S., Gelman, R. (Eds.), The Epigenesis of Mind: Essays on Biology and Cognition. Erlbaum, Hillsdale, NJ, pp. 67–110.

Diamond, A., 2000. Close interrelation of motor development and cognitive

development and of the cerebellum and prefrontal cortex. Child Dev. 71 (1), 11–50.

Doidge, N., 2007. The Brain That Changes Itself: Stories of Personal Triumph from the Frontiers of Brain Science. Penguin Group (USA), Inc., New York, NY.

Edelman, G.M., 1987. Neural Darwinism: The Theory of Neuronal Group Selection. Basic Books, New York, NY.

Enderby, S.F., 1984. The effects of self-produced locomotion on the development of spatial orientation in infancy. Unpublished Honors Thesis, University of Denver, Denver.

Erickson, K.I., Miller, D.L., Weinstein, A.M., Akl, S.L., Banducci, S.E., 2012. Physical activity and brain plasticity in late adulthood: a conceptual review. Ageing Res. 4 (e6), 34–47.

Foreman, N., Orencas, C., Nicholas, E., Morton, P., 1989. Spatial awareness in seven to 11 year old physical handicapped children in mainstream schools. Eur. J. Spec. Needs Educ. 4 (3), 171–179.

Foreman, N., Foreman, D., Cummings, A., Owens, S., 1990. Locomotion active choice and spatial memory in children. J. Gen. Psychol. 117, 354–355.

Foster, E.C., Sveistrup, H., Woollacott, M.H., 1996. Transitions in visual proprioception: a cross-sectional developmental study of the effect of visual flow on postural control. J. Mot. Behav. 28, 101–112.

Freedman, D.L., 1992. Locomotor experience and the deployment of attention to near and distant space. Unpublished Honors Thesis, University of California, Berkeley, Berkeley, CA.

Gesell, A., 1928. Infancy and Human Growth. Macmillan, New York.

Gibson, E.J., 1988. Exploratory behaviour in the development of perceiving, acting, and the acquiring of knowledge. Annu. Rev. Psychol. 39, 1–41.

Gibson, E.J., Pick, A.D., 2000. An Ecological Approach to Perceptual Learning and Development. Oxford University Press, New York.

Gibson, E.J., Schmuckler, M.A., 1989. Going somewhere: an ecological and experimental approach to the development of mobility. Ecol. Psychol. 1, 3–25.

Gibson, J.J., 1966. The Senses Considered as Perceptual Systems. Houghton Mifflin, Boston, MA.

Gibson, J.J., 1979. The Ecological Approach to Visual Perception. Houghton Mifflin, Boston, MA.

Gilmore, R.O., Rettke, H.J., 2003. Four month-olds' discrimination of optic flow patterns depicting different directions of observer motion. Infancy 4, 177–200.

Gilmore, R.O., Hou, C., Pettet, M.W., Norcia, A.M., 2007. Development of cortical responses to optic flow. Vis. Neurosci. 24 (6), 845–856.

Goldfield, E.C., 1995. Emergent Forms: Origins and Early Development of Human Action and Perception. Oxford University Press, Inc., New York, NY.

Gomes da Silva, S., Unsain, N., Mas o, D.H., Toscano-Silva, M., de Amorim, H.A., et al., 2012. Early exercise promotes positive hippocampal plasticity and improves spatial memory in the adult life of rats. Hippocampus 22, 347–358.

Gustafson, G.E., 1984. Effects of the ability to locomote on infants' social and exploratory behaviours: an experimental study. Dev. Psychol. 20 (3), 397–405.

Haith, M., Benson, J., 1998. Infant cognition. In: Kuhn, D., Siegler, R. (Vol. Eds.), Cognition, Perception and Language. Vol. 2. Damon, W. (Series Ed.), Handbook of Child Psychology. John Wiley, New York, pp. 199–254.

Haith, M.M., 1993. Preparing for the 21st century: some goals and challenges for studies of infant sensory and perceptual development. Dev. Rev. 13, 354–371.

Hein, A., Held, R., Gower, E.C., 1970. Development and segmentation of visually controlled movement by selective exposure during rearing. J. Comp. Physiol. Psychol. 73 (2), 181–187.

Held, R., Hein, A., 1963. Movement-produced stimulation in the development of visually-guided behaviour. J. Comp. Physiol. Psychol. 56, 872–876.

Herbert, J., Gross, J., Hayne, H., 2007. Crawling is associated with more flexible memory retrieval by 9-month-old infants. Dev. Sci. 10 (2), 183–189.

Higgins, C.I., Campos, J.J., Kermoian, R., 1996. Effect of self-produced locomotion on infant postural compensation to optic flow. Dev. Psychol. 32, 836–841.

Horobin, K., Acredolo, L.P., 1986. The role of attentiveness, mobility history, and separation of hiding sites on stage IV search behaviour. J. Exp. Child. Psychol. 41 (1), 114–127.

Jouen, F., 1988. Visual-proprioceptive control of posture in newborn infants. In: Amblard, B., Berthoz, A., Clarac, F. (Eds.), Posture and Gait: Development, Adaptation and Modulation. Elsevier Science, Amsterdam, pp. 59–65.

Jouen, F., 1990. Early visual–vestibular interactions and postural development. In: Bloch, H., Bertenthal, B.I. (Eds.), Sensory-Motor Organizations and Development in Infancy and Early Childhood. Martinus Nijhoff, Dordrecht, Netherlands, pp. 199–215.

Jouen, F., Lepecq, J.C., Gapenne, O., Bertenthal, B.I., 2000. Optic flow sensitivity in neonates. Infant Behav. Dev. 23 (3–4), 271–284.

Kermoian, R., Campos, J.J., 1988. A facilitator of spatial cognitive development. Child Dev. 59 (4), 908–917.

Kershner, J.R., 1974. Relationship of motor development to visual-spatial cognitive growth. J. Spec. Educ. 8 (1), 91–101.

Kopp, C.B., Shaperman, J., 1973. Cognitive development in the absence of object manipulation during infancy. Dev. Psychol. 9 (3), 430.

Lee, D.N., 1978. The functions of vision. In: Pick, H.L., Saltzman, E. (Eds.), Modes of Perceiving and Processing Information. Erlbaum Associates, New York.

Lee, D.N., 1980. The optic flow field: the foundation of vision. Philos. Trans. R. Soc. Lond., B, Biol. Sci. 290 (1038), 169–179.

Lee, D.N., Aronson, E., 1974. Visual proprioceptive control of standing in human infants. Percept. Psychophys. 15, 529–532.

Lepecq, J.C., 1990. Self-produced movement, position constancy, and the perceptual-learning approach. In: Bloch, H., Bertenthal, B.I. (Eds.), Sensory-Motor Organizations and Development in Infancy and Early Childhood. Kluwer Academic, Dordecht, Netherlands, pp. 445–453.

Lew, A.R., Hopkins, B., Owen, L.H., Green, M., 2007. Postural change effects on infants' AB task performance: visual, postural, or spatial? J. Exp. Child Psychol. 97, 1–13.

Lishman, J.R., Lee, D.N., 1973. The autonomy of visual kinaesthesis. Perception 2, 287–294.

Maguire, E.A., Gadian, D.G., Johnsrude, I.S., Good, C.D., Ashburner, J., Frackowiak, R.S.J., et al., 2000. Navigation-related structural change in the hippocampi of taxi drivers. Proc. Natl. Acad. Sci. U.S.A. 97, 439–4403.

Maguire, E.A., Woollett, K., Spiers, H.J., 2006. London taxi drivers and bus drivers: a structural MRI and neuropsychological analysis. Hippocampus 16, 1091–1101.

McKenzie, B.E., 1987. The development of spatial orientation in human infancy: what changes?. In: McKenzie, B.E., Day, R.H. (Eds.), Perceptual Development in Early Infancy: Problems and Issues. Lawrence Erlbaum Associates, Hillsdale, NJ, pp. 125–142.

Mix, K.S., Smith, L.B., Gasser, M., 2010. The Spatial Foundations of Language and Cognition. Oxford University Press, Oxford.

Munakata, Y., 1998. Infant perseveration and implications for object permanence theories: a PDP model of the A-not-B task. Dev. Sci. 1 (2), 161–211.

Neisser, U., 1988. Five kinds of self-knowledge. Philos. Psychol. 1 (1), 35–59.

Newcombe, N.S., Frick, A., 2010. Early education for spatial intelligence: why, what, and how. Mind Brain Educ. 4, 102–111.

Odding, E., Roebroeck, M.E., Stam, J.H., 2006. The epidemiology of cerebral palsy: incidence, impairments, and risk factors. Disabil. Rehabil. 28, 183–191.

Parkes, J., White-Koning, M., Dickinson, H.O., Thyen, U., Arnaud, C., Beckung, E., et al., 2008. Psychological problems in children with cerebral palsy: a cross-sectional European study [multicentre study]. J. Child Psychol. Psychiatry 49, 405–413.

Pavlova, M., Sokolov, A., Krägeloh-Mann, I., 2007. Visual navigation in adolescents with early periventricular lesions: knowing where, but not getting there. Cereb. Cortex 17, 363–369.

Piaget, J., 1952. The Origins of Intelligence in Children. International Universities Press, New York.

Piaget, J., 1954. The Construction of Reality in the Child. Basic Books, New York.

Piaget, J., Inhelder, B., 1948. Representation of Space by the Child. Presses Universitaires de France, Paris, France.

Piek, J.P., Dawson, L., Smith, L.M., Gasson, N., 2008. The role of early fine and gross motor development on later motor and cognitive ability. Hum. Mov. Sci. 27, 668–681.

Pirilä, S., van der Meere, J.J., 2010. Cerebral palsy: effects of early brain injury on development. In: Armstrong, C.L., Morrow, L. (Eds.), Handbook of Medical Neuropsychology. Springer, New York, NY, pp. 149–163.

Ploughman, M., 2008. Exercise is brain food: the effects of physical activity on cognitive function. Dev. Neurorehabil. 11 (3), 236–240.

Rakison, D.H., Woodward, A.L., 2008. New perspectives on the effects of action on perceptual and cognitive development. Dev. Psychol. 44 (5), 1209–1213.

Ratey, J.J., 2007. Spark: The Revolutionary New Science of Exercise and the Brain. Little, Brown and Company, New York, NY.

Ritterband-Rosenbaum, A., Christensen, M.S., Kliim-Due, M., Petersen, L.Z., Rasmussen, B., Nielsen, J.B., 2011. Altered sense of agency in children with spastic cerebral palsy. BMC Neurol., 11.

Ritterband-Rosenbaum, A., Christensen, M.S., Nielsen, J.B., 2012. Twenty weeks of computer-training improves sense of agency in children with spastic cerebral palsy. Res. Dev. Disabil. 33, 1227–1234.

Rochat, P., 1992. Self-sitting and reaching in 5- to 8-month-old infants: the impact of posture and its development on early eye–hand coordination. J. Mot. Behav. 24, 210–220.

Rosenbaum, D.A., 2005. The Cinderella of psychology: the neglect of motor control in the science of mental life

and behaviour. Am. Psychol. 60 (4), 308–317.

Schatz, J., Craft, S., White, D., Park, T.S., Figiel, G.S., 2001. Inhibition of return in children with perinatal brain injury. J. Int. Neuropsychol. Soc. 7, 275–284.

Schmuckler, M.A., Gibson, E.J., 1989. The effect of imposed optical flow on guided locomotion in young walkers. Br. J. Dev. Psychol. 7, 193–206.

Sheets-Johnstone, M., 1999. The Primacy of Movement. Benjamins Publishing Co., Amsterdam.

Sherrington, C., 1951. Man on his Nature. The University Press, Cambridge.

Siegel, A.W., White, S.H., 1975. The Development of Spatial Representations of Large-Scale Environments. Academic Press, Inc., New York, NY.

Simms, B., 1987. The route learning ability of young people with spina bifida and hydrocephalus and their able-bodied peers. Zeitschrift für Kinderchirurgie 42, 53–56.

Smith, L.B., Thelen, E., Titzer, R., McLin, D., 1999. Knowing in the context of acting: the task dynamics of the A-Not-B error. Psychol. Rev. 106 (2), 235–260.

Sommerville, J.A., Woodward, A.L., 2010. The link between action production and processing in infancy. In: Grammont, F., Legrand, D., Livet, P. (Eds.), Naturalizing Intention in Action. MIT Press, Cambridge, MA, pp. 67–89.

Spelke, E.S., Kinzler, K.D., 2009. Innateness, learning, and rationality. Child Dev. Perspect. 3, 96–98.

Sperry, R.W., 1952. Neurology and the mind-brain problem. Am. Sci. 40, 291–311.

Stanton, D., Wilson, P.N., Foreman, N., 2002. Effects of early mobility on shortcut performance in a simulated maze. Behav. Brain Res. 136, 61–66.

Stoffregen, T.A., 1985. Flow structure versus retinal location in the optical control of stance. J. Exp. Psychol. Hum. Percept. Perform. 11, 554–565.

Stoffregen, T.A., Schmuckler, M.A., Gibson, E.J., 1987. Use of central and peripheral optic flow in stance and locomotion in young walkers. Perception 16, 113–119.

Straub, K., Obrzut, J.E., 2009. Effects of cerebral palsy on neuropsychological function. J. Dev. Phys. Disabil. 21, 153–167.

Tao, S., Dong, Q., 1997. Referential gestural communication and locomotor experience in urban Chinese infants. Unpublished manuscript, Beijing Normal University, Beijing, China.

Taylor, H.B., Landry, S.H., Barnes, M., Swank, P., Cohen, L.B., Fletcher, J., 2010. Early information processing among infants with and without spina bifida. Infant Behav. Dev. 33, 365–372.

Thelen, E., 2000. Motor development as foundation and future of developmental psychology. Int. J. Behav. Dev. 24 (4), 385–397.

Thelen, E., Smith, L.B., 1994. A Dynamic Systems Approach to the Development of Cognition and Action. MIT Press, Cambridge, MA.

Thelen, E., Smith, L.B., 2006. Dynamic systems theories. In: Lerner, R.M., Damon, W. (Eds.), Handbook of Child Psychology. John Wiley & Sons, Inc., Hoboken, NJ, pp. 258–312.

Thelen, E., Spencer, J.P., 1998. Postural control during reaching in young infants: a dynamic systems approach. Neurosci. Biobehav. Rev. 22, 507–514.

Thelen, E., Schoner, G., Scheier, C., Smith, L.B., 2001. The dynamics of embodiment: a field theory of infant preservative reaching. Behav. Brain Sci. 24, 1–86.

Topál, J., Gergely, G., Miklósi, A., Erdöhegyi, A., Csibra, G., 2008. Infants' perseverative search errors are induced by pragmatic misinterpretation. Science 321, 1831–1834.

Uchiyama, I., Anderson, D.I., Campos, J.J., Witherington, D., Frankel, C.B., Lejeune, L., et al., 2008. Locomotor experience affects self and emotion. Dev. Psychol. 44 (5), 1225–1231.

Varela, F.J., Thompson, E., Rosch, E., 1992. The Embodied Mind: Cognitive Science and Human Experience. The MIT Press, Cambridge, MA.

Warren, R., Wertheim, A.H., 1990. Perception & Control of Self-Motion. Lawrence Erlbaum Associates, Hillsdale, NJ.

Weimer, W.B., 1977. A conceptual framework for cognitive psychology: motor theories of the mind. In: Shaw, R., Bransford, J. (Eds.), Perceiving, Acting and Knowing: Toward an Ecological Psychology. Lawrence Erlbaum Associates, Hillsdale, NJ, pp. 267–311.

Wiedenbauer, G., Jansen-Osmann, P., 2006. Spatial knowledge of children with spina bifida in a virtual large-scale space. Brain Cogn. 62, 120–127.

Wilson, M., 2002. Six views of embodied cognition. Psychon. Bull. Rev. 9 (4), 625–636.

Yan, J.H., Thomas, J.R., Downing, J.H., 1998. Locomotion improves children's spatial search: a meta-analytic review. Percept. Mot. Skills 87, 67–82.

Young, M., 1977. Cognitive Development in Cerebral Palsy Children. University Microfilms International, Ann Arbor, MI.

# PART 5

## Specific Methods of Motor Training for Infants

# Training lower limb performance in early infancy: Support, balance and propulsion

11

Roberta B. Shepherd

## Introduction

The development of the brain and corticospinal tract in the infant with cerebral palsy (CP) may depend on early and varied use of the limbs. A full-term newborn infant in the early weeks of life begins to adapt to and take advantage of a new and gravitational environment, and over the first weeks begins an exploration of the possibilities available. Much of the first two years is spent learning how to balance the body and develop fundamental skills. A review of the anatomical and biomechanical characteristics of the lower limbs makes it clear that their basic action, underlying most of the actions of daily life, is flexion and extension at hips, knees and ankles (Fig. 11.1). When the feet are on the ground, the lower limbs support the body mass, balance it over the base of support, and propel it in the desired direction (Forssberg, 1982).

Simplifying motor function in this way has enabled the development, over the past three decades, of training and exercise guidelines for adult neurological rehabilitation. These programme consist of task-oriented exercises and activities that are focused on muscle activation, contractility and strength, and on developing co-ordination or motor control of the lower limbs as they flex and extend, support, balance and move the body mass in actions such as standing up and sitting down, squatting to pick up an object on the floor and standing up again, walking up and down stairs and slopes (Carr and Shepherd, 2003, 2010). The focus is on developing skill, learning to control body and limbs to produce effective and efficient movements.

DOI: http://dx.doi.org/10.1016/B978-0-7020-5099-2.00011-X

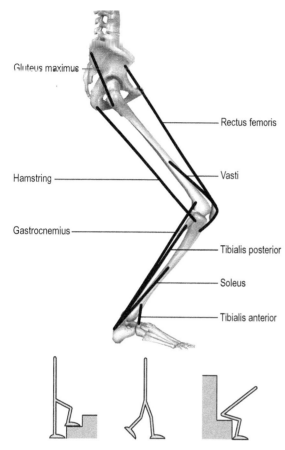

Gluteus maximus

Rectus femoris

Vasti

Hamstring

Gastrocnemius

Tibialis posterior

Soleus

Tibialis anterior

**Figure 11.1** • Diagram showing lower limb segments and eight functional muscle groups affecting segmental movement with feet on the support surface. [Reproduced with permission from Kuo and Zajac (1993) A biomechanical analysis of muscle strength as a limiting factor in standing posture. J Biomech 26:137–150, with permission from Elsevier.]

The exercise guidelines developed for adult neurorehabilitation, since they are developed out of applied biomechanics, functional anatomy and motor learning processes, are also applicable to infants and children with CP, incorporated into play and activity-related exercises (Damiano, 2006; Shepherd, 1995; Ulrich, 2010). However, infants with CP not only experience the effects of a lesion of the central motor systems but also, as they grow, the secondary effects on the musculoskeletal system of poor muscle contractility, weakness and inactivity. These include changes to muscle morphology and function, and to bone structure. The significance of these secondary effects should not be underestimated. Due to recent technological advances and the resultant research, these secondary effects are predictable and this means they may also

be preventable. The alignment of the limbs, muscle morphology, bone structure and shape are dependent on how the infant learns to move, specifically on the stresses provided by the musculature of the limb.

If for example, the hip flexors lose their extensibility and develop contracture the alignment of the lower limb is altered. Figure 11.11C, D illustrates the resultant pattern of movement as the small child with hemiplegic or diplegic CP walks. The crouch gait of children with diplegia is described by Arnold and Delp (2005). Developments in technology are enabling detailed examination of bone structure in children with diplegia, outlining the altered features of long bones (Carriero et al., 2009), and the altered morphology of muscles (see Chapters 6 and 7).

The shape (form or topology) of functional movements (see Fig. 11.8) is dependent on co-operative action from major abductor/adductor and rotator muscles in addition to flexion and extension. The strength and control of basic lower limb movements depends also on muscles within the trunk that, although they do not themselves move the limbs, contribute to lower limb movements by stabilizing the muscle attachments on the pelvis and lumbar spine. Early weight-bearing and lower limb flexion/extension activities provide the stresses critical for stimulating bone growth and density, for development and growth of muscle, and the experiences that will foster the learning processes that underpin motor development.

Targeted training of the lower limbs in infants with CP appears to have been neglected in the literature in comparison to the upper limbs. Chen and colleagues (2002) suggested that this might have resulted from a view that although infants are making purposeful reaching movements with the upper limbs within the early months, the lower limbs appear to be moving spontaneously in random kicking actions until required to perform purposeful weight-bearing activities. This neglect may also be due to the long-held view that upper limb actions are 'fine motor skills' while those of the lower limb, including balancing and locomotion, are 'gross motor skills'. These terms have become meaningless as neuroscience and biomechanics teach us about the complexity and flexibility of motor control mechanisms, particularly those complex and finely tuned balance adjustments that occur as a critical part of our most critical everyday actions.

Effective performance of standing up and sitting down, walking, reaching out for a variety of objects and manipulating them to achieve desired goals in different environments is critical to independent living. Most of our goal-directed motor behaviour is carried out when we are upright, in sitting or standing, and infants need the opportunity to focus on developing a functional linkage between upper and lower limbs (and including the vertebral joints) in the context of these two positions most critical for independence. Emphasis on sitting and standing enables the infant to develop the necessary orienting behaviours and balance mechanisms that enable them to explore and attend to their environment, communicate with others, and to develop the ability to formulate and carry out their goals. In the upright position infants, driven by their need for visual focus, also learn to control their head position. This is necessary for the development of visual acuity, visuomotor control and ability to pay attention, as well as eye contact for communication with others, all of which function together with independent head movement (Chapman, 2002).

It is now recognized that the varied actions practiced by infants as they grow and learn, as they become stronger and develop more control, depend to a large extent on their opportunities, in particular their curiosity, drive and determination, their environment, and the effects of cultural influences within the family on child-rearing practices. Given the opportunity, and encouraged and assisted by parents and siblings, infants practice intensively, exploring the possibilities of crawling, creeping, standing and walking; they push and pull up from prone and supine, squat and stand up on a parent's lap, kneel on one or both legs, cruise sideways along the furniture (Figs 11.2 and 11.3). The more the infant is allowed to explore and experiment with movement, the more he/she learns.

This chapter is focused on the details of intervention: on methods of encouraging and driving the infant's own actions, and on setting up an interesting and challenging environment that enables the infant to practice using the lower limbs to support and balance the body mass. Guidance and constraint are provided when necessary. The infant is encouraged and assisted to be active and to explore, to practice a variety of movements that increase activation, contractility and strength of muscles, as well as preserve muscle extensibility (Fig. 11.2). Whatever the action to be learned, the infant needs to support the body through the lower limbs, balance it throughout the action, and, with many actions including walking and standing

up, propel the body in the desired direction. The aims of intervention are to increase mobility, train functional actions (promote skill learning), and to activate and exercise muscles (for increased contractility, strength, extensibility, intersegmental co-ordination). The aims of prevention are to minimize changes to muscle morphology that may negatively impact functional performance, and to monitor during functional training, and if necessary correct, lower limb alignment that may negatively impact bone (and joint) alignment.

# Part 1: support, balance, propulsion

## Support of upper body over lower limbs

In standing, support is brought about by the generation of the extensor muscle activity necessary to maintain segmental alignment in the presence of gravitational forces working to collapse the limbs. Many mono- and bi-articular muscles that span hip, knee and ankle joints work co-operatively across the three joints to maintain support and to balance the body mass over the thighs and feet (in sitting), feet (in standing) or knees (in kneeling). The co-operative extensor muscle force throughout each limb as we flex and extend hips, knees and ankles in standing and when standing up is illustrated by the 'support moment of force', an algebraic summation of the moments of force acting over the three joints, demonstrated in biomechanical studies of walking (Winter, 1987) and sit-to-stand (Shepherd and Gentile, 1994). Any reduction of extensor force at one joint can be made up for by increased moments of force at the other two joints. Muscles within the trunk that rotate, flex and extend the vertebral joints provide flexibility and stability to the movements of the upper and lower limbs.

## Balance of body mass over base of support

The ability to balance the body mass over the lower limbs enables us to move about under different conditions and for a variety of different goals. Movements that balance us and prevent

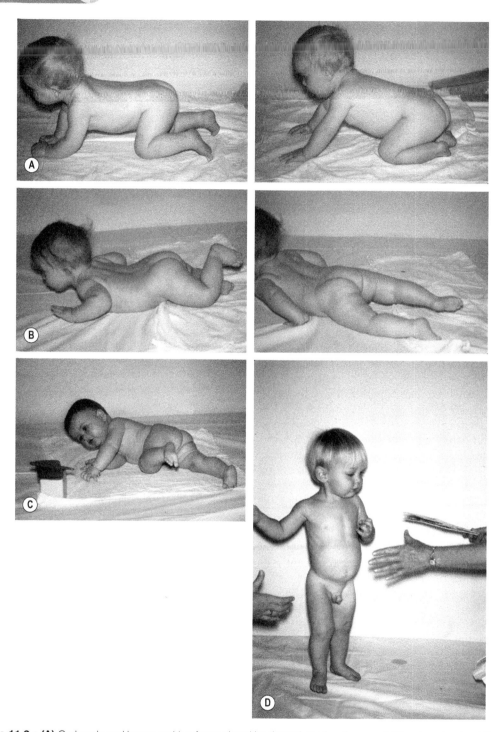

**Figure 11.2 • (A)** On hands and knees rocking forward and backward, testing the possibilities, learning to shift weight. **(B)** In prone, practicing extension of head and spine; progressing along the floor by pulling with arms and pushing with legs. **(C)** Mastery of rolling over involving the whole body working as one unit. **(D)** Just prior to the first independent steps in a forward direction.

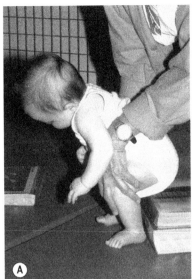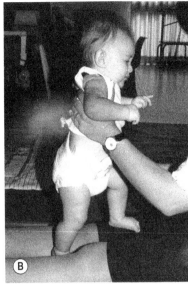

**Figure 11.3** • Two task-specific exercises to stimulate extensor muscle activation, increase extensor muscle strength, and preserve muscle extensibility. **(A)** Assisted sit-stand-sit: some assistance ensures knees are forward (i.e., ankles sufficiently dorsiflexed) with some downward pressure so the infant gets the idea of pushing down through the feet. **(B)** Step up and down on someone's lap. The infant is steadied to prevent a fall but she raises and lowers her body mass herself.

a fall include adduction/abduction and rotation movements at the hips, and movements within the spine, as well as the basic flexion/extension of the hips, knees and ankles, and small movements at the joints of the feet. These movements control the body mass as it moves about over the base of support, ensuring the body's centre of mass (CoM) stays within the base of support. Ongoing neuromotor interactions between our intent (pick up an object from the floor) and information from tactile, pressure and motion sensors (including plantar load receptors in soles of feet, and muscle and tendon receptors), and from vision, anticipate upcoming destabilizations, ensure ongoing musculoskeletal responsiveness throughout the action or a quick enough response to an unexpected perturbation to prevent a fall. The need for motor control is magnified when the base of support is small and when the body's centre of gravity (CoG) is far from the support base, as in walking and standing on one leg.

The mechanical problem of remaining balanced in the presence of the destabilizing forces that occur as we move is a particular challenge to the corticospinal system. Anticipatory and ongoing adjustments, and responses to unexpected perturbations, ensure the body is aligned and balanced over the base of support, stabilizing parts of the body while other parts move, and preventing a fall (Ghez, 1991). Even simple actions such a raising an arm in standing, or taking a deep breath, require initial (anticipatory/preparatory) and ongoing muscle activations. The muscle activations and joint movements (called 'postural adjustments') that balance us as we move about are flexible and vary specifically according to task and context (Belenkii et al., 1967; Cordo and Nashner, 1982; Eng et al., 1992; Smart et al., 2004) (Fig. 11.4). When bearing weight through the lower limbs and learning to stand up and sit down, reach for an object in standing or in sitting, squat to pick up an object, and to walk, balance is always a major focus of the neuromotor system. Once they can stand independently, although with frequent falls, infants practice balancing in standing and taking steps. They often prefer independence when walking, and will take a few steps unaided rather than hold a parent's hand.

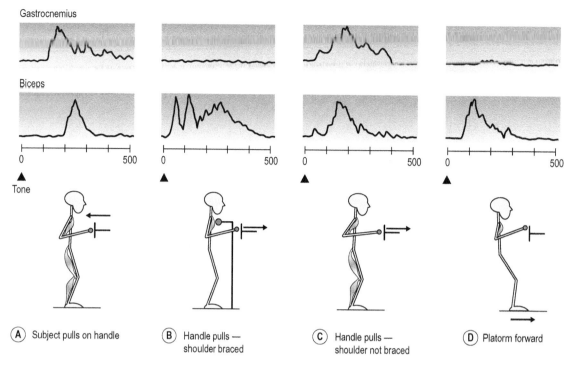

**Figure 11.4 •** An example of the task- and context-specificity of muscle activity. An arm muscle (biceps brachii) and a leg muscle (gastrocnemius) were monitored during different tasks. **(A)** The subject pulls on the handle. **(B)** The subject leans against a chest support, unexpected movement of the handle. **(C)** As in (B), but subject is free standing. **(D)** Unexpected forward movement of the platform. [Adapted with permission from Nashner LM (1983) Analysis of movement control in man using the movable platform. In: Desmedt JE (Ed.), Motor Control Mechanisms in Health & Disease. Raven Press, New York.]

## Propulsion of body mass

Moving the body mass requires the generation and timing of muscle forces to accelerate the body in the desired direction: forward and upward to stand up from a seat and from a squat, more vigorously in jumping vertically and walking fast. Leg extensor muscles increase in strength and ability to generate a powerful contraction as infants practice squatting to standing and sitting to standing (Liao et al., 2007). Calf muscles and hip extensors propel the body mass forward during stance phase in walking. Walking faster requires more powerful muscle contractions to propel the body forward at the end of stance. Infants learn to increase propulsion when they can place their heel down at the end of swing phase and push-off at the end of stance phase. When they start to run a few steps, they demonstrate some difficulty in the control of momentum and may over-run and fall. Figure 11.5 shows the lack of control over horizontal momentum in young children when they stand up

from a seat—even when standing up is independent, the child may take a few steps forward instead of standing still (Cahill et al., 1999).

Gradually, young children start to practice other actions that require the ability to generate and control forceful muscle contractions. Examples include actions in which powerful contractions of calf muscles, hip and knee extensor muscles propel the body mass off the floor, or to jump off a step, and in the vertical jump, long jump, skipping, and hopping on one leg. When the young child practices throwing a ball, she is learning that to throw it a long distance, elbow, shoulder and wrist muscles plus spinal muscles and muscles of the lower limbs must co-operate to produce a powerful action of the upper limb, with shoulder girdle and trunk, in order to propel the ball through the air. When to release the ball is a major problem in the early stages of learning.

In the following section, keep in mind that lower limb skills almost all require the ability to support the body mass, balance it and move it from one place to another.

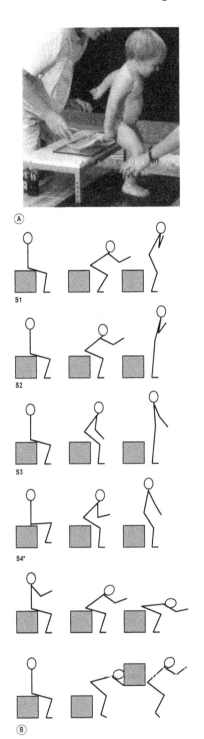

Figure 11.5 • (A) The infant can stand up independently but takes a step forward to regain balance. He has not mastered the action as, on this attempt, he has not controlled the forward momentum of his body produced in the first phase of the action. (B) Stick figure

# Development of lower limb motor skills

This section is a brief account of motor development as it relates to the lower limb. More detailed information is provided in references cited and elsewhere (e.g., Bradley and Westcott, 2006; Piek, 2006; Sutherland, 1997).

Developmental changes in motor function reflect the gradual gaining of skill as an infant practices actions that are rewarding. Although there has been some investigative focus on infant kicking and the development of locomotion, there has been less interest in investigating the development of other lower limb skills in infancy beyond the observational. However, skilled movement of the lower limbs is critical to functional motor performance, and particularly in balancing the body mass, and most actions, including those involving the upper limb, involve the co-ordinated action of many lower limb muscles, crossing several joints.

Our current understanding of motor development is now influenced by experimental findings from biomechanical and electromyographical (EMG) studies. For example, as reaching with the upper limb becomes more efficient and effective, a phase plane plot can demonstrate the gradual changes occurring in joint co-ordination (Fig. 11.6A). A comparative study of the lower limbs as skill develops in sit-to-stand in different age groups is likely to show similar changes occurring over time, reflecting increasing co-ordination of limb segments as the action becomes more skilled (Fig. 11.6B). Studies of kinetics and kinematics illustrate the development of balance control in infants and young children (Roncesvalles et al., 2001), although investigation is typically confined to the infant's response to unexpected support surface movement.

diagrams taken from videotape of six children with CP aged between 4 and 6 years as they stand up from a height-adjusted stool. Note that although the starting position was standardized, the performance varies with each infant. The diagrams show that several infants had difficulty in achieving an erect standing position and maintaining balance. [(A) From Cahill et al. (1999) Intersegmental co-ordination in sit-to-stand: an age cross-sectional study. Physiother Res Internat 4:12–27, with permission from John Wiley and Sons. (B) From McDonald C 1994 A biomechanical analysis of the sit-to-stand movement in children with diplegic cerebral palsy, BAppSc(Hon) thesis, The University of Sydney.]

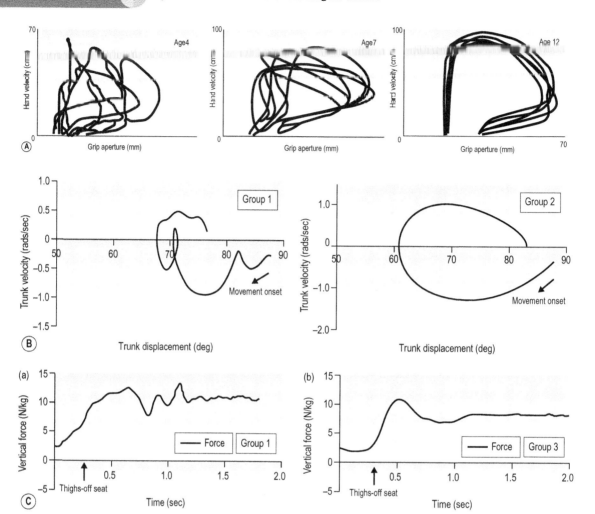

**Figure 11.6 • (A)** Kinematic profiles of prehension at the age of 4, 7 and 12 years. Linear velocity of the hand was plotted against grip aperture in three children, one from each age group, as they reached to pick up an object. Six trials are superimposed for each subject. By the age of 12 years, reaching and opening the hand to grasp is well co-ordinated and the movement of the hand through space is smooth with no deviations. **(B)** A velocity–displacement phase plane plot of trunk (i.e., hip) flexion/extension in standing up in an infant from the youngest group (Group 1) shows typical deviations (interruptions and reversals) indicating lack of ability to co-ordinate a smooth transition from hip flexion to hip extension around thighs-off. Compare this to the plot of an older child in Group 2. **(C)** A representative trial of standing up showing vertical ground reaction forces produced by a child from Group 1 and another from Group 3. The older children (Group 3) showed the distinctive peak around thighs-off similar to adult performance (i.e., skilled), while the younger showed many fluctuations with no distinctive peak. [(A) From Kuhtz-Buschbeck JP et al. (1998) Development of prehension movements in children: a kinematic study Exp Brain Res 122:424–432, with permission from Springer Science + Business Media.] [(B,C) From Cahill et al. (1999) Intersegmental co-ordination in sit-to-stand: an age cross-sectional study. Physiother Res Internat 4:12–27, with permission from John Wiley and Sons.]

Several biomechanical studies have reported the changes as gait matures around 5 years of age (Fossberg, 1985; Sutherland, 1997, 2001, 2002; Sutherland et al., 1980; Whitall et al., 1985), and the data show the stages through which an infant passes en route to skilled performance. Many of the changes taking place are similar to those found in adults as they learn a novel skill: for example, improved balance, smooth co-ordination, increased speed, decreased energy expenditure, increased effectiveness. Sutherland (1997) has noted that 'we must understand the natural history of immature walking in order to define and interpret pathological gait in young children' (p. 163).

The basic motor pattern of lower limb movement referred to earlier is seen in utero, where infants practice flexion and extension of lower limbs, kicking and pushing their feet against the uterine wall (Milani-Comparetti, 1980). After birth they retain this ability to flex and extend their legs. The most obvious active movement of lower limbs in the first months in infancy is kicking in various forms. However, when held in standing, full-term newborn infants can also support the body mass through the feet, flex and extend the lower limbs, and take steps, although the way they do this seems to depend on opportunities provided. Most infants can take a few steps on a treadmill if supported (see Fig. 11.10). Early stepping used to be considered a reflexive movement that would disappear, to be followed later by 'true' walking. However, Zelazo et al. (1983) found that, with practice and experience of walking, infants retained their ability to take steps and their walking improved. Thelen and Cooke (1987) suggested that this ability to walk after a period of 'practice' was due to increased lower limb strength. Evidence also comes from cross-cultural child-rearing studies that advanced walking skill is evident in those societies that give infants the opportunity to walk (see Chapter 1).

Infants continue to experiment with lower limb movement when held upright, sometimes kicking, or flexing and extending hips and knees. Held in standing with feet on a supporting surface they bend and straighten their legs, 'practicing' the basic pattern of intersegmental co-ordination (flexion and extension at hips, knees, ankles) that they will need in many actions significant to daily life (see Annotation A, Fig. A.6). In raising and lowering the body mass over the supporting lower limbs, they gradually gain control until the limb segments can act together as a single functional unit, seen most clearly in standing up from crouch and from a seat. With the foot on the floor, foot, shank and thigh make up the segmental linkage, movement at one joint, by necessity, producing movement of the other joints (see Figs 1.3A, 1.10a, A.9, and A.6).

At around 8–10 months (earlier if they have the opportunity) infants pull themselves to standing of their own volition. They are slower to lower themselves to the floor. This action makes different strength and motor control demands, and lowering the body mass involves eccentric muscle activity (muscles lengthening while contracting), compared to the concentric activity of standing up (muscles shortening as they contract).

As learning progresses, the motor control system appears to use simplifying strategies to 'manage' this segmental linkage, with co-operation between muscle forces produced over the three joints, varying according to the task and the conditions under which it is performed. Variability is a driving force of developmental change, evident in motor development and acquisition of skill throughout life (Dusing and Harbourne, 2010; Fetters, 1991; Hadders-Algra, 2002). Infants gradually co-ordinate the joints of their lower limbs and develop skilfull performance by repetitive but variable practice (Bernstein's 'repetition without repetition'), driven by curiosity and by the opportunities offered by the environment.

Although this chapter is focused on the lower limbs, they do not function in isolation from the rest of the body. In the first few months, infants develop the ability to raise their head in supine and prone and to support the head when picked up. The arms reach out to explore the surroundings and arm and leg movements enable the infant to move about in prone and roll over (Fig. 11.2B, C). A major input to gaining control of head, trunk and limbs is vision: infants are driven to move by what they see around them, and with these exploratory movements they begin to develop and fine-tune an integrated movement system involving body, limbs and head.

## Kicking

Co-ordination patterns of lower limbs in healthy infants are characterized by a coupling among hip, knee and ankle joints in which all joints tend to flex or extend in temporal synchrony (Thelen, 1985). These typically tight couplings change as the infant practices different joint combinations and a 'decoupling' begins as the infant investigates the possibilities during the first few months (Angulo-Kinzler et al., 2002; Jensen et al., 1994).

Since infants before birth practice flexion and extension movements, it is likely that even in the first few weeks of life leg movements are not merely random but also exploratory. It is evident that infants can learn to move their legs to achieve a goal (Thelen, 1994). In early movements and attempts at movement the infant seems to be learning what is possible (see Annotation C). Chen et al. (2002) tested the hypothesis that 4-month-old infants can learn a kicking task that involved interacting with a mobile. The authors noted that 'Infants are capable of shifting the patterns they generate to bring back the responses they want.' (p. 215). Such devices provide examples of how young infants can learn to fine-tune their lower limb (kicking) movements to achieve a goal. They enable the infant to practice independently.

The pattern of kicking movements, particularly their variability, can provide early information about disordered motor control (Jeng et al., 2002). For example, any abnormalities in kicking co-ordination in young infants are observable during general movements testing (Chapter 8). Kinematic analysis of movement patterns enables kicking deficits to be detected as early as 1 month of age in premature low birth weight infants with white matter disorder (Fetters et al., 2004). The information gained from such testing of motor performance should lead to an earlier referral to remedial activity programmes.

## Balancing in sitting and standing

The most critical feature of motor development is the ability to balance the body when moving (e.g., reaching out) in sitting or standing. Some degree of standing balance is generally considered a necessary precursor to locomotor skills (Roncesvalles et al., 2001), but it also underpins virtually all our activities. The development of balance has been investigated in many studies utilizing a movable platform (Brogren et al., 1996; Forssberg and Nashner, 1982; Hirschfeld, 1992; Shumway-Cook and Woollacott, 1985). There has been less investigation of balance mechanisms during other actions. The perturbation studies have demonstrated the muscle activity, joint movements and shifts in CoM (i.e., postural adjustments) under conditions when the child's balance was unexpectedly perturbed, but they give us no information about the complexity of anticipatory or preparatory and ongoing adjustments as the child balances during self-initiated movements.

Studies of balance in adults, however, have examined actions such as reaching in sitting and standing (Eng et al., 1992; Dean and Shepherd, 1997) and raising one leg to take a step (Kirker et al.,

2000). Such studies provide information that can assist exercise planning (Carr and Shepherd, 2003, 2010). Even simple actions like turning the head in standing are characterized by oscillations in the line of gravity that are countered by muscle activity and small, barely detectable movements, usually at ankles and hips (Bouisset and Duchenne, 1994).

Several studies of the role of vision in balancing the body were carried out with children during the 1970s and 1980s (Butterworth, 1986; Butterworth and Hicks, 1977; Lee and Aronson, 1974) showing that vision has a dominant proprioceptive function in developing children as it does in adults. Vision provides critical environmental and positional guidance for the control of all actions, including gait (see Chapter 10). Learning to judge and predict aspects of the environment, such as verticality and horizontality, provides visual cues about where we are in space, and these abilities probably depend on our experience during our own self-initiated movements in the upright position.

There have been few biomechanical investigations of the actions of infants as they learn to gain control over their movements in the first year. However, for an understanding of the mechanisms of balance adjustments (muscle contractions and joint movements) as we move about in sitting and standing we need to know the critical biomechanical features, i.e., movements of the body's CoG within the periphery of the base of support, kinematic and kinetic details of joint movements. *Kinematic* details give us joint angular displacements, linear movement of the limbs through space, and the overall topology of the movement. *Kinetic* analyses, i.e., estimating the forces responsible for an observed movement, yield variables that describe the cause of motion. *Vertical and horizontal ground reaction forces*, tested with a force plate, demonstrate the movements made in order to maintain an imaginary vertical line drawn from the CoG to the ground to remain within the base of support (Winter, 2009) (Fig. 11.7). From electromyographic studies we see the variability of muscle activity underlying a smoothly co-ordinated and skilled action.

## Standing up and sitting down

### Standing up

Getting to the feet independently and without relying on hand use is one of the most significant

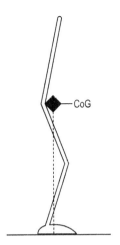

**Figure 11.7** • Schematic of a four-segment model showing the position of the centre of gravity (CoG). The dotted line is used to determine the movement of the CoG in standing.

and physically demanding abilities developed by infants. Although infants get into standing by pulling themselves up from crouch or half-kneeling, gaining the ability to sit independently on a seat, using the lower limbs for support and balance, provides the opportunity to practice standing up without using the hands. Independent sit-to-stand and squat-to-stand are essential to the early practice of independent walking. One of the most difficult mechanical problems to be mastered by infants learning to stand up is the ability to control the destabilizing forces caused by joint movement, particularly the horizontal momentum of the body's CoM that is generated by rapid movement of the upper body forward over the feet (Fig. 11.5).

Angular momentum is created as the erect upper body rotates forward by flexion at the hips. Flexion of the hip changes to extension when the CoG is over the feet and the body mass is propelled vertically into standing. The muscular effort involved in raising the body mass against gravity is minimized in skilled performers by certain strategies. The feet are moved back (Fig. 11.8A), downward and backward pressure is exerted through the feet, as the upper body flexes forward at the hips bringing the weight forward over the feet as a single smooth movement, an example of a linked segment system in action (Fig. 11.8). The speed of this forward movement of the body mass at the hips and ankles creates horizontal momentum of the body mass. The movement

forward is accompanied by active ankle dorsiflexion and vertical pressure downward that stabilizes and holds the shanks forward (dorsiflexed) at the ankles. Calf muscles, hip and knee extensors extend the lower limbs (at ankles, knees, hips) and move the body vertically over the feet and into standing. Fig. 11.8D illustrates the order of muscle onsets during the standing up action (Khemlani et al., 1998). The result is a smooth continuous movement, although one of the most physically demanding of the actions we commonly perform.

## Sitting down

Sitting down appears to be the reverse action to standing up, but there are significant differences that make it particularly difficult for an infant. There are different mechanical constraints as the movement is performed by gravity and controlled by eccentric (lengthening) contractions of the lower limb extensor muscles that slow the descent of the body mass. The limbs flex and, just before the seat is reached, flexion of the trunk at the hips increases and the body mass, moving at the ankles, shifts backward, with the tibialis anterior muscle contracting strongly (Carr and Shepherd, 2010). This is a destabilizing movement, and the balance, muscle and mechanical constraints are considerable. Even when the infant can sit down, he finds it difficult to initiate the descent.

There appear to be few investigations of the stages an able-bodied infant goes through in the first year to learn these two actions or of the mechanical differences between an able-bodied infant and an infant with CP (da Costa et al., 2010). Nevertheless, biomechanical analysis can document clearly the mechanical reasons for poor performance in children with CP compared to able-bodied children (dos Santos et al., 2011; Park et al., 2003; Yonetsu et al., 2009;). A study of standing up (Cahill et al., 1999) involved 18 able-bodied children between the ages of 12 months and 10 years, six in each of three age groups (12–18 months, 4–5 years, 9–10 years). They wore reflective markers and were videotaped as they stood up from a height-adjustable seat that straddled a force plate (see Fig. 11.5A). Cahill and colleagues found infants as young as 13 months could stand up using a similar basic motor pattern to that of adults. However, although the younger children could stand up independently, they appeared to have difficulty understanding the idea of standing up as an end in itself. The authors commented that

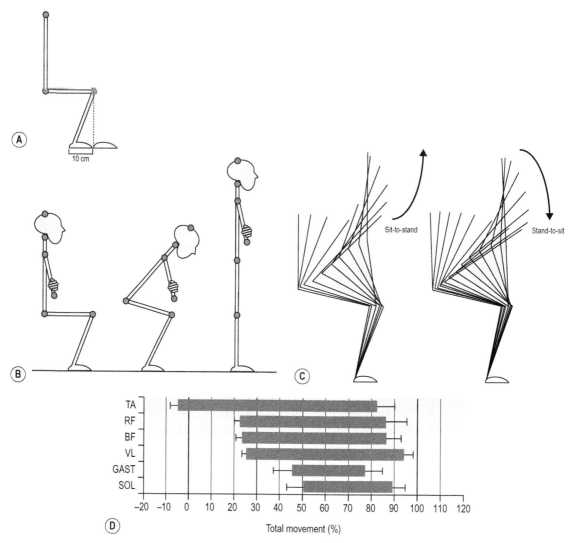

**Figure 11.8 • (A)** Moving the feet back to approximately 75° of ankle plantarflexion decreases the distance the body's centre of mass has to move over the new base of support (the feet) and decreases extensor force generation. Foot position seems to be a major determinant of energy expenditure in sit-to-stand. **(B)** A simplified illustration to show the major kinematic features of sit-to-stand in the sagittal plane. **(C)** Stick figure drawings taken from a biomechanical study of standing up and sitting down showing the topology (shape) of the movement taken from joint displacement data. The young adult subject shows little difference in the topology of standing up compared to sitting down but some differences in joint movement in the eccentric sitting down phase compared to standing up against gravity (concentric). **(D)** Mean and standard error of time-normalized onsets and durations of six lower limb muscles as able-bodied adults stand up at their preferred speed. TA, tibialis anterior; RF, rectus femoris; BF, biceps femoris; VL, vastus lateralis; GAST, gastrocnemius; SOL, soleus. Percentage of total movement: 0%, movement onset; 31%, thighs-off; 100%, movement end. [(A–C) From Carr and Shepherd, 2010 Neurological Rehabilitation. Optimizing Motor Performance, with permission from Elsevier. (D) Adapted from Khemlani M, Carr JH, Crosbie WJ et al. (1998) Muscle synergies and joint linkages in sit-to-stand under two different initial foot positions.Clin Biomech 14:236–246, with permission from Elsevier.]

the children seemed unable to end the movement in quiet standing but either took a few steps forward or went up on their toes, depending on whether vertical or horizontal momentum was the more destabilizing. Older children showed less variability in performance than the younger children (Fig. 11.6B,C). By 4 years of age, children could flex the hips and rotate the upper body further forward and faster, and could end the action in quiet standing.

Developmental trends were evident on the videotapes and in the kinetic and kinematic variables. Movement time, amplitude and peak angular velocity of hip flexion increased with age. Children in the older groups displayed a pattern of ground reaction forces similar to those reported for adults. The youngest reached peak force more slowly, often with fluctuations. Phase plane plots showed the co-ordination of the movement increasing with age and skill level (Fig. 11.6B). The authors suggested that differences in intersegmental co-ordination as the action developed may reflect the child's increasing ability to control horizontal momentum and to balance. The results are of particular interest since they illustrate the changes taking place in a complex action as the infant/child develops skill after learning the basic motor pattern: feet back → push down through feet + flex trunk forward at hips → extend hips, knees, ankles → stand still. Gaining the ability to time joint movements, control muscle forces and balance the body mass throughout the action and from a variety of different seats required a great deal of practice.

Data from another study of children 4- to 6-year-old children with diplegia also showed that they often overbalanced forward as they rose to standing (Fig. 11.5B). In addition, in most trials the children had difficulty producing peak vertical force at thighs-off, which suggests that both generating and timing lower limb extensor muscles forces were difficult (Shepherd and McDonald, 1995). More recently, Park et al. (2003) found increased hip flexion and slowness of movement, with decreased peak knee extensor moment of force and decreased extensor power generation at hips and knees in a group of children with hemiplegia or diplegia.

## Crawling

Transitional quadripedal locomotion on hands and knees or hands and feet, such as crawling, creeping and bear walking (Fig. 1.10B), enables the infant to get about on the floor in the first year, before the muscles are strong enough and attempts at bipedal locomotion are sufficiently balanced for the infant to be independent in standing up and walking. These quadripedal actions may have a significant effect on the development of overall limb co-ordination, linking the upper and lower limbs in ways that may potentiate a child's performance of any actions that involve interactions between all four limbs. Which method the infant prefers seems arbitrary but probably depends on the ground surface available, how often he/she is placed on the ground, and what possibilities the environment offers (Chapman, 2002; Groenen et al., 2010).

Not all infants crawl, and there is evidence from studies of child-rearing practices that suggests that an infant's preferred early locomotion depends on opportunity (Wong, 2009). Infants who are placed on the floor and who have developed the ability to push themselves up on their arms may pull themselves along the floor (Fig. 11.2B). The infant may then get on to hands and knees, rock to and fro (Fig. 11.2A), and crawl. Some children 'bear walk' on hands and feet before they get to their feet and start cruising around the furniture (Fig. 11.9B). There is considerable variability and the action selected seems to depend on opportunity and practice.

One of the few biomechanical studies of crawling (Freedland and Bertenthal, 1994) has described acquisition of a diagonal crawling pattern around 33 and 45 weeks. Variability of timing and some instability are observed at first, and once stability of performance is achieved the infant increases speed. The findings confirm the current view that, rather than being the result of neuromaturational processes, it seems likely that crawling is a learned behaviour contingent upon opportunity and being able to get on to the hands and knees.

## Walking

Locomotor-like behaviour and other movements similar to those seen in newborns have been observed in utero by 15 weeks' post-gestation (de Vries et al., 1982). Thelen and Fisher (1982) showed similarities in newborn infants between the movement pattern seen when kicking in supine and the action of stepping present at birth, but with different mechanical demands. By

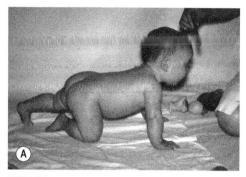

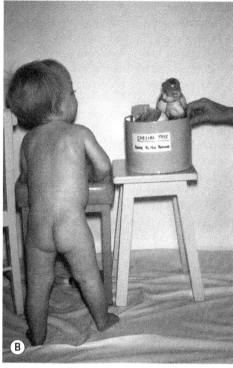

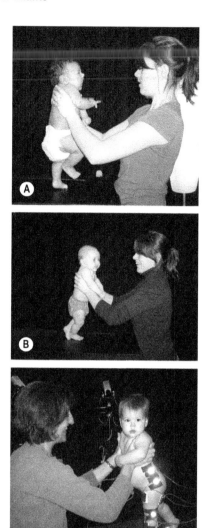

**Figure 11.9 • (A)** Half crawl–half bear walk. **(B)** Walking sideways, probably critical for controlling hip movement in walking. It enables practice of balancing on the feet.

**Figure 11.10 •** Walking for infants on infant treadmill: **(A)** aged 2 months, **(B)** 4 months and **(C)** 9 months.
[From Groenen A et al. (2010) Constraints on early movement: Tykes, togs, and technology. Infant Behav Dev 16–22, with permission from Elsevier.]

the time independent walking commences, the infant already demonstrates the basic locomotor pattern learned from the simple stepping pattern present at birth (Thelen, 1986). Young infants, even pre-walkers aged 4 to 12 months, when placed on a treadmill show similar EMG patterns and interlimb co-ordination as appear in adult walking (Bradley and Westcott, 2006; Pang et al., 2003) (Fig. 11.10).

As noted above, locomotion in the upright position depends on the development of support (weight-bearing), balance and propulsion of the lower limbs. These are the three basic necessities for over-ground progression (Winter, 1987). The study of the basic biomechanics (kinematics, kinetics) and muscle activity of walking in adults provides a framework for understanding the deviations that occur as infants slowly, over many years, develop skill and learn to vary aspects of walking to fit environmental circumstances and task. Knowing the basic biomechanical characteristics also forms a framework for analysis and intervention for individuals with impairments of the neuromuscular system (Fig. 11.11A,B).

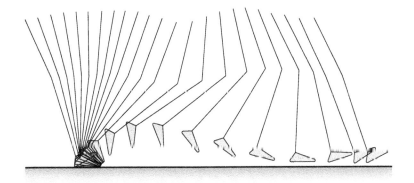

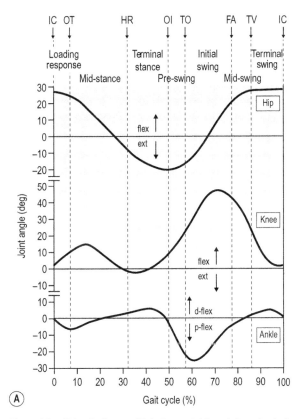

**Figure 11.11A •** Upper: position of the R leg in the sagittal plane at 40 ms intervals during a single gait cycle. Lower: sagittal plane hip, knee, ankle joint angles (degrees) during a single gait cycle. IC, initial contact; OT, opposite toe-off; HR, heel rise; OI, opposite initial contact; TO, toe-off; FA, feet adjacent; TV, tibia vertical. [(A) From Whittle MW (2007) Gait analysis: An introduction 4th ed. with permission from Elsevier.]

There have been several descriptions of the kinematics, kinetics and EMG parameters of gait in children with and without CP (Forssberg, 1985). Before walking independently, the infant 'cruises' the furniture, walking sideways. This has the advantage of providing practice of one of the critical features of walking, its initiation. For example, prior to lifting the left foot to take a step, pressure downward through this foot shifts the body mass to the right, over the stance leg (Kirker et al., 2000).

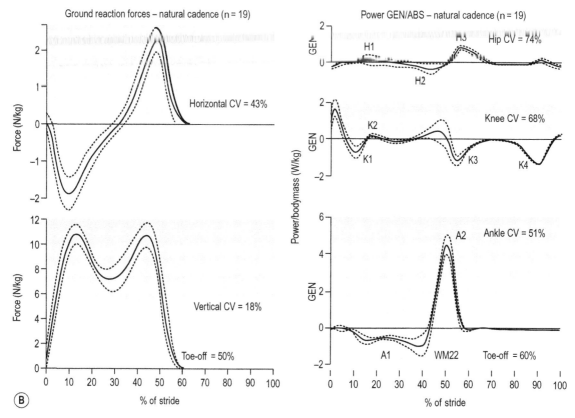

**Figure 11.11B** • Left: averaged horizontal (upper) and vertical (lower) ground reaction forces (GRF). Horizontal GRF has a negative phase in the first half of stance, indicating a slowing down of the body, and a positive phase indicating forward acceleration of the body, during the latter half of stance. Vertical force has the characteristic double hump, the first related to weight-acceptance, the second to push-off. CV, coefficient of variation. Right: ensemble averages of power patterns of able-bodied subjects walking at their preferred cadence plotted over a single gait cycle showing the most important power phases for hip (H), knee (K) and ankle (A); 60% indicates the beginning of swing phase. CV, coefficient of variation.

[(B) From Winter DA (1987) The Biomechanics and Motor Control of Human Gait Waterloo Biomechanics.]

In other words, a step can be taken only when there has been a shift of the body mass in the frontal plane from the stepping leg to the standing leg, a shift that is initiated by the stepping leg. Early attempts at walking show the strain of balancing the body mass and the effects of poor motor control— the infant takes small flat-footed steps with feet apart to give a wider base of support.

Once walking becomes independent (usually between 9 and 18 months), it gradually becomes more effective in achieving the infant's goals and is therefore more skilled. This development occurs as the infant practices in different environments. Increases in strength and balance are integral to the development of mature walking. Balancing through stance phase as the leg extends at the hip over

the dorsiflexing ankle is a particular challenge to stability. Early attempts at walking avoid this action to some extent as the infant moves quickly, takes small steps with feet apart, places the foot down flat at the end of swing and lifts it up without push-off at the start of swing.

As balance in walking improves, the infant carries toys, pushes and pulls trailers, walks on different surfaces, and up and down small steps and inclines, and runs. As infants practice, they develop flexibility of performance. Although walking in varied environments involves the same basic movement pattern (stance phase, swing phase, double stance phase) and similar joint ranges, different environments demand different patterns of muscle force production; for example, the timing of peak

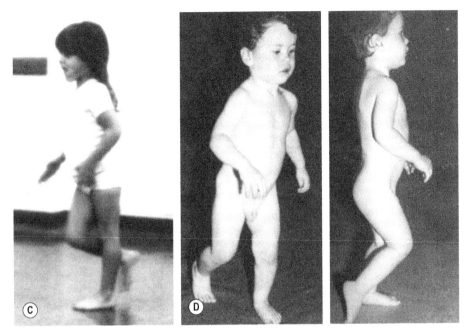

**Figure 11.11C,D** • The little girl on the left with left hemiplegia demonstrates at mid-stance two mechanical effects of calf muscle (soleus) contracture—hyperextended knee due to decreased dorsiflexion, and limited hip extension. Note also the poor control of hip abduction in left stance phase, i.e., her pelvis drops down to the R when she takes weight through her left leg. (D) The boy on the right with diplegia is at the end of stance phase/start of swing phase (i.e., push-off). He demonstrates the mechanical effects of hip flexion contracture and extensor and abductor muscle weakness—internally rotated and adducted hips, and lack of knee and hip extension through stance phase. These effects are more obvious in the lateral view. [(C,D) From Shepherd (1995) Physiotherapy in Paediatrics, with permission from Elsevier.]

forces varies and the type of muscle work differs when walking up and walking down steps and hills (concentric or eccentric; more or less muscle force and energy expenditure). Advanced actions such as jumping (2–3 years), standing on one leg (4 years) and hopping (5 years) take longer before skill is acquired.

The dysfunction stemming from impairments (weakness and dyscontrol) and maladaptive changes to muscle (decreased extensibility) associated with CP become more obvious at the transition between dependent and independent walking. An interesting study carried out 20 years ago, using a treadmill, EMG, motion analysis (for kinematics) and foot contact measures, examined gait immediately before and after the acquisition of independent locomotion in children with and without CP. The children's ages ranged from 9 months to 6 years. The gait pattern of the children with CP was similar initially to that of the able-bodied children. However as walking progressed, they retained some of the characteristics of the infant motor pattern but developed none of the major features of adult gait (dorsiflexion

at heel strike, plantarflexion and hip extension at the end of stance phase, with knee flexion mid-stance) (Leonard et al., 1991; see also Berger et al., 1982, 1984; Berger and Adolph, 2007). It is these major characteristics that should be a focus of early exercise. Training should include exercises for lower limb muscles such as calf muscles and hip extensors (see Figs 11.15–11.24) and walking on a treadmill, since the moving belt tends to drive these aspects of gait.

The change to a more adult pattern of walking normally begins when the child begins to walk independently and continues until 2–4 years of age (Forssberg, 1992). In the infant with CP, the foot is placed flat or on the toes, with premature activation of the calf muscles. In infants with diplegia or hemiplegia, however, when walking becomes independent, calf and hip flexor muscle contractures, if they have not been prevented, may become more evident, together with decreased hip flexion in swing, increased hip internal rotation and adduction and a hyperextended knee through stance phase (Fig. 11.11C,D). Poor activation of calf muscles, in particular, but also weakness and limited hip and knee extension in stance phase, result in weak or absent propulsive force at the end of stance phase.

There have been comparatively few biomechanical studies of gait designed to examine and differentiate the effects of impairments and secondary muscle changes on motor performance in young children with CP (Mayer, 2002; Olney et al., 1990; Tardieu et al., 1982). Gait patterns that continue into childhood and adult life vary depending on the nature of constraints that result from maladaptive musculotendinous changes and joint malformations (Leonard et al., 1991). Modelling studies by Delp et al. (1999) have shown that the major changes to movement of the lower limbs may be linked to hip flexion contracture (see Annotation A, Fig. A.8). This research should stimulate very early and intensive exercise training to strengthen hip extensors and external rotators with exercises and activities targeted to actively stretch the muscles that we anticipate will shorten.

The results of passive movement tests do not predict or inform about the effects of spasticity (stretch reflex hyperactivity) and other impairments on motor performance. However, studies of motor performance that examine biomechanical characteristics and muscle activity have provided useful insights. Crenna (1998, 1999) investigated the effects of hypersensitivity of stretch receptors (muscle spindles) on gait and examined aspects of independent walking in a group of children with CP (average age 7.4 years, with a control group of age-matched able-bodied children). He used EMG of hamstrings and quadriceps muscles and tested biomechanical parameters, including kinematics and kinetics, using a motion analysis system. The unimpaired children showed a positive correlation between the level of motor output and muscle length and/or lengthening velocity during eccentric (lengthening) contractions. In children with diplegia, he found that muscles were active too soon (decreased threshold of lengthening velocity for muscle activation), and with excess force (increased gain of EMG/lengthening velocity relationship). There was a lack of modulation of these timing and force parameters according to walking speed, clonus-like EMG profiles, and increased *mechanical* resistance to joint rotation. The profile

varied with task (walking, hopping, stepping). Eccentric contractions occurring when muscles were decelerating joint rotation were the most frequently affected hamstrings in early stance and late swing, triceps surae in early stance, and quadriceps in late stance.

More recently, van der Krogt and colleagues (2010) set out to quantify dynamic spasticity in 17 children with CP, comparing them with 11 matched able-bodied children. The major finding was an increase in the coupling between muscle–tendon stretch velocity and muscle activity (gastrocnemius medialis, soleus), particularly during swing phase. This explains the commonly observed problem in terminal swing and at foot contact as further elongation of the calf muscles is limited, limiting in turn knee extension and ankle dorsiflexion at foot contact. Muscle length was not reported, so it is possible that the major problem was caused principally by calf muscle contracture associated with secondary (adaptive) stretch reflex hypersensitivity (see Crenna, 1998, 1999).

It is possible that targeted intervention from early infancy aimed at increasing muscle activation, strength and extensibility, and training motor control in task-oriented exercises, as well as minimizing maladaptive changes to muscle (including the development of stretch reflex hyperactivity) would lead to a more appropriate transition to mature walking. This has not been tested. When it is, the methodology used by the above investigators provides a possible model.

## Walking up and down stairs

The biomechanics of these actions have been investigated in adults (Andriacchi et al., 1980), but not in developing infants or young children. Walking up and down stairs is mechanically different from over-ground walking in terms of range of joint movement and magnitude of forces; walking up involves concentric muscle activity, walking down eccentric activity. In young children stairs present difficulty as the stairs are high relative to their leg length. Walking up is usually achieved before walking down. Infants use a variety of methods, including crawling, half-crawling and half-stepping (Fig. 1.10).

Crosbie et al. (2012) investigated associations between the active and passive mechanical properties of the calf muscle in children with CP, together with the spatiotemporal features of their gait on both level ground and over stairs. Twenty-six children with hemiplegia (age range 4–10 years) walked barefoot across a level 10m pathway and a staircase. Walking speed, stride length and cadence were calculated and spasticity, maximum isometric strength, stiffness and hysteresis of the affected side calf muscle were measured. Multiple linear regression indicated that walking speed and stride length were significantly associated with isometric dorsiflexor muscle strength and calf muscle stiffness, while stair ascent and descent speeds were significantly and inversely related to the amount of hysteresis displayed by the calf muscle. Hysteresis is an indicator of the muscle's capacity for elastic recoil and energy release. A high level of hysteresis means that less of the energy applied to muscle to stretch it during loading is returned during unloading. In a recent study it was found to be three times greater in the children with CP compared with able-bodied children (Alhusaini et al., 2010; see Annotation B). The authors point out that reduction in stored elastic energy may contribute to mechanical inefficiencies during weight-bearing activities.

The results demonstrate the considerable influence passive mechanical properties of calf muscle have on walking performance. Given the mechanical similarity between stair walking and the step-up/step-down exercise, it may be that early intervention that includes and persists with this exercise (with variations) and includes other specific strength training exercises and activities that actively stretch the calf muscles may minimize the development of morphological and functional changes to these muscles, and promote more effective and efficient functional performance.

# Part 2: guidelines for activity-based intervention in infancy

Studies of movement in neuroscience and biomechanics are leading to the development of specifically targeted task- or activity-oriented exercise programmes for infants with CP. Such programmes are designed to increase muscle strength, preserve muscle extensibility and stimulate or foster the development of functional motor control in infants who, without intervention,

do not have the necessary muscle strength or co-ordinating ability to initiate more than a few stereotyped and ineffective movement patterns. In these programmes the therapist/parent sets up an environment designed to encourage and 'drive' the actions required and to give clear feedback to the infant about what is effective and what is not. Successful attempts, achieving the goal, are in themselves rewarding. Instead of the therapist and parent controlling the infant's movements, the infant is stimulated to move about and explore the possibilities available, with guidance as required. The emphasis is on an effective action that achieves a goal, with training based on establishing critical biomechanical components (those without which the action cannot be performed), not on the vague concept of movement 'quality' or 'normalization'.

Gaining skills in motor performance requires that the infant not only has the ability to generate muscle forces, but also to time the forces produced by a large number of muscles in order to produce an effective movement. Infants need to incorporate and control the effects of muscle forces along with interactional, intersegmental and gravitational forces. The capacity to do all this enables the muscle system to take advantage of enhancing mechanisms such as the stretch-shortening cycle, in which the stored elastic energy produced by a muscle's forceful eccentric contraction is released when this contraction switches to concentric (Komi, 2000, 2003). Control of complex intersegmental relationships has to be 'learned' through repetitive and challenging practice in order to bring about an effective (as skilled as possible) movement.

# Optimizing support and balance

Balance is defined as the ability to control the body mass relative to the base of support (Ghez, 1991). Terms commonly used in the clinic to refer to balance include postural stability, postural control and postural adjustments. These are general terms that relate to the ability of the body to adjust itself appropriately for effective functional performance. They can be replaced by more accurate descriptors—it is muscle activation and joint movement that enable us to balance and they depend on inputs from movement sensors that include vision and the vestibular system. Balance must maintain a steady state in the presence of gravity; it must anticipate potentially destabilizing effects of self-initiated movements and be adaptive throughout those movements, and must also respond to unexpected perturbations. Balance forms the foundation for all voluntary motor skills (Massion and Woollacott, 1996) and training balanced movement may therefore be the most significant part of rehabilitation (Carr and Shepherd, 2003, 2010). This information has clinical implications even in early infancy. The infant has to experience instability in order to learn how to balance. The therapist and parent create a situation of instability by not holding the infant too firmly when she is in sitting or standing, and by giving her the chance to experience what adjustments are most effective, i.e., best achieve the goal.

Throughout life the ability to balance develops during practice of specific actions and balance adjustments are an integral part of any movement. Therefore balance training itself cannot be separated from movement and cannot be a separate item in a targeted activity programme. Similarly, balance is not testable as a separate entity in clinical investigations. The failure of balance to be understood in this way may be a relic of the time when balance was thought to be the result of reflex mechanisms, automatic responses. Bobath therapy was based on the idea that balance was the result of a 'postural reflex mechanism', which included 'equilibrium reactions' and 'righting reactions' (Bobath, 1971; Bower, 2009)—reactive responses made when the body's CoM is moved by the therapist beyond an individual's limit of stability, causing the person to respond. Treatment included facilitation of these reactions, with the assumption that the effects would transfer or generalize into self-initiated functional actions. There is no theoretical or evidence-based support for these ideas since biomechanical research carried out in the last half of the 20th century clarified the various ways in which an individual balances the body mass prior to and during self-initiated movement, and in response to external perturbations.

Current understanding of balance is that the muscle activations and joint movements involved in balancing the body mass throughout our actions are specific to task and context, and depend on muscle activity and motor control. Tests used in the clinic, however, may assume generalizability from, for example, a greater distance reached in standing (Functional Reach Test) to improved balance in standing when other actions are performed. This assumption has not been tested, but there is no reason why it could not be tested. It is more likely that balance can only be achieved, in either infants or adults, by independent self-initiated practice of a large variety of activities. Effective balance while walking may be inferred from records of change in biomechanical or spatiotemporal parameters over time: for example, reduced width of stance during walking, increased stride length and speed, ability to walk along a straight line. In sit-to-stand, reduced movement of CoG ('steadiness') when standing is reached, approximately equal peak vertical force under each foot and increased speed of movement can be taken to infer more effective balance throughout performance of the action.

Most investigations of balance in both sitting and standing have involved the study of the infant's response to unexpected perturbations (Hedberg et al., 2005; Hirschfeld, 1992) and there has been little investigation in children or adults of the muscle and joint adjustments (or 'postural' adjustments) that occur during self-initiated movement. However, a positive result of the unexpected perturbation studies has been the development of a method of training this aspect of balance. A study of older children investigated the effects of training balance responses on a movable force plate system that subjected the children to unexpected perturbations (Shumway-Cook et al., 2003). The findings showed improvements in the children's ability to recover stability when balance was unexpectedly disturbed, following a period of training with 100 perturbations per day for five days. In a later study (de Graaf-Peters et al., 2007), a group of high-risk infants at corrected age 3 months were allocated to a neurodevelopmental therapy (NDT group or an active self-initiated trial-and-error group. The results suggested that treatments such as NDT that involve substantial amount of handling and provision of support are not effective in improving postural control.

It is very likely that the ability to balance the body mass while moving develops over time according to the infant's opportunities to practice self-initiated actions without support, and this needs further investigation.

Dusing and Harbourne (2010) have highlighted the importance of variability in postural control during development in able-bodied infants, pointing out that variable and adaptive balance control enables exploration of the possibilities available. They discuss the variability of balance control during infant development from the perspective of spontaneous behaviour rather than reactive. They also point out that 'guidance to facilitate normal patterns of postural behaviour' should not be the focus of intervention, but should be replaced by guidance involving verbal or light touch cues to encourage the infant's own explorations.

Parents can provide infants with varied experiences in a variety of positions with decreasing amounts of support. They are shown ways to carry and play with the infant that encourage movements of the head, trunk and upper and lower limbs (Fig. 11.12). Soft materials, including strapping, can constrain a limb from taking up a stereotyped position when in supine and prone and enable reaching or kicking movements to take up different trajectories. Parents help their infant to develop balance in sitting and standing when they sit the infant on the lap or across one leg with feet on the floor, or stand him between their knees and talk, sing and play. Light fingertip support is usually sufficient as the infant moves the body from side to side and back and forth, returning to the erect position (Fig. 11.12A).

## Balancing in sitting

In early infancy, sitting balance is practiced on a parent's lap and sitting on a bench or the floor. As trunk and hip muscles increase in strength, the infant learns to control head and body movement without falling back. By 7–8 months, when infants can sit independently on the floor, and on a seat supported by thighs and feet, and their hands are no longer needed for support, their capacity for exploration becomes more varied. The rate at which independent sitting is achieved seems to depend to some extent on child-rearing practices: that is, on opportunity. The sooner the infant can sit on a small stool, the sooner he can practice reaching out for toys across a table, getting down on to the floor and standing up (Fig. 11.13C). For infants with CP (particularly with hemiplegia and diplegia), sitting on a seat allows early practice of weight-bearing through the feet, standing up, taking a few steps and walking. Early practice of standing up with feet flat on the floor may help preserve extensibility in hip flexors, hamstrings and calf muscles.

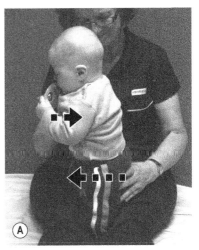

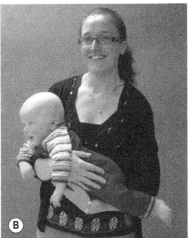

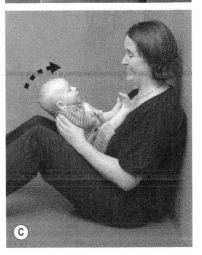

**Figure 11.12** • Holding, moving and playing are particularly important in young infants as they learn to move and control the head and body against gravity.
[From www.physiotherapyexercise.com with permission.]

Two studies on the effects of active balance training during movements performed in sitting showed improvements. In one study (Hadders-Algra et al., 1996), infants aged 5–6 months received three months of daily balance training carried out at home three times a day for five minutes. By 7–8 and 7–9 months of age, when responses to platform perturbation were tested, infants showed an accelerated development of the ability to modulate the degree of ventral muscle contraction to the velocity of the moving platform and to body configuration at perturbation onset. The other study (Sveistrup and Woollacott, 1997) tested the effect of exposure to 100 balance perturbations/day on three consecutive days during pull-to-stand with infants aged 9–11 months. These infants showed an increase in the rate of direction-specific adjustments, and an increase in the distal-to-proximal muscle recruitment.

There has been little investigation of the development of the ability to sit independently on a seat, feet on floor, perhaps because Western-reared babies spend much of their time on the floor. Sitting on the floor may not be a suitable position for an infant who is slow to progress beyond sitting (Fig. 11.13C), or has developed contractures of hamstring muscles (Fig. 11.13A).

## Balancing in standing

Standing at a table or chair allows practice of balancing in standing (Fig. 11.13D). The infant is encouraged to experiment with movement, taking one hand (or both) off the support to reach out to play, to reach down to pick up a toy. At this point, if the opportunity is provided, major practice time can be spent mastering the control of the body over a small base of support (the feet), with constraints placed on the floor to prevent too wide a base, and to keep the feet closer together if necessary. A harness allows this practice if the infant has insufficient balance. Infants are also learning to balance when they practice walking sideways using the furniture for support or, dependent upon an adult and a harness or grab belt for support, take a few steps. Standing practice should involve different foot placements, including one foot a short distance ahead of the other, and stepping movements with one leg in all directions (Fig. A.5A). A harness is a useful aid as it enables independent practice, with self-initiated movement, allowing the infant to stagger but not

to fall (Figs 1.1 and A.10B). It can give varying amounts of support and infants (as well as adults after stroke) can find it a relatively secure way for independent practice that allows them to 'get the idea' of keeping their balance as they move about.

Above are descriptions of some activities that challenge balance. The next few pages describe specific exercises for muscle strength, intersegmental control and extensibility of muscles prone to contracture. The activity-specific exercises described are designed to drive the learning of functional actions that are made up of the same basic biomechanical pattern (Fig. 11.1): i.e., it is assumed, with some evidence, that practice of these basic actions will generalize to improved performance of the actions of which they are a critical part. Practice of these weight-bearing actions is also directed at challenging balance. The therapist keeps this in mind so the infant is not supported any more than is necessary to prevent a heavy fall or to provide specific assistance.

## Functional activities for the lower limbs

Extending the trunk and hips and weight-bearing through the arms in prone is encouraged from earliest infancy. In the first few months, infants need encouragement and assistance to move about in supine and prone (Fig. 11.14A). They must develop the ability to control their head position and a major stimulus is provided by vision and when the infant is upright (Fig. 11.12). The environment can be developed to encourage (drive) head and trunk extension weight-bearing through the arms, reaching out and rolling over (Fig. 11.14B). Experience of bearing weight on hands and knees can be assisted by a harness or 'noodle' that holds the infant's trunk, shoulders and hips off the floor.

The exercises below target the basic flexion–extension movements of the lower limbs that are present from earliest infancy and are major biomechanical characteristics of functional actions performed in daily life (Box 11.1). It is likely that mastering flexion and extension of hips, knees and ankles while supporting and balancing the body mass over the plantigrade feet is critical to an infant's future motor development just as flexion and external rotation of the shoulder, extension of the elbow and wrist and finger extension, and supporting

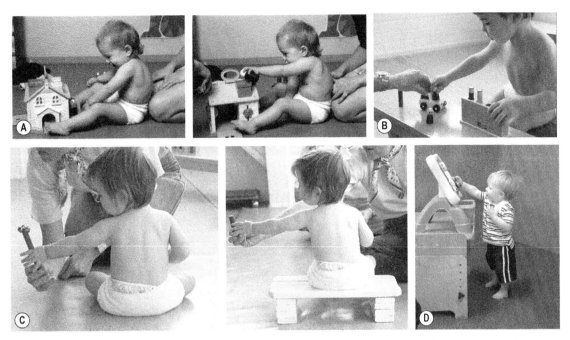

**Figure 11.13 • (A)** This infant with diplegia demonstrates the mechanical and functional effects of increased hamstring stiffness and contracture. She cannot flex her hips sufficiently to sit on the floor. She would have improved concentration and play more effectively if she were to sit on a stool with feet on the floor, as does the boy in **(B)** who can now pay more attention to his games. Both children need exercises to teach actions made up of flexion and extension of hips, knees, ankles, to decrease extensor muscle overactivity, as well as to preserve the extensibility of lower limb muscles (see Figs 11.15 to 11.18). **(C)** The little girl habitually adopts this sitting position when on the floor and although she reaches out toward toys she does not move her body away from the midline. Sitting on a stool with her feet on the floor enables her to use her lower limbs to balance as she shifts her body a little further to the side. **(D)** Learning to balance in standing during self-initiated actions—making preparatory and ongoing adjustments (at joint and muscle levels). [(A–C) From Shepherd (1995) Physiotherapy in Paediatrics, with permission from Elsevier. (D) From www.physiotherapyexercise.com with permission.]

and balancing the body, are the basic actions underlying transport of the hand in reaching actions.

## Kicking

Parents can demonstrate the kicking action to the infant by using passive movements if necessary, with appropriate encouragement to copy actively, both legs kicking together or alternately. Kicking a mobile has been described in several investigations and interactive devices are in development (Chen et al., 2002; Fetters et al., 2004; Thelen, 1994) (see Annotation C). Such a device must be developed for clinical use since it would enable the infant to practice a variety of leg movements independently, offers an interesting challenge and provides mental as well as physical stimulus. An

infant who is slow to move the legs may be more likely to take up kicking when half-lying or in supine if she is also experiencing other lower limb actions such as crouch or sit-to-stand.

## Raising and lowering the body mass

The weight-bearing actions below are aimed at stimulating muscle activation since weakness and diminished force production are sequelae of the neural lesion. The exercises are task-related and target motor control, muscle contractility, strength and extensibility. They train the basic lower limb actions of raising and lowering the body mass over the feet and stimulate learning processes associated with development of motor control. It may be

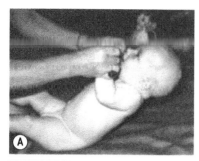

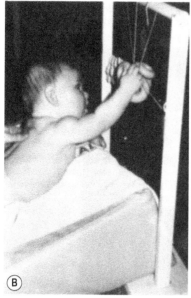

**Figure 11.14 • (A)** Infant aged 3 months: exercise to train neck and trunk flexor muscles. **(B)** Training extensor muscles during play. Eye contact is critical at this early stage as visual attention drives movement, particularly movement of the head.
[From Shepherd (1995) Physiotherapy in Paediatrics, with permission from Elsevier.]

## Box 11.1

### Basic lower limb actions in infancy

- Kicking
- Raising and lowering the body mass with feet on the floor:
  - Squat-stand-squat
  - Sit-stand-sit to and from a seated position
  - Stepping up and stepping down
- Bipedal locomotion:
  - Overground walking- sideways along wall/bench, forwards, carrying objects, pushing a cart
  - Stair walking: up and down
  - Slope walking: up and down

---

As discussed in the Introduction, exercise effects tend to be specific to task and context, with the greatest changes occurring in the training exercise itself. However, there is also evidence that transfer of the training effect can occur between actions that share similar biomechanical characteristics (see Chapter 1 and Annotation A). Exercises such as step ups, heels raise and lower, standing up and sitting down, and squats strengthen weak lower limb muscles concentrically and eccentrically, using body weight resistance, and can improve segmental limb control. They take advantage of the specificity principle in that they provide similar functional stresses to many common actions. Muscles are exercised in an action pattern that shares common dynamic characteristics with many everyday actions. In particular, these exercises train the ability of extensor muscles to switch from shortening (concentric) to lengthening (eccentric) contractions in muscles spanning more than one joint (e.g., biceps femoris, gastrocnemius), as well as single-joint muscles such as gluteus maximus and soleus. In addition, they require contraction of other muscles that play a synergic role in controlling the limb and balancing the body mass.

All of these activities target balance, as none can be performed independently without balance. They are performed with focus on the foot/feet placed firmly on the floor, and they should be as challenging as possible (i.e., increasing the load to be lifted and lowered and the number of repetitions, and increasing the difficulty over time). The hip, knee and ankle muscles are exercised throughout the range required by these actions in daily life. The aims are to preserve functional muscle lengths (minimize

possible that increasing the demands on muscles to contract in the first few weeks after birth may act as a stimulant to corticomotor tract development and this hypothesis needs testing. Guidance or manipulation of the exercise environment can ensure that muscles at risk of contracture are exercised through the fullest range. These actions can be trained and practiced concurrently from earliest infancy. As a general rule, an action to be learned should be practiced in its entirety since one component of the action depends on preceding components. The required physiological and biomechanical control mechanisms involved in any action can only be organized during practice of that action.

or prevent muscle contracture development), exercise (strengthen) lower limb extensor muscles in both concentric and eccentric mode, and to train co-ordination of the lower limbs. Motor learning focus is on a basic lower limb pattern, and developing a flexibility of performance that will enable the infant to be successful in a variety of different environments and scenarios as she grows and develops.

Early emphasis is on preserving calf muscle length, particularly single-joint soleus muscle. Practice of the following actions with attention to foot position and weight-bearing may, in infants with diplegia or hemiplegia, minimize development of soleus muscle contracture, which, even in the early months, can have a widespread effect on the position of the lower limb in standing and sitting. For example, if the ankles cannot be placed at approximately 75° in sitting it will be difficult for the infant to stand up, and to maintain standing and balance (see Fig. 1.2). A foot frame to hold the foot/feet plantigrade while exercising/practicing may be necessary (Fig. A.3); standing on a backward sloping wedge or on parent's knee stretches the calf muscles actively when the infant is encouraged to raise and lower the heels.

The exercises below are practiced with 'maximum repetitions' with no breaks, in sets of three, with a short break between sets. Of course this is an ideal and the details are adapted as they depend on the infant's acceptance and ability. A counter is a useful aid for a child to count repetitions once he understands numbers. In infants, repetitive practice is organized during play; for example, standing up from a seat to take a toy and then sitting down to put it on the floor, several times (see Figs 11.17, 11.18, 11.21, 11.24). Exercises are practiced as often as possible to increase muscle activation capacity and ability to generate necessary muscle force. Exercises should be difficult enough to present a challenge, while still being possible. Enabling variability in performance as the infant catches sight of something interesting is also important so the infant develops the capacity to vary movements when necessary: that is, when a goal or the environment demand it.

The incentive to perform particular actions is provided by toys and objects of suitable size and varied interest. Interactive aids are being developed that add incentive, feedback and challenge to even young infants in the early stages of their motor development (see Chapter 15 and Annotation C). Interactive devices and those that can constrain specific movements to their natural kinematic

patterns will enable an intensity of practice that is otherwise not practical for families. Therapists who have used manipulating and handling techniques for many years to help stimulate desirable movement patterns will change the focus to a more training model, minimizing their own control of the action, and passing control on to the infant with minimal hands-on from themselves: setting up natural environmental constraints, using soft splinting and their own fingertip control to guide the infant's performance. As Damiano points out in Chapter 9 'manipulating and handling techniques...may have actually restricted learning in that they also compensated for rather than addressed the deficits that prevented the child from doing the task him or herself and did not allow the child to develop [and use] accurate intrinsic feedback'.

## Step up and down exercise

Hip, knee and ankle extensor muscles are trained to work co-operatively, concentrically and eccentrically to raise and lower the body mass (Fig. 11.15). In stepping up forwards, the ankle dorsiflexors and lower limb extensors are exercised *concentrically* as they move the body mass forward and up over the front foot on the step, then lengthen *eccentrically* as the body mass is lowered on to the back leg. In stepping up sideways, the abductor muscles of the standing leg are producers of hip abduction/extension force if the hip is held in an extended position, for example with light strapping. Forces are normally distributed evenly over the three joints when stepping up and down in a forward direction, and are more concentrated at the knee in lateral step ups (Agahari et al., 1996).

Load is supplied by body weight, and the amount of muscle strength required can be progressed by raising step height, or, in an older infant, by adding small weights to a vest with pockets (see Liao et al., 2007). The exercise can also be practiced in a harness that gives the infant freedom to move (and to stumble) while preventing a fall.

Performance is progressed as infants grow and develop (Fig. 11.15B), until they can incorporate the action into walking over obstacles and climbing stairs (see Figs 11.18D, 11.23 and 11.24B,C). Stepping down forwards is also encouraged as soon as possible. The action makes different biomechanical and muscle demands and is necessary for stair descent (see Fig. 11.18D).

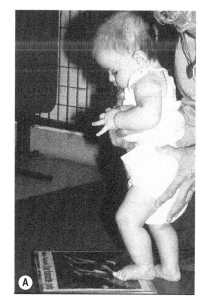
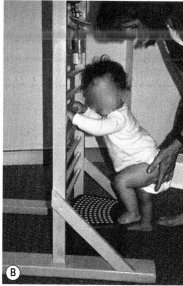
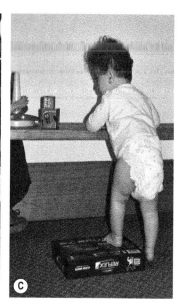

**Figure 11.15** • Step up and down exercises in the sagittal plane. **(A)** This young infant needs assistance but is getting the idea of stepping up and down on one leg. **(B)** This 13-month-old girl supports herself on the rails as she steps up and down; only fingertip assistance for balance from the therapist/parent is necessary. The environment has been set up to offer many possibilities for exploration. She is encouraged to step up and play with objects higher up the railings. The height of the step is progressively increased as her extensor muscle strength increases. **(C)** Step up and down in the frontal plane. She also practices lateral step ups and is learning to control her ability to raise and lower her body mass through a variety of different actions.

[(A) From Shepherd (1995) Physiotherapy in Paediatrics, with permission from Elsevier.]

## EXERCISE: STEP UP AND DOWN IN SAGITTAL PLANE

Start with one foot on a small step or the infant puts her foot on the step herself. With encouragement and a little pressure forward, the infant steps up and down, i.e., her body moves forward and up over the left foot, then back and down, stepping back and forth several times if possible (Fig. 11.15A, B).

### CHECK

- Organize the environment to provide several incentives for the infant to move
- Place the foot on the step if necessary
- Ensure the knee moves forward over the foot before the upward movement
- Hold the knee gently to keep it forward and to stabilize the foot on the step during the action if necessary
- Align the right knee/hip in extension with the foot on the floor; assist the movement forward and up
- Do not take all of the infant's weight; use gentle pressure forward at the hips if necessary

## EXERCISE: STEP UP AND DOWN IN FRONTAL PLANE

Place the foot of the affected leg on a small step or let the infant place the foot on the step herself. The body is shifted sideways, up and down or she will progress along the bench, stepping up and down where necessary (Fig. 11.15C).

### CHECK

- Organize the environment to provide several incentives for movement
- Place the foot on the step or demonstrate the action if necessary
- The knee should move forward over the foot before the upward movement
- Hold the left knee gently to keep it forward and the foot on the step if necessary
- Do not hold the infant up; use fingertip control, a grab belt or harness if necessary
- The infant can also walk sideways along the bench, bending the right hip and knee to step down with the left foot.

## Crouching-squatting

Crouching and squatting are necessary actions throughout life, e.g., to pick up objects from the floor when standing. Infants can normally stand up from a sitting position on the floor through a squat using hands for support, and squatting is a common position for playing on the floor (see Annotation A, Fig. A.9). In very young infants, the action needs assistance, but if held appropriately the infant can do repetitive squat-to-stands (Figs 11.16 and 11.17). If the infant tends to stiffen the legs in standing, repetitive squats up and down through a small range can be practiced, preventing full extension until the stiffening ceases; the therapist might turn this into a sing-song routine—up and down, down and up. It is necessary at first to hold the lower legs and to steady the infant but assistance should be as little as possible. The infant can practice the action by reaching down to pick up (or touch) an object (Fig. 11.18 A–C). The depth of squat can be modified, with the object placed on a stool or on the floor. Until balance is acquired the infant can practice in a harness that allows him to squat down and stand up. At first it may be more difficult for an infant to flex hips, knees and ankles and lower the body mass into a squat, as it involves eccentric muscle contractions. Gentle pressure behind or in front of the knees may initiate the flexion action.

Attention to foot position is essential if calf muscles are to be stretched. If the feet are not flat on the floor the infant may need to wear shoes on a foot frame that holds the feet flat during the exercises (see Fig. A.3).

### EXERCISE: SQUATTING-CROUCHING

- Start with infant in the squat position.
- Provide incentives to stand up from the squat; set up the environment to encourage the action, e.g., hands on table or in parent's hands and pulling up into standing.
- Increase flexibility of performance by having the infant combine squat-to-stand with sit-to-stand.
- In the squat position, set up the surroundings so the infant can play in this position, encourage a shift from sitting to squat and standing.
- Infant needs to get the idea of the movement and the possibilities for play.

## Weight-bearing calf muscle exercises

Ankle plantarflexors are critical muscles in all actions performed while bearing weight through the feet, but they are prone to increasing stiffness and contracture, and they should be exercised actively through range as early as possible in infancy (Hampton et al., 2003; Olney et al., 1990). The length of gastrocnemius and, particularly, soleus should be a major focus of prevention from a very early age. Calf muscles provide power and energy for propulsion in the stance phase of walking, particularly when walking up a slope, and they generate faster walking speeds (Olney et al., 1986; Winter, 1989). With the dorsiflexor muscles, they contribute to ankle stability

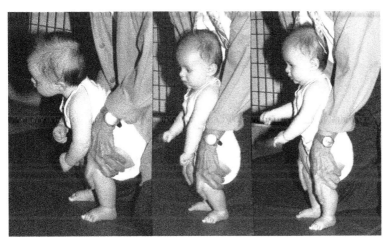

**Figure 11.16** • Left hemiplegia. This 3-month-old infant is practicing repetitive crouch-stand with some support. Nursery rhymes or counting make it a game. [From Shepherd (1995) Physiotherapy in Paediatrics, with permission from Elsevier.]

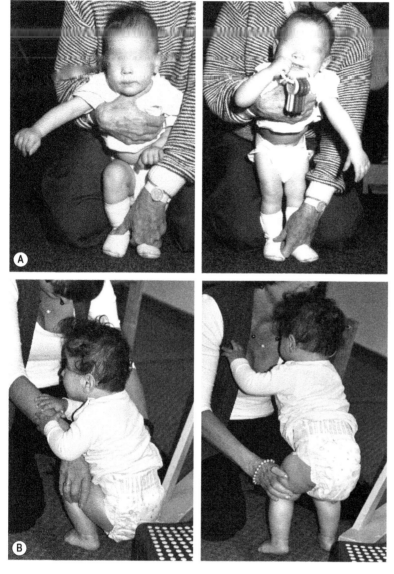

**Figure 11.17** • Crouch–stand–crouch. **(A)** He crouches to pick up the keys, then stands up to put them on the table. Pressure was applied down through his feet so he got the idea of bending and straightening his legs by pushing through his feet. **(B)** At 13 months, she needs only gentle pressure down through her legs to help her stand up, and gentle pressure behind her knees helps her to initiate flexion to descend into crouch.
[(A) From Shepherd (1995) Physiotherapy in Paediatrics, with permission from Elsevier.]

in standing, and assist in balancing the body mass over the base of support, with movements that take place at the ankles and hips in standing. The step up and down, squatting and sit-to-stand exercises described here all involve active lengthening of calf muscles through almost full range if the infant can perform the action (Figs 11.17 and 11.18). The feet must be placed appropriately with heels on the floor. The actions may have to be performed in a small range (constrained) until the heels can remain on the ground. If this is not possible, the feet should be held flat to the floor by some means (see Figs A.3 and 11.17) and periods of active stretching during heels raise and lower limb exercise can be interspersed with passive stretches while bearing weight through the legs (Fig. 11.19).

Zhao et al. (2011) have recently published evidence that controlled passive ankle stretching driven by a servomotor and controlled by a digital signal processor plus resisted (assisted if necessary) active exercise to the calf muscles can result in elongation of muscle fascicles, reduced pennation angle and fascicular stiffness, decreased tendon length and increased Achilles tendon stiffness. The authors suggest that in vivo examinations of muscles and tendon mechanical properties can increase our understanding of exercise-induced changes in muscle and facilitate development of more effective

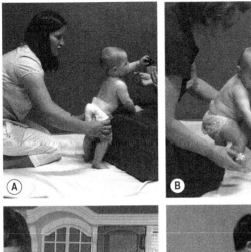

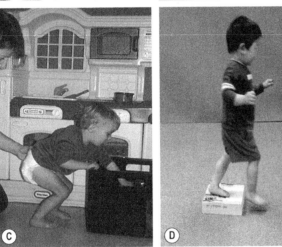

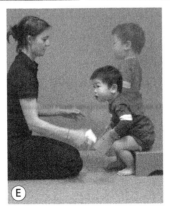

**Figure 11.18** • Exercises/games to train lower limb control. **(A)** Practicing standing—the 'coach' gives him the idea of extending his hips; then she should remove her hands so he can initiate the necessary movements himself as he reaches up (extending hips) to take the toy. **(B)** Squatting to pick up the toy. **(C)** Squatting to take a toy out of the box. **(D)** Flexion/extension as he steps on to and off a book placed as part of an obstacle-walking trail. **(E)** Sit stand sit with the left foot placed further back to 'force' the weaker left leg to bear weight. [(A, B, D, E) From www.physiotherapyexercise.com with permission.]

treatments. A recent study (Forrester et al., 2011) of a robotic device that involved the individual actively dorsiflexing-plantarflexing the ankle to operate a computer game resulted in improved ankle control (faster, smoother movements), increased walking velocity and more even support through the paretic limb. Although the subjects were adults after stroke, a version of this device may assist infants to

obtain better control of the ankle movements so critical to motor development.

The *heels raise and lower exercise* in Figures 11.19 and 11.20 starts with ankles in maximum dorsiflexion. Raising the body mass from a dorsiflexed position in the heels raise action exercises the calf muscles concentrically as they plantarflex the ankle as the heels are lowered,

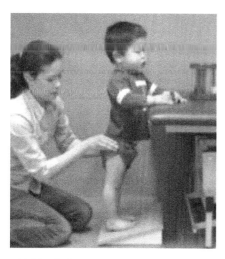

**Figure 11.19** • Calf muscle exercise. The infant stands on a wedge to play (passive stretch of calf muscles + co-ordination of lower limb joints); raises and lowers his heels for a maximum number of repetitions (active stretch to calf muscles + co-ordination of lower limb joints); and also exercises his dorsiflexor muscles. [From www. physiotherapyexercise.com with permission.]

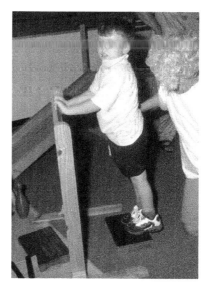

**Figure 11.20** • Heels raise and lower exercise. One of the workstations in a circuit-training class. The boy lowers his heels to the floor then lifts them to the plantigrade position, with maximum number of repetitions. The objective is to strengthen, actively stretch and train calf muscles specifically for push-off at the end of stance phase.

and eccentrically as the heels are lowered. It is preferable that the infant raises the heels only to the plantigrade position if they have a tendency to go up on their toes. The exercise actively stretches the eccentrically contracting calf muscles when the heel is lowered and the foot is dorsiflexed. It is therefore important for preserving the calf muscle length critical for push-off in gait and in the performance of many weight-bearing actions, including sit-to-stand.

This exercise is useful for training motor control throughout the limb, since the mechanics and motor control processes of the action are surprisingly complex. Prior to rising on to the toes in standing, the body moves forward. Swinging the upper body forwards and dorsiflexing the ankles brings the body mass forward over the feet; the quadriceps contracts prior to the plantarflexors to counter the knee flexion force arising from the bi-articular gastrocnemius contraction as the body weight is raised (Diener et al., 1992). This apparently simple action is probably effective in training intersegmental control of the hip, knee and ankle.

The *forward step down exercise* puts a maximum stretch on calf muscles of the supporting leg and trains eccentric control of extensor muscles of that leg, particularly quadriceps (Fig. 11.18D).

These are difficult actions to train in an infant but should be attempted as part of play whenever

the possibility arises. Standing on a parent's knee, for example, is relatively simple with a very young infant. Heels raise and lower can be done on two legs or on one, with the infant held in standing by a grab belt or by holding clothing.

## EXERCISE: STRETCHING AND STRENGTHENING CALF MUSCLES

### Heels raise and lower

- Forefoot on small step, heels on floor, ankle(s) in dorsiflexion
- Raise heel(s) to plantigrade
- Hip(s) and knee(s) extended throughout
- Use fingertip control to keep the hips forward (extended)
- Standing on parent's leg, feet in dorsiflexion

### Forward step downs

- Start with both feet on the step, infant steps down and forward, then back and up
- Include steps in a walking route (Fig. 11.18D)
- Use a grab belt if necessary

### Standing to play

- Infant stands on a wedge with feet in dorsiflexion during table play
- The stretch is both passive and active as the infant moves about

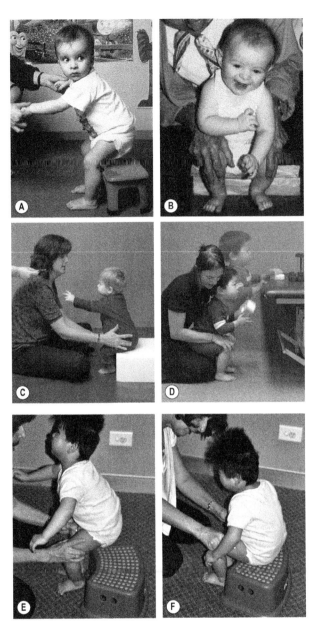

**Figure 11.21** • Sit-to-stand exercise. **(A)** Compare the shape of this boy's attempt to stand up with the shape in Fig. 11.8B. He has diplegia and has extended his knees and hips prematurely. His feet are not placed optimally; his knees are not sufficiently forward and his upper body is not flexed at the hips. He should not practice like this as it may be too hard to unlearn later. Instead, he should practice repetitive up and downs with his knees held forward until he has the idea of moving his weight forward over his feet on his own. As he progresses a toy can be placed on the seat before he sits down. This allows practice of sitting down to touch the toy with his bottom, then stand up, and it makes him work hard at the point of most difficulty. **(B)** A 4-month-old practices with assistance at the knees. Note feet have been placed in the optimal position. **(C)** The therapist steadies the infant as he does not yet have the ability to balance throughout the action. **(D)** The therapist moves the infant's knee (and body mass) forward to show him what he must do. **(E, F)** This little boy needs assistance to initiate knee flexion for sitting down. [(A, B) from Shepherd (1995) Physiotherapy in Paedatrics, with permission from Elsevier. (C, D) From www.physiotherapyexercise.com with permission.]

## Standing up and sitting down

Normative biomechanics provides the basis for recognizing the mechanical reasons for poor performance of standing up and sitting down in children with CP. Standing up requires major force generation from hip, knee and ankle extensors, principally from quadriceps, as well as the ability to control both angular momentum caused by the trunk flexing forward at the hips, and horizontal and vertical linear momentum of the CoM. The able-bodied child can only master the action when she has acquired the ability to balance and to vary the goal, probably towards the end of the second year.

The action, if performed with many repetitions, can become an exercise to increase muscle strength and control of the limbs, as well as a vehicle for learning how to stand up and sit down while remaining in balance (Fig. 11.21; see Fig. A.1). If muscles are weak, seat height is increased so less muscle force is required. As muscles become stronger, seat height is lowered and repetitions are increased to improve endurance (see Fig. A.5D). In infants with hemiplegia, the foot of the paretic limb can be 'forced' to bear weight during the action by placing it further back than the non-paretic foot before movement starts, making sure the heel is on the floor (Fig. 11.18E). If necessary, gentle pressure down and back can be given through the knee to maintain the heel on the floor. Infants with hemiplegia spontaneously shift the foot of the stronger leg back before attempting to stand up. If so, a solid block can constrain this foot so that it is cannot be moved back, forcing the weaker leg to take more weight.

Common problems in infants and children with diplegia or hemiplegia as they attempt to stand up include an inability to: (1) move both feet back sufficiently—Figure 11.21A shows what happens when the feet are too far forward; (2) time peak knee and hip extensor forces—in this figure the infant has extended the hips and knees too soon.

Calf muscle contracture interferes with foot position and prevents the shank from dorsiflexing at the ankle and this exercise is another method of preserving calf muscle extensibility. In sitting down, an infant with CP may have difficulty initiating the eccentric contraction of the extensor muscles, particular the quadriceps, and, once initiated, to control the descent, including the movement of body mass back to the seat, which requires sufficient strength and control of dorsiflexor muscles to steady the body as it moves backward (Fig. 11.21E,F).

Studies of adults after stroke following similar guidelines have shown positive effects (Britten et al., 2008; Cheng et al., 2001; Dean et al., 2000; Monger et al., 2002). Two studies of young children have shown significant improvement in sit-to-stand performance after periods of training based on these guidelines. Blundell et al. (2003), in a study with children aged 3–8 years, found that a four-week group circuit-training programme for the lower limbs, which included repetitive sit-to-stand practice, significantly increased lower limb muscle strength and sit-to-stand performance (see Figs A.3 and A.5).

Liao et al. (2007) found that a programme of standing up and sitting down training, following similar strength training guidelines and progressively increasing load with a weighted vest, had a positive effect on the performance of sit-to-stand in a group of children aged 5–12 years. After six weeks training the children could lift a significantly greater load into standing and back to sitting, i.e., the strength of the action had increased. The Physiological Cost Index (working heart rate – resting heart rate/walking speed (m/minute) showed a decrease in energy cost in a walking test, so the exercise may also have increased endurance and cardiorespiratory fitness. There was no increase in quadriceps strength tested isometrically. It is not clear at what angle the test was done, but given the fact that strength gains are specific to the action being practiced, one would not expect an isometric test with the knee in, for example, full extension, to reflect strength of the muscles at approximately 90°, which is the angle at which peak moment of force is generated at the knee (Carr and Shepherd, 2010). Furthermore, it can be argued that both hip and knee extensor forces peak at thighs-off and it is therefore inappropriate to test the quadriceps independently of hip extensors, as has been demonstrated recently (Yoshioka et al., 2012).

## EXERCISE: STANDING UP, SITTING DOWN

- Start with feet flat on floor. Set the seat height appropriate for leg length, ankle angle at approximately 75°, upper body erect
- Try for a 'natural' speed (not too slow)
- Provide incentives for the infant to stand up and sit down, e.g., reaching up to a toy to encourage standing up, sitting down to put it on the floor
- Use a grab strap to prevent a fall if necessary
- In sitting, the infant practices reaching far forward for a toy on the floor or on a table (flexing the hips). This gives the idea of shifting weight forward on to the feet

## Walking

It is important to note that an infant will only learn to walk if there is opportunity to practice walking. Previous sections have described exercises that are designed to develop strength in lower limb muscles and to train co-ordination of the lower limb but early practice of stepping and cruising around furniture and of balancing the body mass over the feet in standing are critical for infants to become effective walkers. Self-produced locomotion may be critical in infancy for its organizing effects on the motor control system (Berthenthal and Campos, 1990; see Chapter 10). Organization of the environment to encourage kicking in young infants may also assist, since the movements involved are similar to walking (Thelen and Cooke, 1987).

## Walking sideways

The knees are normally kept relatively extended when walking sideways; so, for some infants with CP, wraparound soft splints may be necessary to keep the knees from collapsing into flexion, make the action possible, and give the infant the idea of the optimum way to move (Fig. A.10). Shifting weight from foot to foot in a lateral direction is an important action to practice, as it involves the abductor/adductor muscles as prime movers, and the hip flexors/extensors must work co-operatively to ensure a lateral movement at the hips: that is, so that the leg moves directly sideways without excessive flexion (Fig. 11.22).

## Over-ground walking

In early walking practice, the infant can practice the action when pushing a cart (Fig. 11.23A); when he is walking free, his parent may use a grab strap or harness to steady him and prevent a fall. Particular difficulties should be noted. Children usually need special exercise to encourage hip flexion in swing

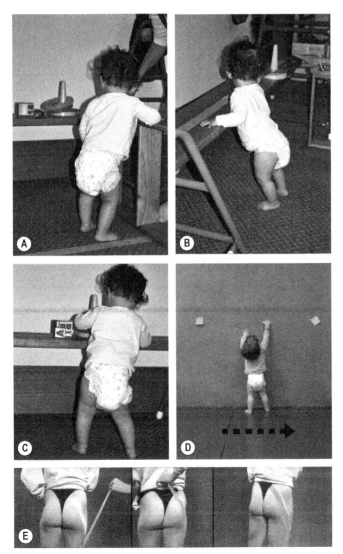

**Figure 11.22 • (A–C)** A series of pictures showing practice of independent walking sideways, using hands for support when she needs to for balance. **(D)** A game for encouraging walking sideways. **(E)** Strapping may encourage hip extension/abduction by limiting internal rotation and adduction. Note the direction of the pull. [(D) From www. physiotherapyexercise.com with permission. (E) With permission from J. McConnell.]

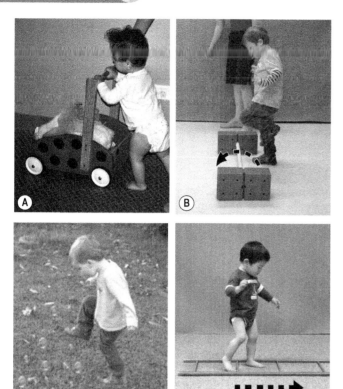

**Figure 11.23 ● (A)** Practicing walking. As the infant gets the idea of pushing the trolley, adding items to the trolley can make it harder to push, so she can exercise her upper and lower limb muscles. **(B)** Increasing hip flexion by walking over an obstacle course and **(C)** by stamping on bubbles. **(D)** Developing effective balance by walking between the rungs of a ladder. [(B–D) From www.physiotherapyexercise.com with permission.]

phase (e.g., marching on the spot lifting knees high; Fig. 11.23B,C) and extension in stance phase. A tendency to flex and internally rotate the hips can be minimized by strapping from the thigh over the hip in a posterolateral direction to encourage extension and external rotation (Fig. 11.22E). The strapping may stimulate the muscles to contract more forcefully. Infants with hemiplegia may walk with more even strides when constrained by walking between the rungs of a ladder placed on the floor, or over small objects (Fig. 11.23D). Walking on a treadmill at an average speed may 'drive' more even strides and this effect may transfer to over-ground walking, although this has not been tested.

*Walking up hill (slope)* (Fig. 11.24A) requires the production of more muscle force and, if practiced intensively, is a way to increase muscle strength as well as cardiorespiratory capacity. It also requires extensibility of the calf muscles and hip flexors in particular. *Walking down hill* requires eccentric work for quadriceps and hip extensor muscles and extensibility of hip flexors in particular.

*Stair ascent/descent:* an infant who is too small for stairs can practice stepping up and down on small steps to learn the basic action and the balance constraints (Figs 11.3B and 11.15).

*Step up and down and heels raise and lower exercises* described above aim to strengthen muscles within an appropriate range for walking, increase the ability to generate forceful (propulsive) concentric contraction of calf muscles from a dorsiflexed position and hip extensors, to train limb control including the switch from concentric to eccentric contractions, and to preserve muscle length.

The exercises described in this section should be practiced with as many repetitions and variations in goal and environment as possible and with continuing challenge. Of course, the number of repetitions will be variable with infants, and the ability to turn these exercises into play and for them to be sufficiently repetitive and intensive is a challenge for parent and therapist. Modifying the environment and choosing the right time to exercise are also critical factors. Placement of

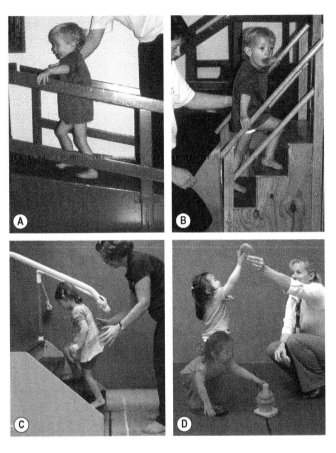

**Figure 11.24 •** (A) Practicing on a hill helps preserve extensibility of ankle plantarflexors; strengthens hip, knee, ankle extensors. (B) Stair ascent/descent: after some practice, when he has the idea of what to do, he should try not to hold on. (C) She now needs to move a little faster by pushing down with each leg as she climbs the stairs. This will also improve her ability of balance; the stairs are relatively high for her. (D) Balance training: she practices reaching and stretching out while maintaining a squat, and standing up while reaching and stretching up. [(C, D) From www.physiotherapyexercise.com with permission.]

objects to 'force' a narrower or a wider base, an increase in hip flexion, or a particular action, are modifiers of the infant's locomotor pattern, with the added advantage of providing feedback for the infant (whether his action was successful, or not) and requiring his full attention (Fig. 11.23).

Playing games that increase propulsion of the body forward or upward—running, jumping, hopping on one leg—should start as soon as practical. Jumping can be practiced in a harness or holding on to a hand or a handrail. Jumping down from a small step or over a line on the floor can be practiced quite early. The infant needs to be able to follow instructions or copy a demonstration. The major instruction to get them started is to bend the knees, then jump down.

## Treadmill walking

A treadmill provides an opportunity for an infant to practice stepping and walking in interesting and challenging conditions, the moving belt maximizing the extent of hip extension and ankle dorsiflexion which set up a necessary condition for the limb to shift into swing phase (Figs 11.10 and A.12). Treadmill and over-ground walking have similar basic biomechanical characteristics (Arsenault et al., 1986), and the moving belt can 'force' critical aspects of performance such as plantarflexion at the end of stance phase (at push-off). The belt carries the stance leg into extension at the hip and dorsiflexion at the ankle at the end of stance phase, a movement that is difficult for children with diplegia and hemiplegia because of muscle weakness and contracture. Extension at the hip and plantarflexion at the ankle normally drives the body mass forward during stance phase and, because it stretches the hip flexors, optimizes flexion (pull-off) of the hip at the start of the swing phase. The moving belt in this way promotes the rhythmic, cyclical and propulsive action of the lower limbs.

The results of a recent review of treadmill training suggest that it is feasible across a wide range of ages and functional abilities in children with CP (Willoughby et al., 2009). No infants were included. The review noted positive effects on walking speed over short distances and on functional actions, particularly in children who were more severely affected.

Use of partial body weight support from a harness (see Fig. 1.1A), by decreasing the muscle force needed, enables the child with muscle weakness and poor control to practice walking until they have stronger leg muscles and can walk on the treadmill without the harness. For infants it may be better to use the harness as a way of preventing a fall. However, with a small treadmill a parent can provide assistance (see Fig. 11.10). Richards et al. (1997) reported a study of four children aged 19–27 months who were trained on a treadmill. They received no extra training of walking. None was an independent walker at the start. As the children improved they received less body weight support and speed of the belt was increased.

It is reasonable to assume that treadmill practice increases leg muscle strength and lower limb motor control. A randomized controlled study of infants with Down syndrome (aged under 12 months at entry to the study) reported that infants in the experimental group who practiced walking on a treadmill demonstrated accelerated independent walking acquisition compared with controls (Ulrich et al., 2001). An earlier study had shown that infants with Down syndrome aged 7–11 months were able to take alternating steps on the treadmill several months before they began to walk independently (Ulrich et al., 1992). Independent walking requires the ability to balance and the treadmill may not allow for balance improvement unless wearing a harness enables the infant to walk without holding on to the handrail. Independent over-ground walking and treadmill walking practice aided by some form of harness or grab belt or held by a parent (Fig. 11.10; see Fig. A.10B), may accelerate the development of balanced walking. For older children, harnessed apparatus such as Litegait™ (Fig. 1.1B) can be used to practice over ground walking.

Treadmill walking may also act as an important modulator of leg muscle reflexes. Hodapp et al. (2009) tested a group of children, all functional walkers) aged 5–15 years with Gross Motor Function Classification System (GMFCS) from 1–3 out of 5. The children had TM training for 10 minutes/day over 10 consecutive days.

Soleus Hoffman (H) reflexes were tested during treadmill walking before and after the last session. The training led to a significant improvement in velocity. Soleus reflexes were almost completely depressed during swing phase, as in able-bodied subjects, reflecting an improvement toward a more functionally useful walking pattern, and these physiological changes, according to the authors, might reflect task-specific plasticity of the central nervous system.

A low level of aerobic capacity and physical fitness is common in children with CP, particularly those who locomote via mobility aids. Treadmill walking, progressed by increasing slope and speed, can increase endurance, strength and fitness if practiced sufficiently according to guidelines. Poor cardiorespiratory fitness, decreased work capacity and higher oxygen uptake are commonly reported in children. Rose et al. (1990) found that energy expenditure (oxygen uptake, heart rate) measured at a given walking speed was three times higher in children aged 7–16 years with CP than in able-bodied children. In 1991 they described and tested an Energy Expenditure Index (EEI) to quantify children's walking energy levels (Rose et al., 1991). Norman et al. (2004), following an investigation of the EEI test, suggested that it may be a useful clinical indicator of oxygen consumption at self-paced ambulation speeds in children with diplegia. Nsenga et al. (2012) have recently tested another method of judging oxygen uptake (a combination of a six-minute walk test with gas collection) that can easily be used in clinical practice, a method they found to be valid and reliable.

One significant difference between treadmill and over-ground walking lies in the visual inputs available. Over-ground walking is normally controlled in part by optic flow: as the infant walks forward, the visual environment changes, moving backward relative to the infant. This input does not occur on the treadmill but could be available using a virtual reality system that is currently being investigated (Rahman et al., 2011) (see Chapters 10 and 12).

In summary, training of an action such as walking or standing up involves practice of the action itself, with task-oriented exercises that incorporate similar dynamic characteristics to the action, in order to learn the motor control parameters. Research into movement dynamics indicates that the control system normally utilizes simplifying strategies as a means of controlling the many degrees of freedom inherent in the body's segmental linkage (Zatsiorsky et al., 2000). This information enables us to plan a programme of training incorporating exercises that increase muscle force generation and that are likely to transfer into improved performance of several similar actions, as well as specific training of the action to be learned.

## Concluding comments

It is generally recognized that exercise and training are the preferred interventions for infants and children with CP when inadequate muscle activation, muscle weakness and poor motor control are the principal motor impairments. Given the serious effects of secondary changes to the neuromusculoskeletal system, it seems obvious that specific exercises also have the potential to minimize or even prevent the most disabling of these. Both strength and motor control are required for the infant with CP to achieve effective and efficient functional abilities. But what are these exercises and what is involved in training? What do the children actually do and what part does the therapist (as teacher) play? Investigations of the effects of exercise and training programmes typically do not give much detail of what the infant does, for how long or at what intensity. To report in a research paper that intervention included an exercise programme or that exercises were given intensively is not informative. We need studies such as that of Liao et al. (2010) who tested the physiological and functional effects of weight training incorporated into task-specific practice of one functional activity, sit-to-stand. Sufficient detail is given to allow the experiment to be replicated.

There are many different kinds of exercise and different exercises achieve different effects. There is a long history of investigations into the specificity of exercise to strengthen muscles and train motor skill learning, and guidelines for both have been described for adult neurological rehabilitation for many years (see Chapter 1; Carr and Shepherd, 2000, 2003, 2010; Gentile, 2000). More recently there has been a growing research interest in different forms of exercise in the fields of sports and exercise science and in physiotherapy. Jensen et al. (2005) discuss the specific effects of exercises to increase strength and exercises to train skill acquisition, pointing out that the two forms of exercise are likely to be most effective in the promotion of skill acquisition when carried out in the same programme.

The exercises in this chapter have been developed from scientific information about human movement. They are task- and context-specific and they are based on current knowledge of musculoskeletal anatomy and functional biomechanics, methods of stimulating motor learning and motor control. These fields of study play a critical role in evaluation and planning, and in the process of intervention. The guidelines and figures included here demonstrate what the infant should do and how the therapist and family as 'teacher' may enable and actually drive the process of skill acquisition. The exercises described may also increase muscle contractility and force production, preserve muscle length and minimize deformity, but these hypotheses remain to be tested. Future studies will also test whether or not specified exercise/training programmes are associated with brain and neuromotor changes, as has been shown to occur in adults after stroke (e.g. Enzinger et al., 2009; Acerra et al., 2011). Future developments will include technological aids to enable small infants to practice independently in a stimulating environment, and to provide ongoing assistance to parents and siblings who play a large part in developing the infant's potential at home.

## References

Acerra, N., Vidoni, E., Wessell, B., et al., 2011. Does task-specificity matter for motor sequence learning after stroke? Insights from fMRI. Physiother 97 (Suppl.), S1.

Agahari, I., Shepherd, R.B., Westwood, P.A., 1996. A comparative evaluation of lower limb forces in two variations of the step exercises in able-bodied subjects.

In: Lee, M. Gilleard, W., Sinclair, P., et al. (Eds.), First Australasian Biomechanics Conference, Sydney, Australia p. 94–95.

Alhusaini, A.A.A., Crosbie, J., Shepherd, R.B., et al., 2010. Mechanical properties of the plantarflexor musculotendinous unit during passive dorsiflexion in children with cerebral palsy

compared with typically developing children. Dev. Med. Child Neurol. 52, e101–e106.

Andriacchi, T.P., Andersson, G.B.J., Fermier, R.W., et al., 1980. A study of lower limb mechanics: a study of stair climbing. J. Bone Jt Surg. 62A, 749–757.

Angulo-Kinzler, R.M., Ulrich, B., Thelen, E., 2002. Three-month-old infants can select specific leg motor solutions. Motor Control 6, 52–68.

Arnold, A.S., Delp, S.L., 2005. Computer modelling of gait abnormalities in cerebral palsy: application to treatment planning. Theor. Issues in Ergon. Sci 6, 305–312.

Arsenault, A.B., Winter, D.A., Martenuik, R.G., et al., 1986. Treadmill walking versus walkway locomotion in humans: an EMG study. Ergonomics 29, 665–676.

Belenkii, V.E., Gurfinkel, V.S., Paltsev, R.I., 1967. On the elements of voluntary movement control. Biofizika 12, 135.

Berger, S., Adolph, K.E., 2007. Learning and development in infant locomotion. In: von Hofsten, C., Rosander, K. (Eds.), From Action to Cognition Elsevier, Amsterdam, pp. 237–255.

Berger, W., Quintern, J., Dietz, V., 1982. Pathophysiology of gait in children with cerebral palsy. Electroencephalogr. Clin. Neurophysiol. 53, 38–41.

Berger, W., Horstman, G., Dietz, V., 1984. Tension development and muscle activation in the leg during gait in spastic hemiparesis: independence of muscle hypertonia and exaggerated stretch reflexes. J. Neurol. Neurosurg. Psychiatry 47, 1029–1033.

Berthenthal, B.I., Campos, J.J., 1990. A systems approach to the organising effects of self-produced locomotion during infancy In: Rovee-Collier, C. Lipsitt, C.L. (Eds.), Advances in Infancy Research, 6. Ablex, Norwood, NJ, pp. 1–60.

Blundell, S.W., Shepherd, R.B., Dean, C.M., et al., 2003. Functional strength training in cerebral palsy: a pilot study of a group circuit training class for children aged 4–8 years. Clin. Rehabil. 17, 48–57.

Bobath, B., 1971. Abnormal Postural Reflex Activity Caused by Brain Lesions. Heinemann, London.

Bouisset, S., Duchenne, J.-L., 1994. Is body balance more perturbed by respiration in seating than in standing posture? NeuroReport 5, 957–960.

Bower, E., 2009. Finnie's Handling the Young Child with Cerebral Palsy at Home, fourth ed. Elsevier, Oxford.

Bradley, N.S., Westcott, S.L., 2006. Developmental aspects of motor control in skill acquisition. In: Campbell, S. (Ed.), Physical Therapy for Children A Comprehensive Reference for Pediatric Practice, third ed. WB Saunders, Philadelphia.

Britten, E., Harris, N., Turton, A., 2008. An exploratory randomised controlled trial of assisted practice for improving sit-to-stand in stroke patients in the hospital setting. Clin. Rehabil. 22, 458–468.

Brogren, E., Hadders-Algra, M., Forssberg, H., 1996. Postural control in children with spastic muscle activity during perturbations in sitting. Dev. Med. Child Neurol. 138, 379–388.

Butterworth, G., 1986. Some problems in explaining the origins in movement control. In: Wade, M.G., Whiting, H.T.A. (Eds.), Motor Development in Children. Problems of Coordination and Control Martinus Nijhoff, Dordrecht, pp. 23–32.

Butterworth, G., Hicks, L., 1977. Visual perception and postural stability in infancy: a developmental study. Perception 6, 255.

Cahill, B.M., Carr, J.R., Adams, R., 1999. Intersegmental co-ordination in sit-to-stand: an age cross-sectional study. Physiother. Res. Int. 4, 12–27.

Carr, J.H., Shepherd, R.B. (Eds.), 2000. Movement Science. Foundations for Physical Therapy in Rehabilitation, second ed. Aspen, Rockville MD.

Carr, J.H., Shepherd, R.B., 2003. Stroke Rehabilitation. Guidelines for Exercise and Training to Optimize Motor Skill. Butterworth-Heinemann, Oxford.

Carr, J.H., Shepherd, R.B., 2010. Neurological Rehabilitation: Optimizing Motor Performance, second ed. Butterworth-Heinemann, Oxford.

Carriero, A., Zavatsky, A., Stebbins, S., et al., 2009. Correlation between lower limb bone morphology and gait characteristics in children with spastic diplegic cerebral palsy. J. Pediatr. Orthop. 29, 73–79.

Chapman, D., 2002. Context effects on the spontaneous leg movements

of infants with spina bifida. Pediatr. Phys. Ther. 14, 62–73.

Chen, Y.P., Fetters, L., Holt, K.G., et al., 2002. Making the mobile move: constraining task and environment. Infant. Behav. Dev. 25, 195 220.

Cheng, P.-T., Wu, S.-H., Liaw, M.-Y., 2001. Symmetrical body-weight distribution training in stroke patients and its effect on fall prevention. Arch. Phys. Med. Rehabil. 82, 1650–1654.

Cordo, P.J., Nashner, L.M., 1982. Properties of postural adjustments associated with rapid arm movements. J. Neurophysiol. 47, 287–302.

Crenna, P., 1998. Spasticity and spastic gait in children with cerebral palsy. Neurosci. Biobehav. Rev. 22, 571–578.

Crenna, P., 1999. Pathophysiology of lengthening contractions in human spasticity: a study of the hamstring muscles during locomotion. Pathophysiology 5, 283–297.

Crosbie, J., Alhusaini, A.A., Dean, C.M., Shepherd, R.B., 2012. Plantarflexor muscle and spatiotemporal gait characteristics of children with hemiplegic cerebral palsy: an observational study. Dev. Neurorehabil. 15, 114–118.

da Costa, C.S.N., Savelsbergh, G., Rocha, N.A., 2010. Sit-to-stand movement in children: a review. J. Mot. Behav. 42, 127–134.

Damiano, D.L., 2006. Activity, activity, activity: rethinking our physical therapy approach to cerebral palsy. Phys. Ther. 86, 1534–1540.

Dean, C.M., Shepherd, R.B., 1997. Task-related training improves performance of seated reaching tasks after stroke: a randomised controlled trial. Stroke. 28, 722–728.

Dean, C.M., Richards, C.L., Malouin, F., 2000. Task-related circuit training improves performance of locomotor tasks in chronic stroke: a randomised controlled pilot trial. Arch. Phys. Med. Rehabil. 81, 409–417.

de Graaf-Peters, V.B., Blauw-Hospers, C.H., Dirks, T., et al., 2007. Development of postural control in typically developing children and children with cerebral palsy: possibilities for intervention? Neurosc. Biobehav. Rev. 31, 1191–1200.

Delp, S.L., Hess, W.E., Hungerford, D.S., et al., 1999. Variation of rotational arms with hip flexion. J. Biomech. 23, 493–501.

De Vries, J.I.P., Visser, G.H.A., Prechtl, H.F.R., 1982. The emergence of fetal behavior: 1. Qualitative aspects. Early Human Dev. 7, 301–322.

Diener, H.-C., Dichgans, J., Guschlbauer, 1992. The coordination of posture and voluntary movement in patients with cerebellar dysfunction. Mov. Disord. 7, 14–22.

dos Santos, A.N., Pavao, S.L., Rocha, N.A.F., 2011. Sit-to-stand movement in children with cerebral palsy: a critical review. Res. Dev. Disabil. 32, 2243–2252.

Dusing, S.C., Harbourne, R.T., 2010. Variability in postural control during infancy: implications for development, assessment, and intervention. Phys. Ther. 90, 1838–1849.

Eng, J.J., Winter, D.A., Patla, A.E., et al., 1992. Role of the torque stabiliser in postural control during rapid voluntary arm movement. In: Woollacott, M., Horak, F. (Eds.), Posture and Gait: Control Mechanisms. University of Oregon Books, Portland, OR.

Enzinger, C., Dawes, H., Johansen-Berg, H., et al., 2009. Brain activity changes associated with treadmill training after stroke. Stroke 40, 2460–2467.

Fetters, L., 1991. Measurement and treatment in cerebral palsy: an argument for a new approach. Phys. Ther. 71, 244.

Fetters, L., Chen, Y.P., Jonsdottir, J., et al., 2004. Kicking coordination captures differences between full-term and premature infants with white matter disorder. Hum. Move. Sci. 22, 729–749.

Forrester, L.W., Roy, A., Krebs, H.I., et al., 2011. Ankle training with a robotic device improves hemiparetic gait after a stroke. Neurorehabil. Neural Repair 25, 369–377.

Forssberg, H., 1982. Spinal locomotor functions and descending control. In: Sjolund, B., Bjorklund, A. (Eds.), Brain Stem Control of Spinal

Mechanisms. Elsevier Biomedical Press, New York.

Forssberg, H., 1985. Ontogeny of human locomotor control 1: infant stepping, supported locomotion and transition to independent locomotion. Exp. Brain Res. 57, 480–493.

Forssberg, H., 1992. Evolution of plantigrade gait: is there a neuronal correlate? Dev. Med. Child Neurol. 34, 920–925.

Forssberg, H., Nashner, L.M., 1982. Ontogenetic development of posture control in man: adaptation to altered support and visual conditions during stance. J. Neurosci. 2, 545–552.

Freedland, R.L., Bertenthal, B.I., 1994. Developmental changes in interlimb coordination: transition to hands-and-knees crawling. Psychol. Sci. 5, 26–32.

Gentile, A.M., 2000. Skill acquisition. Action, movement and neuromotor processes. In: Carr, J.H., Shepherd, R.B. (Eds.), Movement Science. Foundations for Physical Therapy in Rehabilitation, second ed. Aspen, Rockville, MD, pp. 111–180.

Ghez, C., 1991. Posture. In: Kandel, E.R., Schwartz, J.H., Jessell, T.M. (Eds.), Principles of Neural Science, third ed. Appleton & Lange, Norwalk, CT.

Groenen, A., Kruijsen, A.J.A., Mulvey, G.M., et al., 2010. Constraints on early movement: tykes, togs, and technology. Infant Behav. Dev., 16–22.

Hadders-Algra, M., 2002. Variability in infant motor behavior: a hallmark of the healthy nervous system. Infant Behav. Dev. 25, 133–151.

Hadders-Algra, M., Brogren, E., Forssberg, H., 1996. Training affects the development of postural adjustments in sitting infants. J. Physiol. 493, 289–298.

Hampton, D.A., Hollande, K.W., Engsberg, J.R., 2003. Equinus deformity as a compensatory mechanism for ankle plantarflexor weakness in cerebral palsy. J. Appl. Biomechan. 19, 325–339.

Hedberg, A., Carlberg, E., Forssberg, H., et al., 2005. Development of postural adjustments in sitting position during the first half year of life. Dev. Med. Child Neurol. 47, 312–320.

Hirschfeld, H., 1992. Postural control: acquisition and integration during development. In: Forssberg, H., Hirschfeld, H. (Eds.), Movement Disorders in Children. Karger, Basel, pp. 199–208.

Hodapp, M., Vry, J., Mall, V, et al., 2009. Changes in soleus H-reflex modulation after treadmill training in children with cerebral palsy. Brain 132 (Pt 1), 37–44.

Jeng, S.F., Chen, L.C., Yau, K.I., 2002. Kinematic analysis of kicking movements in preterm infants with very low birth weight and full-term infants. Phys. Ther. 82, 148–159.

Jensen, J.L., Ulrich, B.D., Thelen, E., et al., 1994. Adaptive dynamics of the leg movement patterns of human infants: 1. The effects of posture on spontaneous kicking. J. Mot. Behav. 26, 303–312.

Jensen, J.L., Marstrand, P.C.D., Nielsen, J.B., 2005. Motor skill training and strength training are associated with different plastic changes in the central nervous system. J. Appl. Physiol. 99, 1558–1568.

Khemlani, M., Carr, J.H., Crosbie, W.J., et al., 1998. Muscle synergies and joint linkages in sit-to-stand under two different initial foot positions. Clin. Biomech. 14, 236–246.

Kirker, S.G.B., Simpson, D.S., Jenner, J.R., et al., 2000. Stepping before standing: hip muscle function in stepping and standing balance after stroke. J. Neurol. Neurosurg. Psychiatry 68, 458–464.

Komi, P.V., 2000. Stretch–shortening cycle: a powerful model to study normal and fatigued muscle. J. Biomech. 33, 1197–1206.

Komi, P.V., 2003. Stretch-shortening cycle. In: Komi, P.V. (Ed.), Strength and Power in Sport, second ed. Blackwell Science, London, pp. 184–202.

Kuhtz-Buschbeck, J.P., Stolze, H., Boczek-Funcke, A., et al., 1998. Kinematic analysis of prehension movements in children. Behav Brain Res. 93, 131–141.

Kuo, A.D., Zajac, F.E., 1993. A biomechanical analysis of muscle strength as a limiting factor in standing posture. J. Biomech. 26, 137–150.

Lee, D.N., Aronson, E., 1974. Visual proprioceptive control of standing in human infants. Percept. Psychophys. 15, 529.

Leonard, C.T., Hirschfeld, H., Forssberg, H., 1991. The development of independent walking in children with cerebral palsy. Dev. Med. Child Neurol. 33, 567–577.

Liao, H.-F., Liu, Y.-C., Liu, W.-Y., et al., 2007. Effectiveness of loaded sit-to-stand resistance exercise for children with mild spastic diplegia: a randomized clinical trial. Arch. Phys. Med. Rehabil. 88, 25–31.

Massion, J., Woollacott, M., 1996. Normal balance and postural control. In: Bronstein, A.M., Brandt, T., Woollacott, M. (Eds.), Clinical Aspects of Balance and Gait Disorders. Edward Arnold, London, pp. 1–18.

Mayer, M., 2002. Clinical neurokinesiology of spastic gait. Bratial. Lek. Listy 103 3-1.

Milani-Comparetti, A., 1980. Pattern analysis of normal and abnormal development: the fetus, the newborn, the child. In: Slaton, D.S. (Ed.), Development of Movement in Infancy. University of South Carolina Press, Chapel Hill, SC.

Monger, C., Carr, J.H., Fowler, V., 2002. Evaluation of a home-based exercise and training program to improve sit-to-stand in patients with chronic stroke. Clin. Rehabil. 16, 361–367.

Norman, J.F., Bossman, S., Gardner, P., et al., 2004. Comparison of the energy expenditure index and oxygen consumption index during self-paced walking in children with spastic diplegia cerebral palsy and children without physical disabilities. Pediatr. Phys. Ther. 16, 206–211.

Nsenga, A.L., Nsenga, A.L., Shephard, R.J., et al., 2012. The six-minute walk test in children with cerebral palsy GMFCS level I and II: validity, reproducibility and training effects. Arch. Phys. Med. Rehabil. in press.

Olney, S.J., Monger, T.N., Costigan, P.A., 1986. Mechanical energy of walking of stroke patients. Arch. Phys. Med. Rehabil. 67, 92–98.

Olney, S.J., MacPhail, H.E.A., Hedden, D., et al., 1990. Work and power in hemiplegic cerebral palsy gait. Phys. Ther. 70, 431–438.

Pang, M.Y., Lam, T., Yang, J.F., 2003. Infants adapt their stepping to repeated trip-inducing stimuli. J. Neurophysiol. 90, 2731–2740.

Park, E.S., Park, C.I., Kim, D.Y., et al., 2003. The characteristics of sit-to-stand transfer in young children with spastic cerebral palsy based on kinematic and kinetic data. Gait Posture 17, 43–49.

Piek, J., 2006. Infant Motor Development. Human Kinetics, New York.

Rahman, S.A., Rahman, A., Shaheen, A.A., 2011. Virtual reality use in motor rehabilitation of neurological disorders: a systematic review. Middle-East J. Sci. Res. 7, 63–70.

Richards, C.L., Malouin, F., Dumas, F., et al., 1997. Early and intensive treadmill locomotor training for young children with cerebral palsy: a feasibility study. Pediatr. Phys. Ther. 9, 158–165.

Roncesvalles, M.N.C., Woollacott, M.H., Jensen, J.L., 2001. Development of lower extremity kinetics for balance control in infants and young children. J. Mot. Behav 33, 180–192.

Rose, J., Gamble, J.G., Burgos, A., et al., 1990. Energy expenditure index of walking for normal children and for children with cerebral palsy. Dev. Med. Child Neurol. 32, 333–340.

Rose, J., Gamble, J.G., Lee, J., et al., 1991. The energy expenditure index: a method to quantitate and compare walking energy expenditure for children and adolescents. J. Pediatr. Orthop. 11, 571–578.

Shepherd, R.B., 1995. Physiotherapy in Paediatrics, third ed. Butterworth-Heinemann, Oxford.

Shepherd, R.B., Gentile, A.M., 1994. Sit-to-stand: functional relationships between upper body and lower limb segments. Hum. Move. Sci. 13, 817–840.

Shepherd, R.B., McDonald, C.M., 1995. A biomechanical analysis of sit-to-stand in children with diplegic cerebral palsy. In: Hakkinen, K. (Ed.), Abstracts of XVth Congress of International Society of Biomechanics. University of Jyvaskla, Jyvaskla, Finland.

Shumway-Cook, A., Woollacott, M., 1985. The growth of stability: postural control from a developmental perceptive. J. Mot. Behav. 17, 131.

Shumway-Cook, A., Hutchinson, S., Kartin, D., et al., 2003. Effect of balance training on recovery of stability in children with cerebral palsy. Dev. Med. Child Neurol. 45, 59i–602.

Smart, L.J., Mobley, B.S., Otten, E.W., et al., 2004. Not just standing there: the use of postural coordination to aid visual tasks. Hum. Mov. Sci. 22, 769–780.

Sutherland, D., 1997. Review paper. The development of mature gait. Gait Posture 6, 163–170.

Sutherland, D.H., 2001. The evolution of clinical gait analysis part I: kinesiology EMG. Gait Posture 14, 61–70.

Sutherland, D.H., 2002. The evolution of clinical gait analysis part II: kinematics. Gait Posture 16, 159–179.

Sutherland, D.H., Olshen, R., Cooper, L., et al., 1980. The development of mature gait. J. Bone Jt Surg. 62A, 336–353.

Sveistrup, H., Woollacott, M.H., 1997. Practice modifies the developing automatic postural response. Exp. Brain Res. 114 (1), 33–43.

Tardieu, C., de l Tour, H., Bret, M.D., et al., 1982. Muscle hypoextensibility in children with cerebral palsy. 1. Clinical and experimental observations. Arch. Phys. Med. Rehabil. 63, 97–102.

Thelen, E., 1985. Developmental origins of motor coordination: leg movements in human infants. Dev. Psychobiol. 18, 1–22.

Thelen, E., 1986. Treadmill-elicited stepping in 7-month-old infants. Child Dev. 57, 1498–1506.

Thelen, E., 1994. Three-month-old infants can learn task-specific patterns of interlimb coordination. Psychol. Sci. 5, 280–285.

Thelen, E., Cooke, D.W., 1987. Relationship between newborn stepping and later walking: a new interpretation. Dev. Med. Child Neurol. 29, 380–393.

Thelen, E., Fisher, D.M., 1982. Newborn stepping: an explanation for a 'disappearing reflex'. Dev. Psychol. 18, 760–775.

Ulrich, B.D., 2010. Opportunities for early intervention based on theory, basic neuroscience, and clinical science. Phys. Ther. 90, 1868–1880.

Ulrich, B.D., Ulrich, D.A., Collier, D., 1992. Alternating stepping patterns: hidden abilities of 4-month-old infants with Down syndrome. Dev. Med. Child Neurol. 34, 233–239.

Ulrich, D.A., Ulrich, B.D., Angulo-Kinzler, R.M., et al., 2001. Treadmill training of infants with Down syndrome: evidence-based development outcomes. Pediatrics 108, E84.

van der Krogt, M.M., Doorenbosch, C.A., Becher, J.G., Harlaar, J., 2010. Dynamic spasticity of plantar flexor muscles in cerebral palsy gait. J. Rehabil. Med. 42 (7), 656–663.

Whitall, J., Clark, J.E., Phillips, S.J., 1985. Interaction of postural and oscillatory mechanisms in the development of interlimb coordination of upright bipedal locomotion. Paper presented at North American Society for the Psychology of Sport and Physical Activity, Long Beach, Mississippi.

Willoughby, K.L., Dodd, K.J., Shields, N., 2009. A systematic review of the effectiveness of treadmill training for children with cerebral palsy. Disabil. Rehabil. 31, 1971–1979.

Winter, D.A., 1987. The Biomechanics and Motor Control of Human Gait. University of Waterloo Press, Waterloo Ont.

Winter, D.A., 1989. Coordination of motor tasks in human gait. In: Wallace, S.A. (Ed.), Perspectives on the Coordination of Movement. North Holland, New York, pp. 329–363.

Winter, D.A., 2009. Biomechanics and Motor Control of Human Movement, fourth ed. John Wiley & Sons, New York.

Wong, K., 2009. Crawling may be unnecessary for normal child development. Scient. Am. 30 June.

Yonetsu, R., Nitta, O., Surya, J., 2009. "Patternizing" standards of sit-to-stand movements with support in cerebral palsy. NeuroRehabilitation 25, 289–296.

Yoshioka, S., Nagano, A., Hay, D.C., et al., 2012. The minimum required force for a sit-to-stand task. J. Biomech. 45, 699–705.

Zatsiorsky, V.M., Li, Z.M., Latash, M.L., 2000. Enslaving effects in multi-finger force production. Exper. Brain Res. 131, 187–195.

Zhao, H., Wu, Y-N., Hwang, M., et al., 2011. Changes of calf muscle–tendon biomechanical properties induced by passive stretching and active-movement training in children with cerebral palsy. J. Appl. Physiol. 11, 435–442.

# Annotation C
## Kick start: using the mobile infant learning paradigm to promote early leg action

Linda Fetters

## Infants are dynamically changing

Human infants experience continual and profound changes in all systems during the first year of life. They begin to master control of their bodies in relation to the world while their central and peripheral nervous systems, as well as their musculoskeletal system, are in dynamic development.

## Development requires exploration

Mastery of action during this dynamic development is achieved through extensive exploration and discovery (Adolph et al., 1993; Gibson, 1988, 1997; Gibson and Pick, 2000). Mastery of action is a process that relies on extensive practice and the variability that accompanies practice. The creative research of Adolph et al. (2003) suggests that emerging walkers explore their limits of balance and locomotion through practice of more than six hours a day, walking the equivalent of 29 football fields. Skilled action depends as much on error as is does on successful achievement of the chosen goals (Fetters, 2010). Overshooting or undershooting when reaching for a toy affords information to the infant, not only about the location of the toy but also about the forces necessary to successfully grab the toy.

## Altered development for the infant and child with cerebral palsy

These dynamic processes of development are altered for the infant and child with cerebral palsy (CP), and this alteration has serious consequences for development. The limited exploration that is typical for the child with cerebral palsy reduces the available variability that is essential to the discovery and mastery of action. These constraints on variability have serious consequences on all systems. Children with cerebral palsy are smaller and weigh less than typically developing children (Campbell et al., 1989). The tissues of the musculoskeletal system are altered, leading to reduced contractibility, weaker muscles and potential contractures (Lieber and Bodine-Fowler, 1993; Lieber and Fridén, 2002) (see Chapter 6).

Compromised systems also constrain exploration through space for children with CP, which has potential impact on perceptual, social and cognitive development. Thelen and Smith (1994) describe the development of meaning and cognition by stating 'Meaning has its origins in actions and is made manifest—created—in real time and through activity (p. 323)'. Development of the embodied mind (Johnson, 1987; Thelen, 2000) is indeed compromised for the child with constraints on action development such as the child with CP.

## Early intervention is essential

The earliest intervention possible provides the best opportunity to change the developmental trajectory for all of these systems. Early intervention not only promotes the development of leg action but also promotes the neural foundations for this action. Eyre et al. (2000, 2001) (see Chapter 2) have demonstrated the critical importance of maintaining cortical inputs for the development of spinal circuits that maintain leg movements. Lesions of either the brain or spinal cord during fetal and neonatal development dramatically alter the formation and function of sensorimotor pathways. Lesions of the brain or spinal cord during critical periods of development lead to increased levels of cell death in the damaged pathways that alter the competitive dynamics, resulting in the retention of aberrant pathways (Bayatti et al., 2008). Evidence now exists that the corticospinal system is already active and shaping spinal circuits by the late prenatal period, but that these dynamics are derailed by pre- to postnatal insults (Eyre et al., 2000). Therapeutic interventions that motivate movement are potential substrates for driving these circuits during their most dynamic phase of plasticity.

We are developing an intervention to promote leg action during the very first weeks and months after birth. Our research seeks to understand the development of the control of leg action in order to use this foundational knowledge to inform the earliest possible intervention to improve leg action for infants at risk for CP. We have developed a line of research investigating the earliest leg movements of infants born full term (FT) and infants born prematurely who are at high risk for the development of CP. Infants born prematurely with very low birth weight (VLBW; less than 1,500 grams or about 3 lbs), specifically those with white matter abnormalities, are at increased risk for CP, in particular spastic diplegia and other types of cerebral palsy (Spittle et al., 2011). Infants and children with spastic diplegia have reduced lower extremity movement, movement in atypical patterns, and delayed onset of mobility including walking.

Although it is typically thought that the hands are the first to explore and bring the world into view for infants, Thelen and colleagues suggest that exploration with the feet actually precedes exploration with the hands (Galloway and Thelen, 2004; Galloway et al., 2002; Heathcock and Galloway, 2009). The quality and quantity of lower extremity (LE) movement are critical for the development of mobility. Independent mobility enables the toddler to freely engage in self-directed learning through independent exploration of the environment. Mobility through the environment has been demonstrated to enhance socialization, perception and cognition for the developing infant, with an increase in each of these developmental domains with onset of crawling and walking (Bertenthal et al., 1984; Herbert et al., 2007).

One emergent property of typically developing leg action is the selective control of segments of the leg. We have demonstrated that this selective control is aberrant in prematurely born VLBW infants with white matter disorder (WMD) (Fetters et al., 2004) and other research groups have demonstrated the importance of selective control for independent locomotion in older children with CP (Fowler and Goldberg, 2009). Our work and the work of others support that the more dominant newborn synergies of total lower extremity flexion and total lower extremity extension are replaced with more selective control of segments with, for example, the hip joint moving into extension and the knee joint moving into flexion (Fetters et al., 2004; Heriza, 1988; Jeng et al., 2004; Vaal et al., 2000). Creeping, crawling, moving into sitting or standing and walking all require this disassociation of segments as selective control emerges. During infancy, these joint combinations have been described as moving from the dominant newborn in-phase interjoint coupling to a more out-of-phase interjoint coupling (Heriza, 1988; Thelen et al., 1983). An in-phase movement of the legs is characterized by all joints, hip, knee and ankle, moving in flexion or all joints

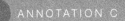

moving in extension. These phase transitions have been studied using kinematics and kinetics. Using kinematics, the emergence of out-of-phase coupling is seen to begin with the hip–ankle joints at 1 to 2 months of age, followed by the hip–knee and knee–ankle joints over the next few months (Jeng et al., 2002; Piek, 1996).

## Early intervention through contingency learning

This selective control of the legs is occurring during the period in which infants are discovering that their actions have consequences in the environment: that is, they discover the relationship between their actions and an environmental event. This relational learning is referred to as the learning of contingencies. The learning of contingencies occurs very early, as infants learn the connections between their actions and the effects of their actions on the world (Goldfield et al., 1993; Milewski and Siqueland, 1975; Siqueland and DeLucia, 1969). For example, 1-month-old infants demonstrate the ability to modify their sucking frequency to maintain the visual presence of a slide of a coloured shape (Milewski and Siqueland, 1975) and even to use sucking to effect the amount of luminance in a slide presentation (Siqueland and DeLucia, 1969). In a now classic study, Goldfield et al. (1993) demonstrated that 8-month-old infants learn to bounce at the resonant frequency of a baby-bouncer suspended by a spring. After a period of exploration characterized by high variability, infants learned to produce longer bouts of bouncing with a concomitant decrease in bounce amplitude and period variability. Exploration in contingency studies such as this is typically captured through measures of variability such as standard deviations. Improvement of performance and learning are then characterized as actions with reduced variability.

We know very little, however, about the characteristics of the exploratory *processes* associated with learning contingencies in the first months of life; it is unclear if exploration is a relevant parameter in learning, and, if it is, how exploration actually affects learning. Previous research with infants has sought to investigate the behaviours that immediately precede learning. For example, significant correlations have been found between the amount of familiarization decrement (lack of sustained levels of sucking to maintain a visual image) that occurs during the acquisition phase of a learning experiment and the amount of response recovery when a novel stimulus is introduced (Milewski and Siqueland, 1975). More recently, the effect of immediate previous kicking experience of one leg in a learning paradigm was seen to increase the rate of learning by the other leg (Angulo-Kinzler, 2001). Thus, performance in a learning paradigm may be influenced by prior experience, but this tells us little about the specific characteristics of the prior behaviour and its relation to learning. In particular, although the importance of exploratory actions in infant learning has been stressed by many authors, and the reduction in variability after a period of exploration has been documented, there is scant data supporting a causal relationship between exploration and learning or data detailing the necessary amount or timing of the exploratory actions adequate for learning.

## Contingency learning in prematurely born infants

We have combined the concepts and processes of contingency learning with an intervention to promote out-of-phase development in early kicking. We, like other research groups (Angulo-Kinzler, 2001; Angulo-Kinzler et al., 2002; Chen et al., 2002), have previously established that infants as young as 3–4 months of age who are tethered to a musical mobile can learn the contingency between their leg movements and the activation of the mobile, and that by increasing their leg movements they can increase activity in a musical mobile. In our laboratory, we have established that infants *not* physically tethered to the mobile can activate the mobile by pushing on a pressure transducer that activates a musical mobile. Infants were placed supine on a mat for testing. A plastic plate was mounted over a pressure transducer within the kicking range of each supine infant. We then shaped their leg selective movement by changing the positioning of their legs in relation to the force plate. Infants were positioned such that in order to contact the plate, a leg action including hip flexion and knee extension was required; this is a relatively 'out-of-phase' movement. The kicking pattern changed from a less mature pattern, termed an 'in-phase pattern' with infants using total flexor or extensor movements when they were not in contact with the plate, to a more mature pattern, termed an 'out-of-phase pattern' with infants combining flexion and extension in order to keep the mobile active when the plate was contacted. We and others (Fetters et al., 2004, 2010; Vaal et al., 2002) have previously demonstrated that the immature, in-phase pattern discriminates, as early as 1 month of age, between premature infants with VLBW and WMD and comparison infants without WMD. Our work demonstrates that infants can increase the quantity of leg movements but more importantly that we can change the amount of selective control they demonstrate.

In the next step in our research, we integrated the motor control research on the development of selective movements in the legs with the research on early contingency learning in order to develop a new intervention learning paradigm. Infants learn selective control of leg movements while exploring the immediate environment but without tethering their legs or having them kick a tangible target. Our research includes both FT and premature VLBW infants in an experiment that links leg movements to the rotation of a musical mobile. We are hoping to change not only the frequency of leg action but also the amount of selective control demonstrated by both groups of infants. In our paradigm, when an infant moves her foot above a specified virtual threshold, a musical mobile rotates, thus creating a reward for the specific leg action. The virtual threshold is created through our motion analysis co-ordinate system and the threshold is unique to the kicking state space of each infant. We define the kicking state space just before the contingent learning paradigm begins: that is, during baseline we determine where each infant typically kicks and then we set the threshold at the mean value of this state space. Once the threshold has been determined (two minutes of baseline kicking), we activate the paradigm such that each time an infant moves either leg above the threshold, the mobile activates for three seconds. In order to keep the mobile turning and the music playing, the infant must continually cross the threshold (Fig. C.1). The threshold is at first defined only in the vertical ($z$) dimension. After infants learn the threshold, we will add a horizontal component to the threshold, meaning that the infant will need to achieve flexion with extension in the leg (out-of-phase movement) in order to activate the mobile.

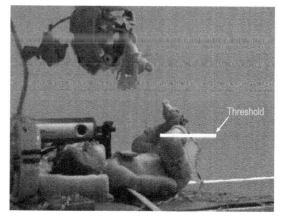

**Figure C.1** • A 3-month-old, full-term infant activating the musical mobile by crossing the virtual threshold.

## Understanding the dynamics

Our research is also aimed at understanding the control of muscle forces as the mobile contingency is learned. Control of actions to explore with the feet and kick with the legs requires not only the generation of active muscle forces but also the anticipation and control for the effects of gravity and for the reactive and passive forces that are generated as a result of their active muscle force generation (Jeng et al., 2002; Latash, 1996; Schneider and Zernicke, 1992). We have developed the method to estimate the 3D dynamics from complete 3D kinematic (including all joint motions) and anthropometric data. We have applied this method to the investigation of the contribution of the intersegmental dynamics of infant kicks and the emergence of selective control.

Using kinetics, we have an understanding of the control of emergent forces within the leg across joints that are combined to produce a kicking motion. Schneider and Zernicke (1992) made an important contribution to the understanding of infant limb dynamics, but their analysis has not been applied to the emergence of selective control of the limbs. One additional limitation is that their analysis included a 2D analysis of the dynamics, although a 3D dynamic analysis is necessary to advance our understanding of control during infancy. More specifically, we are interested in furthering the understanding of how infants learn to co-ordinate gravitational, interactive and active muscle forces to produce selective leg action.

## Intervention programmes and future research using contingency-based learning

Our goal is for infants at risk for lower extremity movement disorders to increase the frequency of kicking and to improve the amount of kicking in developmentally appropriate patterns. We have abundant evidence that children with CP have atypical muscle tissue, potential contractures and are weak. We do not know the exact mechanisms for these changes in the muscular apparatus. We do know that the spinal cord begins to make rapid changes when the central nervous system is damaged, producing atypical outputs to muscles. We can hypothesize that this atypical nervous output will have consequences on the integrity of muscles and other tissues in the legs. We suggest that encouraging a more typical kicking repertoire early and often, using a full range of concentric and eccentric muscle activity, could support the maintenance of healthy muscular tissue. This could potentially avoid contracture and promote strength from the very beginnings of life (see Chapter 11).

Once we have developed and demonstrated that this intervention paradigm can effectively change the quantity and quality of leg actions for prematurely born infants, we will apply the paradigm to other infants with congenital developmental problems such as infants with myelomeningocele or Down syndrome. Infants in both of these groups have decreased leg movement at birth that are associated with reduced later mobility, including walking (Lloyd et al., 2010; Schoenmakers et al., 2005). With appropriate modifications for the upper extremity actions, we believe we can also use this intervention with infants with brachial plexus injuries and hemiplegic CP.

To date, all of our research has been conducted in a laboratory setting using motion analysis technology and other sophisticated instrumentation. However, in order to provide an intervention that is of sufficient intensity to support true motor learning, infants need intensive practice of the exploratory and contingent leg actions. As a consequence, we are developing a novel technology-based therapeutic solution that can be implemented within the home environment to encourage infants on a frequent and daily basis to engage in independent exploration of their leg movements and control an object of interest. A key novel aspect of this work is the development of a computational model of reward-based learning that accounts for infants learning the contingent kicking task, and the use of this model to develop automatic and *individualized* intervention protocols that maximize LE kicking patterns. It is through parent-friendly, home-based and very early intervention that we believe infants will gain the necessary practice to make important changes to the movement patterns that will be critical for later mobility.

## References

Adolph, K.E., Vereijken, B., Shrout, P., 2003. What changes in infant walking and why. Child Dev. 74, 475–497.

Aldoph, K.E., Eppler, M.A., Gibson, E.J., 1993. Crawling versus walking infants' perception of affordances for locomotion over sloping surfaces. Child Dev. 64, 1158–1174.

Angulo-Kinzler, R.M., 2001. Exploration and selection of intralimb coordination patterns in 3-month-old infants. J. Mot. Behav. 33, 363–376.

Angulo-Kinzler, R.M., Ulrich, B., Thelen, E., 2002. Three-month-old infants can select specific leg motor solutions. Motor Control 6, 52–68.

Bayatti, N., Moss, J.A., Sun, L., et al., 2008. A molecular neuroanatomical study of the developing human neocortex from 8 to 17 postconceptional weeks revealing the early differentiation of the subplate and subventricular zone. Cereb. Cortex 18, 1536–1548.

Bertenthal, B.I., Campos, J.J., Barrett, K.C., 1984. Self-produced locomotion: an organizer of emotional, cognitive, and social development in infancy. In: Emde, R.N., Harmon, R.J. (Eds.), Continuities and Discontinuities in Development. Plenum, New York, pp. 175–210.

Campbell, S., Wilhelm, I., Slaton, D., 1989. Anthropometric characteristics of young children with cerebral palsy. Pediatr. Phys. Ther. 1, 105–108.

Chen, Y., Fetters, L., Holt, K.G., Saltzman, E., 2002. Making the mobile move: constraining task and environment. Infant Behav. Dev. 25, 195–220.

Eyre, J.A., Miller, S., Clowry, G.J., Conway, E.A., Watts, C., 2000. Functional corticospinal projections are established prenatally in the human foetus permitting involvement in the development of spinal motor centres. Brain 123, 51–64.

Eyre, J.A., Taylor, J.P., Villagra, F., Smith, M., Miller, S., 2001. Evidence of activity-dependent withdrawal of corticospinal projections during human development. Neurology 57, 1543–1554.

Pattersoj by 2010. Perspective on variability in the development of human action. Phys. Ther. 90, 1860–1867.

Fetters, L., Chen, Y.P., Jonsdottir, J., Tronick, E.Z., 2004. Kicking coordination captures differences between full-term and premature infants with white matter disorder. Hum. Mov. Sci. 22, 729–748.

Fetters, L.S.I., Chen, Y., Kubo, M., Tronick, E.Z., 2010. Spontaneous kicking in full-term and preterm infants with and without white matter disorder. Dev. Psychobiol. 52, 524–536.

Fowler, E.G., Goldberg, E.J., 2009. The effect of lower extremity selective voluntary motor control on interjoint coordination during gait in children with spastic diplegic cerebral palsy. Gait Posture 29, 102–107.

Galloway, J.C., Thelen, E., 2004. Feet first: object exploration in young infants. Infant Behav. Dev. 27, 107–112.

Galloway, J.C., Heathcock, J., Bhat, A., Lobo, M., 2002. Feet reaching: the interaction of experience and ability in full-term infants. J. Sport Exerc. Psychol. 24, 57.

Gibson, E.J., 1988. Exploratory behavior in the development of perceiving acting and the acquiring of knowledge. Annu. Rev. Psychol. 39, 1–41.

Gibson, E.J., 1997. An ecological psychologist's prolegomena for perceptual development: a functional approach. In: Goldring, Z. (Ed.), Evolving Explanations of Development: Ecological Approaches to Organism–Environment Systems. APA, Washington DC, pp. 23–45.

Gibson, E.J., Pick, A.D., 2000. An ecological approach to perceptual development An Ecological Approach to Perceptual Learning and Development. Oxford University Press, New York, pp. 14–25.

Goldfield, E.C., Kay, B.A., Warren, W.H., 1993. Infant bouncing: the

assembly and tuning of action systems. Child Dev. 64, 1128–1142.

Heathcock, J.C., Galloway, J.C., 2009. Exploring objects with feet advances movement in infants born preterm: a randomized controlled trial. Phys. Ther. 89, 1027–1038.

Herbert, J., Gross, J., Hayne, H., 2007. Crawling is associated with more flexible memory retrieval by 9-month-old infants. Dev. Sci. 10, 183–189.

Heriza, C.B., 1988. Comparison of leg movements in preterm infants at term with healthy full-term infants. Phys. Ther. 68, 1687–1693.

Jeng, S.F., Chen, L.C., Yau, K.-I.T., 2002. Kinematic analysis of kicking movements in preterm infants with very low birth weight and full-term infants. Phys. Ther. 82, 148–159.

Jeng, S.-F., Chen, L.-C., Tsou, K.-I., Chen, W.J., Lou, H.-J., 2004. Relationship between spontaneous kicking and age of walking attainment in preterm infants with very low birth weight and full-term infants. Phys. Ther. 84, 159–172.

Johnson, M., 1987. The Body in the Mind: The Bodily Basis of Meaning, Imagination, and Reason. Chicago University Press, Chicago, IL.

Latash, M., 1996. The Bernstein problem: how does the central nervous system make its choices?. In: Latash, M., Turvey, M. (Eds.), Dexterity and Its Development. Lawrence Erlbaum Associates, Inc. Marwah, NJ, pp. 277–303.

Lieber, R.L., Bodine-Fowler, S.C., 1993. Skeletal muscle mechanics: implications for rehabilitation. Phys. Ther. 73, 844–856.

Lieber, R.L., Fridén, J., 2002. Spasticity causes a fundamental rearrangement of muscle–joint interaction. Muscle Nerve 25, 265–270.

Lloyd, M., Burghardt, A., Ulrich, D.A., Angulo-Barroso, R., 2010. Physical activity and walking onset in infants with Down syndrome. Adapt. Phys. Activ. Q. 27, 1–16.

Milewski, A.E., Siqueland, E.R., 1975. Discrimination of color and pattern

novelty in one-month human infants. J. Exp. Child Psychol. 19, 122–136.

Piek, J., 1996. A quantitative analysis of spontaneous kicking in two-month-old infants. Hum. Mov. Sci. 15, 707–726.

Schneider, K., Zernicke, R.F., 1992. Mass, center of mass and moment of inertia estimates for infant limb segments. J. Biomech. 25, 145–148.

Schoenmakers, M.A., Uiterwaal, C.S., Gulmans, V.A., Gooskens, R.H., Helders, P.J., 2005. Determinants of functional independence and quality of life in children with spina bifida. Clin. Rehabil. 19, 677–685.

Siqueland, E.R., DeLucia, C.A., 1969. Visual reinforcement of nonnutritive sucking in human infants. Science 165, 1144–1146.

Spittle, A.J., Cheong, J., Doyle, L.W., et al., 2011. Neonatal white matter abnormality predicts childhood motor impairment in very preterm children. Dev. Med. Child Neurol. 53, 1000–1006.

Thelen, E., 2000. Grounded in the world: developmental origins of the embodied mind. Infancy 1, 3–28.

Thelen, E., Smith, L.A., 1994. Dynamic Systems Approach to the Development of Cognition and Action. Massachusettes Institute of Technology, Cambridge, MA.

Thelen, E., Ridley-Johnson, R., Fisher, D.M., 1983. Shifting patterns of bilateral coordination and lateral dominance in the leg movements of young infants. Dev. Psychobiol. 16, 29–46.

Vaal, J., van Soest, A.J., Hopkins, B., Sie, L.T.L., van der Knaap, M.S., 2000. Development of spontaneous leg movements in infants with and without periventricular leukomalacia. Exp. Brain Res. 135, 94–105.

Vaal, J., Knoek van Soest, A., Hopkins, B., Sie, L.T.L., 2002. Spontaneous leg movements in infants with and without periventricular leukomalacia: effects of unilateral weighting. Behav. Brain Sci. 129, 83–92.

# Treadmill training in early infancy: sensory and motor effects

# 12

Caroline Teulier, Marianne Barbu-Roth, David I. Anderson

## CHAPTER CONTENTS

When newborn infants are supported in an upright position with their feet contacting a flat surface they will make co-ordinated stepping movements that are very similar in character to those of an older child or adult (Andre-Thomas and Autgaerden, 1966; Peiper, 1963; Zelazo, et al., 1972). The activity bears such striking similarity to the mature form of independent walking that it is generally viewed as the appropriate starting point for studying the development of upright locomotion. That starting point may be even earlier, given that human fetuses as young as 13–14 weeks gestational age will produce alternating steps while somersaulting in the uterus (de Vries et al., 1982). These seemingly precocious stepping behaviours highlight two important questions for the development of independent locomotion: (1) how does mature locomotion emerge from early stepping; and (2) how important is it to maintain and promote early stepping to improve later locomotion?

From a clinical standpoint, the challenge is to determine whether and how the earlier-appearing stepping patterns can be progressively guided into functional patterns of locomotion when the integrity of the musculoskeletal and nervous systems is compromised by disease or trauma. It is somewhat surprising that although locomotion is one of the most extensively studied skills in motor development (Bernstein, 1967; Dominici et al., 2011; Forssberg, 1985; McGraw, 1940; Shirley, 1931; Sutherland et al., 1980; Thelen and Smith, 1994), experimental discoveries on infant stepping are only now being integrated into clinical practice (Teulier et al., 2009; Ulrich et al., 2001). We argue that there is a pressing need to implement these discoveries at a much faster rate so that the odds of acquiring independent locomotion are improved for the millions of children worldwide who suffer from some form of locomotor disability.

The goal of the current chapter is to examine whether treadmill-induced stepping might be used to promote functional mobility in infants with cerebral palsy (CP). While no evidence currently exists to support the efficacy of treadmill stepping for infants with CP, an impressive body of evidence gathered on typically developing infants and infants with other neurological disorders shows that treadmill stepping practice can hasten the onset of independent walking and improve the quality of gait. We will review this evidence and discuss how researchers are currently augmenting and varying perceptual information during training to further enhance the efficacy of the treadmill stepping paradigm. These modifications to the paradigm are providing opportunities to initiate training interventions at earlier and earlier ages and in more ecological settings. Based on the scientific community's increasing understanding of the early plasticity in neural and behavioural systems, as well as its appreciation of the widespread nature of critical periods in perceptual and motor development, we argue that early interventions may be essential to ensuring the infant with CP reaches his or her motoric potential.

## The birth of the infant treadmill stepping paradigm

The infant treadmill stepping paradigm emerged in the context of a theoretical debate about the most appropriate explanation for the disappearance of newborn stepping. One of the most curious features of early stepping is its disappearance at around 2–3 months of age followed by its reappearance shortly before the onset of independent walking (McGraw, 1932, 1940, 1945). The ontogeny of stepping is a classic example of the U-shaped character of several developmental phenomena (Strauss, 1982). Because

the stepping pattern has traditionally been viewed as a primitive reflex, controlled by simple circuits in the brainstem and spinal cord, its disappearance and reappearance was attributed to maturation of cortical brain areas that suppressed the reflex temporarily before bringing it back under voluntary control (Fiorentino, 1981; Forssberg, 1985; McGraw, 1945; Peiper, 1963). This belief was seriously challenged by the fascinating discovery that practicing stepping not only prevented it from disappearing but also increased the quantity of stepping and led to an earlier onset of independent walking (Andre-Thomas and Autgaerden, 1966; Peiper, 1963; Zelazo et al., 1972).

A series of ingenious experiments conducted by Esther Thelen and her colleagues ultimately debunked the notion that stepping's disappearance was attributable to cortical maturation. The series of experiments began with a simple observation—that despite the impressive similarity between the kinematic features and muscle activation patterns underlying supine kicking and stepping, supine kicking did not disappear, whereas stepping did (Thelen et al., 1981). Assuming that stepping and kicking were basically the same behaviours expressed in different postural contexts, Thelen wondered why the brain would inhibit the behaviour in one context but not the other. The rapid accumulation of leg fat mass relative to muscle mass at the time stepping disappeared proved to be the pivotal discovery in overturning the cortical maturation hypothesis (Thelen and Fisher, 1982). It became obvious that the legs simply became too heavy to lift when the infant was supported in an upright position. The most compelling evidence to support this argument was that stepping could be inhibited if small weights were added to the infant's legs and that infants who had stopped stepping could be made to step again if their heavy legs were buoyed in a tank of water (Thelen et al., 1984).

The treadmill stepping paradigm was born in the context of the experiments described above. Thelen and colleagues discovered that they could also induce stepping to reappear by supporting the infant on a moving treadmill belt (Thelen, 1986; Thelen and Ulrich, 1991; Thelen et al., 1987). Moreover, and of great importance for clinicians, the steps induced in typically developing infants on the treadmill were more mature than those seen when the infant was supported with their feet touching a stationary surface. Notably, a greater degree of hip extension is observed on the treadmill and often infants show the heel-to-toe progression characteristic of adult walking (Thelen and Smith, 1994; Thelen and Ulrich, 1991; Jensen et al.,1994). These discoveries all emerged from experiments that were originally designed to test Thelen's explanation for the disappearance of the stepping pattern.

## Plasticity and adaptability of the stepping pattern

The treadmill stepping paradigm has revealed a high degree of adaptability in the infant stepping pattern. Stepping shows a level of sophistication and contextually adapted modulation when leg movements are mechanically driven by the treadmill that belies its original reputation as a rigidly stereotyped spinal reflex. For example, the legs can maintain a stable phase relation even when each leg is placed on separate treadmills running at different speeds from each other (Thelen and Smith, 1994; Thelen et al., 1987; Yang et al., 2005). In addition, the pattern has been shown to adapt to repeated perturbations (Pang et al., 2003) and to scale to the speed of the treadmill (Lamb and Yang, 2000). Furthermore, sideways and backward stepping have been elicited, with both scaled to treadmill speed (Lamb and Yang, 2000), and the individual legs have been driven to step in different directions when two treadmill belts are moved in opposite directions (Yang et al., 2004).

Plasticity in the stepping pattern is the feature that makes stepping an ideal target for clinical intervention. Moreover, the degree of responsiveness in the pattern to variations in treadmill parameters opens exciting new avenues for using the treadmill to train early infant locomotion.

## Continuity from stepping to walking

The evidence described in the preceding paragraph provides some insight into the stepping pattern's plasticity. However, the primary evidence for plasticity comes from the early experiments in which infants were given stepping practice for extended periods of time. Those experiments demonstrated clearly that stepping would not disappear if it was practiced and, more importantly, that practice led to an earlier onset of independent walking (Andre-Thomas and Autgaerden, 1966; Peiper, 1963; Zelazo

et al., 1972). The latter finding provides particularly strong support for continuity in locomotor development from the earliest stepping movements to the emergence of independent walking. More recent support has been provided by researchers who have used sophisticated neural modelling to argue that the basic patterns of lumbosacral motor neuron activity seen in neonatal stepping are retained in adult walking, even though new patterns are also evident (Dominici et al., 2011). Despite the obvious similarities between stepping and walking, however, it is abundantly clear that the two are not isomorphic.

The research to date suggests strongly that stepping is an important, and probably necessary, precursor to walking, but two caveats have to be kept in mind. First, the underlying electromyographic patterns and movement kinematics are much more variable in early stepping than mature walking. Healthy infants produced a wide variety of muscle activation combinations and timings when stepping on a treadmill, even though decreases in co-contraction suggest an increase in muscular co-ordination over time (Teulier et al., 2012). This finding implies that the earliest locomotor patterns do not simply reflect the output of a stereotyped central pattern generator (CPG). Second, walking is far more demanding than stepping. For example, supported stepping places no demands on balance and steering, no demands on movement planning and initiation, no demands on monitoring the external layout, and only minimal (though adjustable) demands on strength. Nevertheless, as a precursor to independent walking, the stepping pattern is highly amenable to clinical intervention.

To understand what can be accomplished with treadmill stepping interventions, as well as their limitations, it is helpful to further examine the demands on independent walking and further delineate the differences between stepping and walking. The analysis will also help to clarify the range of different variables that need to be addressed in interventions designed to promote motor development. The analysis begins with a brief summary of Newell's model of constraints on behaviour (Newell, 1984, 1986).

## Constraints on the development of walking

Drawing on the seminal works of Kugler et al. (1980, 1982) as well as Higgins (1977), Newell

(1986) argued that all motor behaviour emerges from the interaction of constraints from three broad sources: the individual's body; the tasks in which individuals participate; and the environment. The myriad of constraints channel movement dynamics and specify what sources of information are likely to be most useful in the control of action.

## Individual constraints

With respect to walking, the capacity to generate alternating limb movements, sufficient strength to support the body and generate propulsive force, and balance have been identified as important individual constraints, though it is important to realize that a new skill like walking will be influenced by a range of perceptual, affective, attentional, motivational, postural, anatomical, and physiological variables interacting in a particular context (Thelen and Smith, 1994; Thelen and Ulrich, 1991).

The constraints can be viewed as important substrates of skillful walking that, if weak or missing, might be the target of interventions to promote walking. Sufficient strength and balance, in particular, are often considered key contributors to independent walking (Thelen and Smith, 1994). Adolph et al. (1998) also identified strength as an important contributor to the development of hands-and-knees crawling. Infants who had engaged in several weeks of belly crawling prior to the onset of hands-and-knees crawling mastered hands-and-knees crawling much faster than infants who had skipped belly crawling altogether. Belly crawling presumably 'shored up' the prerequisites, e.g., strength, that were necessary for proficient hands-and-knees crawling.

## Task constraints

Task constraints and environmental constraints are often given far less attention in the organization of behaviour than individual constraints. However, they are just as important. Task constraints in walking would largely involve the locomotor goals that the child sets itself. These goals change of course as the child becomes a more competent walker. Choices of places to go, for example, increase exponentially as walking skill improves. Task constraints also involve the rules associated with tasks. The young child need not conform to any formal rules when first learning to walk, though

the older child must, particularly when navigating city streets, where a number of rules are in place to protect pedestrian traffic.

## Environmental constraints

Environmental constraints represent the final class of constraints from which behaviours emerge. These constraints include the field of external forces (such as gravity) in which all movements are made as well as the social and cultural forces that shape the activities we choose to participate in as well as the manner in which we express those choices (Gentile 1987). All movements represent a blend of internal forces that are generated through muscular contraction and external forces that surround the individual. Gravity is the most pervasive external force that influences the character of a movement—witness the dramatic changes in gait that occur when astronauts 'walk' on the surface of the moon—though inertial forces, frictional forces, and various reaction forces will also heavily influence the character of a movement. The most obvious environmental constraints, however, include the physical features of the environment because movements are organized relative to these features.

Gentile (1987, 2000) has provided a particularly clear description of the environmental constraints that impose themselves on movement dynamics. She has coined the term *regulatory conditions* to describe the physical features of the environment to which movements must conform if they are to be successful. In the case of walking, important regulatory conditions include the size of the surface on which walking occurs, its slope, its solidity, and its texture. People walk very differently on a slippery surface like ice, for example, than on a textured surface like concrete. Any variations in the regulatory conditions force some form of adaptation or reorganization of the movement pattern. This point is crucially important because the regulatory conditions will vary in an infinite number of ways. Consequently, in a task like walking, the motor system is continually challenged to come up with adaptations that accommodate to changing regulatory conditions. This notion highlights how important the processing of sensory information is during functional locomotion. We will return to this point later in the chapter when we discuss ways to enhance the efficacy of treadmill training.

The point of this primer on constraints has been to reinforce the complexity associated with learning and performing an ostensibly simple task like walking. That complexity needs to be given careful consideration in the development of interventions designed to promote independent walking. While it is clear from the earlier discussion that treadmill stepping is remarkably adaptable to contextual variations in the way the treadmill belt moves, functional locomotion is far more demanding. Moreover, adaptations in gait require continuous monitoring of the environment and one's relation to it to ensure that the locomotor goal is achieved and that it is achieved efficiently. As such, the demands on attention are far greater during independent walking than they are during supported stepping. With these points in mind, it is possible to design interventions that progressively challenge the infant to acquire the prerequisite skills and capacities to engage in functional locomotion. The primary goal of interventions should be to develop the substrates of independent locomotion, provide opportunities to integrate these substrates into functional patterns, and systematically expose the patterns to contextual variations to promote the development of flexible locomotor strategies. In addition, where possible, the infant should be exposed to the sources of perceptual information that will be available during independent locomotion.

## When should interventions start?

Having established the goals for treadmill training interventions, we now turn to the important question of when interventions should be started. Discussions about the most appropriate times to initiate motor skill learning have historically been couched relative to the critical periods and readiness concepts (Anderson et al., 2012). The critical period concept originated in embryology, where the embryo's ultimate form was shown to be exquisitely sensitive to the timing of developmental disruptions (Spemann, 1938; Stockard, 1921). Critical periods are now well-established phenomena in embryological development and nearly every parent is familiar with the notion that teratogens (external agents) will have widely different effects depending on the timing of exposure. The period of most rapid growth or differentiation of an organ or system is generally considered the most susceptible time (Moore and Persaud, 1998).

The most widely cited example of a critical period in mammalian development concerns the visual system. Hubel and Wiesel (1970) demonstrated that surgical closure of one eye during a brief period after birth causes a severe visual impairment in species such as cats and monkeys when the eye is later reopened. Critical periods have been demonstrated for auditory development, tactile development, and motor and neuromuscular development in the rat (Jamon and Serradj, 2009). A special issue of *Developmental Psychobiology* maintains that critical periods in human sensory development are pervasive (Maurer, 2005).

Though critical periods in human development have most often been discussed relative to neurological development, particularly as it pertains to the perceptual systems, an experiment by Walton et al. (1992) suggests that they are equally present in other physiological systems. Using tail suspension to simulate weightlessness, they discovered a critical period in rat locomotor development during which unloading of the weight-bearing limbs caused permanent disruptions to swimming and walking. Jamon and Serradj (2009) have reviewed the effects of exposure to hypo- and hypergravity and confirmed that muscular development is highly sensitive to disruptions in the normal forces on the limbs during early postnatal development. For example, rats reared in hypergravity showed marked changes in the contractile and morphological properties of their muscles. Their review also showed that altered gravity has significant effects on the development of the vestibular system during a critical period in development. Given the number of different components from which independent locomotion is assembled, each with its own developmental trajectory, it is likely that multiple critical periods exist in the development of locomotion.

This brief discussion of critical periods suggests that interventions should be initiated as early as possible to enable infants with disabilities to achieve their locomotor potential. When combined with our increasing understanding of the plasticity in early neurological systems, the case for early interventions is even more compelling (Ulrich, 2010). In the remaining sections of this chapter, we will highlight how the treadmill paradigm has been used to promote the development of independent walking. In addition, we will describe recent discoveries about the sophistication of early perception–action coupling that can be used to enhance the effectiveness of treadmill training and potentially allow interventions to begin even earlier.

## Can treadmill interventions promote independent walking in clinical populations?

Researchers have increasingly used treadmill interventions (Fig. 12.1) to promote locomotion in clinical populations over the last 10 years, particularly for infants with Down syndrome (DS). In contrast, no such intervention has been published on infants with CP or at risk for CP. Most of the studies designed to improve mobility in children with CP have used other approaches and/or they were initiated after infancy (for reviews see Damiano and DeJong 2009; Valentin-Gudiol et al., 2011). In this section, we focus on three aims: (1) to describe the currently known benefits of treadmill training for infants without CP; (2) to discuss these findings relative to what is currently known about motor development in infants with CP; and (3) to explore how early treadmill interventions might be used to promote independent locomotion in children with CP.

The first treadmill intervention with a clinical population was published in 2001 by Ulrich and colleagues following Thelen's finding that after one month of treadmill training, typically developing infants increased the quantity and quality (more alternating steps) of their stepping responses (Vereijken and Thelen 1997). In the Ulrich et al. (2001) study, 32 infants with DS were assigned to a control or intervention group. The treadmills were lent to the parents so that they could deliver the intervention in their own homes. This is an important detail because implicating parents in their child's motor development benefits the development of the parent–infant relationship and allows the physical therapist to focus more on the infant's specific physical needs in the context of the intervention. In addition, the infants can receive more stimulation and training that benefits neuromotor function. Ulrich's main finding was that infants in the intervention group walked independently 101 days earlier on average than infants in the control group, with only eight

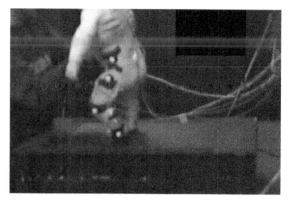

**Figure 12.1** • A 9-month-old infant stepping on a treadmill.

minutes of training per day for five days a week over the course of approximately 10 months (the intervention was pursued until the onset of walking). Infants who did the intervention walked at around 19.9 months of age, which is quite early for a population that usually learns to walk at around 24 months of age. This outcome was also preceded by a faster development of other motor skills like standing and walking with help.

Subsequent studies showed that the infants with DS could be made to walk even earlier (by 19.2 months of age) and with more alternating steps if the duration and intensity (increased treadmill belt speed) of the training was increased and weights were selectively attached to the ankles as the infants took progressively more steps (Ulrich et al., 2008; Wu et al., 2007). Infants who received high-intensity (HI) treadmill training also engaged in more high-intensity activity and less low-intensity activity outside of the intervention period than infants who were given lower-intensity (LI) training (Angulo-Barroso et al., 2008a). Spending more time in high-level physical activity is a gauge of motor development but also a contributor to motor development because it increases the number of experience-dependent processes that can be recruited to further developmental change.

## Treadmill interventions can have lasting effects

The benefits seen in the Wu et al. (2007) study were retained even 15 months after the end of the intervention, highlighting that treadmill interventions can have a long-lasting effect on activity levels and neuromotor development. Besides the earlier onset of walking and the higher level of physical activity, the quality of gait also remained better after the intervention. This criterion is important because many populations with neuromotor developmental delay develop walking patterns that are highly energetically costly (Bell and Davies, 2010), patterns that can later hinder the capacity to use independent locomotion to accomplish activities of everyday living (Palisano et al., 2010). After three months of walking experience the HI group showed better gait parameters overall (like increased average velocity, step width, stride time, stance time, and dynamic base), and, especially, longer stride lengths than the LI group (Wu et al., 2007). Within six months after training, the HI group was also better at adapting their stepping to cross an obstacle. The infants were able to quickly adjust their last three steps to prepare for obstacle clearance, whereas it took much longer for the LI group to preferentially use a stepping strategy than a crawling strategy to negotiate the obstacle. However, both groups were adept at making appropriate locomotor adjustments after more experience with locomotion (Wu et al., 2008).

These aforementioned findings are important because they show that progressively challenging (compared to a consistent challenge) interventions designed to improve treadmill stepping show transfer to more ecological contexts. In this case, the transfer was in the form of fast and flexible adaptation when crossing an obstacle. As the treadmill is often seen as task-specific practice for stepping and walking, these findings clearly highlight that reinforcing stepping in one context facilitates the child's ability to adapt her own individual constraints to task/environmental constraints (clearing the obstacle). Finally, after 15 months, the group that received the HI intervention walked at a higher velocity and cadence and produced a lower double support time than the group that received LI training. Nevertheless, the gaits of both groups improved over the first year of walking experience and foot rotation asymmetry was also reduced (Angulo-Barroso et al., 2008b). Though no follow-up longer than 15 months post-intervention has been published, we at least know that children around 3 years of age continue to benefit from their early treadmill training in terms of their level of physical activity, their quality of gait, and their ability to adapt locomotion to environmental features.

## Can infants with cerebral palsy benefit from treadmill training?

Because few published early interventions for infants with CP or at risk for neuromotor delays (ND) are available compared to interventions with older CP children (Damiano and DeJong, 2009; Valentin-Gudiol et al., 2011), it is hard to evaluate how effective treadmill interventions might be for such infants over the first years of life.

Recently, Angulo-Barroso et al. (2010) described the developmental trajectory of the stepping pattern in infants with CP from 6 to 23 months of age. Their study showed that infants who were later diagnosed with CP did not step as well as their peers with ND on the treadmill (e.g., fewer alternating steps, more toe contact) and had a lower level of physical activity, both of which were associated with a later onset of walking. Even though the sample was small, the study provides some insight into the specific constraints associated with the CP population. The study clearly shows that the developmental trajectory of stepping is similar for typically developing children and children who later were diagnosed as having CP, though the stepping response was depressed in the latter children (Fig. 12.2). Hence, it appears that infants with CP have the capacity to produce alternating steps but are delayed in doing so. From Figure 12.2, we can also see that infants at risk for ND also seem to be slightly behind their typically developing peers, though caution is needed in interpreting the figure because the data for the three groups were taken from different studies (Angulo-Barroso et al., 2010; Teulier et al., 2009; Thelen and Ulrich, 1991).

Data from an earlier study showed that premature infants at low risk for ND responded in a similar way to typically developing infants on the treadmill (Davis et al., 1994). Overall, these results are clinically relevant and provide added support to the idea that early interventions could be used to improve functional motor skills like walking. Finally, a trend has been reported showing that the amount of time spent in low-level physical activity is related to a later walking onset. In contrast, a high level of physical activity is related to an earlier walking onset in infants with ND and CP, similar to what has been observed in infants with DS (McKay and Angulo-Barroso, 2006), reinforcing again the potential value of early intervention.

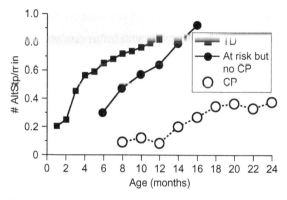

**Figure 12.2** • Development of alternating stepping without training for three populations: infants with CP; infants at risk for CP but not diagnosed with CP; and infants with typical development (TD).

## An early treadmill intervention with infants at risk for CP

A case study by Bodkin et al. (2003), which looked at one infant at risk for ND, suggests that treadmill interventions might be effective for this population. Similar to previous studies highlighting the developmental trajectory of infants at risk for ND, Bodkin's infant was able to increase his stepping response over several months of treadmill intervention, although he struggled to produce any steps at 5 to 6 months of age. This is not too surprising as typically developing infants also struggle to produce many alternating steps at around 2 to 3 months of age (Fig. 12.2). Hence, the delay in motor development in this population might reflect the depressed response seen in younger typically developing infants, when muscles are weak and infants lack the strength to overcome the increasing weight of the lower limb. More data are clearly needed to verify this conclusion and to determine whether there are windows of opportunity for initiating treadmill stepping interventions to improve gait in children with CP or at risk for ND.

## A treadmill intervention on older children with CP

Cherng et al. (2007) and Richards et al. (1997) worked with 2 to 7-year-old children ($n = 8$ and $n = 4$, respectively) and showed that, similar to what has been shown in infants with DS, the use of body weight-supported treadmill training improved the children's gait characteristics (increased stride length and decreased percentage of the gait cycle spent in double limb support) as well as other aspects of motor function. Again, the sample size is small and children had already learned to ambulate in one study; however, the findings suggest that some of the treadmill training benefits seen in other clinical populations could generalize to children with CP. Clearly, more studies are needed, with larger sample sizes, long-term follow-up of participants to determine whether they are formally diagnosed as having CP, and randomized controlled trials to ascertain with certainty the potential benefits of early supported treadmill interventions for children with CP.

## Can treadmill training have negative effects?

Negative effects of early treadmill training are yet to be reported in the literature (Damiano and DeJong 2009). Moreover, Ulrich et al. (2001) reported no changes in anthropometric characteristics (crown–heel length, thigh and calf lengths, thigh and calf circumferences, foot length and width, thigh, calf, umbilicus, skinfold, and body weight) between the group of infants with DS that received the treadmill intervention five times per week for around 10 months and the control group that was not supported on the treadmill and only received their usual physical therapy twice a week. This finding highlights that treadmill interventions can be implemented without negatively impacting the infant's morphological characteristics, possibly because infants self-select how much of their body weight they can or want to support when placed on the treadmill. Of course, it is important to note that a researcher or physiotherapist taught the parents how to hold the baby on the treadmill. Consequently, the benefits associated with having the family involved in the therapeutic intervention can be realized with appropriate supervision from qualified professionals.

## Important considerations when deciding to use treadmill training

To maximize the effectiveness of treadmill training, a few considerations need to be highlighted. The first concerns the inclusion criteria used to accept infants into a study. Given that treadmill interventions with DS infants have required that infants be capable of independent sitting or taking at least six steps on the treadmill (Ulrich et al., 2001, 2008), we should question what criteria would be most appropriate for infants at risk for ND given how little we know about their stepping trajectory over the first six months of life. The second consideration concerns the training design, including parameters such as treadmill speed and duration of training. Again, it is hard to make recommendations because of lack of data. Angulo-Barroso et al. (2010) used a belt speed of 20 cm/second, whereas Bodkin et al. (2003) used 15 cm/second. The literature suggests that infants are capable of adapting quite well to different speeds, but tend to struggle with higher speeds, particularly at younger ages (Thelen and Ulrich, 1991). Consequently, it would be wise to raise speed over time. Speeds ranging from 4 cm/second for infants as young as 1 month old to 30 cm/second for infants older than 12 months of age have proven to be effective (Teulier et al., 2009; Ulrich et al., 2008).

The duration of training can also be increased over time consistent with the infant's ability to respond to the treadmill. Usually, the duration is increased once the infant has reached a threshold of 10 or more steps produced per minute (Ulrich et al., 2008); this criterion has also been used to determine when to increase treadmill speed during the intervention (Moerchen et al., 2011; Ulrich et al., 2008). Here it is important to highlight that the goal of a treadmill intervention is not to elicit automatic responses but to prepare the body to learn how to walk by developing the underlying neural and musculoskeletal substrates used in walking. Creating an infant-centred intervention that adjusts to the individual's constraints and rate of progress is most likely to promote the 'good variability' that enables flexible adaptation to environmental constraints during independent walking. Finally, adaptability can be heightened even further by creating contexts that simulate the flows of perceptual information experienced during independent walking. Though this recommendation has not yet been widely implemented, we believe that it can enhance the effectiveness of treadmill interventions significantly.

# A more ecological approach to treadmill training

One criticism of treadmill training is how dissimilar walking on a treadmill is with everyday locomotion.

As mentioned earlier, to understand what can and cannot be accomplished with treadmill stepping interventions it is helpful to examine the demands associated with independent walking. Once those demands are understood, it becomes clear that treadmill interventions should attempt to mimic the ecological context in which natural locomotion occurs as closely as possible. While it is impossible to make treadmill locomotion identical with walking in a natural environment, it is possible to increase their similarity by: (1) increasing proprioceptive feedback (tactile and visual); (2) varying perceptual input by varying surface characteristics and the presence or absence of obstacles, for example; (3) modifying individual constraints such as leg or foot weight; and (4) exposing the infant to stimuli that have hedonic qualities or that are associated with the goals that normally drive locomotion.

# The importance of proprioception during natural locomotion

To adapt their locomotor patterns to variable environments, mobile organisms need a constant flow of information about the external layout, about their own movements, and about the relation between their movements and the layout. The vestibular system, the somatosensory system (e.g., receptors in muscles, joints, and the skin) and the visual system provide most of this information. However, some of the most important sources of information are either non-existent or only partially available during treadmill walking. For example, because the head and body are not translated forward during treadmill walking, the tactile feedback associated with the propulsive forces under the foot, the vestibular feedback, and the visual feedback are quite different from that experienced during over-ground walking. This is particularly obvious when one considers the lack of optic flow (see Chapter 10 for a more detailed discussion of optic flow) experienced during treadmill walking. Aside from the small and typically unpatterned belt of the treadmill, the individual does not experience optic flow during treadmill walking. Despite these problems, however, researchers are discovering clever ways to enhance the perceptual information available during treadmill walking.

# When can infants use visual information to regulate stepping?

Researchers have traditionally assumed that a newborn's visual system is too immature at birth to provide them with useful information for controlling actions. Recent discoveries suggest, however, that the traditional assumptions are false. For example, reasoning that vision is the predominant perceptual system used by most mobile species to regulate locomotion, Barbu-Roth et al. (2009) exposed 3-day-old infants to terrestrial optic flow (a *visual treadmill*) to see if it would have any effect on the newborn stepping pattern. The newborns were suspended above a white surface onto which was projected a static black-and-white checkerboard, a rotating black-and-white pin wheel, or a black-and-white checkerboard that translated toward the infant (Fig. 12.3). The infants were suspended above the surface to permit the legs to move freely and to remove the tactile feedback presumed necessary to elicit the stepping pattern. Remarkably, the infants stepped significantly more when the checkerboard moved toward them, simulating forward displacement, than in the other conditions. We speculated that the neonates experienced a sense of self-motion and stepped in order to match the visual and kinaesthetic consequences of movement.

The coupling between vision and stepping suggests that the neonate is biologically prepared at birth to use vision to control locomotion. The finding further strengthens arguments for the continuity between newborn stepping and independent locomotion. Moreover, the finding suggests that newborn stepping might be controlled at a higher level than the brainstem/spinal cord and so might be responsive to a much wider range of stimuli than previously imagined.

Recently, we performed a pilot study that suggests the coupling between vision and stepping might be quite sophisticated. When 15 newborns were exposed to optic flows that simulated forward translation (Barbu-Roth et al., 2009) or backward translation, they took a similar number of air steps. However, the condition simulating forward locomotion elicited more alternating steps (more mature locomotion) than the condition simulating backward translation (Barbu-Roth et al., 2008). These findings suggest a surprising precociousness in the coupling between vision and stepping.

The relevance of the Barbu-Roth et al. (2009) findings to the treadmill training paradigm has already been examined. For example, Moerchen and Saeed (2009) exposed young (2–5 months of age) and older (7–10 months of age) infants to a terrestrial optic flow while they were stepping on a treadmill. The optic flow was created by painting a

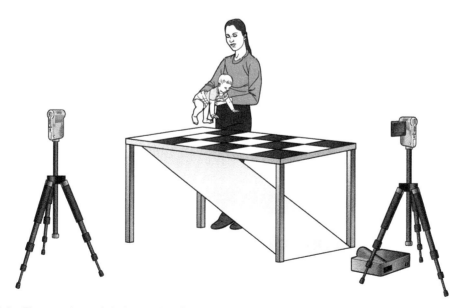

**Figure 12.3** • The experimental design used by Barbu-Roth et al. (2009).

checkerboard pattern on the treadmill belt. Infants took more steps, took more alternating steps, and looked more at the treadmill belt when exposed to the patterned belt than either a black or white belt. So, not only did the patterned belt capture the infants' attention but also it increased the amount of stepping as well as the quality of the co-ordination between the two legs during stepping. These findings are important because they provide the first preliminary evidence that stimulating the infant visually can enhance the effectiveness of treadmill stepping interventions.

Clinically, visual stimulation has recently been added to a treadmill study on infants with spina bifida. Ulrich and colleagues used the same checkerboard pattern on the treadmill belt as Moerchen and Saeed (2009) to see if it would enhance stepping in 2- to 10-month-old infants with spina bifida (with lesions at the lumbar or sacral level). The authors only examined the immediate effect of visual stimulation, rather than extended effects over the course of an intervention. Nevertheless, the results showed that by simply adding visual flow to a 30-second treadmill trial, infants increased the numbers of steps produced on the treadmill, especially between 7 and 10 months of age (Pantall et al., 2011). In addition, the increase in stepping was accompanied by an increase in certain characteristics of muscle activity, such as burst frequency (Pantall et al., 2012). Consequently, these results are highly encouraging in terms of the potential long-term benefits to be gained from adding visual stimulation to treadmill interventions.

Two main conclusions can be drawn from the aforementioned studies. First, visual stimulation alone can elicit stepping at birth (i.e., tactile information from the foot contacting a surface is not necessary). This visual air stepping paradigm could be highly appropriate for stimulating leg movements in young infants. It could be also a highly effective technique for stimulating alternating stepping in older infants who have difficulty supporting their own weight and/or pushing their legs against a surface. Air stepping is much easier than stepping on a surface because the infant's legs do not encounter resistance in the air. The second conclusion is that vision seems to have an additive effect on tactile (treadmill) stepping in older infants, such that more steps and higher-quality steps are produced when the two sources of information are combined. This finding encourages us to test whether newborns will also respond with more steps and higher-quality steps when the two sources of information are combined. In addition, we are exploring how modifying tactile feedback might further enhance the response seen in newborns and older infants when visual and tactile feedback are combined.

## Modifying tactile feedback: does the treadmill surface influence stepping?

As we stated in the introduction, treadmill interventions can start very early in life given that neonates are able to step on a solid surface. An interesting question, then, is will different surfaces elicit different stepping rates and different types of steps and, if so, what surface is most effective. Until now, treadmill belts have been made of the same type of resistant rubber. However, this surface is not necessarily conducive to eliciting the most functional types of steps. In a recent study, we tested the effect of adding a high friction, adhesive material to the surface of the treadmill belt (Pantall et al., 2011, 2012). Again, this study only examined the immediate adaptation of the infants to the modified sensory stimulation and it focused on 2–10-month-old infants with spina bifida. Compared to the normal treadmill belt, increasing friction significantly increased the quantity and quality of steps taken by the infants, including an increase in the vertical displacement of each step and modification of gastrocnemius activation.

Are the surfaces that work well for older infants also likely to work well for younger infants, particularly neonates? This is an interesting question because newborns are a special population. Before birth, newborns were stepping in the visco-elastic environment of their mother's womb. The uterine wall is very different from the solid surface of a treadmill. While it is impossible to reproduce this environment on a treadmill, it is possible to approximate it. For example, a silicon lining on the treadmill belt would provide a surface that is much closer to the uterine wall than the current treadmill belt. Another potentially valuable idea would be to alternate different types of surfaces to begin the process of adapting the infant's stepping response to the range of surfaces that will ultimately be experienced during independent walking.

## Motivational factors

Humans are motivated to move for many different reasons. However, in new crawlers and walkers, one of the most powerful reasons is likely the immediate rewards that stem from their interactions with people and objects in far space. While treadmill training does not allow infants to move freely across the terrain, opportunities nevertheless exist to use hedonically valued objects or people to enhance the infant's motivation to step. This has already been done in many of the studies discussed earlier, where the parents and experimenters were always encouraging infants to step on the treadmill. Although the effects of encouragement were not directly manipulated and tested, we speculate that they must have played some role in motivating infants to step on the treadmill. We could also imagine that presenting a toy to grasp in front of the treadmill would also enhance an infant's motivation to step. To be effective as an incentive, the distance of the toy would need to be adjusted so that the infant could experience success at attaining the toy. The distance between the infant and the toy could be increased as the infant's stepping became more co-ordinated and she became capable of moving along the treadmill belt.

Other consequences of independent locomotion can also motivate infants to continue exercising their skills. Chapter 10 has documented the range of spatial-cognitive changes that take place because of the experiences infants have when they move from place to place. Those experiences motivate infants to continue to explore their environment. Even though treadmill stepping limits the range of those experiences, the infant can still be motivated by them to explore their movement possibilities on the treadmill. Zelazo et al. (1972) have reported such effects during the daily training of newborns to step on a rigid surface. They note: 'it was shown that by 4 weeks an infant learns to control his environment. Walking movements produce spatial, visual and kinesthetic-tactile changes in his world, and these accompanying sensory changes may serve as the inherent reward that reinforces walking' (p. 315). In a subsequent paper, Zelazo was more specific, identifying two factors that potentially motivated the infants to continue stepping: (1) the increasing amount of time spent in a posture that was more and more vertical; and (2) the increasing freedom to move the head and eyes when vertical

to sample more interesting visual stimuli (Zelazo 1983). These observations, while still conjectural suggest that infants with CP or at risk for ND, particularly those who have difficulty controlling their head and maintaining an upright posture, could be motivated to step on a treadmill by the simple rewards associated with being upright and capable of visually scanning the environment. More importantly, treadmill interventions could lead to important improvements in head and body posture.

## Conclusions

In this chapter, we have described how neonatal stepping could be used as the starting point to train future walking, especially in clinical populations. As neonates do not step frequently or with regular patterns, we described treadmill interventions as good candidates to maintain and progressively increase locomotor skill from birth to the emergence of independent walking. The key to promoting functional walking is to maximize motor output (without overloading the infant), by stimulating movement mechanically and via different sensory inputs, and to create the largest possible repertoire of adaptable motor responses and strategies. Of course, a range of strategies can be used to promote independent locomotion and overall motor development, including, for example, the use of air stepping with a visual treadmill.

In conclusion, the seemingly precocious stepping behaviours of neonates provide an excellent illustration of the developmental processes, wherein the substrates of skilled action are seen in fragmented and primitive form well before the skill becomes functional. Much of the developmental process then is characterized by the elaboration, differentiation, and inter-co-ordination of these fragments into a functional whole. Understanding how these primitive behavioural forms contribute to mature behaviours is one of the major challenges for developmental research (Brumley and Robinson, 2010). The treadmill stepping paradigm continues to advance our understanding of how development takes place while helping countless children with disabilities to develop independent locomotion. Continued collaboration between clinicians and researchers is needed to further our understanding of the developmental puzzle and to improve interventions for children with disabilities.

# References

Adolph, K.E., Vereijken, B., Denny, M.A., 1998. Learning to crawl. Child Dev. 69 (5), 1299–1312.

Anderson, D.I., Magill, R.A., Thouvarecq, R., 2012. Critical periods, sensitive periods, and readiness for motor skill learning. In: Williams, A.M., Hodges, N.J. (Eds.), Skill Acquisition in Sport, second ed. Taylor and Francis, London.

Andre-Thomas, Y., Autgaerden, S., 1966. Locomotion from Pre- to Post-Natal Life. Spastics Society and William Heinemann, London.

Angulo-Barroso, R., Burghardt, A.R., Lloyd, M., Ulrich, D.A., 2008a. Physical activity in infants with Down syndrome receiving a treadmill intervention. Infant Behav. Dev. 31 (2), 255–269.

Angulo-Barroso, R.M., Wu, J., Ulrich, D.A., 2008b. Long-term effect of different treadmill interventions on gait development in new walkers with Down syndrome. Gait Posture 27 (2), 231–238.

Angulo-Barroso, R.M., Tiernan, C.W., Chen, L.C., Ulrich, D., Neary, H., 2010 Spring. Treadmill responses and physical activity levels of infants at risk for neuromotor delay. Pediatr. Phys. Ther. 22 (1), 61–68.

Barbu-Roth, M., Anderson, D., Provasi, J., Desprès, A., Streeter, R., Schleihauf, R., 2008. Neonatal Stepping in relation to approaching and receding terrestrial optic flows. ISIS (International Society for Infant Studies), Vancouver, Canada.

Barbu-Roth, M., Anderson, D.I., Despres, A., Provasi, J., Cabrol, D., Campos, J.J., 2009. Neonatal stepping in relation to terrestrial optic flow. Child Dev. 80 (1), 8–14.

Bell, K.L., Davies, P.S., 2010. Energy expenditure and physical activity of ambulatory children with cerebral palsy and of typically developing children. Am. J. Clin. Nutr. 92 (2), 313–319.

Bernstein, N.A., 1967. The Co-Ordination and Regulation of Movements. Pergamon Press, Oxford.

Bodkin, A.W., Baxter, R.S., Heriza, C.B., 2003. Treadmill training for an infant born preterm with a grade III intraventricular hemorrhage. Phys. Ther. 83 (12), 1107–1118.

Brumley, M.R., Robinson, S.R., 2010. Experience in the perinatal development of action systems. In: Blumberg, S., Freeman, J.H., Robinson, S.R. (Eds.), Oxford Handbook of Developmental Behavioural Neuroscience. Oxford University Press, New York.

Cherng, R.J., Liu, C.F., Lau, T.W., Hong, R.B., 2007. Effect of treadmill training with body weight support on gait and gross motor function in children with spastic cerebral palsy. Am. J. Phys. Med. Rehabil. 86 (7), 548–555.

Damiano, D.L., DeJong, S.L., 2009. A systematic review of the effectiveness of treadmill training and body weight support in pediatric rehabilitation. J. Neurol. Phys. Ther. 33 (1), 27–44.

Davis, D.W., Thelen, E., Keck, J., 1994. Treadmill stepping in infants born prematurely. Early Hum. Dev. 39 (3), 211–223.

de Vries, J.I.P., Visser, G.H.A., Prechtl, H.F.R., 1982. The emergence of fetal behaviour. 1. Qualitative aspects. Early Hum. Dev. 7, 21.

Dominici, N., Ivanenko, Y.P., Cappellini, G., d'Avella, A., Mondi, V., Cicchese, M., et al., 2011. Locomotor primitives in newborn babies and their development. Science 334 (6058), 997–999.

Fiorentino, M.R., 1981. A Basis for Sensorimotor Development—Normal and Abnormal: The Influence of Primitive, Postural Reflexes on the Development and Distribution of Tone. Thomas, Springfield, IL.

Forssberg, H., 1985. Ontogeny of human locomotor control. I. Infant stepping, supported locomotion and transition to independent locomotion. Exp. Brain Res. 57 (3), 480–493.

Gentile, A.M., 1987. Skill acquisition: action, movement, and neuromotor processes. In: Carr, J.H., Shepherd, R.B. (Eds.), Movement Science: Foundations for Physical Therapy in Rehabilitation. Aspen, Rockville, MD, pp. 93–154.

Gentile, A.M., 2000. Skill acquisition: action, movement, and neuromotor processes. In: Carr, J.H., Shepherd, R.B. (Eds.), Movement Science: Foundations for Physical Therapy in Rehabilitation, second ed. Aspen, Rockville, MD, pp. 111–187.

Higgins, J.R., 1977. Human Movement: An Integrated Approach. C. V. Mosby, St. Louis, MI.

Hubel, D.H., Wiesel, T.N., 1970. The period of susceptibility to the physiological effects of unilateral eye closure in kittens. J. Physiol. 206 (17), 419.

Jamon, M., Serradj, N., 2009. Ground-based researches on the effects of altered gravity on mice development. Microgravity Sci. Technol. 21, 10.

Kugler, P.N., Kelso, J.A.S., Turvey, M.T., 1980. On the concept of coordinative strucutres as dissipative structures: I. Theoretical lines of convergence. In: Stelmach, G.E., Requin, J. (Eds.), Tutorials in Motor Behavior. North-Holland, Amsterdam, pp. 3–47.

Kugler, P.N., Kelso, J.A.S., Turvey, M.T., 1982. On the control and co-ordination of naturally developing systems. In: Clark, J.E., Kelso, J.A.S. (Eds.), The Development of Movement Control and Co-ordination. John Wiley & Sons, Chichester, UK.

Jensen, J.L., Schneider, K., Ulrich, B.B., Zernicke, R.F., Thelen, E., 1994. Adaptive dynamics of the leg movement patterns of human infants: II. Treadmill stepping in infants and adults. J. Mot. Behav. 26, 313–324.

Lamb, T., Yang, J.F., 2000. Could different directions of infant stepping be controlled by the same locomotor central pattern generator? J. Neurophysiol. 83 (5), 2814–2824.

Maurer, D., 2005. Introduction to the special issue on critical periods reexamined: evidence from human sensory development. Dev. Psychobiol. 46, 163–183.

McGraw, M.B., 1932. From reflex to muscular control in the assumption of an erect posture and ambulation in the human infant. Child Dev. 3, 291–297.

McGraw, M.B., 1940. Neuromuscular development of the human infant as exemplified in the achievement of erect locomotion. J. Pediatr. 17, 21.

McGraw, M.B., 1945. The Neuromuscular Maturation of the Human Infant. Hafner, New York.

McKay, S.M., Angulo-Barroso, R.M., 2006. Longitudinal assessment of leg motor activity and sleep patterns in infants with and without Down syndrome. Infant Behav. Dev. 29 (2), 153–168.

Moerchen V.A., Saeed M., 2009. Patterned treadmill belt as optic flow: prelocomotor infants respond with organized stepping. Society for Research in Child Development biannual meeting, 2009; Denver, CO.

Moerchen, V.A., Habibi, M., Lynett, K.A., Konrad, J.D., Hoefakker, H.L., 2011 Spring. Treadmill training and overground gait: decision making for a toddler with spina bifida. Pediatr. Phys. Ther. 23 (1), 53–61.

Moore, K.L., Persaud, T.V.N., 1998. The Developing Human: Clinically Oriented Embryology, sixth ed. W.B. Saunders, Philadelphia, PA.

Newell, K.M., 1984. Physical constraints to the development of motor skills. In: Thomas, J.R. (Ed.), Motor Development during Preschool and Elementary Years. Burgess, Minneapolis, MN.

Newell, K.M., 1986. Constraints on the development of coordination. In: Wade, M.G., Whiting, H.T.A. (Eds.), Motor Development in Children: Aspects of Coordination and Control. Nijhoff, Dordrecht, pp. 341–360.

Palisano, R.J., Hanna, S.E., Rosenbaum, P.L., Tieman, B., 2010. Probability of walking, wheeled mobility, and assisted mobility in children and adolescents with cerebral palsy. Dev. Med. Child Neurol. 52 (1), 66–71.

Pang, M.Y.C., Lam, T., Yang, J.F., 2003. Infants adapt their stepping to repeated trip-inducing stimuli. J. Neurophysiol. 90, 9.

Pantall, A., Teulier, C., Smith, B.A., Moerchen, V., Ulrich, B.D., 2011. Impact of enhanced sensory input on treadmill step frequency: infants born with myelomeningocele. Pediatr Phys Ther 23 (1), 42–52.

Pantall, A., Teulier, C., Ulrich, B.D., 2012. Changes in muscle activation patterns in response to enhanced sensory input during treadmill stepping in infants born with myelomeningocele. Hum. Mov. Sci. 31 (6), 1670 1687.

Peiper, A., 1963. Cerebral Function in Infancy and Childhood. Consultants Bureau, New York.

Richards, C.L., Malouin, F., Dumas, F., Marcoux, S., Lepage, C., Menier, C., 1997. Early and intensive treadmill locomotor training for young children with cerebral palsy: a feasibility study. Pediatr. Phys. Ther. 9, 7.

Shirley, M.M., 1931. The first two years: a study of twenty-five babies Locomotor Development, vol. 1. The University of Minnesota Press, Minneapolis, MN.

Spemann, H., 1938. Embryonic Development and Induction. Yale University, New Haven, CT.

Stockard, C.R., 1921. Developmental rate and structural expression: an experimental study of twins, 'double monsters' and single deformities, and the interaction among embryonic organs during their origin and development. Am. J. Anat. 28, 160.

Strauss, S., 1982. U-Shaped Behavioural Growth. Academic Press, New York.

Sutherland, D.H., Olshen, R., Cooper, L., Woo, S.L.Y., 1980. The development of mature gait. J. Bone Joint Surg. 62, 17.

Teulier, C., Smith, B.A., Kubo, M., Chang, C.L., Moerchen, V., Murazko, K., et al., 2009. Stepping responses of infants with myelomeningocele when supported on a motorized treadmill. Phys. Ther. 89 (1), 60–72.

Teulier, C., Sansom, J.K., Muraszko, K., Ulrich, B.D., 2012. Longitudinal changes in muscle activity during infants' treadmill stepping. J. Neurophysiol. 108 (3), 853–862.

Thelen, E., 1986. Treadmill-elicited stepping in seven-month-old infants. Child Dev. 57 (6), 1498–1506.

Thelen, E., Fisher, D.M., 1982. Newborn stepping: an explanation for a 'disappearing reflex.' Dev. Psychol. 18, 15.

Thelen, E., Smith, L.B., 1994. A dynamic systems approach to the development of cognition and action. MIT Press, Cambridge, MA.

Thelen, E., Ulrich, B.D., 1991. Hidden skills: a dynamic systems analysis of treadmill stepping during the first year. Monogr. Soc. Res. Child Dev. 56 (1), 1 98. (discussion 99 104).

Thelen, E., Bradshaw, G., Ward, J.A., 1981. Spontaneous kicking in month-old infants: manifestation of a human central locomotor program. Behav. Neural Biol. 32, 8.

Thelen, E., Fisher, D.M., Ridley-Johnson, R., 1984. The relationship between physical growth and a newborn reflex. Infant Behav. Dev. 7, 479–493.

Thelen, E., Ulrich, B.D., Niles, D., 1987. Bilateral coordination in human infants: stepping on a split-belt treadmill. J. Exp. Psychol. Hum. Percept. Perform. 13 (3), 405–410.

Ulrich, B.D., 2010. Opportunities for early intervention based on theory, basic neuroscience, and clinical science. Phys. Ther. 90 (12), 1868–1880.

Ulrich, D., Ulrich, B.D., Angulo-Kinzler, R.M., Yun, J., 2001. Treadmill training of infants with Down syndrome: evidence-based developmental outcomes. Pediatrics 108 (5), 84–93.

Ulrich, D.A., Lloyd, M.C., Tiernan, C.W., Looper, J.E., Angulo-Barroso, R.M., 2008. Effects of intensity of treadmill training on developmental outcomes and stepping in infants with Down syndrome: a randomized trial. Physical. Therapy. 88 (1), 114–122.

Valentin-Gudiol, M., Mattern-Baxter, K., Girabent-Farres, M., Bagur-Calafat, C., Hadders-Algra, M., Angulo Barroso, R.M., 2011. Treadmill interventions with partial body weight support in children under six years of age at risk of neuromotor delay. Cochrane Database Syst. Rev. (12), CD009242.

Vereijken, B., Thelen, E., 1997. Training infant treadmill stepping: the role of individual pattern stability. Dev. Psychobiol. 30 (2), 89–102.

Walton, K.D., Lieberman, D., Llinás, A., Begin, M., Llinás, R.R., 1992. Identification of a critical period for motor development in neonatal rats. Neuroscience 51, 4.

Wu, J., Looper, J., Ulrich, B.D., Ulrich, D.A., Angulo-Barroso, R.M., 2007. Exploring effects of different treadmill interventions on walking onset and gait patterns in infants with Down syndrome. Dev. Med. Child Neurol. 49 (11), 839–845.

Wu, J., Ulrich, D.A., Looper, J., Tiernan, C.W., Angulo-Barroso, R.M., 2008. Strategy adoption and locomotor adjustment in obstacle clearance of newly walking toddlers with Down syndrome after different treadmill interventions. Exp. Brain Res. 186 (2), 261–272.

Yang, J.F., Lam, T., Pang, M.Y., Lamont, E., Musselman, K., Seinen, E., 2004. Infant stepping: a window to the behaviour of the human pattern generator for walking. Can. J. Physiol. Pharmacol. 82 (8–9), 662–674.

Yang, J.F., Lamont, E.V., Pang, M.Y., 2005. Split-belt treadmill stepping in infants suggests autonomous pattern generators for the left and right leg in humans. J. Neurosci. 25 (29), 6869–6876.

Zelazo, P.R., 1983. The development of walking: new findings and old assumptions. J. Mot. Behav. 15 (2), 99–137.

Zelazo, P.R., Zelazo, N.A., Kolb, S., 1972. 'Walking' in the newborn. Science 176 (32), 314–315.

# Very early upper limb interventions for infants with asymmetric brain lesions

# 13

Roslyn Boyd, Micah Perez, and Andrea Guzzetta

The main focus of early intervention for infants with asymmetric brain lesions who may progress to classification of unilateral cerebral palsy (UCP) is very early and accurate detection of the brain lesion, followed by provision of an enriched environment and training to maximize upper limb function during critical periods of development. The challenge for clinicians and researchers are the limited quantitative tools available to identify the problem and measure progress as well as the paucity of evidence for efficacy of very early upper limb rehabilitation. In this book chapter we will: (1) focus on the current knowledge of critical periods of early upper limb development and the potential neural correlates; (2) summarize the evidence for efficacy of current interventions; and (3) explore new options for early stimulation of the damaged cortex to achieve better symmetry of upper limb motor development. Lessons learned from our clinical trials of intensive upper limb interventions in school-aged children with UCP, including the impact of dose, density and components of training on neuroplasticity, will be discussed in light of the implications for training the young infant with an asymmetric brain lesion in the first two years of life.

# The problem

Infants with early asymmetric brain injury are at high risk of developing congenital hemiplegia as a result of presumed prenatal, perinatal or postnatal brain injury (Cioni et al., 1999). The underlying injuries usually consist of periventricular white matter damage (e.g. periventricular leukomalacia or venous infarctions), cortical and/or deep grey matter damage (e.g. arterial ischaemic stroke) and, less frequently, brain malformations of one hemisphere (e.g. focal cortical dysplasia or unilateral schizencephaly). Congenital hemiplegia is the most common type of cerebral palsy (CP), with a prevalence of 1 in 1300 live births (Wiklund and Uvebrant, 1991). These infants have impaired upper limb motor function and can experience difficulties participating in activities of daily life (e.g. feeding, play and self-care). There are, broadly speaking, two common clinical presentations of asymmetric brain lesions: early or delayed. Early presentation consists of perinatal onset of neurological symptoms, or seizures, or reduced movement at 24 to 48 hours post-birth with verification on cranial ultrasound and/or magnetic resonance imaging (MRI) of the presence of a unilateral or asymmetric brain lesion. Specific imaging protocols may be needed for the diagnosis in the early phases, such as diffusion MRI to identify an acute stroke in the first hours or days (Huppi, 2002). In a delayed presentation, the infant may have an initially uncomplicated perinatal course and may not show signs of stroke or asymmetric brain injury until three to seven months of age when unilateral weakness and early hand preference start to manifest (Golomb et al., 2001; Lynch and Nelson, 2001).

# Definitive diagnosis of hemiplegia

The current most predictive tools for early diagnosis of CP are a combination of brain MRI at term and a general movements (GMs) assessment in the fidgety period (Spittle et al., 2009). Specifically, GMs at 1 month and 3 months post-term age are highly associated with white matter abnormalities on MRI at term age (Spittle et al., 2009). The GMs assessment is a well-validated and reliable tool, and is more sensitive at predicting CP than other motor assessments used in infancy (Noble and Boyd, 2011; Spittle et al., 2008). Neuromotor assessments utilized in the neonatal period have strong validity to detect CP in infants born preterm on criterion assessments at 12 months corrected age (such as the Bayley Developmental Scales II and III); moderate evaluative validity (on the Test of Motor Impairment, TIMP), as well as prediction of minor motor difficulties using the GMs (Hadders-Algra et al., 2004; Noble and Boyd, 2011). The classification of early writhing GMs is abnormal although asymmetries are not yet visible, while asymmetry of fidgety GMs around 12 weeks post-term can be the first definitive clinical sign of hemiplegia (Cioni et al., 2000; Guzzetta, 2010; Guzzetta et al., 2003).

Very early detection of hemiparesis frequently requires serial evaluation of subtle signs of interlimb differences or asymmetries in muscle resistance to passive movement, muscle stiffness, upper limb reaching (both spontaneous and purposeful), and grasp strength (Heathcock et al., 2008). Both bimanual and unimanual reaching with early strong hand preference at four to six months of age can be considered to be a strong sign of early hemiplegia (Golomb et al., 2001). Studies of infants who have sustained an early perinatal stroke from 4 to 7 months corrected age have suggested that until reach to grasp behaviours have emerged, an asymmetry may not be clearly evident so that a hemiparesis may not be confirmed (Duff and Charles, 2004; Duff and Gordon, 2003).

# Critical periods of typical upper limb motor development

Upper limb skills of typically developing infants generally develop in several stages: (1) discovering the hand; (2) visually regarding the hand; (3) visually exploring objects in space; (4) swiping at objects; (5) contacting objects; (6) ineffectively grasping objects; and (7) developing prehensile movements to better grasp objects (White and Held, 1966). These stages of prehension are not consecutive and often overlap (Table 13.1). Prior to the onset of reach, infants have been observed to demonstrate prehensile movements that provide multimodal input about their upper limb function within their environment and sensorimotor experiences that provide early motor programmes for upper limb control (Eyre et al., 2001; Thelen and Smith, 1994; von Hofsten and Ronnqvist, 1993). Grasping involves the shaping and co-ordinated movements of fingers and rotation of the wrist in a manner that anticipates the size, shape and physical features of the target object (Jeannerod, 1997).

All the components of prehension, including visual regard, reach, grasp, manipulation, pulling, pushing objects and release, can be impacted by an early brain lesion. In typically developing infants hand preference is strong initially and often varies (e.g. Corbetta and Thelen, 1996; Fagard, 1998). Handedness in infants can be observed when they undertake bimanual tasks (Fagard and Marks, 2000). Switching hand preference while manipulating an object happens early in motor development, prior to 6 months of age (Fagard and Lockman, 2005). There

**Table 13.1  Presumed timing of development of reaching, grasping and releasing in infants**

| General motor skill | Specific upper limb motor skill | Proposed time point (post-term months) |
|---|---|---|
| Reaching | • Visually attending to objects carefully while reaching ineffectively<br>• Demonstrating finger, eye and hand adjustments to better contact objects<br>• Reaching objects in a controlled manner | • 1–3 months<br><br>• 4 months<br><br>• 6 months |
| Grasping | • Reflexively grasping objects<br>• Beginning to use a voluntary palmar grasp with both hands<br>• Beginning to grasp with the preferred hand<br>• Using a pincer grasp<br>• Using a controlled grasp | • Birth to 4 months<br>• 3 months<br><br>• 5 months<br>• 9 months<br>• 14 months |
| Releasing | • Having a basic ability to release objects from grasp<br>• Demonstrating controlled release of objects | • 12–14 months<br>• 18 months |
| Bimanual co-ordination | • Demonstrating reaching, grasping and releasing skills that are well co-ordinated and controlled | • 18 months |

Sources: Gallahue and Ozmun (2002); Thelen et al. (1993); and von Hofsten et al. (1998).

is evidence that fine motor skills such as reaching, grasping and releasing develop at variable and often overlapping time points (see Table 13.1).

At 5 months of age, typically developing infants demonstrate preparatory forearm rotation and hand pre-shaping based on a toy's position, shape and size, which leads to successful grasping (von Hofsten et al., 1998). Infants with early asymmetric brain damage and visual deficits can start to develop maladaptive prehensile skills such as asymmetric reaching, increased forearm pronation, ineffective opening and pre-shaping of the hand to the toy. These maladaptive prehensile skills result in inefficient manipulation (such as contacting and grasping toys) and difficulty releasing objects.

# Cortical reorganization after an early brain lesion: a critical window

There is some evidence to suggest that for infants with early brain lesions, important phases of sensorimotor reorganization occur during their first year of life (Eyre et al., 2007). After a brain lesion has occurred, development of the damaged cortex is compromised and its remaining contralateral corticospinal (CS) pathways that connect the damaged cortex to the impaired upper limb stop developing (Eyre et al., 2007). Eventually, the synaptic space that these pathways initially occupied is taken over by the more active ipsilateral pathways (which connect the intact cortex to the impaired upper limb) (Eyre et al., 2007). Both sets of CS pathways compete for synaptic space, which results in the ipsilateral CS pathway outgrowing the contralateral CS pathway. As a consequence, two main types of brain reorganization can be observed after early asymmetric brain injuries. Ipsilesional reorganization (i.e., reorganization occurring within some spared cortical tissue of the damaged hemisphere) allows for the motor cortex of the damaged hemisphere to become reconnected to the spinal cord, and is usually what is seen in adults following stroke. Contralesional organization (i.e., reorganization occurring in the undamaged cortex) is based on existing ipsilateral motor projections remaining intact, instead of becoming retracted within the first months of life.

This specific alternative type of reorganization is possible if the lesion occurs early in development (Staudt et al., 2004). It allows the undamaged cortex to directly control both upper limbs and often involves the dissociation of the primary sensory and motor pathways (Guzzetta et al., 2009; Thickbroom et al., 2001), resulting in limited upper limb functional activity (Staudt et al., 2004). On these grounds, the first three to six months of life following an asymmetric brain lesion appear to be a critical window of opportunity for very early intervention. This intervention could be aimed at maintaining cortical motor control within the impaired hemisphere by activating the damaged sensorimotor (SM) cortex (Eyre et al., 2007), and thus enhancing its competitive ability to develop alongside the intact SM cortex, as well as ameliorating the effects of the lesion on upper limb motor activity (Eyre et al., 2007). A crucial role in predicting the type of functional reorganization is influenced by the degree of involvement of the CS tract. A perilesional reorganization can be unachievable in the case of a massive destruction of the CS tract of one hemisphere. Nevertheless, when some sparing of the tract is present, some other factors are likely to come into play, and early intervention can have the potential to shape cortical reorganization and potentially ameliorate the eventual outcome (Fig. 13.1).

A recent review of studies in a feline model provides support for the initiation of prehensile training in infants before six months of age (Martin et al., 2011). The authors have highlighted the close correlation between the activity of the CS tracts and the strength of the synaptic connections with spinal motor circuits. This supports the hypothesis that early brain damage might initiate a vicious cycle in which damaged CS tracts are competitively disadvantaged for maintaining spinal synapses, resulting in secondary reductions in these connections (Martin et al., 2011). More recently, the same group has tested the ensuing hypothesis that targeted activation of the spared CS tracts should lead to functional improvement, by exploring the effects of early intervention in cats with primary motor cortex (M1) inactivation (Friel et al., 2012). Three experimental groups were studied. In the first group, the limb ipsilateral to inactivation was restrained, forcing use of the contralateral impaired limb, for the month following the inactivation (early restraint alone group with no training of the impaired limb). In the second group, the early restraint was supplemented with daily training of a reaching task with the contralateral forelimb (early restraint + training). In the third group, both restraint and training were postponed to feline adolescence (late restraint + training). Outcome was measured at three levels

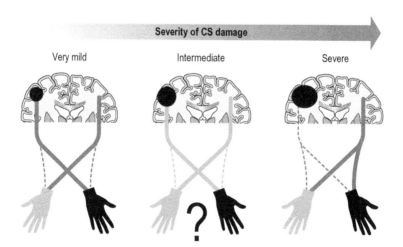

**Figure 13.1** • Diagrammatic representation of ipsilesional versus contralesional reorganization following an asymmetric brain lesion and impact on upper limb function. The extent of primary motor cortex (M1) damage can be the strongest predictor of the type of reorganization in case of very mild (left) or very severe (right) injuries. When M1 damage is of intermediate size (centre), the type of motor reorganization can be harder to predict and is likely to be significantly influenced by intervention.

by analysing: (1) CS tract spinal connections; (2) M1 motor maps; and (3) motor performance. Interestingly, restraint alone was able to restore CS tract connectivity yet failed to impact on M1 motor maps or motor function, while late training impacted on both CS tract connectivity and motor maps (however, it failed to induce significant functional recovery). The only intervention resulting in all three measures of outcome was the one based on early restraint combined with training. Altogether these findings suggest that in order to achieve significant motor improvement, a complex network of integrated functions of the CS system needs to be re-established, which targets intervention at multiple hierarchical levels.

The importance of a multilevel network in the reorganization of the CS system has been suggested by recent work in humans with congenital hemiplegia. Evidence from advanced diffusion imaging has suggested that the developing connectivity and symmetry of the thalamocortical pathways connecting M1 with the motor thalamus is at least as important as the symmetry of the CS tracts for upper limb unimanual capacity and bimanual co-ordination in children with congenital hemiplegia (Rose et al., 2011). Our group studied 16 children with congenital hemiplegia, of whom nine were classified as having periventricular leukomalakia and seven were classified as having predominantly deep grey matter lesions, according to the Krägeloh-Mann qualitative scheme (Krägeloh-Mann and Horber, 2007). Advanced diffusion imaging utilizing the HARDI model (high angular diffusion imaging) was performed to elucidate the symmetry in the CS (motor) and the thalamocortical (sensorimotor) tracts (Fig. 13.2, Table 13.2). Surprisingly, the sensorimotor thalamic tracts were more significantly correlated with paretic hand functions than were the CS tracts. These data suggest that functional outcome is not only related to the integrity of the CS tract (the final output) but rather to the integrity of a wider neural integrated network. Our data also support the concept that the motor system requires feedback from sensory systems to shape the development of the motor cortex and efferent motor pathways (Eyre et al., 2007; Rose et al., 2011). To date, upper limb rehabilitation has focused primarily on interventions to promote activation of the motor tracts with little regard to the preservation and balance of input to the sensory tracts.

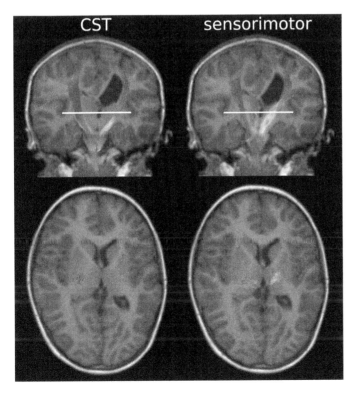

**Figure 13.2** • Advanced diffusion imaging utilizing the HARDI model. Top left is motor cortex (pre- + post-central) to brainstem through the posterior limb of the internal capsule (PLIC), top right is motor cortex (pre- + post-central) to brainstem through the thalamus. Bottom row shows cross-sectional area of the same tracts as above at the level of PLIC/thalamus. (Please refer to colour plate section)

**Table 13.2 Corticothalamic tract (CTT) pathways were more highly correlated with baseline hand function than corticospinal tract (CST) pathways**

| AI [(C − I)/(C + I)] | Jebsen | MUUL | AHA |
|---|---|---|---|
| CST | 0.39 | −0.23 | −0.35 |
| CTT | 0.80* | −0.67* | −0.62* |

CTT, corticothalamic corticospinal tract; CST, corticospinal tract; AI, asymmetry index; Jebsen, Jebsen–Taylor hand function test; MUUL, Melbourne unilateral upper limb assessment; AHA, assisting hand assessment
*Significant correlation at $p < 0.001$.

# Current evidence for early upper limb interventions for infants with hemiplegia

Upper limb rehabilitation for school-aged children with hemiplegia focuses on improving unimanual and bimanual function and enhancing participation (World Health Organisation, 2001). Our recent meta-analysis of all non-surgical interventions (Sakzewski et al., 2009) provided evidence for modest improvements in unimanual and bimanual co-ordination using various models of constraint-induced movement therapy (CIMT) (Hoare et al., 2010), bimanual intensive training (Charles and Gordon, 2006), a combination of CIMT and bimanual training (Aarts et al., 2011), and adjunctive use of intramuscular botulinum toxin A (BoNT-A) injections combined with upper limb training (Hoare et al., 2010).

While early interventions for infants at risk of developing congenital hemiplegia are considered to be very important, the reality is that rehabilitation programmes commonly do not commence until six months of age (Eyre et al., 2007). This may be due to a delayed diagnosis, for those infants not showing early acute signs of brain damage, or to a lack of consensus on the safety and efficacy of early interventions, both of which prevent early intervention from being included in service programmes. To date, no review has investigated the efficacy, feasibility, compliance and impact of upper limb interventions in improving upper limb motor development specifically for infants and young children aged less than 3 years with early brain injury. A recent systematic review of non-surgical interventions (including modified CIMT,

bimanual training, goal-directed occupational therapy (OT) and occupational performance-based OT) has examined the efficacy for improvements in unimanual capacity of the impaired limb, bimanual co-ordination and the amount and quality of hand use in randomized clinical trials for infants and toddlers up to 2.5 years of age with asymmetric brain lesions (Perez et al., unpublished data). In three systematic reviews and 17 randomized clinical trials only six per cent of the 1446 participants with unilateral CP were aged less than 2.5 years.

In this systematic review nine randomized controlled trials (RCTs) used modified constraint-induced movement therapy (mCIMT, modified for a paediatric population) in samples including infants up to 2.5 years of age (Aarts et al., 2010; Al-Oraibi and Eliasson, 2011; DeLuca et al., 2006; Eliasson et al., 2011; Facchin et al., 2011; Smania et al., 2009; Taub et al., 2011; Wallen et al., 2011; Xu et al., 2011, ) with the total dose varying from 16 hours to 210 hours. Four studies of mCIMT (Aarts et al., 2010; Al-Oraibi et al., 2011; Eliasson et al., 2011; Wallen et al., 2011) found a small treatment effect on bimanual co-ordination for CIMT compared with control groups (OT, physiotherapy [PT], neurodevelopmental therapy [NDT]). Only one study found that mCIMT effects were sustained for the treatment group at 17 weeks follow-up in an ecologically delivered programme of constraint with activity-based practice (Eliasson et al., 2011). One study of CIMT found a clinically important change post-treatment for amount of use and quality of movement using constraint of the unimpaired limb with a cast and shaping to train the impaired limb (DeLuca et al., 2006).

Four RCTs used intramuscular botulinum toxin A (BoNT-A) injections for forearm muscles with spasticity interfering with function as an adjunct to goal-directed training (Kanellopoulos et al., 2009; Lowe et al., 2007; Olesch et al., 2010; Wallen et al., 2007). As yet, safety and efficacy of intramuscular BoNT-A is not determined for use in infants with congenital hemiplegia less than 2 years of age. The potential for adverse events (although short acting and reversible), as well as muscle weakness and atrophy in school-aged children (Barber et al., 2011; Gough et al., 2005), promotes caution for the use of neuromuscular blockage of the overactive muscles in young infants with asymmetric brain lesions under two years of age.

In our systematic review, none of the study populations solely comprised participants under

2.5 years of age (Perez et al., unpublished data). Seven of the 17 RCTs reported adverse events, some of which were thought to be associated with the intervention, including tolerating CIMT (Wallen et al., 2011), physical symptoms that may have been associated with BoNT-A injections or the conscious sedation (Wallen et al., 2007). As it was not possible to separate the number of adverse events related to participants under the age of 3 years, the feasibility and compliance of these interventions for this younger age group is unclear. The existing evidence suggests small effects of CIMT with activity-based practice and shaping to improve unimanual capacity and bimanual co-ordination (Perez et al., unpublished data).

## Potential early interventions for infants with asymmetric brain lesions

There are several promising very early interventions for infants with asymmetric brain lesions that focus either on (1) bilateral stimulation of hand function; (2) modified constraint-induced movement therapy; and (3) action observation training. To date, there are no published randomized trials to confirm the efficacy and feasibility of these interventions in infants.

## Early bilateral stimulation of reaching and grasping with motor and sensory components

Traditional approaches to early upper limb training such as NDT have focused on bimanual delivery of sensory stimulation (stroking, tactile stimulation) and either equal presentation of toys to both upper limbs or increased presentation to the impaired side. Few studies have ensured equal stimulation of both limbs in a controlled manner and have tended to focus on additional stimulation with visual, tactile stimulation and object presentation on the impaired side (Al-Whaibi and Eyre, 2008). While bimanual grasp of an object emerges in the typically developing infant from three months post-term, bimanual co-ordination of objects may not mature until 18 months post-term. This provides a challenge for delivery of bimanual training as developed in older children with congenital hemiplegia, whereby the nature of the task and objects require bimanual

use with varying amounts of use of the impaired hand as an assisting hand (Charles and Gordon, 2006; Gordon et al., 2005; Sakzewski et al., 2009). In the young infant, equal presentation of toys to both upper limbs and the bilateral facilitation of reaching and grasping are considered to be an important component to develop early motor representations in the brain. The unimpaired hand is thought to act as a template for the development of reaching in the impaired hand (Utley and Sugden, 1998). The challenge is to deliver equal training for the infant with an asymmetric brain lesion where overcompensation with the unimpaired hand and increased lateralization of the motor cortex can lead to maladaptive plasticity. The challenge remains as to how to stimulate the damaged sensorimotor cortex before volitional movement develops (before three months) to ensure equal input to development of both the motor and sensory pathways.

## Infant modified constraint-induced movement therapy

Considerable experience and evidence has been determined for various models of a child-friendly modified form of CIMT for school-aged and preschool-aged children (down to 18 months corrected age) (Eliasson et al., 2011; Hoare et al., 2009). Various constraints have been utilized for the unimpaired hand, including a glove with rigid insert (Eliasson et al., 2011; Sakzewski et al., 2009), a sling (Aarts et al., 2010; Charles and Gordon, 2005, 2006), gentle manual restraint (Naylor and Bower, 2005), and rigid plaster casts (Taub et al., 2004; Willis et al., 2002). Our comprehensive meta-analysis has not demonstrated superior effects for 24 hour use of the rigid cast over 21 days (Taub et al., 2004; Willis et. al., 2002) compared with shorter doses of constraint of the unimpaired hand with a glove (six hours per day for 10 days) (Sakzewski et al., 2009). In children under 18 months with an asymmetric brain lesion, we propose the use of a more child-friendly mitt that enables some gross assistance with the gloved hand in bimanual tasks and limits manipulation of the unimpaired hand, while still enabling some training of bimanual tasks (Fig. 13.3A).

Vigorous debate has ensued regarding the type of constraint and the dose of intervention required; however, the type and intensity of accompanying training of the impaired limb appears to be more critical to success (Gordon et al., 2011). Activity-

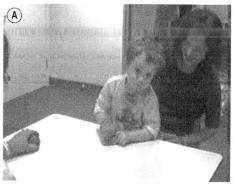

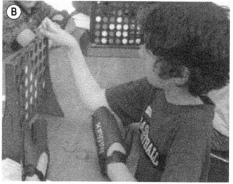

**Figure 13.3 •** Two examples of modified constraint-induced movement therapy suitable for young children with congenital hemiplegia using **(A)** a soft material mitten on the unimpaired hand to constrain the manipulative abilities of the dominant hand and to shift the role of manipulation to the more impaired hand or **(B)** a glove with rigid insert accompanied by group activity-based practice.

based practice in the context of ecologically friendly environments such as the preschool (Eliasson et al., 2011) and home (Wallen et al., 2011) or in intensive day camps (Bonnier et al., 2006) and with motivating themes (Boyd et al., 2010a; Sakzewski et al., 2009) appear to be key ingredients to successful training of unimanual capacity and compliance with the constraint (Gilmore et al., 2010). Our own study, the 'INCITE' trial, employed a novel circus theme during the activity-based day camps to ensure practice with the 'just right challenge' and minimal frustration with the constraint (glove) (Fig. 13.2B), achieving high study retention (Boyd et al., 2010b; Gilmore et al., 2010; Sakzewski et al., 2009).

A major consideration for current approaches of CIMT and bimanual therapy (BIM) for children with UCP is that dosage of intervention vary between 60 to 120 hours of training (Boyd et al., 2010b; Taub

et al., 2004). Recently we have concluded two single blind (investigator masked) matched pairs (children were matched for age, gender, side of hemiplegia and unimanual capacity) then randomized in a comparison trial directly comparing mCIMT (with a glove and intensive activity-based practice) with an equal dose of bimanual training (BIM) where the activities all demanded equivalent use of both hands (Boyd et al., 2010a). These trials directly comparing equal dosages of a block of mCIMT or BIM in the same environment provide evidence for the differential effects on unimanual capacity and bimanual performance (Sakzewski et al., 2011a); there are similar effects on translation to enhanced participation in goal areas and improvements in quality of life (Sakzewski et al., 2011b, 2012), features of best responders (Sakzewski et al., 2011c), and the long-term retention of these effects at 12 months after delivery (Sakzewski et al., 2011d).

In a related study, our team has also addressed the question as to whether sufficient effect might be achieved at lower dosages of intensive upper limb training (total dose of 30 hours compared to 60 hours) (Boyd et al., 2010b). In comparing the efficacy of two intensities of mCIMT and BIM on unimanual capacity and individualized goals, we hypothesized that half the dose of training would still have 75% effect and would therefore be more feasible. These studies of school-aged children with CP provide important information that 'half the dose may not be enough, and double the dose may be too much'. The question of the size of the therapy pill in young infants with asymmetric brain lesions is a critical one.

In infants under 2 years of age, modifications have been proposed to reduce the period of constraint down to a few hours per day (Eliasson et al., 2005), to vary the type of constraint including gentle manual guidance (Naylor and Bower, 2005) or a padded glove (Eliasson et al., 2005); to ensure the type of accompanying training is activity based (Eliasson et al., 2005); or shaping (Taub et al., 2004). Recent studies in a feline model, however, suggest caution in constraining the unimpaired limb and consideration of the impact in development of the CS projections (Martin et al., 2011). Early use of CIMT may lead to increased lateralization of the CS projections with greater chance of contralesional reorganization (see Fig. 13.1). The limitations of CIMT in the young infant include reduced sensory feedback from the unimpaired hand, reduced active use of the unimpaired hand with limitation for its use as a template for developing motor control in the impaired hand, as well as limitations in the development of bimanual grasp. An alternative may be the use of either gentle manual constraint of the unimpaired hand during motor training (toy presentation combined with sensory stimulation) or the use of short periods of a material mitten on the unimpaired hand to reduce the manipulative abilities of the unimpaired hand (see Fig. 13.3), thereby enabling a more infant-friendly form of modified CIMT. To date, none of these methods have been tested in adequately powered clinical trials with infants. A further consideration is the provision of evidence to determine the impact of early modified constraint on the development of both CS projections and spinothalamic projections.

## Early action observation training

Action observation therapy (AOT) is a recently developed intervention that has been shown to improve upper limb motor function in adults with chronic stroke (Ertelt et al., 2007), and is being investigated in school-aged children with UCP (Sgandurra et al., 2011). Intervention is based on action observation, whereby new motor skills can be learned by observing motor actions. AOT is a rehabilitative methodology that combines the observation of daily actions with physical training of the observed actions, to reinforce the activation of motor areas (Ertelt et al., 2007). An example of this is watching video sequences of goal-directed upper limb actions in daily life activities, followed by repetitive practice of the observed actions with the impaired upper limb (see Sgandurra et al., 2011 for an example in school-aged children with congenital hemiplegia). This process appears to be facilitated by the mirror neuron system (MNS). It has been proposed that the MNS codes for the execution of motor actions, which implies that: (1) there are pre-existing motor representations in the motor cortex of hand movements; and (2) the ability to match the physical features of an object with appropriate hand movements in order to grasp the object effectively is innate (Murata et al., 1997; Rizzolatti and Luppino, 2001; Rizzolatti et al., 1988).

Recent evidence suggests that this mechanism is present from birth, and yet little is known about its role in motor development (Lepage and Theoret, 2007). Use of AOT in school-aged children with congenital hemiplegia (Sgandurra et al., 2011) and

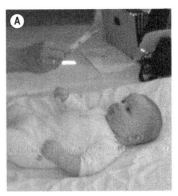

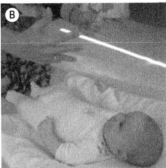

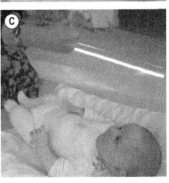

Figure 13.4 • Examples of (A) action observation training (AOT) and (B, C) toy observation training (TOT) in the upper limb baby early action observation training (UP-BEAT) study.

adults following stroke (Ertelt et al., 2007) provides promising results for the recovery of unimanual capacity accompanied by brain reorganization. Our group has commenced an infant modified version called upper limb baby early action observation training (UP-BEAT, Australian Research Council grant DP110104292). The feasibility, efficacy and neural correlates of AOT are being compared in a sham control randomized clinical trial of infants with asymmetric brain lesions and typically developing infants (Fig. 13.4).

In animal and human adult studies, AOT has been shown to be an effective method to increase cortical excitability of the sensorimotor cortex. Based on the hypothesis that the same activation can be induced in young infants, we predict that a training based on movement observation (very early observation of grasping, Fig. 13.4A), coupled with actual hand motor activity (contacting the toy, and later grasping and reaching), will enhance the excitability of the sensorimotor cortex, will accelerate the maturation of the CS tracts as well as the shaping of spinal motor circuits. This will potentially result in the modification of various quantitative and qualitative measures of grasping and reaching behaviours (e.g., the age at onset of reaching, frequency, symmetry, movement properties, grip power), both in healthy infants and in those with congenital brain damage.

A sham control study design is being used for the RCT, in consideration that it would be unethical to give no intervention to an at-risk population. The sham control will consist of a standard intervention that does not include the active component of the intervention for the treatment group (toy presentation with no observation of grasping, Fig. 13.4B,C). Infants with an asymmetric brain lesion (e.g., arterial stroke, venous infarction, intraventricular haemorrhage or periventricular leukomalacia) that have been identified through a neonatal ultrasound or neonatal MRI are entered into the study. Parents of the active training or AOT group will repeatedly show the infant a grasping action on a set of toys, presented in random order (Fig. 13.4A). Parents of the standard care or toy observation training (TOT) group will show the infant the same set of toys, also presented in random order, without demonstrating the grasping action (Fig. 13.4B,C). This study will determine if AOT can influence the early development of reaching and grasping of typically developing infants and improve the upper limb motor activity of infants with asymmetric brain lesions. Very early intervention should also be combined with current upper limb training methods (e.g., unimanual and bimanual activity-based training) as soon as infants can reach voluntarily, to reinforce the growth and connectivity of cortical pathways and consolidate learning of upper limb motor skills. Based on the hypothesis that the same activation can be elicited in infants, it is predicted that AOT will enhance the excitability of the SM cortex, accelerate the maturation of the CS tract and the shaping of

spinal motor circuits. While AOT training in infants is still undergoing experimental confirmation it is hoped that it will offer an opportunity to stimulate the damaged motor cortex during that first critical period (birth to 4 months) to minimize asymmetries in development of the CS tracts.

## Adjunctive therapies

For infants with asymmetric brain lesions, there is currently no evidence for safety or efficacy for the use of adjunctive interventions such as intramuscular injections of BoNT-A, splints for assistance, casting to stretch muscles with contracture and/or the use of neoprene thumb splints or taping to assist or provide feedback for overactive movements (i.e., thumb in palm) as utilized in school-aged children with hemiplegia. There is developing evidence that pharmacological interventions may have very negative effects on the developing neuromuscular system, so that use of BoNT-A in the very young infant should be viewed with extreme caution (Barber et al., 2011; Gough et al., 2005). Adjunctive interventions which immobilize the hand and arm, reduce sensory feedback, limit activity-based practice, bimanual co-ordination and restrict the development of motor maps should also be viewed with caution.

## Translation into the real world

To date, few clinical trials of mCIMT and BIM in school-aged children with UCP have measured outcomes until 12 months follow-up with positive benefits for the continued improvement in upper limb activity (Sakzewski et al., 2011d). Our large single blind randomized trial directly comparing mCIMT with activity-based practice to an equal dose of intensive bimanual training (where all tasks required bimanual co-ordination) led to differential improvements in activity limitations (Sakzewski et al., 2011d). Children in each arm of the RCT 'gained what they trained' in that while both programmes were effective, CIMT had a differential effect on unimanual capacity and BIM improved bimanual co-ordination (Sakzewski et al., 2011d). These improvements translated to reductions in participation restrictions only in goal areas selected by the child that were context-specific (Sakzewski et al., 2011b). There are some promising effects of improvements in domains of quality of life, with both models of intensive upper limb training providing evidence that an intensive activity-based training can have more global benefits (Sakzewski et al., 2012). Our INCITE trial also provided the first evidence for the differential effect of CIMT compared to BIM to improve neuroplasticity, confirmed on both transcranial magnetic stimulation (TMS) and functional MRI (fMRI) (Boyd et al., 2012). These series of studies confirm that mCIMT is best at 'turning on the motor cortex and improving unimanual capacity'; however, it should be followed by BIM to consolidate these effects into improvements in bimanual co-ordination which encompass at least 75% of daily hand use.

The next challenge is to provide upper limb training programmes that are able to be translated into the home for continued incremental practice at high intensities. Optimal brain plasticity occurs when interventions incorporate the following key elements: (1) intensive task-oriented repetition; (2) incremental challenges with increasing difficulty; and (3) the presence of motivators or rewards (Nudo, 1999; Nudo et al., 1996). Web-based multimodal training programmes such as 'Mitii®: Move it to improve it' provide promising data for improvements in manual ability combined with physical and cognitive challenge for school-aged children with UCP (Bilde et al., 2011), see Chapter 15. Programmes such as Mitii, which provide a multimodal approach with multi-system incremental challenges at high intensity, are more likely to drive neuroplasticity and have lasting benefits. Web-based training can provide expertise from centrally based virtual trainers to enable progressive incremental challenge of daily training in the home. New environmental training mats and toys with sensors for measurement and provision of visual, auditory and tactile stimulation are currently being developed, which if linked via cable to an internet-linked camera will enable training and monitoring in the home with external expert advice. These web-delivered or monitored training environments offer new opportunities for prehensile training of young infants at home at high intensities, with incremental challenge and frequent expert feedback. The efficacy of these approaches are currently being tested in randomized trials.

# Future directions

Very early training of prehensile skills for young infants with signs of hemiplegia is likely to be beneficial as it can take advantage of neural plasticity associated with skill development before learned non-use, musculoskeletal impairments or ineffective behaviours can develop. An important consideration in testing the efficacy of new interventions to improve manipulative skills is the role of neural recovery alone, or whether recovery is augmented by the specific training provided. Randomized clinical trials with a sham control are therefore essential. There are some lessons learned from our studies of school-aged children with UCP regarding the type (model), intensity, use of incremental challenges, motivation and the task relatedness of training which need to be explored to determine the components of success in infants with asymmetric brain lesions.

The small numbers of infants detected very early highlights the need for comprehensive multi-site trials to examine the efficacy of new prehensile training models for young infants with asymmetric brain lesions. An important consideration is the measurement of neural correlates to determine the positive or negative plasticity accompanying changes in prehensile development.

# References

Aarts, P.B., Jongerius, P.H., Geerdink, Y.A., van Limbeek, J., Geurts, A.C., 2010. Effectiveness of modified constraint-induced movement therapy in children with unilateral spastic cerebral palsy: a randomized controlled trial. Neurorehabil. Neural. Repair 24, 509–518.

Aarts, P.B., Jongerius, P.H., Geerdink, Y.A., van Limbeek, J., Geurts, A.C., 2011. Modified constraint-induced movement therapy combined with bimanual training (mCIMT-BiT) in children with unilateral spastic CP: how are improvements in arm-hand use established? Res. Dev. Disabil. 32, 271–279.

Al-Oraibi, S., Eliasson, A.C., 2011. Implementation of constraint-induced movement therapy for young children with unilateral cerebral palsy in Jordan: a home-based model. Disabil. Rehabil. 33, 2006–2012.

Al-Whaibi, R., Eyre, J., 2008. Environmental cues influence hand movement from 1 month of age: implications for therapy following perinatal stroke. Dev. Med. Child Neurol. 50 (s114), 14.

Barber, L., Hastings-Ison, T., Baker, R., Barrett, R., Lichtwark, G., 2011. Medial gastrocnemius muscle volume and fascicle length in children aged 2 to 5 years with cerebral palsy. Dev. Med. Child Neurol. 53, 543–548.

Bilde, P., Kliim-Due, M., Rasmussen, B., Petersen, L.Z., Petersen, T.H., Nielsen, J.B., 2011. Individualized, home-based interactive training of cerebral palsy children delivered through the internet. BMC Neurol. 11, 1–9.

Bonnier, B., Eliasson, A.C., Krumlinde-Sundholm, L., 2006. Effects of constraint induced movement therapy in adolescents with hemiplegic cerebral palsy: a day camp model. Scand. J. Occup. Ther. 13, 13–22.

Boyd, R., Sakzewski, L., Ziviani, J., Abbott, D.F., Badawy, R., Gilmore, R., et al., 2010a. INCITE: a randomised trial comparing constraint induced movement therapy and bimanual training in children with congenital hemiplegia. BMC Neurol. 10, 1–15.

Boyd, R.N., Provan, K., Ziviani, J., Sakzewski, L., 2010b. Comparison of dosage of constraint induced movement therapy versus bimanual training for children with congenital hemiplegia—is half the dose enough? Dev. Med. Child Neurol. 52 (s5), 25.

Boyd, R.N., Sakzewski, L., Guzzetta, A., Rose, S., 2012. Relationship between structural brain connectivity and treatment response following intensive upper limb training in congenital hemiplegia. Dev. Med. Child Neurol. 53 (s5), 49.

Charles, J., Gordon, A.M., 2005. A critical review of constraint induced movement therapy and forced use in children with hemiplegia. Neural Plast. 12, 245–261.

Charles, J., Gordon, A.M., 2006. Development of hand-arm bimanual intensive training (HABIT) for improving bimanual coordination in children with hemiplegic cerebral palsy. Dev. Med. Child Neurol. 48, 931–936.

Cioni, G., Sales, B., Paolicelli, P.B., Petacchi, E., Scusa, M.F., Canapicchi, R., 1999. MRI and clinical characteristics of children with hemiplegic cerebral palsy. Neuropediatrics 30, 249–255.

Cioni, G., Bos, A.F., Einspieler, C., Ferrari, F., Martijn, A., Paolicelli, P.B., et al., 2000. Early neurological signs in preterm infants with unilateral intraparenchymal echodensity. Neuropediatrics 31, 240–251.

Corbetta, D., Thelen, E., 1996. The developmental origins of bimanual coordination: a dynamic perspective. J. Exp. Psychol. 22, 502–522.

DeLuca, S.C., Echols, K., Law, C.R., Ramey, S.L., 2006. Intensive pediatric constraint-induced therapy for children with cerebral palsy: randomized, controlled, crossover trial. J. Child Neurol. 21, 931–938.

Duff, S.V., Charles, J., 2004. Enhancing prehension in infants and children: fostering neuromotor strategies. Phys. Occup. Ther. Pediatr. 24, 129–172.

Duff, S.V., Gordon, A.M., 2003. Learning of grasp control in children with hemiplegic cerebral palsy. Dev. Med. Child Neurol. 45, 746–757.

Eliasson, A.-C., Krumlinde-Sundholm, L., Shaw, K., Wang, C., 2005. Effects of constraint-induced movement therapy in young children with hemiplegic cerebral palsy: an adapted model. Dev. Med. Child Neurol. 45, 357–359.

Eliasson, A.-C., Shaw, K., Berg, E., Krumlinde-Sundholm, L., 2011. An ecological approach of constraint induced movement therapy for 2–3-year-old children: a randomized control trial. Res. Dev. Disabil. 32, 2820–2828.

Ertelt, D., Small, S., Solodkin, A., Dettmers, C., McNamara, A., Binkofski, F., et al., 2007. Action observation has a positive impact on rehabilitation of motor deficits after stroke. Neuroimage 36, T164–T173.

Eyre, J., Taylor, J., Villagra, F., Smith, M., Miller, S., 2001. Evidence of activity-dependent withdrawal of corticospinal projections during human development. Neurology 57, 1543–1554.

Eyre, J., Smith, M., Dabydeen, L., Clowry, G.J., Petacchi, E., Battini, R., et al., 2007. Is hemiplegic cerebral palsy equivalent to amblyopia of the corticospinal system? Ann. Neurol. 62, 493–503.

Facchin, P., Rosa-Rizzotto, M., Visona Dalla Pozza, L., Turconi, A.C., Pagliano, E., Signorini, S., et al., 2011. Multisite trial comparing the efficacy of constraint-induced movement therapy with that of bimanual intensive training in children with hemiplegic cerebral palsy. Am. J. Phys. Med. Rehabil. 90, 539–553.

Fagard, J., 1998. Changes in grasping skills and the emergence of bimanual coordination during the first year of life. In: Connolly, K.J. (Ed.), The Psychobiology of the Hand. Mac Keith Press, London.

Fagard, J., Lockman, J.J., 2005. The effect of task constraints on infants' (bi)manual strategy for grasping and exploring objects. Infant. Behav. Dev. 28, 305–315.

Fagard, J., Marks, A., 2000. Unimanual and bimanual tasks and the assessment of handedness in toddlers. Dev. Sci. 3, 137–147.

Friel, K.M., Chakrbarty, S., Kuo, H.-C., Martin, J.H., 2012. Using motor behaviour during an early critical period to restore skilled movement after damage to the corticospinal motor system during development. J. Neurosci. 32, 9265–9276.

Gallahue, D.L., Ozmun, J.C., 2002. Understanding Motor Development: Infants, Children, Adolescents, Adults, fifth ed. McGraw-Hill, New York.

Gilmore, R., Ziviani, J., Sakzewski, L., Shields, N., Boyd, R., 2010. A balancing act: experience of modified constraint induced therapy for children with hemiplegia. Dev. Neurorehabil. 13, 88–94.

Golomb, M.R., MacGregor, D.L., Domi, T., et al., 2001. Presumed pre- or perinatal arterial ischemic stroke: risk factors and outcomes. Ann. Neurol. 50, 163–168.

Gordon, A.M., Charles, J., Wolf, S.L., 2005. Methods of constraint induced movement therapy for children with hemiplegic cerebral palsy: development of a child-friendly intervention for improving upper extremity function. Arch. Phys. Med. Rehabil. 86, 837–844.

Gordon, A.M., Hung, Y.C., Brandao, M., Ferre, C.L., Kuo, H.-C., Friel, K., et al., 2011. Bimanual training and constraint-induced movement therapy in children with hemiplegic cerebral palsy: a randomized trial. Neurorehabil. Neural Repair 25, 692–702.

Gough, M., Fairhurst, C., Shortland, A.P., 2005. Botulinum toxin and cerebral palsy: time for reflection? Dev. Med. Child Neurol. 47, 709–712.

Guzzetta, A., 2010. Mirror neurons and congenital cerebral lesions. In: Riva, D., Njiokiktjien, C. (Eds.), Localization of Brain Lesions and Developmental Functions. John Libbey Eurotext

Guzzetta, A., Mercuri, E., Rapisardi, G., et al., 2003. General movements detect early signs of hemiplegia in term infants with neonatal cerebral infarction. Neuropediatrics 34, 61–66.

Guzzetta, A., Pizzardi, A., D'Acunto, M.G., Belmonti, V., Romeo, D., Roversi, M.F., et al., 2009. Early development of hand motor function in infants with neonatal cerebral infarction. Dev. Med. Child Neurol. 51, 78.

Hadders-Algra, M., Mavinkurve-Groothuis, A.M.C., Groen, S.E., Stremmelaar, E.F., Martijn, A., Butcher, P.R., 2004. Quality of general movements and the development of minor neurological dysfunction at toddler and school age. Clin. Rehabil. 18, 287–299.

Heathcock, J.C., Lobo, M., Galloway, J.C., 2008. Movement training advances the emergence of reaching in infants born at less than 33 weeks of gestational age: a randomized clinical trial. Phys. Ther. 88, 310–322.

Hoare, B.J., Wasiak, J., Imms, C., Carey, L., 2009. Constraint-induced movement therapy in the treatment of the upper limb in children with hemiplegic cerebral palsy (review). Cochrane Database Syst. Rev.

Hoare, B.J., Wallen, M.A., Imms, C., Villanueva, E.B.R.H., Carey, L., 2010. Botulinum toxin A as an adjunct to treatment in the management of the upper limb in children with spastic cerebral palsy (UPDATE). Cochrane Database Syst. Rev. [Online].

Huppi, P., 2002. Advances in postnatal neuroimaging: relevance to pathogenesis and treatment of brain injury. Clin. Perinatol. 29, 827–856.

Jeannerod, M., 1997. Neural substrates for object-oriented actions. The Cognitive Neuroscience of Action. Blackwell Publishers Inc. Malden, MA.

Kanellopoulos, A.D., Mavrogenis, A.F., Mitsiokapa, E.A., Panagopoulos, D., Skouteli, H., Vrettos, S.G., et al., 2009. Long lasting benefits following

the combination of static night upper extremity splinting with botulinum toxin A injections in cerebral palsy children. Eur. J. Phys. Rehabil. Med. 45, 501–506.

Krägeloh-Mann, I., Horber, V., 2007. The role of magnetic resonance imaging in elucidating the pathogenesis of cerebral palsy: a systematic review. Dev. Med. Child Neurol. 49 (2), 144–151.

Lepage, J.F., Theoret, H., 2007. The mirror neuron system: grasping others' actions from birth? Dev. Sci. 10, 513–523.

Lowe, K., Novak, I., Cusick, A., 2007. Repeat injection of botulinum toxin A is safe and effective for upper limb movement and function in children with cerebral palsy. Dev. Med. Child Neurol. 49, 823–829.

Lynch, J.K., Nelson, K.B., 2001. Epidemiology of perinatal stroke. Curr. Opin. Pediatr. 13, 499–505.

Martin, J.H., Chakrabarty, S., Friel, K.M., 2011. Harnessing activity-dependent plasticity to repair the damaged corticospinal tract in an animal model of cerebral palsy. Dev. Med. Child Neurol. 53 (Suppl.), 9–11.

Murata, A., Fadiga, F., Fogassi, L., Gallese, V., Raos, V., Rizzolatti, G., 1997. Object representation in the ventral premotor cortex (area F5) of the monkey. J. Neurophysiol. 78, 2226–2230.

Naylor, C.E., Bower, E., 2005. Modified constraint induced movement therapy for young children with hemiplegic cerebral palsy. Dev. Med. Child Neurol. 53, 365–369.

Noble, Y., Boyd, R., 2011. Neonatal assessments for the preterm infant up to 4 months corrected age: a systematic review. Dev. Med. Child Neurol. 54, 129–139.

Nudo, R., 1999. Recovery after damage to motor cortical areas. Curr. Opin. Neurobiol. 9, 740–747.

Nudo, R.J., Milliken, G.W., Jenkins, W.M., Merzenich, M.M., 1996. Use-dependent alterations of movement representations in primary motor cortex of adult squirrel monkeys. J. Neurosci. 16, 785–807.

Olesch, C.A., Greaves, S., Imms, C., Reid, S.M., Graham, H.K., 2010. Repeat botulinum toxin-A injections in the upper limb of children with hemiplegia: a randomized controlled

trial. Dev. Med. Child Neurol. 52, 79–86.

Rizzolatti, G., Luppino, G., 2001. The cortical motor system. Neuron 31, 889–901.

Rizzolatti, G., Camarda, R., Fogassi, M., Gentilucci, M., Luppino, G., Matelli, M., 1988. Functional organisation of inferior area 6 in the macaque monkey: II. Area F5 and the control of distal movements. Exp. Brain Res. 71, 491–507.

Rose, S., Guzzetta, A., Pannek, K., Boyd, R.N., 2011. MRI structural connectivity, disruption of primary sensorimotor pathways, and hand function in cerebral palsy. Brain Connectivity 1, 309–316.

Sakzewski, L., Ziviani, J., Boyd, R., 2009. Systematic review and meta-analysis of therapeutic management of upper-limb dysfunction in children with congenital hemiplegia. Pediatrics 123, e1111–e1122.

Sakzewski, L., Ziviani, J., Boyd, R.N., MacDonnell, R., Abbott, D., Jackson, G., 2011a. Randomized trial of constraint-induced movement therapy and bimanual training on activity outcomes for children with congenital hemiplegia. Dev. Med. Child Neurol. 53, 313–320.

Sakzewski, L., Ziviani, J., Abbott, D.F., MacDonnell, R.A., Jackson, G.A., Boyd, R.N., 2011b. Participation outcomes in a randomized trial of 2 models of upper-limb rehabilitation for children with congenital hemiplegia. Arch. Phys. Med. Rehabil. 92, 531–539.

Sakzewski, L., Ziviani, J., Abbott, D.F., MacDonnell, R.A., Jackson, G.A., Boyd, R.N., 2011c. Best responders after intensive upper limb training for children with unilateral cerebral palsy. Arch. Phys. Med. Rehabil. 92, 578–584.

Sakzewski, L., Ziviani, J., Abbott, D.F., MacDonnell, R.A.L., Jackson, G.D., Boyd, R.N., 2011d. Equivalent retention of gains at 1 year after training with constraint-induced or bimanual therapy in children with unilateral cerebral palsy. Neurorehabil. Neural Repair 25, 664–671.

Sakzewski, L., Carlon, S., Shields, N., Ziviani, J., Ware, R., Boyd, R.N., 2012. Impact of intensive upper limb rehabilitation on quality of life: in a randomised trial for children with unilateral cerebral palsy. Dev. Med. Child Neurol. 54, 415–423.

Sgandurra, G., Ferrari, A., Cossu, G., Guzzetta, A., Biagi, L., Tosetti, M., et al., 2011. Upper limb children action-observation training (UP-CAT): a randomised controlled trial in hemiplegic cerebral palsy. Bio. Med. Central Neurol. 11, 1–19.

Smania, N., Aglioti, S.M., Cosentino, A., Camin, M., Gandolfi, M., Tinazzi, M., et al., 2009. A modified constraint-induced movement therapy (CIT) program improves paretic arm use and function in children with cerebral palsy. Eur. J. Phys. Rehabil. Med. 45, 493–500.

Spittle, A.J., Doyle, L.W., Boyd, R.N., 2008. A systematic review of the clinimetric properties of neuromotor assessments for preterm infants during the first year of life. Dev. Med. Child Neurol. 50, 254–266.

Spittle, A.J., Boyd, R.N., Inder, T.E., Doyle, L.W., 2009. Predicting motor development in very preterm infants at 12 months' corrected age: the role of qualitative magnetic resonance imaging and general movements assessments. Pediatrics 123, 512–517.

Staudt, M., Gerloff, C., Grodd, W., Holthausen, H., Niemann, G., Krägeloh-Mann, I., 2004. Reorganization in congenital hemiparesis acquired at different gestational ages. Ann. Neurol. 56, 854–863.

Taub, E., Ramey, S.L., DeLuca, S., Echols, K., 2004. Efficacy of constraint-induced movement therapy for children with cerebral palsy with asymmetric motor

impairment. Pediatrics 113, 305–312.

Taub, E., Griffin, A., Uswatte, G., Gammons, K., Nick, J., Law, C.R., 2011. Treatment of congenital hemiparesis with pediatric constraint-induced movement therapy. J. Child Neurol. 26, 1163–1173.

Thelen, E., Smith, L.B. (Eds.), 1994. A Dynamic Systems Approach to the Development of Cognition and Action. MIT Press, Cambridge, MA.

Thelen, E., Corbetta, D., Kamm, K., Spencer, J., Schneider, K., Zernicke, R.F., 1993. The transition to reaching: mapping intention and intrinsic dynamics. Child Devel. 64, 1058–1098.

Thickbroom, G.W., Byrnes, M.L., Archer, S.A., Nagarajan, L., Mastaglia, F.L., 2001. Differences in sensory and motor cortical organisation following brain injury early in life. Ann. Neurol. 49, 320–327.

Utley, A., Sugden, D., 1998. Interlimb coupling in children with hemiplegic cerebral palsy during reaching and grasping speed. Dev. Med. Child Neurol. 40, 396–404.

von Hofsten, C., Ronnqvist, L., 1993. The structuring of neonatal arm movements. Child Dev. 64, 1046–1057.

von Hofsten, C., Vishton, P., Spelke, E.S., Feng, Q., Rosander, K., 1998. Predictive action in infancy: tracking and reaching for moving objects. Cognition 67, 255–285.

Wallen, M., O'Flaherty, S.J., Waugh, M.A., 2007. Functional outcomes of intramuscular botulinum toxin

type A and occupational therapy in the upper limbs of children with cerebral palsy: a randomized controlled trial. Arch. Phys. Med. Rehabil. 88, 1–10.

Wallen, M., Ziviani, J., Naylor, O., Evans, R., Novak, I., Herbert, R.D., 2011. Modified constraint-induced therapy for children with hemiplegic cerebral palsy: a randomized trial. Dev. Med. Child Neurol. 11, 1–9.

White, B.L., Held, R., 1966. Plasticity of sensorimotor development in the human infant. In: Rosenblith, J.F., Allinsmith, W. (Eds.), The Causes of Behavior: Readings in Child Development and Educational Psychology. Allyn and Bacon, Boston, MA.

Wiklund, L.M., Uvebrant, P., 1991. Hemiplegic cerebral palsy. Correlation between CT morphology and clinical findings. Dev. Med. Child Neurol. 33, 512–523.

Willis, J.K., Morello, A., Davie, A., Rice, J.C., Bennett, J.T., 2002. Forced use treatment of childhood hemiparesis. Pediatrics 110, 94–96.

World Health Organisation. 2001. International Classification of Functioning, Disability and Health. WHO, Geneva. Retrieved from: <http://www.who.int/classifications/icf/en/>.

Xu, K., Wang, L., Mai, J., He, L., 2011. Efficacy of constraint-induced movement therapy and electrical stimulation on hand function of children with hemiplegic cerebral palsy: a controlled clinical trial. Disabil. Rehabil. 34, 337–346.

# Constraint-induced therapy and bimanual training in children with unilateral cerebral palsy

Andrew M. Gordon

## CHAPTER CONTENTS

Unilateral cerebral palsy (CP), characterized by motor impairments mainly lateralized to one side, is among the most common subtypes of cerebral palsy, accounting for 30–40% of new cases (Himmelman et al., 2005). Through much of the last century the motor impairments, especially in the upper extremity (UE), were thought to be static with little potential for rehabilitation. Thus, rehabilitation efforts largely focused on minimizing impairments (e.g., reducing spasticity, preventing contractures). In fact, as recent as two decades ago, studies suggested that individuals with CP could reduce unwanted motor activity or spasticity with visual tracking or biofeedback, but that they had little ability to learn appropriate motor commands for skilled behaviours (Neilson et al., 1990; O'Dwyer and Neilson, 1988). Our own initial work studying prehensile force control reinforced this view, suggesting that children with CP retain infantile co-ordination strategies (Eliasson et al., 1991). However, subsequent research provided two separate lines of evidence that these impairments are actually *not static*.

First, developmental studies of children with CP have shown that motor function does develop. For example, as children with CP get older, global motor function has been shown to improve (Rosenbaum et al., 2002). Development of hand function also occurs. For example, the longitudinal development of bimanual UE use in children with unilateral CP was recently studied (Holmefur et al., 2010). Children were followed for more than four years with the assisting hand assessment (AHA), a Rasch-based measure that describes how effectively the affected UE is used as a non-dominant assist during bimanual activities (Krumlinde-Sundholm and Eliasson, 2003; Krumlinde-Sundholm et al., 2007). Bimanual proficiency was found to improve during the course of development, but the rate of development and the time point of subsequent plateau depended on the initial level at 18 months of age. Specifically, children with unilateral CP with better bimanual function in early childhood developed bimanual skills and reached their plateau more quickly than children with worse initial bimanual function. It is interesting to note that the development of bimanual UE use differs from that of the lower extremity in CP (Rosenbaum et al., 2002), where children with milder impairments reach their limit later. In a separate 13-year follow-up study in children with CP starting at the age of 6–8 years, improvements in hand function were also seen with age (Eliasson et al., 2006). Specifically, the time to complete items on the Jebsen–Taylor Test of Hand Function (JTTHF) (Jebsen et al., 1969) improved in all children, and grip force co-ordination during manipulation improved over the 13-year period. Thus, motor functions of both upper and lower limbs do develop, although these two general types of skills seem to develop and plateau differently.

A second line of evidence that motor function is not static in CP comes from studies on the effects of extended practice that have demonstrated that motor performance does improve with practice (Jarus and Gutman, 2001). In one study, children with CP were asked to repeatedly lift an object of a given weight 25 times (Gordon and Duff, 1999). Even though the learning of object properties used for force scaling was considerably slower than in typically developing children, impairments in manipulative capabilities and force regulation during object handling were partially ameliorated with this extended practice. This can be seen in Figure 14.1, which shows the load-force rate as a function of practice during consecutive lifts of objects weighing 200 g and 400 g. Unlike the typically developing children who show higher rates of force increase for the heavier object on the fifth trial, the rates of force increase are similar for the two weights at the same time point. However, after extended practice (20 to 25 lifts), higher rates of force increase are seen for the heavier object. This suggests that the initial impaired performance, at least in part, may be due to lack of use of the more affected UE and that there is residual motor capacity. In fact, this suggests that many impairments in motor control previously documented may be due to the fact that insufficient practice was provided (i.e., investigators were looking at the early stages of motor learning rather than motor control processes). Similarly, in-hand manipulation (Eliasson et al., 2003) and postural control (Shumway-Cook et al., 2003) have been found to improve with practice. These findings suggest

that intensive practice may provide a window of opportunity for improvement. It is increasingly being recognized that reduction of spasticity alone (i.e., by the use of botulinum toxin) does not improve function (Rameckers et al., 2009), and that motor learning-based treatments and exercise provided with sufficient intensity have the potential to improve motor function in CP (Ahl et al., 2005; Gorter et al., 2009; Ketelaar et al., 2001; Verschuren et al., 2009). As in adults (Wu et al., 2000), children with CP may benefit more from practice with concrete tasks (van der Weel et al., 1991). For children with CP, experiences can be made concrete by using objects that are irresistible to pick up, i.e., the concrete component is provided by the environmental organization tied to instructions. Motor learning in this case may be enhanced by ensuring the task and object provide feedback on the effects of performance, as well as feedback from the therapist and higher-level cognitive strategies to achieve better performance levels (Gordon and Magill, 2012; Thorpe and Valvano, 2002).

It is important to note that some methods of optimizing learning may not be applicable for those children with potential higher-level cognitive and proprioceptive impairments. Slower feedback processing even in typically developing children can result in information overload, which could interfere with learning. Thus, one would imagine they would benefit from intermittent feedback. However, such reduced feedback has been found to be less beneficial than constant feedback after every trial in children (Sullivan et al., 2008). Children, especially those with impaired sensory processing, may require increased feedback to update internal representations. Gradual reduction of feedback may be detrimental to learning in children (Sullivan et al., 2008). Feedback may therefore need to be withdrawn more gradually.

Despite potential differences in motor learning strategies and capabilities, developmental studies and studies of motor learning in children with CP contradict traditional clinical assumptions that motor impairments in CP are static, and instead indicate that UE performance in children with CP may improve with practice and development. More importantly, these findings imply that hand function in particular may well be amenable to treatment, in particular with intensive practice. So what are the best models for delivery of intensive practice schedules?

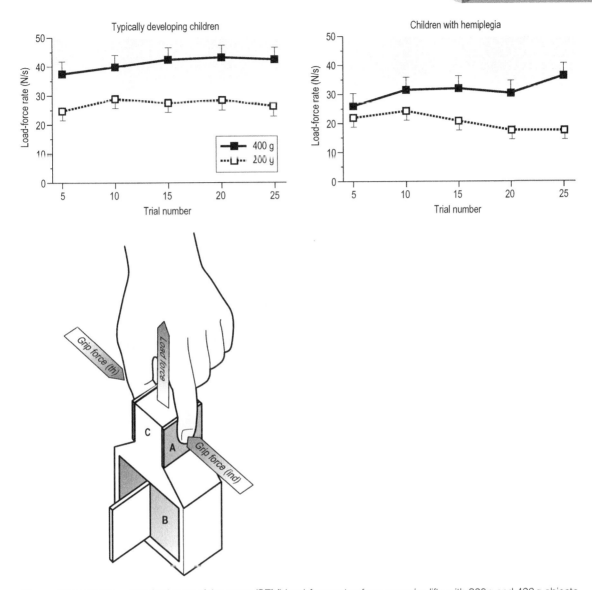

**Figure 14.1** • Mean ± standard error of the mean (SEM) load-force rates for successive lifts with 200 g and 400 g objects as a function of trials for typically developing children (*n* = 15) and children with hemiplegia (*n* = 15). Note the large differences in the load-force rates for the control children during all blocks and small initial differences which increase across blocks for the children with hemiplegia. (A, forces transducers; B, exchangeable weight; C, position sensor)
[Modified from Gordon AM, Duff SV. Fingertip forces during object manipulation in children with hemiplegic cerebral palsy. I: anticipatory scaling. Dev Med Child Neurol. 1999;41(3):166–175, with permission from John Wiley and Sons.]

## Task-oriented training

Unlike neuromuscular re-education treatments that traditionally focused on impairment-level disablement, task-oriented training focuses on the effectiveness and efficiency of motor performance in specific actions rather than on correction of movement patterns or prevention of compensations.

Activity limitations are an important aspect of CP (Bax et al., 2005). Task-oriented training can be considered a motor learning (or goal-directed) approach to rehabilitation (Carr and Shepherd, 1989; Trombly, 1995; Winstein and Wolf, 2009) (see Chapters 1 and 11). This method of treatment is based on integrated models of motor learning and motor control and behavioural neuroscience.

Focus is on participation and skill acquisition, and involves targeted physical and mental activity. An important component is the active problem solving described earlier. The associated behavioural demands of the tasks and motor skill training may result in cortical reorganization (Plautz et al., 2000) underlying concurrent functional outcomes. For optimal efficacy, the training must be challenging, with progressively increasing behavioural demands, and involve active participation. Skilled training in animals shows increased plasticity of UE cortical representations, whereas unskilled training did not (Kleim et al., 1998). At least beyond a certain point, time on task may be less important than what is practiced.

Although evidence for functional and task-oriented training is accumulating, evidence for other treatments such as neurodevelopmental therapy (NDT) is more limited. An evidence report for the American Academy of Cerebral Palsy and Developmental Medicine concluded: 'there was not consistent high-level evidence that NDT improved motoric responses, slowed or prevented contractures, or that it facilitated more normal motor development or functional motor activities' (Butler and Darrah, 2001).

Next we provide two examples of contemporary UE task-oriented treatments that further incorporate motor learning principles: constraint-induced movement therapy and functional bimanual training.

# Constraint-induced movement therapy

There was a strong rationale from motor learning and neuroscientific studies underlying the application of intensive practice-based models to human UE rehabilitation (see, for example, Taub and Shee, 1980, Tower, 1940). Early attempts included 'forced use' in adult stroke patients, whereby the less-affected UE was restrained to passively induce practice of the more affected UE (Wolf et al., 1989). Subsequent attempts incorporated principles of psychology (shaping, whereby movements are reinforced using successive approximations) and motor learning to elicit active practice of the more affected UE, evolving to what is now known as 'constraint-induced movement therapy' (Taub and Wolf, 1997). Constraint-induced movement therapy (CIMT) has been studied extensively in

adult hemiparetic stroke patients, where there is strong evidence of efficacy (see, for example, Wolf et al., 2006, 2008).

## Constraint-induced therapy in children with unilateral CP

CIMT has not been studied in the paediatric population nearly to the same extent that it has in adults with unilateral CP. Nevertheless, since our initial case study more than a decade ago (Charles et al., 2001), there have been nearly 70 studies of CIMT, including 27 randomized controlled trials (RCTs) as of April 2012. Thus, CIMT has been tested more than any other type of UE training approach. Since children are not as easily motivated to perform activities of daily living or part practice for sustained periods of time in the way that adults are, the overall approach must be adapted to focus on age-appropriate activities that sustain interest for long periods. The protocol used for adults, with a cast on the less-affected UE and training for three weeks has been used in children (Taub et al., 2004, 2007). It has been suggested that deviations from this protocol result in compromised intensity (Taub et al., 2007). However, effect sizes used for comparison were performed on different measures, none of which were validated for use in this population. Without building on each other in a rigorous fashion, modifications have been made that include restraint type, restraint duration, therapy duration, dose frequency, and providers without building on each other. The study designs, age of participants and outcome measures also differ greatly across studies. While overall there is increasing evidence of efficacy irrespective of these differences (Gordon, 2011; Hoare et al., 2007; Huang et al., 2009; Sakzewski et al., 2009), the diversity of protocols makes it nearly impossible to compare across studies to determine the effect of various models. This greatly limits the clinician's ability to implement a model of CIMT that suits the local environment and meets the needs of children and families. These factors are reviewed below.

## Age of CIMT participants

Knowing the optimal age to conduct CIMT is an important consideration for children, families and providers. The mean age of children in the majority of studies ranges from 2 to 7 years. However, studies have included children as young as 7 months (Taub et al., 2004) to teenagers (Gordon et al., 2006; Sakzewski et al., 2011a). Given the very early age in which brain damage occurs in CP, one would think that there is tremendous potential for recovery (Kennard, 1936) and that 'earlier treatment is better.' While there may indeed be certain windows of opportunity that could lead to better outcome, it is now understood that plasticity is more complicated than that. There is only one specific study examining age (Gordon et al., 2006). No difference between outcomes in children aged 4 to 8 years and with those aged 9 to 13 years was found, as seen in Figure 14.2, which shows similar changes in the JTTHF in both age groups. However, it may well be that the older children had greater attention and motivation, and thus worked harder for the same gains. In a modified study of restraint schedules, Eliasson et al. (2005) found that in children aged 1.5 to 4 years, the older children actually made greater gains than the younger ones. Sakzewski et al. (2011a) showed the same relationship between age and outcome in children aged 5 to 16 years. Yet, other studies have shown the opposite (Eliasson et al., 2005; Hoare et al., 2013).

Despite the discrepancies, there is neuroanatomical data in the developing infant and kitten to suggest that the best time to start treatments eliciting movements of the more affected UE such as CIMT may well be earlier than studied to date. Unilateral damage to cortical motor areas results in a failure of the affected corticospinal tract (CST) to secure and maintain normal terminations in the spinal cord (Eyre et al., 2007; see Martin et al., 2011). Termination of the CST in the spinal cord requires activity-dependent competition between the two sides of the developing motor system. During normal development, the CST initially projects bilaterally from both motor cortices at birth, and is pruned into the mature contralateral projection pattern seen in adults during the first few years of life (Eyre et al., 2001). Damage to one side of the motor cortex, as occurs often in unilateral CP, results in aberrant organization of the motor system, with the damaged side failing to establish normal CST connections. Concurrently, the undamaged/less-damaged CST maintains excessive bilateral projections that invade the normal

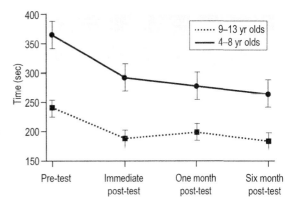

**Figure 14.2** • Mean ± SEM time to complete the six timed items (writing excluded) of the Jebsen–Taylor test of hand function for the younger (n = 12) and older (n = 8) age groups at each testing session. Faster times correspond with better performance. [Modified from Gordon AM, Charles J, Wolf SL. Efficacy of constraint-induced movement therapy on involved-upper extremity use in children with hemiplegic cerebral palsy is not age-dependent. Pediatrics 2006;117:e363–373, with permission from the American Academy of Pediatrics.]

termination zone of the contralateral spinal cord. A non-invasive brain stimulation technique, transcranial magnetic stimulation (TMS), has been used to study the integrity of the CST in children with unilateral CP (Eyre et al., 2001, 2007; Staudt et al., 2004) (see Chapters 2 and 3). Initially after the neurological insult, the CST from the damaged hemisphere is readily excitable by TMS, indicating connectivity to the spinal cord. The excitability of the damaged CST decreases in a time-dependent fashion, even years after the initial damage. Concurrently, the hemisphere contralateral to the damage increases in excitability. Specifically, the ipsilateral stimulation response is heightened, suggesting a strengthening of these projections. The strengthening of ipsilateral CST connections is believed to be a consequence of activity-dependent competition between the two hemispheres—the more active side 'wins out' over the less active (damaged) side (Eyre et al., 2007; Martin et al., 2011).

Consistent with this TMS data, neuroanatomical and behavioural studies in a feline model of unilateral CP indicate that behavioural deficits that emerge with unilateral CP are caused by aberrant organization of the CST that appears to increase with maturation (Martin et al., 2011). Balancing activity of the two hemispheres immediately after unilateral brain trauma by pharmacologically decreasing activity of the uninvolved side, restores motor function, normal anatomical connectivity of the CST and the motor representational map in primary motor cortex (Martin et al., 2011). This model points to the importance of increasing activity of the involved UE, a principle incorporated into both CIMT and bimanual training (see below). It encourages very early training of the affected UE to balance activity between the two sides before the less-affected CST 'outcompetes' the affected CST for synaptic space in the spinal cord. The time window for restoring CST connectivity by balancing activity may be rather narrow, occurring at a very young age. However, the converse is also true: restricting movement of the less-affected UE for long periods of time would disrupt the normal development of the CST, potentially resulting in impaired function of the better hand. Thus, restriction of the less-affected UE should be done in moderation at an early age. Modified schedules with just two hours per day of CIMT have been shown to be effective (Eliasson et al., 2005, 2011; Wallen et al., 2011). An important point is that CIMT should not be viewed as a one-time opportunity whereby the less-affected UE is restrained as much as possible (e.g., with a cast) and the highest possible intensity is provided regardless of age. In fact, there is increasing evidence that CIMT can be provided multiple times during development without reducing the magnitude of subsequent change (Fig. 14.3) (Charles and Gordon, 2007; Gordon et al., 2011).

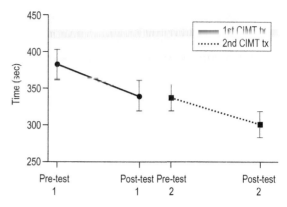

**Figure 14.3** • Mean ± SEM time to complete the six timed items (writing excluded) of the Jebsen–Taylor test of hand function immediately before (pre-test 1) and after (post-test 1) the first intervention, and immediately before (pre-test 2) and after (post-test 2) the second intervention one year later. Faster times on the Jebsen–Taylor test correspond to better performance. Note that gains are retained one year after the initial CIMT intervention, and the times improve further after the second intervention.

[Modified from Gordon AM, Schneider JA, Chinnan A, Charles JR. Efficacy of a hand-arm bimanual intensive therapy (HABIT) in children with hemiplegic cerebral palsy: a randomized control trial. Dev Med Child Neurol. 2007;49:830–838, with permission from John Wiley and Sons.]

the diversity of treatments and the fact that there are no direct comparison studies, there is no evidence to suggest that one type of restraint is more effective than another in eliciting better affected UE outcomes. Thus, comfort and safety should be a key factor in restraint selection.

## Restraint type

Restraints used during CIMT include plaster casts worn full time (Case-Smith et al., 2012; Taub et al., 2004, 2011), slings (Charles et al., 2001, 2006; Gordon et al., 2006, 2011), splints (Brandão et al., 2010; Park et al., 2009), and mitt/gloves (Eliasson et al., 2005, 2011; Hoare et al., 2013; Sakzewski et al., 2011a). The cast restricts all movement and does not allow the participant choice to remove it. The other types of restraint allow movement of the less-affected UE (and in the case of a splint or mitt, the restrained UE could be used as an assist). These restraints could be removed by an unco-operative child, although few reports of this occurring exist. In our experience with over 80 children participating in CIMT with a sling, only one (an 8-year-old girl with behavioural problems) refused to wear the restraint. Despite

## Ingredients of CIMT

Despite the large number of CIMT studies, overall, little description is typically provided about the specific movements and activities practiced, largely because of the space constraint of journals. Methodology papers mainly focus on information about RCT designs and procedures (Aarts et al., 2010; Boyd et al., 2010; Facchin et al., 2009) although some treatment details are provided. Early CIMT models (Case-Smith et al., 2012; Taub et al., 2004) involved shaping (called 'part practice' in the motor learning literature), which involves approaching a behavioural objective (task) in small steps by successive approximation (Skinner, 1968). The task is made more challenging as the child improves, taking into consideration their abilities. Other models simply involve engaging the children in play and functional activities (Bonnier et al., 2006;

Eliasson et al., 2005) without regard to shaping, and in many studies this is not specified. There have not been any studies that examined the roles of specific ingredients such as shaping in children with CP, but nearly all studies suggest efficacy. Since all CIMT approaches involved practice of motor activities, intensity of training may well be more important than ingredients (how practice is provided), at least at the high intensity CIMT is normally provided.

The choice of activities to engage children in is important. To engage the child in active intervention and to maintain their attention and effort, we established a battery of motor activities that elicit the general movement behaviours of interest that includes a range of functional and play activities (Gordon et al., 2005). The activities are age-appropriate and can all be performed unimanually. Activities are selected by considering: (1) joint movements with pronounced deficits; (2) joint movements that therapists believe have greatest potential of improving performance; and (3) child preference for activities that have similar potential for improving identified movements. Therapists usually begin with a quick task which results in successful completion to build confidence. The task is made progressively more challenging as the child's performance improves by requiring greater speed or accuracy, additional movement repetitions or performance-sensitive adaptations. We adapt task constraints to allow success, and remove them as skill improves using specific criteria. Age-specific structured feedback (knowledge of results) is provided to motivate the child. Nevertheless, whether such structured interventions are advantageous over just play and functional practice with less structure is not known.

Table 14.1 illustrates the types of activities we have used for children aged 3.5 years and above, with examples of targeted movements and how the constraints are graded to vary the difficulty. There are eight categories, consisting of board games (e.g., Candyland®, Monopoly®), card games (e.g., Old Maid®, Uno®), manipulative games (e.g., Don't Break the Ice®, Battleship®), puzzles, arts and crafts (e.g., drawing, painting), functional tasks (e.g., eating, dressing), full upper extremity motor activities (e.g., throwing a large ball, Scatch®), and video gaming (Gordon and Okita, 2010). We view the choice of specific activities as less important than the movements they elicit. For example, board games could be used to encourage

wrist supination and extension, precision grasp and grasp maintenance. Video gaming consoles (such as the Nintendo Wii®) can be used to induce full UE movements and to challenge postural control (especially if seated on a fitness ball).

## Duration of CIMT

The length of CIMT programmes varies widely from two to ten weeks, with restraint use ranging from 40 (Xu et al., 2012) to more than 1000 (Sung et al., 2005) hours, and active training time from zero (Willis et al., 2002) to 126 (Case-Smith et al., 2012; Taub et al., 2004) hours. Intensive 'camp models' lasting two to three weeks (approximately six hours/day) are often used for school-aged children, since this makes it possible to conduct a programme during school holidays (Charles et al., 2006; Gordon et al., 2011; Sakzewski et al., 2011a). For children below 4 years of age, more distributed practice models (about two hours/day) for six to eight weeks have been applied in the children's daily environment (Eliasson et al., 2005). The choice of distributed practice for small children is a practical issue since hours of daily training is not feasible in young children. It should be pointed out that there does not seem to be a relationship between intensity and efficacy, but it is difficult to compare across studies, as mentioned above, given the diversity of procedures and outcome measures. One study compared three hours versus six hours of daily CIMT, with no difference in efficacy (Case-Smith et al., 2012), but the restraint (cast) was worn 24/7, so the added 'passive' practice may have washed out any potential differences.

## CIMT providers

Studies of CIMT have employed a variety of individuals of different backgrounds. These include parents and/or teachers (Eliasson et al., 2005, 2011), physical/occupational therapists (Aarts et al., 2010; Hoare et al., 2013; Sakzewski et al., 2011a; Taub et al., 2004, ) and undergraduate/graduate students trained and supervised by physical/occupational therapists (Charles et al., 2006; Gordon et al., 2011). One study performed an ad hoc analysis of the outcomes of participants who received CIMT from a physical/occupational therapist versus those who received it from non-clinicians (Gordon et al., 2011), and found no

**Table 14.1 CIMT activities**

| Activity category | Targeted movements | Graded constraints |
|---|---|---|
| Board games | Supination, wrist extension, precision grasp, maintaining grasp through changes in spatial orientation | Active wrist extension—position deck of cards to elicit wrist extension and grade difficulty by changing position of deck |
| Card games | Supination, precision grasp | Precision grasp—less difficult when cards are bevelled on deck for easier grasp. Increase difficulty by not bevelling the cards |
| Functional tasks | Wrist extension, supination and pronation | Supination and pronation—for turning key in lock, vary starting position of key to grade from using only supination to using both supination and pronation |
| Whole upper extremity | Shoulder flexion, shoulder abduction, shoulder external rotation, wrist extension | Shoulder flexion—elicit shoulder flexion by moving child from easier position stabilized against a wall, to free standing position that requires more control |
| Manipulative games | Finger individuation, precision grasp, wrist extension, modifying grasp to accommodate various objects | Precision grasp—to increase difficulty provide child with increasingly smaller or more complex objects to manipulate |
| Puzzles | In-hand manipulation, precision grasp, release accuracy | Release accuracy—once competency in releasing puzzle pieces is attained, increase difficulty by introducing a puzzle with smaller pieces |
| Arts and crafts | Supination, precision grasp, maintaining grasp through changes in spatial orientation | Maintaining grasp—begin child at an easier level with a built-up brush, and increase difficulty by removing assist. Smaller brushes can be introduced |
| Video gaming | Wrist supination and extension, shoulder flexion, shoulder abduction dexterity, shoulder external rotation | Wrap controller with tape, sit on fitness ball |

differences in outcomes (Fig. 14.4). However it should be noted that the non-clinicians were trained and supervised by clinicians, and clinicians had to adhere only to the study protocol rather than using any additional skills, which may have minimized differences between groups. Nevertheless, it provides an economically feasible model to maintain one-on-one treatment.

## Outcome measures

More than 40 outcome measures have been used across the 70 studies (for a review see Klingels et al., 2010). Outcome measures should reflect what is trained (unimanual dexterity) and what will contribute the most to daily function (bimanual hand use), ideally including real-world assessment. One of the most widely used unimanual dexterity measures has been the AHA (Aarts et al., 2010; Charles et al., 2006; Eliasson et al., 2005, 2011; Gordon et al., 2011; Hoare et al., 2013; Krumlinde-Sundholm et al., 2003, 2007; Sakzewski et al., 2011a). It is validated for use in this population, and in our opinion, is the gold standard outcome measure for UE treatments in this population (Gordon, 2007). If adapted as the 'one common measure', future studies could be compared to each other.

## Limitations of CIMT

Despite showing considerable potential (Gordon, 2011; Hoare et al., 2007; Huang et al., 2009; Sakzewski et al., 2009), a number of conceptual problems have been noted in applying it to children that need consideration. First, CIMT

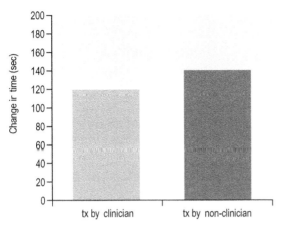

**Figure 14.4** • Comparison of CIMT/bimanual training improvement on the Jebsen–Taylor test of hand function when provided by a clinician (physical/occupational therapist, *n* = 8) versus a trained caregiver (*n* = 34). [Data plotted from Gordon, AM, Hung, YC, Brandao, M, et al. Bimanual training and constraint-induced movement therapy in children with hemiplegic cerebral palsy: a randomized trial. Neurorehabilitation and Neural Repair 2011; 25: 692–702, with permission from Sage Publishers.]

was developed to overcome 'learned non-use' in adults with unilateral stroke and to promote use of the limb rather than skill. But adults who lose UE function are often highly motivated to regain previously learned functional behaviours, and can adhere to boring, repetitive tasks for long periods. In contrast, children must overcome '*developmental disuse*', whereby they may have never learned how to effectively use their more affected UE during many tasks. Thus, treatments must be developmentally focused and must take into account the importance of motor learning.

Second, in older children, restraining a child's less-affected extremity (especially with casts) is potentially invasive since it is the parent choosing for the child to participate rather than the child themselves. The task difficulty must be carefully graded to avoid frustration. CIMT in the adult (24/7) form is not suitable for young or severely impaired children. The less-affected side is still developing in children, and as mentioned above early restriction of UE use on one side during a developmental critical period could reduce the topographic distribution, branch density, and density of presynaptic boutons on the side of restricted use (Martin et al., 2011). Thus, a greatly modified protocol is required in young children.

Finally, CIMT focuses only on training unimanual dexterity, which does not greatly influence functional independence and quality of

life in children with unilateral CP as they have a well-functioning (dominant) hand (Sköld et al., 2004) to perform unimanual tasks. CIMT lacks specificity of training for how the hand will be used once the restraint is removed. Specificity of training would suggest training it to be an effective non-dominant assisting hand during *bimanual activities*. Children with unilateral CP have impairments in spatial and temporal co-ordination of the two hands (Gordon and Steenbergen, 2008; Hung et al., 2004, 2010; Utley and Steenbergen, 2006), as well as global impairments in motor planning (Steenbergen et al., 2009). Constraint therapies cannot address these problems without a transfer protocol (Taub et al., 2007), and thus generalization of training may not apply. Furthermore, problem solving may be limited, given the reduced degrees of freedom.

## Bimanual therapy in children with unilateral CP

From a functional perspective, principles of practice specificity (Thorndike, 1914) would suggest that the best way to achieve improved bimanual control would be to practice bimanual co-ordination directly rather than rely on potential transfer. Recently, a child-friendly form of task-oriented intensive functional training, hand–arm bimanual intensive therapy (HABIT) was developed (Charles and Gordon, 2006). HABIT aims to improve the amount and quality of involved UE use during bimanual tasks. HABIT is based on: (1) basic sciences delineating mechanisms of hand impairments in CP; (2) our intuition that the key ingredient in CIMT is practice intensity; and (3) specificity of training. Thus, HABIT retains the intensive structured practice of CIMT, but engages the child in bimanual activities rather than relying on use of a restraint to encourage use of the more affected UE. Typically it is provided in day-camp environments of six hours/day for 10 to 15 days (i.e., 60–90 hours). Activities that necessitate co-ordination of both UEs are employed. Table 14.2 lists the types of activities we have used, with examples of targeted movements and how the constraints are graded to vary the difficulty. Additional activities for even younger children can be found in a recent review (Greaves et al., 2012).

It is important to note that bimanual training is one of many tools employed by occupational and

**Table 14.2 HABIT activities**

| Activity category | Type of involved hand use | Graded constraints |
| --- | --- | --- |
| Manipulative games and tasks | Stabilizer, manipulator, active/passive assist, symmetrical and asymmetrical movements | Changing spatial and temporal constraints of the task, for symmetrical tasks increasing frequency task is completed within a fixed time period |
| Card games | Stabilizer, manipulator, active/passive assist, symmetrical and asymmetrical movements | Changing spatial and temporal constraints of the task, for symmetrical tasks increasing frequency task is completed within a fixed time period |
| Video games | Manipulator, active assist, symmetrical movements | Changing temporal constraints of task, sit on fitness ball, taping grip |
| Functional tasks | Stabilizer, manipulator, active/passive assist, symmetrical and asymmetrical movements | Stabilizer, manipulator, active/passive assist, symmetrical and asymmetrical movements |
| Whole upper extremity | Stabilizer, manipulator, active/passive assist, symmetrical and asymmetrical movements | Stabilizer, manipulator, active/passive assist, symmetrical and asymmetrical movements, use of fitness ball |
| Arts and crafts | Stabilizer, manipulator, active/passive assist, symmetrical and asymmetrical movements | Stabilizer, manipulator, active/passive assist, symmetrical and asymmetrical movements, placing items on Dycem, building up objects with tape |

physical therapists (Eliasson, 2007; Hoare et al., 2010). However, HABIT differs from common rehabilitation practice in significant ways. The *intensity* of HABIT is much higher than that of most therapies, providing abundant practice using principles of motor learning as well as of neuroplasticity, whereby neuroplastic changes are induced by increasing task complexity and reward (Kleim et al., 2002; Nudo, 2003). It is also more structured than most therapy, as described below, combining ingredients from CIMT (e.g., shaping) and clear rules about activity selection and skill progression.

To date, several efficacy studies have been conducted. A small randomized controlled trial of HABIT was conducted on 20 children with unilateral CP between the ages of 3.5 and 14 years (Gordon et al., 2007). Children who received HABIT had improved scores on the AHA, while those in the treatment control (delayed treatment) group received usual and customary care. Frequency of UE use, measured with accelerometers, increased for the children who received HABIT. Interestingly, the improvement in the amount of use of the involved UE did not correlate with the improvement in AHA scores,

indicating quality and quantity of movement may change (and be maintained) independently.

In a subsequent, small quasi-randomized study, we compared a group of ten children who received 60 hours of HABIT to a group that received 60 hours of CIMT (Gordon et al., 2005, 2008). Overall, we found similar changes in manual dexterity (JTTHF), quality of bimanual hand use (AHA) and amount of movement (accelerometry) in each group. (This was the first reported evidence that it is the treatment intensity that makes CIMT efficacious, since there are no benefits when compared to another treatment of equal intensity.) We subsequently followed this up with a larger randomized clinical trial of HABIT and CIMT (Gordon et al., 2011). Forty-two children between the age of 3.5 and 10 years were randomized (stratified by hand severity and age) to receive 90 hours of either HABIT or CIMT. Our primary outcome was unimanual dexterity (JTTHF) and quality of bimanual hand use (AHA) (see above). Secondary measures also included goal attainment scale (GAS) (Kiresuk et al., 1994) to quantify progress on one functional and one play goal defined by caregivers and/or participants. Goal appropriateness was determined based on age and current abilities and scaled by a physical therapist.

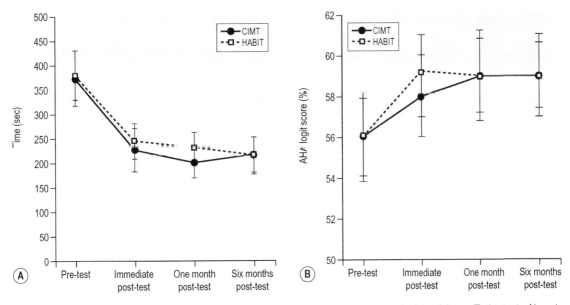

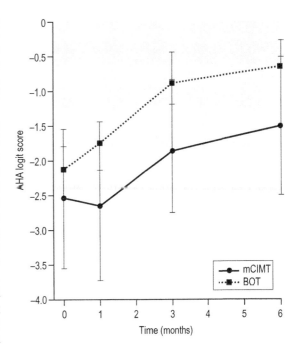

Figure 14.5 • **(A)** Mean ± SEM time to complete the six timed items (writing excluded) of the Jebsen–Taylor test of hand function. Faster times correspond to better performance. **(B)** Mean ± SEM scaled logit scores on the AHA; higher scores represent better performance. [Modified from Gordon, AM, Hung, YC, Brandao, M, et al. Bimanual training and constraint-induced movement therapy in children with hemiplegic cerebral palsy: a randomized trial. Neurorehabilitation and Neural Repair 2011; 25: 692–702, with permission from the American Academy of Pediatrics.]

The goals were practiced up to 30 minutes/day, but the individual working with the child decided how much training (if at all) to provide within the 30-minute limit based on the child's interest. The CIMT group was not able to practice bimanual goals, and instead practiced unimanual components of movements making up the goal.

Consistent with the earlier study (Gordon et al., 2008), both groups of participants had similar significant changes in the JTTHF and AHA (Fig. 14.5) which were retained for the six months the participants were followed. Thus, these findings are in agreement that intensity is the key factor for these variables. Similar findings have been shown for other large randomized clinical trials comparing bimanual training to CIMT (Facchin et al., 2011; Saklzewski et al., 2011a, 2011b, 2011c). For example, in another comparison study, Hoare et al. (2013) conducted an RCT of 34 children (aged 18 months to 6 years) with unilateral CP receiving modified CIMT plus botulinum toxin A (BoNT-A) or bimanual therapy plus BoNT-A. The comparison group (n = 17) received BoNT-A and BOT. All children received individual 45–60 minute treatment sessions twice a week for eight weeks. Children in the CIMT group were required to complete three hours of home training each day, while the bimanual group was encouraged to do the same. There was

Figure 14.6 • Assisting hand assessment mean ± SEM at baseline, one, three and six months of training with modified constraint-induced movement therapy and bimanual training. [Modified from Hoare B, Imms C, Villanueva E, Rawicki HB, Matyas T, Carey L. Intensive therapy following upper limb botulinum toxin A injection in young children with unilateral cerebral palsy: a randomized trial. Dev Med Child Neurol. 2013;55:238–247, with permission from John Wiley and Sons.]

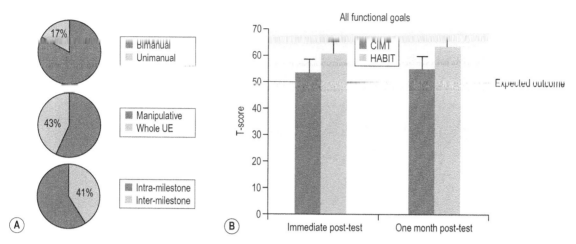

**Figure 14.7 • (A)** Goals selected by children with unilateral CP and/or their caregivers. **(B)** Goal attainment scale score (GAS). A score of 50 means the goal was achieved. Scores above 50 mean goal achievement exceeded expectation. [Data plotted from Gordon, AM, Hung, YC, Brandao, M, et al. Bimanual training and constraint-induced movement therapy in children with hemiplegic cerebral palsy: a randomized trial. Neurorehabilitation and Neural Repair 2011; 25: 692–702.].

no evidence of a difference in the effectiveness of modified CIMT or bimanual training on the AHA (Fig. 14.6), quality of upper extremity skills test, paediatric evaluation of disability inventory, Canadian occupational performance measure or GAS. The investigators concluded that following spasticity reduction with botulinum toxin A CIMT was not more effective than bimanual training for improving UE impairment or activity level outcomes.

The results of goal attainment, however, suggest treatment specificity (Gordon et al., 2011). The majority of goals were bimanual (remaining goals: unimanual with paretic hand), again emphasizing the importance of bimanual skills (Fig. 14.7A). Both the CIMT and HABIT groups achieved or exceeded their expected goal performance. However, the HABIT group made greater progress on their goals than the CIMT group. Nearly 20% of the identified goals were not practiced in either group due to children's interest changing. Interestingly, however, these unpracticed goals also improved, with greater improvement for the participants in the HABIT group (Fig. 14.7B). This suggests that the skills they acquired during HABIT may have allowed faster learning via transfer from training of specific tasks to improvement in similar but unpracticed tasks. In a separate study of goal achievement using the Canadian occupational performance measure (COPM) (Carswell et al., 2004; Law et al., 1990) and self-care performance using the paediatric evaluation of disability inventory

(PEDI) (Haley et al., 1992), children with CP received HABIT or CIMT (Brandão et al., 2012). Both groups showed significant improvements on self-care performance (PEDI functional skills and independence) and progress on goals (COPM satisfaction and performance), but caregivers of children who received HABIT reported perceiving greater improvements on goal performance. Thus, practicing goals, which is more easily done in bimanual training since most goals involve two hands, leads to better goal performance.

It is unknown whether CIMT or bimanual training affects the spatiotemporal co-ordination of the two hands. Thus, we examined the kinematics of a bimanual task in 20 children with unilateral CP who received HABIT or CIMT (Hung et al., 2010). To assess bimanual co-ordination, participants were asked to open a drawer with one hand and manipulate its contents with the other hand while the movement kinematics was recorded (Wiesendanger and Serrien, 2004). There were improvements in both groups, but greater improvements in bimanual co-ordination for the HABIT group was indicated by more movement overlap (the percentage of time with both hands engaged in the task) and better interlimb synchronization (reduced time between each hand completing the task goals) (Fig. 14.8). These findings suggest that bimanual training improves the spatial-temporal control of the two hands, and are also in agreement with the principle of practice specificity.

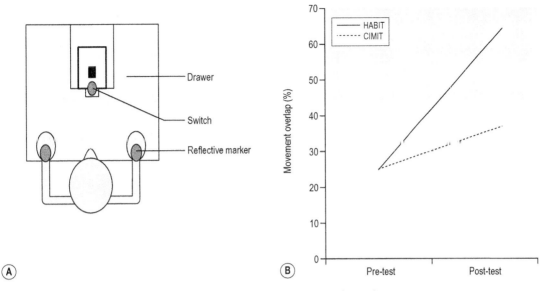

**Figure 14.8 •** Co-ordination of two hands during a bimanual drawer-opening task. [Modified from Hung YC, Charles J, Gordon AM. Influence of accuracy constraints on bimanual coordination during a goal-directed task in children with hemiplegic cerebral palsy. Exp Brain Res 2010; 201: 421–428, from Springer Science + Business Media.].

# Alternative models of training delivery

Providing 90 hours of training over 15 days in a day-camp model is expensive, and participation (e.g., transportation) can be a burden to caregivers. Furthermore, as mentioned above, six hours per day is not feasible for younger children. Thus, we developed a home-based HABIT (H-HABIT) (Ferre et al. unpublished data), and sought to determine whether caregivers can be trained as primary trainers, and whether hand function improves in young children, as has been shown for CIMT (e.g., Eliasson et al., 2005, 2011; Wallen et al., 2011). Thus far we have conducted H-HABIT in four children between the ages of 33 and 54 months in home-based settings. Therapy was provided by caregivers for two hours/day, five days/week, for nine weeks (90 hours). Daily logs were used to track compliance and measure difficulty of fulfilling the two hours each day. The parental stress index—short form (PSI-SF) was used to measure changes in psychosocial dynamics of the caregiver—child dyad. Video observations of H-HABIT were behaviourally scored to examine the quality of the intervention.

All children completed the 90 hours of H-HABIT. Scored video observations indicated children spent on average ~40% of the time with the affected hand in contact with an object. AHA scaled logit scores improved 2.1 points ($p < 0.005$). There were no changes in the PSI-SF, indicating no change in parental stress. These preliminary results suggest that caregivers can effectively be trained to work with their children without increasing parental stress and that home-based interventions can lead to improvements in hand function. Using caregivers as the primary providers of intensive bimanual therapy in a home-based setting might be a cost-effective alternative to expensive day camps, and make available intensive bimanual practice for children below 4 years of age.

# When should CIMT or bimanual training be used?

While there appears to be some evidence of treatment specificity, overall both CIMT and bimanual training lead to improvements in UE function. Nevertheless, there may be different scenarios where one method would be advantageous (Table 14.3). For example, our results (Gordon et al., 2011), and the results of others (Facchin et al., 2011, Sakzewski et al., 2011a–c), suggest either CIMT or bimanual training could be used to elicit improvements in manual dexterity and bimanual performance. Thus, they could be used interchangeably. Bimanual training appears

**Table 14.3 Criteria for selection of CIMT or bimanual training**

| Criteria | CIMT | Bimanual training |
|---|---|---|
| Dexterity | X | X |
| Bimanual assist quality | X | X |
| Frequency of use | X | X |
| Function (goals) | | X |
| Co-ordination of two hands | | X |
| Mild hemi | | X |
| Severe hemi | | X |
| Reduce impairments | X | |
| Behavioural problems | ? | |
| Restraint tolerance problems | | X |
| Low IQ | ? | |
| Diversity of activities | | X |
| Short duration available | ? | |
| Lack of 1:1 child/interventionist ratio | X | |
| Ease of administering | X | |

to be better for achieving bimanual goals (Gordon et al., 2011; Brandão et al., 2012) and bimanual co-ordination (Hung et al., 2010). However, the opposite may well be true for improving unimanual goals or co-ordination, or in reducing unimanual motor impairments (e.g., wrist extension) because CIMT allows more control over how the affected UE is used. One can hypothesize that bimanual training may be better for a child with mild impairments (i.e., who already possesses good manipulation skills but shows developmental disuse during bimanual activities). Bimanual training may also be better for a child with an inability to grasp (where the choice of activities with CIMT would be very limited) since tasks can be graded such that the involved UE can be used as a passive assist to start (e.g., stabilizing paper on the desk while writing). Bimanual training would also be a viable alternative for a child who does not tolerate

the restraint. In contrast, if there is insufficient staffing (less than a 1:1 therapist-child ratio), the restraint used in CIMT could reduce compensation with the less-affected UE, and would be easier to administer. Bimanual training likely provides greater diversity of activities, and is potentially less invasive than CIMT. Nevertheless, bimanual training is much more difficult for interventionists to execute because they must continually anticipate how the child will attempt to compensate and shape the environment accordingly (i.e., always be one step ahead). However, in our experience, bimanual activities are generally more motivating, since activities are generally more salient and may be selected to maximize interest (e.g., video games). Such motivational and social aspects of types of practice are important in the design of interventions (Ochsner and Lieberman, 2001).

CIMT and HABIT are not mutually exclusive, and could be performed back-to-back with sufficient intensity (Aarts et al., 2010). It is worth noting that the advantages seen for HABIT in our RCT (Gordon et al., 2011) may well be due to the conduct of these treatments in a scientific environment that is carefully controlled to prevent loss of treatment fidelity. The hybrid approach whereby CIMT is followed up with bimanual training (Aarts et al., 2010; Case-Smith et al., 2012; Taub et al., 2007) might eliminate any advantage of bimanual training in isolation. Cohen-Holzer et al. (2011) examined one hour of CIMT followed by five hours of bimanual training each day for 10 days. Significant improvements were seen on the AHA, JTTHF, PEDI and grip strength. Whether these combined treatments are better than either individual treatment (Gordon, 2011) has yet to be tested.

# Conclusions

The introduction and subsequent study of CIMT to the paediatric population shifted the landscape of UE paediatric rehabilitation by eliciting thinking about the importance of treatment intensity. The results across a large number of studies now suggest that children with CP can benefit from both CIMT and intensive bimanual training. The specific ingredients that prove to be beneficial or the dose responses are not known, but it is likely that one key ingredient is treatment intensity, i.e., the more practice the better. The results of the studies to date suggest that it is important to put the training goal first, and then choose the appropriate protocol to meet those goals. Although there is more evidence supporting the efficacy of CIMT, here we provide evidence that training bimanual skills can improve bimanual functional skills. Our view is that they can be used interchangeably, depending on the child's needs and therapeutic goals over the long course of treatment. While large improvements can result from such intensive training, the underlying sensory and motor impairments still persist, and these treatments should be integrated with, rather than replace, other long-term paediatric care treatments.

Unfortunately many of the studies of such treatments are redundant. To progress knowledge in the field, agreed-upon standardized measures should be used, and protocols should be designed to carefully manipulate one variable at a time.

Key questions include optimal dosing amount and schedules, which children are likely to respond, whether restraint type (or use at all) matters, the effect of training environments, combined treatments versus CIMT or bimanual training in isolation, and when and how often to repeat treatments. Perhaps, most importantly, adapting these treatments to infants at risk of developing unilateral CP may be the key to minimizing the development of neural and muscular mal-adaptations and optimizing the use of the affected upper limb (Gordon, 2010).

# Acknowledgements

This work was supported by the Thrasher Research Fund.

# References

Aarts, P.B., Jongerius, P.H., Geerdink, Y.A., van Limbeek, J., Geurts, A.C., 2010. Effectiveness of modified constraint-induced movement therapy in children with unilateral spastic cerebral palsy: a randomized controlled trial. Neurorehab. Neural Repair 24, 509–518.

Ahl, L.E., Johansson, E., Granat, T., Carlberg, E.B., 2005. Functional therapy for children with cerebral palsy: an ecological approach. Dev. Med. Child Neurol. 47, 613–619.

Bax, M., Goldstein, M., Rosenbaum, P., Leviton, A., Paneth, N., Dan, B., et al., 2005. Executive Committee for the Definition of Cerebral Palsy, Proposed definition and classification of cerebral palsy, April 2005. Dev. Med. Child Neurol. 47, 571–576.

Bonnier, B., Eliasson, A.C., Krumlinde-Sundholm, L., 2006. Effects of constraint-induced movement therapy in adolescents with hemiplegic cerebral palsy: a day camp model. Scand. J. Occup. Ther. 13, 13–22.

Boyd, R., Sakzewski, L., Ziviani, J., Abbott, D.F., Badawy, R., Gilmore, R., et al., 2010. INCITE: a randomised trial comparing constraint induced movement therapy and bimanual training in children with congenital hemiplegia. BMC Neurol. 10, 4.

Brandão, M., Mancini, M.C., Vaz, D.V., Pereira de Melo, A.P., Fonseca, S.T., 2010. Adapted version of constraint-induced movement therapy promotes functioning in children with cerebral palsy: a randomized controlled trial. Clin. Rehabil. 24, 639–647.

Brandão, M.B., Gordon, A.M., Mancini, M.C., 2012. Functional impact of constraint-therapy and bimanual training in children with cerebral palsy. Am. J. Occup. Ther. 66 (6), 672–681.

Butler, C., Darrah, J., 2001. Effects of neurodevelopmental treatment (NDT) for cerebral palsy: an AACPDM evidence report. Dev. Med. Child Neurol. 43, 778–790.

Carr, J., Shephert, R.B., 1989. A motor learning model for stroke rehabilitation. Physiotherapy 75, 372–380.

Carswell, A., McColl, M.A., Baptiste, S., Law, M., Polatajko, H., Pollock, N., 2004. The Canadian occupational performance measure: a research and clinical literature review. Can. J. Occup. Ther. 71, 210–222.

Case-Smith, J., DeLuca, S.C., Stevenson, R., Ramey, S.L., 2012. Multicenter randomized controlled trial of pediatric constraint-induced movement therapy: 6-month follow-up. Am. J. Occup. Ther. 66, 15–23.

Charles, J., Gordon, A.M., 2006. Development of hand–arm bimanual intensive training (HABIT) for improving bimanual coordination in children with hemiplegic cerebral palsy. Dev. Med. Child Neurol. 48, 931–936.

Charles, J., Lavinder, G., Gordon, A.M., 2001. The effects of constraint induced therapy on hand function in children with hemiplegic cerebral palsy. Ped. Phys. Ther. 13, 68–76.

Charles, J.R., Gordon, A.M., 2007. A repeated course of constraint-induced movement therapy results in further improvement. Dev. Med. Child Neurol. 49, 770–773.

Charles, J.R., Wolf, S.L., Schneider, J.A., Gordon, A.M., 2006. Efficacy of a child-friendly form of constraint-induced movement therapy in hemiplegic cerebral palsy: a randomized control trial. Dev. Med. Child Neurol. 48, 635–642.

Cohen-Holzer, M., Katz-Leurer, M., Reinstein, R., Rotem, H., Meyer, S., 2011. The effect of combining daily restraint with bimanual intensive therapy in children with hemiparetic cerebral palsy: a self-control study. NeuroRehabilitation 29, 29–36.

Eliasson, A.C., 2007. Bimanual training for children with unilateral CP—is this something new? Dev. Med. Child Neurol. 49, 806.

Eliasson, A.C., Gordon, A.M., Forssberg, H., 1991. Basic coordination of manipulative forces of children with cerebral palsy. Dev. Med. Child Neurol. 33, 659–668.

Eliasson, A.C., Bonnier, B., Krumlinde-Sundholm, L., 2003. Clinical experience of constraint induced movement therapy in adolescents with hemiplegic cerebral palsy—a day camp model. Dev. Med. Child Neurol. 45, 357–359.

Eliasson, A.C., Krumlinde-Sundholm, L., Shaw, K., Wang, C., 2005. Effects of constraint-induced movement therapy in young children with hemiplegic cerebral palsy: an adapted model. Dev. Med. Child Neurol. 47, 266–275.

Eliasson, A.C., Forssberg, H., Hung, Y.C., Gordon, A.M., 2006. Development of hand function and precision grip control in individuals with cerebral palsy: a 13-year follow-up study. Pediatrics 118, 1226–1236.

Eliasson, A.C., Shaw, K., Berg, E., Krumlinde-Sundholm, L., 2011. An ecological approach of constraint induced movement therapy for 2–3-year-old children: a randomized control trial. Res. Dev. Disabil. 32, 2820–2828.

Eyre, J.A., Taylor, J.P., Villagra, F., Smith, M., Miller, S., 2001. Evidence of activity-dependent withdrawal of corticospinal projections during human development. Neurology 57, 1543–1554.

Eyre, J.A., Smith, M., Dabydeen, L., et al., 2007. Is hemiplegic cerebral palsy equivalent to amblyopia of the corticospinal system? Ann. Neurol. 62, 493–503.

Facchin, P., Rosa-Rizzotto, M., Turconi, A.C., Pagliano, E., Fazzi, E., Stortini, M., GIPCI Study Group, 2009. Multisite trial on efficacy of constraint-induced movement therapy in children with hemiplegia: study design and methodology. Am. J. Phys. Med. Rehabil. 88, 216–230.

Facchin, P., Rosa-Rizzotto, M., Visonà Dalla Pozza, L., Turconi, A.C., Pagliano, E., Signorini, S., GIPCI Study Group, 2011. Multisite trial comparing the efficacy of constraint-induced movement therapy with that of bimanual intensive training in children with hemiplegic cerebral palsy: postintervention results. Am. J. Phys. Med. Rehabil. 90, 539–553.

Gordon, A.M., 2007. Invited commentary, measuring 'activity limitation' in individuals with unilateral upper extremity impairment. Dev. Med. Child Neurol. 49, 245.

Gordon, A.M., 2010. Two hands are better than one: bimanual skill development in children with hemiplegic cerebral palsy. Dev. Med. Child Neurol. 52, 315–316.

Gordon, A.M., 2011. To constrain or not to constrain, and other stories of intensive upper extremity training for children with unilateral cerebral palsy. Dev. Med. Child Neurol. 53 (S4), 56–61.

Gordon, A.M., Duff, S.V., 1999. Fingertip forces during object manipulation in children with hemiplegic cerebral palsy. I: anticipatory scaling. Dev. Med. Child Neurol. 41 (3), 166–175.

Gordon, A.M., Magill, R.A., 2012. Motor learning: application of principles to pediatric rehabilitation. In: Campbell, S., Linden, V., Palisano, R. (Eds.), Physical Therapy for Children. Elsevier, Saunders, Philadelphia, PA.

Gordon, A.M., Okita, S.Y., 2010. Augmenting pediatric constraint-induced movement therapy and bimanual training with video gaming. Technol. Disabil. 22, 179–191.

Gordon, A.M., Steenbergen, B., 2008. Bimanual coordination in children with cerebral palsy. In: Eliasson, A.C., Burtner, P. (Eds.), Improving Hand Function in Children with Cerebral Palsy: Theory, Evidence, and Intervention. Mac Keith Press, London, pp. 160–175.

Gordon, A.M., Charles, J., Wolf, S.L., 2005. Methods of constraint-induced movement therapy for children with hemiplegic cerebral palsy: development of a child-friendly intervention for improving upper-extremity function. Arch. Phys. Med. Rehabil. 86, 837–844.

Gordon, A.M., Charles, J., Wolf, S.L., 2006. Efficacy of constraint-induced movement therapy on involved-upper extremity use in children with hemiplegic cerebral palsy is not age-dependent. Pediatrics 117, e363–e373.

Gordon, A.M., Schneider, J.A., Chinnan, A., Charles, J.R., 2007. Efficacy of a hand–arm bimanual intensive therapy (HABIT) in children with hemiplegic cerebral palsy: a randomized control trial. Dev. Med. Child Neurol. 49, 830–838.

Gordon, A.M., Chinnan, A., Gill, S., Petra, E., Hung, Y.C., Charles, J., 2008. Both constraint-induced movement therapy and bimanual training lead to improved performance of upper extremity function in children with hemiplegia. Dev. Med. Child Neurol. 50, 957–958.

Gordon, A.M., Hung, Y.C., Brandao, M., Ferre, C.L., Kuo, H.-C., Friel, K., et al., 2011. Bimanual training and constraint-induced movement therapy in children with hemiplegic cerebral palsy: a randomized trial. Neurorehabil. Neural Repair 25, 692–702.

Gorter, H., Holty, L., Rameckers, E.E., Elvers, H.J., Oostendorp, R.A., 2009. Changes in endurance and walking ability through functional physical training in children with cerebral palsy. Pediatr. Phys. Ther. 21, 31–37.

Greaves, S., Imms, C., Krumlinde-Sundholm, L., Dodd, K., Eliasson, A.C., 2012. Bimanual behaviours in children aged 8–18 months: a literature review to select toys that elicit the use of two hands. Res. Dev. Disabil. 33, 240–250.

Haley, S.M., Coster, W.J., Ludlow, L.H., et al., 1992. Pediatric Evaluation of Disability Inventory (PEDI). New England Medical Center Hospitals, Boston, MA.

Himmelmann, K., Hagberg, G., Beckung, E., Hagberg, B., Uvebrant, P., 2005. The changing panorama of cerebral palsy in Sweden. IX. Prevalence and origin in the birth-year period 1995–1998. Acta Paediatr. 94, 287–294.

Hoare, B., Imms, C., Carey, L., Wasiak, J., 2007. Constraint-induced movement therapy in the treatment of the upper limb in children with hemiplegic cerebral palsy: a Cochrane Systematic Review. Clin. Rehabil. 21, 675–685.

Hoare, B.J., Imms, C., Rawicki, H.B., Carey, L., 2010. Modified constraint-induced movement therapy or bimanual occupational therapy following injection of Botulinum toxin-A to improve bimanual performance in young children with hemiplegic cerebral palsy: a randomised controlled trial methods paper. BMC Neurol. 10, 58.

Hoare, B., Imms, C., Villanueva, E., Rawicki, H.B., Matyas, T., Carey, L., 2013. Intensive therapy following upper limb botulinum toxin A injection in young children with unilateral cerebral palsy: a randomized trial. Dev. Med. Child Neurol. 55, 238–247.

Holmefur, M., Krumlinde-Sundholm, L., Bergstrom, J., Eliasson, A.C., 2010. Longitudinal development of hand function in children with unilateral cerebral palsy. Dev. Med. Child Neurol. 52, 352–357.

Huang, H.H., Fetters, L., Hale, J., McBride, A., 2009. Bound for success: a systematic review of constraint-induced movement therapy in children with cerebral palsy supports improved arm and hand use. Phys. Ther. 89, 1126–1141.

Hung, Y.C., Charles, J., Gordon, A.M., 2004. Bimanual coordination during a goal-directed task in children with hemiplegic cerebral palsy. Dev. Med. Child Neurol. 46, 746–753.

Hung, Y.C., Charles, J., Gordon, A.M., 2010. Influence of accuracy constraints on bimanual coordination during a goal-directed task in children with hemiplegic cerebral palsy. Exp. Brain Res. 201, 421–428.

Jarus, T., Gutman, T., 2001. Effects of cognitive processes and task complexity on acquisition, retention, and transfer of motor skills. Can. J. Occup. Ther. 68, 280–289.

Jebsen, R.H., Taylor, N., Trieschmann, R.B., Trotter, M.J., Howard, L.A., 1969. An objective and standardized test of hand function. Arch. Phys. Med. Rehabil. 50, 311–319.

Kennard, M.A., 1936. Age and other factors in motor recovery from precentral lesions in monkeys. Am. J. Physiol. 115, 138–146.

Ketelaar, M., Vermeer, A., Hart, H., van Petegem-van Beek, E., Helders, P.J., 2001. Effects of a functional therapy program on motor abilities of children with cerebral palsy. Phys. Ther. 81, 1534–1545.

Kiresuk, T.J., Smith, A., Cardillo, J.E., 1994. Goal Attainment Scaling: Applications, Theory, and Measurement. Lawrence Erlbaum Associates, Hillsdale, NJ.

Kleim, J.A., Barbay, S., Nudo, R.J., 1998. Functional reorganization of the rat motor cortex following motor skill learning. J. Neurophysiol. 80, 3321–3325.

Kleim, J.A., Barbay, S., Cooper, N.R., Hogg, T.M., Reidel, C.N., Remple, M.S., et al., 2002. Motor learning-dependent synaptogenesis is localized to functionally reorganized motor cortex. Neurobiol. Learn. Mem. 77, 63–77.

Klingels, K., Jaspers, E., Van de Winckel, A., De Cock, P., Molenaers, G., Feys, H., 2010. A systematic review of arm activity measures for children with hemiplegic cerebral palsy. Clin. Rehabil. 24, 887–900.

Krumlinde-Sundholm, L., Eliasson, A.C., 2003. Development of the assisting hand assessment: a Rasch-built measure intended for children with unilateral upper limb impairments. Scand. J. Occup. Ther. 10, 16–26.

Krumlinde-Sundholm, L., Holmefur, M., Kottorp, A., Eliasson, A.C., 2007. The assisting hand assessment: current evidence of validity, reliability, and responsiveness to change. Dev. Med. Child Neurol. 49, 259–264.

Law, M., Baptiste, S., McColl, M., Opzoomer, A., Polatajko, H., Pollock, N., 1990. The Canadian occupational performance measure: an outcome measure for occupational therapy. Can. J. Occup. Ther. 57, 82–87.

Martin, J.H., Chakrabarty, S., Friel, K.M., 2011. Harnessing activity-dependent plasticity to repair the damaged corticospinal tract in an animal model of cerebral palsy. Dev. Med. Child Neurol. 53 (Suppl. 4), 9–13.

Neilson, P.D., O'Dwyer, N.J., Nash, J., 1990. Control of isometric muscle activity in cerebral palsy. Dev. Med. Child Neurol. 32, 778–788.

Nudo, R.J., 2003. Functional and structural plasticity in motor cortex: implications for stroke recovery. Phys. Med. Rehabil. Clin. N. Am. 14 (Suppl.), S57–S76.

Ochsner, K.N., Lieberman, M.D., 2001. The emergence of social cognitive neuroscience. Am. Psychol. 56, 717–734.

O'Dwyer, N.J., Neilson, P.D., 1988. Voluntary muscle control in normal and athetoid dysarthric speakers. Brain 111, 877–899.

Park, E.S., Rha, D.W., Lee, J.D., Yoo, J.K., Chang, W.H., 2009. The short-term effects of combined modified constraint-induced movement therapy and botulinum toxin injection for children with spastic hemiplegic cerebral palsy. Neuropediatrics 40, 269–274.

Plautz, E.J., Milliken, G.W., Nudo, R.J., 2000. Effects of repetitive motor training on movement representations in adult squirrel monkeys: role of use versus learning. Neurobiol. Learn. Mem. 74, 27–55.

Rameckers, E.A., Speth, L.A., Duysens, J., Vles, J.S., Smits-Engelsman, B.C., 2009. Botulinum toxin-A in children with congenital spastic hemiplegia does not improve upper extremity motor-related function over rehabilitation alone: a randomized controlled trial. Neurorehabil. Neural Repair 23, 218–225.

Rosenbaum, P.L., Walter, S.D., Hanna, S.E., Palisano, R.J., Russell, D.J., Raina, P., et al., 2002. Prognosis for gross motor function in cerebral palsy: creation of motor development curves. JAMA 288, 1357–1363.

Sakzewski, L., Ziviani, J., Boyd, R., 2009. Systematic review and meta-analysis of therapeutic management of upper-limb dysfunction in children with congenital hemiplegia. Pediatrics 123, 1111–1122.

Sakzewski, L., Ziviani, J., Abbott, D.F., Macdonell, R.A., Jackson, G.D., Boyd, R.N., 2011a. Randomized trial of constraint-induced movement therapy and bimanual training on activity outcomes for children with congenital hemiplegia. Dev. Med. Child Neurol. 53, 313–320.

Sakzewski, L., Ziviani, J., Abbott, D.F., Macdonell, R.A., Jackson, G.D., Boyd, R.N., 2011b. Participation outcomes in a randomized trial of two models of upper-limb rehabilitation for children with congenital hemiplegia. Arch. Phys. Med. Rehabil. 92, 531–539.

Sakzewski, L., Ziviani, J., Boyd, R.N., 2011c. Best responders after intensive upper-limb training for children with unilateral cerebral palsy. Arch. Phys. Med. Rehabil. 92, 578–584.

Shumway-Cook, A., Hutchinson, S., Kartin, D., Price, R., Woollacott, M., 2003. Effect of balance training on recovery of stability in children with cerebral palsy. Dev. Med. Child Neurol. 45, 591–602.

Skinner, B., 1968. The Technology of Teaching. Appleton-Century-Crofts, New York.

Sköld, A., Josephsson, S., Eliasson, A.C., 2004. Performing bimanual activities: the experiences of young persons with hemiplegic cerebral palsy. Am. J. Occup. Ther. 58, 416–425.

Staudt, M., Gerloff, C., Grodd, W., Holthausen, H., Niemann, G., Krageloh-Mann, I., 2004. Reorganization in congenital hemiparesis acquired at different gestational ages. Ann. Neurol. 56, 854–863.

Steenbergen, B., Crajé, C., Nilsen, D.M., Gordon, A.M., 2009. Motor imagery training in hemiplegic cerebral palsy: a potentially useful therapeutic tool for rehabilitation. Dev. Med. Child Neurol. 51, 690–696.

Sullivan, K.J., Kantak, S.S., Burtner, P.A., 2008. Motor learning in children: feedback effects on skill acquisition. Phys. Ther. 88, 720–732.

Sung, I.Y., Ryu, J.S., Pyun, S.B., Yoo, S.D., Song, W.H., Park, M.J., 2005. Efficacy of forced-use therapy in hemiplegic cerebral palsy. Arch. Phys. Med. Rehabil. 86, 2195–2198.

Taub, E., Shee, L.P., 1980. Somatosensory deafferentation research with monkeys: implications for rehabilitation medicine. In: Ince, L.P. (Ed.), Behavioral Psychology in Rehabilitation Medicine: Clinical Applications. Williams and Wilkins, Baltimore and London, pp. 371–401.

Taub, E., Wolf, S.L., 1997. Constraint-induced (CI) movement techniques to facilitate upper extremity use in stroke patients. Top. Stroke Rehabil. 3, 38–61.

Taub, E., Ramey, S.L., DeLuca, S., Echols, K., 2004. Efficacy of constraint-induced movement therapy for children with cerebral palsy with asymmetric motor

impairment. Pediatrics 113, 305–312.

Taub, E., Griffin, A., Nick, J., Gammons, K., Uswatte, G., Law, C.R., 2007. Pediatric CI therapy for stroke induced hemiparesis in young children. Dev. Neurorehabil. 10 (1), 3–18.

Taub, E., Griffin, A., Uswatte, G., Gammons, K., Nick, J., Law, C.R., 2011. Treatment of congenital hemiparesis with pediatric constraint-induced movement therapy. J. Child Neurol. 26, 1163–1173.

Thorndike, E.L., 1914. Educational Psychology: Briefer Course. Columbia University Press, New York.

Thorpe, D.E., Valvano, J., 2002. The effects of knowledge of performance and cognitive strategies on motor skill learning in children with cerebral palsy. Pediatr. Phys. Ther. 14, 2–15.

Tower, S.S., 1940. Pyramidal lesion in the monkey. Brain (Lond) 63, 36–90.

Trombly, C., 1995. Clinical practice guidelines for post-stroke rehabilitation and occupational therapy practice. Am. J. Occup. Ther. 49, 711–714.

Utley, A., Steenbergen, B., 2006. Discrete bimanual co-ordination in children and young adolescents with hemiparetic cerebral palsy: recent findings, implications and future research directions. Pediatr. Rehabil. 9, 127–136.

van der Weel, F.R., van der Meer, A.L., Lee, D.N., 1991. Effect of task on movement control in cerebral palsy: implications for assessment and therapy. Dev. Med. Child Neurol. 33, 419–426.

Verschuren, O., Ketelaar, M., Gorter, J.W., Helders, P.J., Takken, T., 2009. Relation between physical fitness and gross motor capacity in children and adolescents with cerebral palsy. Dev. Med. Child Neurol. 51, 866–871.

Wallen, M., Ziviani, J., Naylor, O., Evans, R., Novak, I., Herbert, R.D., 2011. Modified constraint-induced therapy for children with hemiplegic

cerebral palsy: a randomized trial. Dev. Med. Child Neurol. 53, 1091–1099.

Wiesendanger, M., Serrien, D.J., 2004. The quest to understand bimanual coordination. Prog. Brain Res. 143, 491–505.

Willis, J.K., Morello, A., Davie, A., Rice, J.C., Bennett, J.T., 2002. Forced use treatment of childhood hemiparesis. Pediatrics 110, 94–96.

Winstein, C.J., Wolf, S.L., 2009. Task-oriented training to promote upper extremity recovery. In: Stein, J., Harvey, R., Macko, R., Winstein, C.J., Zorowitz, R. (Eds.), Stroke Recovery and Rehabilitation. Demos Medical Publishing, New York.

Wolf, S.L., Lecraw, D.E., Barton, L.A., Jann, B.B., 1989. Forced use of hemiplegic upper extremities to reverse the effect of learned nonuse among chronic stroke and head-injured patients. Exp. Neurol. 104, 125–132.

Wolf, S.L., Winstein, C.J., Miller, J.P., et al., 2006. Effect of constraint-induced movement therapy on upper extremity function 3 to 9 months after stroke: the EXCITE randomized clinical trial. JAMA 296, 2095–2104.

Wolf, S.L., Winstein, C.J., Miller, J.P., Thompson, P.A., Taub, E., Uswatte, G., et al., 2008. Retention of upper limb function in stroke survivors who have received constraint-induced movement therapy: the EXCITE randomised trial. Lancet Neurol. 7, 33–40.

Wu, C., Trombly, C.A., Lin, K., Tickle-Degnen, L., 2000. A kinematic study of contextual effects on reaching performance in persons with and without stroke: influences of object availability. Arch. Phys. Med. Rehabil. 81, 95–101.

Xu, K., Wang, L., Mai, J., He, L., 2012. Efficacy of constraint-induced movement therapy and electrical stimulation on hand function of children with hemiplegic cerebral palsy: a controlled clinical trial. Disabil. Rehabil. 34, 337–346.

# Interactive technologies for diagnosis and treatment in infants with cerebral palsy

# 15

Jens Bo Nielsen

The necessity of early diagnosis and intensive long-lasting training of children with cerebral palsy (CP) has been argued elsewhere in this book and is in my opinion not disputable. However, nothing comes for free and both early diagnosis and early treatment cost money. Health welfare expenditures are rising throughout the world with every new advance in diagnosis and treatment forcing doctors and politicians to make unpleasant decisions about what to diagnose and what to treat unless we find ways of making cheaper diagnoses and cheaper treatments. And we have to face the reality: What really costs money is manpower. It is the human resources that we have to put into early diagnosis and early treatment that are the real limiting factors. We may argue that children with cerebral palsy should be diagnosed some years earlier and receive more intensive treatment for many more years than what is the case now, but unless we minimize the human resources (doctors, therapists) required, we will be met by administrators, insurance companies and politicians who fail to find the money, and all the good ideas that we have may never see the light of day. In my opinion,

there is therefore no doubt that we will need to find ways of using technology to supplement some of the human resources involved in diagnosis and treatment. I believe that there is a huge potential that has not been exploited sufficiently in the past, but which becomes more and more difficult to ignore with the increasing economic pressure from increasing health care expenditures, on the one hand, to the explosion of computer, internet and smartphone technologies that offer themselves as intelligent (and cheap) solutions, on the other. There is in my mind no doubt that we will see an explosion in intelligent interactive technologies for diagnosis and treatment within the next five to ten years, not only in the field of neurology but also throughout health care. In this chapter I will highlight a few of the possibilities which have already been tested or are about to be tested and which are directly relevant in relation to ensuring efficient and relatively low cost early diagnosis and treatment of children with cerebral palsy.

## Early diagnosis: a role for technology?

CP is sufficiently rare, even in very premature infants, to make a specific diagnosis necessary before initiating any treatment. Imaging techniques such as serial cranial ultrasound and magnetic resonance imaging certainly provide efficient means of screening for brain damage in premature children (DeVries et al., 2011; Milligan, 2010), but are not feasible or affordable for the larger group of infants born at term, although it is in this group the largest number of infants with CP is found (Krägeloh-Mann and Cans, 2009). There is also only a limited relation between observations from brain imaging and the clinical abnormalities in individual infants with a large number of false-positive (early lesions compensated by later plastic changes) and false-negative (especially the multiple smaller lesions caused by oxygen deficits) findings (Bax et al., 2006; Korzeniewski et al., 2008). Although the relatively rare severe brain lesions are usually noticed early after birth, the much more frequent smaller lesions that produce less apparent cognitive, sensory or motor deficits are often not detected until the child is several years old. This means months and years without proper treatment. What can we do to improve this? One way may be to implement early diagnosis based on the general movement assessment system introduced by Prechtl and co-workers (Einspieler et al., 1997; Prechtl et al., 1993) (see Chapter 8). Several studies have demonstrated that this assessment has a very high predictive value and may be applied to infants as young as three months (Cioni et al., 1997; Einspieler et al., 1997; Guzzetta et al., 2003; Hadders-Algra, 2004). However, one practical problem is that the assessment requires a trained and experienced clinician or therapist who needs to observe the child for a relatively long time either in real life or on a video recording under standardized circumstances. This has prevented the system from being introduced on a larger scale for screening of infants.

A solution to this problem may be to use computer algorithms that are now very powerful to analyse video recordings of the children and detect possible abnormalities in their movement pattern. This would help to minimize the time that clinicians or therapists would need to spend on healthy infants and instead focus their attention on infants who have been identified by the computer algorithm as having diminished or abnormal movement. This would also guarantee a certain level of quality and reproducibility in the diagnosis. Such automatized computer diagnostic systems have already been developed and tested (Adde et al., 2009, 2010; Karch et al., 2010, 2012). The systems do show promise but there are still technical challenges that need to be overcome. One is that optimal tracking of movements requires 3D motion analysis that until recently had been expensive and complex to work with in practice, especially due to the necessity of

placing markers on the infant and calibration of the system. With the recent development in interactive gaming technologies (Kinect from Microsoft and similar), 3D cameras and motion analysis software that do not require markers have become very cheap. This opens up the possibility of a large-scale automatized screening system with video recordings that can be obtained in the home of the infant and transferred to a central health care unit, through the internet, where a diagnosis can be facilitated by automatized computer algorithms. The race has already started for making this come true.

# Early treatment: a role for interactive technologies?

One of the challenges to initiation of early treatment in CP is to ensure sufficiently intensive training for a sufficiently long time. The amount of training that can be offered through individual therapeutic sessions as part of public health systems is insufficient to drive neuroplastic changes (Lang et al., 2009) and significant functional improvements will therefore have to rely on intensive high-quality training conducted by the families in their own home (Katz-Leurer et al., 2009; Lang et al., 2009) and guided by a well-trained clinical movement scientist and therapist. But how do we ensure sufficient high quality in the training if it is conducted without the supervision of an appropriately trained therapist? How do we ensure that training is made progressively challenging as the infant matures and masters new skills? And, probably most important, how do we ensure that the child and the families remain motivated and continue training as intensively and for as long time as required?

One of the answers to these questions may be to develop interactive technologies for supervised training at home (Bilde et al., 2011; Napolitano et al., 2003; van den Berg et al., 2006). One such system (Move it to improve it; MiTii) has been developed at the Helene Elsass Center in Copenhagen, Denmark, and is now being tested in randomized controlled studies in Denmark and Australia. A feasibility and proof of principle study on a sample of nine children in the age group 6–12 years was recently published (Bilde et al., 2011). The training system is based on individualized interactive computer training modules delivered

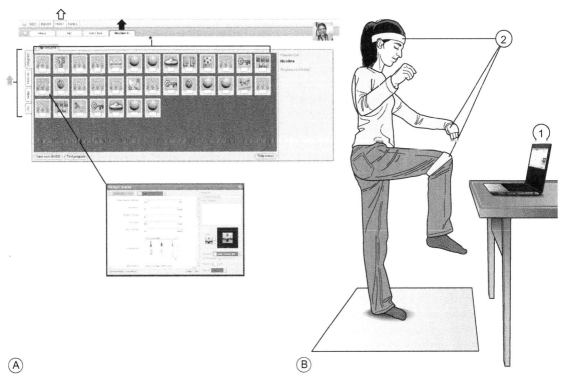

**Figure 15.1** • The MiTii training system. **(A)** Illustration made from screenshots of MiTii. The individual settings are made and progressively modified in the editing window. The first step in editing is to choose the group of patients (open arrow). The next step is to select the individual client details (solid black arrow). Each individual training programme is made up of a sequence of exercises. The different exercises are represented by icons that can be moved around freely to accomplish the optimal individual sequence. The full programme covers from 30–45 minutes (asterisk). In subjacent layers the editing screens offer possibilities for visual feedback from the patients in training, showing intensity and training time from the previous day, week, month or the total training course. This feedback information is obtained automatically on line. A basic case record system is provided to store personal patient information (grey arrow). A double click on each of the icons opens up a new window (seen here as the overlay on the screen). where the range of parameters for each individual exercise—speed, number of repetitions, placing of target and pick-up area on screen, seize of objects, time to react, etc.—can be set. A special database makes it easy to change the graphics for the exercise, e.g., pictures from the patient's own daily life can be uploaded to the database. Changes in the graphic environments are normally performed once a week as it provides excellent motivation. If needed, a video can be uploaded with the exercise giving the therapist a possibility to show, in advance, what the patient is asked to do. The video will automatically play in advance of the exercise. Other parameters to be modified include disturbances, i.e., graphic animations that challenge the attention of the person in training, and time bombs that bring pressure to finishing the exercise in a predetermined space of time. **(B)** MiTii at work in a home environment. The hardware necessary comprises a computer (1) with a webcam and an internet connection. Elastic bands (2) are placed around the head, on the wrists, the knees, the elbows or wherever the therapists find it to meet the requirements. The colour of the elastic band is what controls MiTii. Thus, the therapists may decide which part of the body they want to act as interface to the webcam. These settings can be changed from game to game within the daily programme or over time as the training develops. [Reprinted with kind permission of the Helene Elsass Center.]

through the internet directly to the child's home (Fig. 15.1) (Bilde et al., 2011).

To motivate the child, the training modules consist of small interactive 'computer games' where the child has to solve a cognitive problem or decode visual information and then make appropriate movements that are detected by the web camera and used as a controller of the 'game', providing the child with immediate feedback of the success of their behaviour (Fig. 15.1). At the same time the information from the web camera may be used by the therapist to monitor the progress of the child and adjust the level of the training accordingly. This may also help the therapist to identify when the child loses interest in the training and contact the family in order to encourage and motivate continuing training. With this approach it has been possible to make children with CP train for 30–45 minutes every day for 20 weeks and, unsurprisingly, this has beneficial effects for both their motor and cognitive abilities (Bilde et al., 2011). The ongoing randomized controlled studies are likely to confirm the feasibility of delivering and supervising training in the home in this way and thus stimulate a more widespread use of this approach to guide and motivate self-training.

Interactive computer game-like training modules delivered at home through the internet may work well for children who are able to interact with the computer, but what about younger infants and newborns? Although infants may be limited in their conscious explicit understanding of external stimuli and information, there is an abundance of studies showing that infants show amazing capabilities of learning to interact with and control their environment including computers (Cuevas and Bell, 2010; Luo, 2011). A fundamental basis of development of motor and cognitive skills in infants is their own interaction with the environment, enabling them to learn the possibilities and limitations of their own body and motor system (Wolpert et al., 2011). Interaction with other people and, especially, parents is naturally central for this development, but there is also reason to believe that interactive computer technology may be used to deliver focused training of specific skills for the infants at an early age. Monitoring of the behaviour of the infant, either through movement detectors or video cameras, may provide means by which specific movements and behaviour may be rewarded immediately by a computer and thereby facilitated. A stimulating (enriched) environment may be provided with the use of touch-sensitive toys that respond with sounds, light or movement when the infant grasps or kicks them and video screens and sound systems that are controlled by the activity of the infant (Chen et al., 2002) (Annotation C). The internet provides a means by which such an electronic training system could

be controlled and supervised at a distance by a therapist, similar to the system described above for older children. A larger European project headed by Paolo Dario and Giovanni Cioni, with the aim of developing and evaluating such a training system for premature children in the age group 3–6 months, was initiated in 2011 and is expected to be finished in 2014.

# Delivering and monitoring training by satellite: going small and interactive with smartphone technology

The recent advances in smartphone technology also offer possibilities of delivering individualized training on a daily basis and thus help families to follow and maintain training programmes. Smartphone applications (apps) are already available that can send customized daily reminders to perform specific exercises, and the movement-sensitive technology in the smartphones (GPS, accelerometers, gyroscope) may be used to monitor and keep track of the training. The technology offers obvious possibilities for therapists to produce tailor-made training programmes for children and their families, deliver them automatically on a daily basis, obtain information of the progress of the training through feedback delivered to an internet homepage and use this information to adjust the training according to the progress of the child. Although such a system would provide clear advantages over the existing training programmes that the family usually receives, written on a piece of paper or even as a purely oral communication, this type of smartphone application is not yet available. However, with the present rate of introduction of new smartphone applications there is no doubt that this is only a matter of time. There is reason to be optimistic. Technology used in the right way may be the friend we need to solve the problem of providing efficient training of our youngest ones.

# Acknowledgements

I am grateful to the Ludvig and Sara Elsass Foundation for financial support.

# References

Adde, L., Helbostad, J.L., Jensenius, A.R., Taraldsen, G., Støen, R., 2009. Using computer-based video analysis in the study of fidgety movements. Early Hum. Dev. 85 (9), 541–547.

Adde, L., Helbostad, J.L., Jensenius, A.R., Taraldsen, G., Grunewaldt, K.H., Støen, R., 2010. Early prediction of cerebral palsy by computer-based video analysis of general movements: a feasibility study. Dev. Med. Child Neurol. 52 (8), 773–778.

Bax, M., Tydeman, C., Flodmark, O., 2006. Clinical and MRI correlates of cerebral palsy: the European Cerebral Palsy Study. JAMA 296 (13), 1602–1608.

Bilde, P.E., Kliim-Due, M., Rasmussen, B., Petersen, L.Z., Petersen, T.H., Nielsen, J.B., 2011. Individualized, home-based interactive training of cerebral palsy children delivered through the Internet. BMC Neurol. 11, 32.

Chen, Y.-P., Fetters, L., Holt, K.G., Saltzman, E., 2002. Making the mobile move: constraining task and environment. Infant Behav. Dev. 25 (2), 195–220.

Cioni, G., Ferrari, F., Einspieler, C., Paolicelli, P.B., Barbani, M.T., Prechtl, H.F., 1997. Comparison between observation of spontaneous movements and neurologic examination in preterm infants. J. Pediatr. 130 (5), 704–711.

Cuevas, K., Bell, M.A., 2010. Developmental progression of looking and reaching performance on the A-not-B task. Dev. Psychol. 46 (5), 1363–1371.

deVries, L.S., van Haastert, I.C., Benders, M.J., Groenendaal, F., 2011. Myth: cerebral palsy cannot be predicted by neonatal brain imaging. Semin. Fetal Neonatal Med. 16 (5), 279–287.

Einspieler, C., Prechtl, H.F., Ferrari, F., Cioni, G., Bos, A.F., 1997. The qualitative assessment of general movements in preterm, term and young infants—review of the methodology. Early Hum. Dev. 50 (1), 47–60.

Guzzetta, A., Mercuri, E., Rapisardi, G., Ferrari, F., Roversi, M.F., Cowan, F., et al., 2003. General movements detect early signs of hemiplegia in term infants with neonatal cerebral infarction. Neuropediatrics 34 (2), 61–66.

Hadders-Algra, M., 2004. General movements: a window for early identification of children at high risk for developmental disorders. J. Pediatr. 145 (2 Suppl.), S12–S18.

Johnson, M.H., 1994. Visual attention and the control of eye movements in early infancy. Atten. Perform. 15, 291–310.

Karch, D., Wochner, K., Kim, K., Philippi, H., Hadders-Algra, M., Pietz, J., et al., 2010. Quantitative score for the evaluation of kinematic recordings in neuropediatric diagnostics. Detection of complex patterns in spontaneous limb movements. Methods Inf. Med. 49 (5), 526–530.

Karch, D., Kang, K.S., Wochner, K., Philippi, H., Hadders-Algra, M., Pietz, J., et al., 2012. Kinematic assessment of stereotypy in spontaneous movements in infants. Gait Posture 36 (2), 307–311. (Epub 2012 Apr 13).

Katz-Leurer, M., Rotem, H., Keren, O., Meyer, S., 2009. The effects of a 'home-based' task-oriented exercise programme on motor and balance performance in children with spastic cerebral palsy and severe traumatic brain injury. Clin. Rehabil. 23, 714–724.

Korzeniewski, S.J., Birbeck, G., DeLano, M.C., Potchen, M.J., Paneth, N., 2008. A systematic review of neuroimaging for cerebral palsy. J. Child Neurol. 23 (2), 216–227.

Krägeloh-Mann, I., Cans, C., 2009. Cerebral palsy update. Brain Dev. 31 (7), 537–544.

Lang, C.E., Macdonald, J.R., Reisman, D.S., Boyd, L., Jacobson Kimberley, T., Schindler-Ivens, S.M., et al., 2009. Observation of amounts of movement practice provided during stroke rehabilitation. Arch. Phys. Med. Rehabil. 90, 1692–1698.

Luo, Y., 2011. Three-month-old infants attribute goals to a non-human agent. Dev. Sci. 14 (2), 453–460.

Milligan, D.W., 2010. Outcomes of children born very preterm in Europe. Arch. Dis. Child. Fetal Neonatal Ed. 95 (4), F234–F240.

Napolitano, M.A., Fotheringham, M., Tate, D., Sciamanna, C., Leslie, E., Owen, N., et al., 2003. Evaluation of an internet-based physical activity intervention: a preliminary investigation. Ann. Behav. Med. 25, 92–99.

Prechtl, H.F., Ferrari, F., Cioni, G., 1993. Predictive value of general movements in asphyxiated fullterm infants. Early Hum. Dev. 35 (2), 91–120.

van den Berg, M.H., Ronday, H.K., Peeters, A.J., le Cessie, S., van der Giesen, F.J., Breedveld, F.C., et al., 2006. Using internet technology to deliver a home-based physical activity intervention for patients with rheumatoid arthritis: a randomized controlled trial. Arthritis Rheum. 55, 935–945.

Wolpert, D.M., Diedrichsen, J., Flanagan, J.R., 2011. Principles of sensorimotor learning. Nat. Rev. Neurosci. 12 (12), 739–751.

# Index

*Note*: Page numbers followed by *"f"*, *"t"* and *"b"* refer to figures, tables, and boxes, respectively.

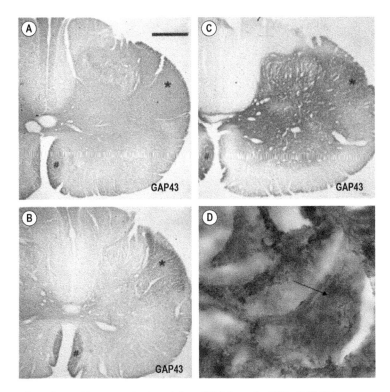

**Figure 2.2** • Horizontal sections of human spinal cord C$_{5-6}$. **(A)** 24 weeks PCA. GAP43 immunoreactivity is widespread in white and grey matter. **(B)** 27 weeks PCA. Corticospinal tracts are the only major axon tracts expressing GAP43 from which weaker immunoreactivity extends into the intermediate grey matter. **(C)** 31 weeks PCA. Immunoreactivity is also now intense in the intermediate grey matter and present in motoneuronal pools and dorsal horn. **(D)** 35 weeks PCA. Section counterstained with cresyl violet. #, Nissl stained motoneuronal cell body; arrow, GAP43 expressing varicose axons. Motoneuron cell bodies are closely apposed by GAP43 immunoreactive varicose axons. (A–C), Scale bar, 500 μm. Stars mark the lateral and the anterior corticospinal tracts. (D) Scale bar, 20 μm.

[From Eyre J, Miller S, Clowry G, Conway E, Watts C. Functional corticospinal projections are established prenatally in the human foetus permitting involvement in the development of spinal motor centres. Brain. 2000;123:51–64, reprinted by permission of Oxford University Press.]

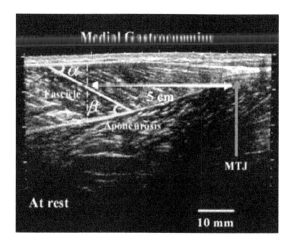

**Figure 6.9** • Longitudinal ultrasonic images of the medial gastrocnemius muscle at rest. The skin is on the top of the image, and the left side corresponds to proximal. The muscle tendon junction represented the musculo-tendon (muscle aponeurosis) junction. α and β are the posterior and anterior pennation angles, respectively.

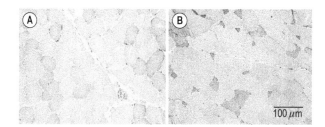

**Figure 6.12** • Muscle fiber morphology is abnormal in spastic muscle. Light micrograph of a muscle obtained from a 19-year-old hemiplegic boy. **(A)** Non-spastic extensor carpi radialis brevis muscle. Histochemical stain of the NADH oxidative enzyme that labels fiber type I and type IIA dark, and type IIB lighter. **(B)** Spastic flexor carpi ulnaris muscle. Note the spastic muscle demonstrates greater fiber size variability. [Micrographs courtesy of Dr Eva Pontén, Karolinska Institute, Stockholm, Sweden.]

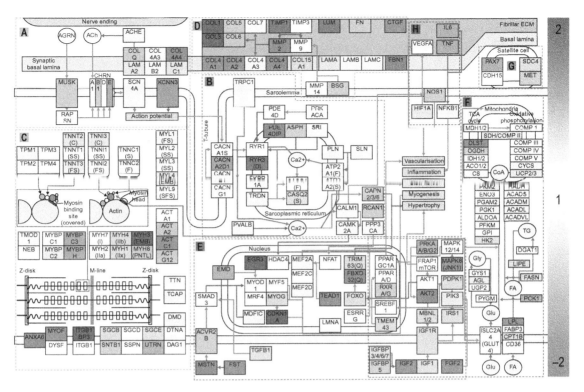

**Figure 6.14** • Linked map of functional muscle gene networks. Color is determined by the expression ratio (CP/typically developing). Gray expression represents transcripts not present on the chip or below present threshold. Green connectors represent activation and red connectors represent inhibition in the direction of the arrow. Pathways represented are: A, neuromuscular junction; B, excitation contraction coupling; C, muscle contraction; D, extracellular matrix; E, muscle signaling; F, inflammation; G energy metabolism; H, satellite cells.

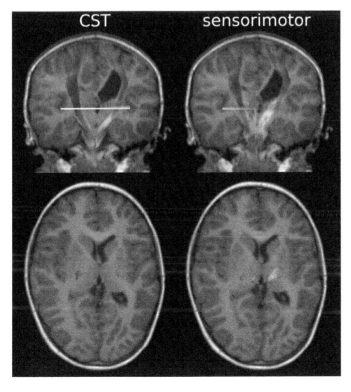

**Figure 13.2** • Advanced diffusion imaging utilizing the HARDI model. Top left is motor cortex (pre- + post-central) to brainstem through the posterior limb of the internal capsule (PLIC), top right is motor cortex (pre- + post-central) to brainstem through the thalamus. Bottom row shows cross-sectional area of the same tracts as above at the level of PLIC/thalamus.

Printed and bound by CPI Group (UK) Ltd, Croydon, CR0 4YY

03/10/2024

01040360-0006